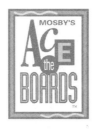

MOSBY'S
ACE the
BOARDS
™

Pathology

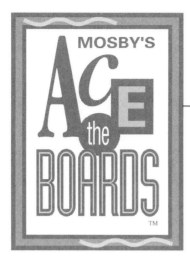

MOSBY'S
USMLE *step* 1
REVIEWS

John Wurzel, M.D.
Associate Professor

James G. Caya, M.D.
Professor of Pathology,
Adjunct Professor of Ophthalmology

Eugene M. Hoenig, M.D.
Professor Emeritus

Department of Pathology and Laboratory Medicine,
Temple University School of Medicine,
Philadelphia, PA

Robert William Coupland, M.D.
Director, Department of Laboratory Medicine,
Cross Cancer Institute;
Associate Professor,
Department of Laboratory Medicine and Pathology,
University of Alberta,
Edmonton, Alberta

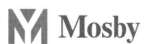 Mosby

St. Louis Baltimore Boston Carlsbad Chicago Naples New York Philadelphia Portland
London Madrid Mexico City Singapore Sydney Tokyo Toronto Wiesbaden

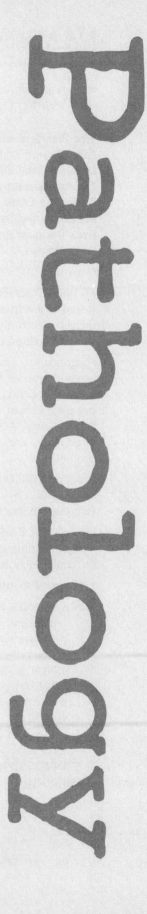

Pathology

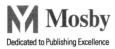

Mosby

Dedicated to Publishing Excellence

A Times Mirror Company

Vice President and Publisher *Anne S. Patterson*
Editor *Emma D. Underdown*
Developmental Editor *Christy Wells*
Project Manager *Dana Peick*
Production Editor *Jeffrey Patterson*
Manufacturing Supervisor *Karen Boehme*
Book Designer *Amy Buxton*
Cover Design *Stacy Lanier/AKA Design*

Printed in the United States of America
Composition by Graphic World, Inc.
Printing/binding by Plus Communications

Mosby-Year Book, Inc.
11830 Westline Industrial Drive
St. Louis, Missouri 63146

Library of Congress Cataloging-in-Publication Data

Mosby's USMLE reviews—pathology / John Wurzel . . . [et al.].
  p. cm. — (Ace the boards)
  1. Pathology—Outlines, syllabi, etc. 2. Pathology—Examinations, questions, etc. I. Wurzel, John. II. Series.
  [DNLM: 1. Pathology—examination questions. QZ 18.2 M894 1997]
 RB32.M67 1997
 616.07′076—dc20
 DNLM/DLC
 for Library of Congress   96-44703
                      CIP

ISBN 0-8151-9276-2 (IBM)
ISBN 0-8151-9428-5 (MAC)

97 98 99 00 / 9 8 7 6 5 4 3 2 1

PREFACE

Pathology is the study of disease. Its concerns are etiology (cause); pathogenesis (how the disease develops in response to the etiologic agent or agents); chemical, morphological, and associated functional alterations; and the relationship between these changes and the clinical features. In some sense, every physician is a student of pathology and knowledge of pathology underlies all of medical practice. Of perhaps more immediate concern to second year medical students is the importance of pathology in standardized examinations. *ACE Pathology* should help students who have successfully completed a pathology course to consolidate and extend their understanding of the field in order to prepare them for standardized examinations and for their subsequent clinical careers. *ACE Pathology* reflects the authors' experiences as teachers of pathology and as practicing pathologists with rather diverse areas of clinical expertise. We emphasize the morphology of disease, but also include as much other basic and clinical laboratory information as is practical.

ACE Pathology is part of a Mosby's ACE the Boards USMLE Step 1 review series and shares many important pedagogic features with other ACE books.

- The most pertinent information is concisely presented in an easy to access, bulleted outline format.
- Numerous black and white photographs of specimens and photomicrographs, as well as two color illustrations and diagrams enhance understanding.
- Icons highlight critical information and facilitate efficient study.

- The layout allows the reader to insert notes while studying other sources, thereby consolidating review in one convenient place.
- Single best answer and matching questions reinforce the utility of the information and enable the student to prepare for the National Boards and other standardized examinations.
- Perforated answer sheets allow the reader to tear out the answers and place them next to the questions for timely and effective feedback.
- The computer diskette provides hundreds of categorized questions in addition to those in the book, permitting additional practice and providing instant feedback for correct and incorrect answers.

We hope that you will find this book useful in preparing both for your examinations and for your future clinical careers.

ACKNOWLEDGMENTS

We wish to thank Emma Underdown for enlisting our participation in this project and providing guidance during its early phases, as well as Christy Wells and Natalie Gehl for helping us see this book through to a successful completion. We acknowledge the thousands of medical students we have taught for the insights they have provided, and, in particular, the student reviewers of this book, Mel Herd, Ph.D., Anna Monias, and Katrina Acosta. Finally, we thank our families for their patience and support.

Test-Taking Strategies

Suzanne F. Kiewit, M.Ed.

To perform well on the USMLEs, it is imperative that you begin with a **plan.** Preparation time is at a premium, so you will want to be as efficient and effective as possible by planning well.

MONTHS AHEAD OF THE EXAM

- Sit down with a blank calendar and block in your commitments: classes, final exams, scheduled events.
- Include time for activities of daily life: eating, sleeping, exercising, socializing, banking, maintaining your home, and so forth.
- The remaining time is available for study/review.
- Determine an orderly approach to the material you need to cover that fits your particular set of needs (e.g., subject-by-subject approach, systems approach, pathologic state approach).
- Assign the remaining time to content areas. This is done in various ways: material covered freshman year first, easiest first, least comfortable material first, detailed subjects last, whatever. Your plan should reflect your goal: to maximize your score.
- Establish a warm-up, which may consist of breaking the tension in major muscle groups (neck rolls, shoulder rolls, etc.), a quick visualization of you performing successfully, or a brief meditation. Practicing this warm-up routine before each of your study sessions will make it a familiar activity that helps you learn effectively, as well as take exams effectively.
- Designate time at the end of your study period for panoramic review. Depending on your needs, that might be a week or just several days before the exam.
- Plan for feedback on your efforts. Schedule time for answering questions on the material you are reviewing and for taking at least one mock comprehensive exam.
- Do the comprehensive exam midway through your study period so that you can refine your efforts to reflect the degree of your performance.

DAYS AHEAD OF THE EXAM

- Divide each day into thirds: morning block, afternoon block, and evening block.

- Consider the time of day that is most productive for you and do the most difficult or least favorite material at that time.
- Assign more blocks of study to those areas requiring the most review to reach a comfortable knowledge level.
- A popular way to use blocks is to pair subjects or materials. For instance, pair strong content with weaker content so that you are not always in the position of not knowing material (which would invite negative feelings or ineffectiveness). Or pair a conceptual subject with a detail subject, such as physiology with anatomy, so that you are not always doing the same kind of thinking (this invites positive effort).
- Use your most productive blocks of time for actual study/review. Use the nonpeak times for reinforcement of material covered or feedback by answering questions on material that you have covered.

Planning the Blocks

- Once you determine time allocations for each content area and an orderly approach that fits your needs and goals, you want to specify what you plan to do during each block.
- Be specific as to content area, material to study, and task; for example, MICRO: review chart on viruses; PHYS: answer questions on renal; and so forth.
- Each study block will last approximately 3 to 4 hours. To be most efficient and effective, plan to take a 5- or 10-minute break every hour. If you are having difficulty getting into the study mode, plan to study for 25 minutes, then take a 5-minute break. Reserve longer breaks for switches between subjects. Get up and move around on breaks.

BEFORE THE EXAM

Knowing about the USMLEs helps demystify them. In general, the USMLE exams are a 2-day, four-book examination. Approximately 3 hours are allotted per exam book. Each day you will complete one book of about 200 items in the morning and another book in the afternoon.

In each exam book, questions are organized by question type, not content. Specific directions precede each set of questions. Only two question formats are used: one-best-answer multiple choice items (which typically come first on the exam) and matching items (toward the end of the exam). Students have reported that one-best-answer items make up the bulk of the exam (70% to 75%) and negatively stemmed items make up only 10% to 15% of the questions (Bushan, Le, and Amin, 1995). Matching sets, which make up about 15% to 20% of the items, may include short leading lists or long leading lists of up to 26 items from which to choose.

From year to year there may be variations in the organization and presentation of both content and item formats. It would be wise to read the National Board of Medical Examiners' *General Instructions* booklet, which you will receive when you register. This booklet contains descriptions of content, item format, and even a set of practice items. Be certain you read this booklet and familiarize yourself with the questions.

You can further maximize exam performance by taking control. Adults tend to perform better when they feel that they have a measure of control. For the USMLE it is easy to feel out of control. You are told what time to arrive, where to go, what writing instrument to use, when to break the seal, and so on. You want to assume control of as many aspects as possible to maximize your performance:

STUDY Follow the sage advice of planning your work and working your plan to maintain satisfactory preparation with regard to study.

SLEEP Get a good night's rest. Sleep needs vary, but 6 hours is usually minimum. Try to get the appropriate amount of sleep that you require.

NUTRITION Maintain proper nutrition during both study time and exam time. Eat breakfast. Choose foods that help keep you on an even energy level. Eat light lunches on exam days. If you have a favorite food and can take it with you, treat yourself.

MEDICATION It may be cold, flu, or allergy season. Take no medications that may make you drowsy.

CLOTHING Heating and cooling systems are rarely balanced enough to suit everyone. Wear articles of clothing that can be added or removed as necessary. Strive for personal comfort.

READINESS Develop physical, mental, emotional, and psychologic readiness for the exam. Keep your thoughts about the exam and your preparation efforts running positively. You must believe that *you can do this!*

ARRIVAL Plan to arrive as close to the designated time as possible and still allow yourself sufficient time to check in. Keep to yourself so that other people's anxieties will not affect you. Take care of personal needs. Find your seat.

ACCLIMATION Settle in and get comfortable. Take several deep breaths. . .RELAX. A relaxed mind thinks better than a tense one—it's that old "fight-or-flight" syndrome. Do your warm-up routine to help you relax.

ATTENTION Pay attention to the proctor. Complete all identification material as required. Read all instructions carefully. Ask for clarification as needed. Do not open your booklet until told to do so. After you are told to break the seal, quickly glance through the whole test to see how it is set up and how questions are organized. Again, you want to take control of the situation. A quick review eliminates surprises and allows you to develop a plan.

DURING THE EXAM

Plan Your Approach

There are numerous approaches to answering questions. Answer questions in the order that appeals to you. Doing the easier ones first may give a psychologic boost; however, the ones you skip may stay on your mind and cloud your thinking.

Another approach is to answer each question in sequence. Start with the first one in the section with which you begin and fill in an answer for each question. Do not leave any blanks! The theory behind this is that if you spend any time at all on an item, you should mark your best response at that time and go on. If you are not certain of your choice, mark "R" in the test booklet for review and return to it later as you have time.

Some students plan to do the matching items first. Matching items are the last set of questions in the booklets. If you prefer matching items, this is a reasonable plan because it helps you get started with items about which you feel confident. It is also reasonable because matching items are not good items on which to guess if you run short of time. **You** must decide the order in which you want to do the questions.

Complete the Bubble Sheet or Answer Card Carefully

There are two schools of thought on this matter. One is to fill in the bubble sheet **item by item** as you go. This method minimizes transcription errors. The other method is **block transfer.** Complete a logical chunk of questions in the test booklet (one or two pages) and then transfer responses to the bubble sheet. Be sure that the last question number on the page is the last numeral you blacken. This method saves time and offers a mini–mental break at the end of each block. Such minibreaks help decrease fatigue during a long exam. Choose the method that will work for you and *practice* it as you take prep questions.

Budget Your Time

If only the allotted time and the number of questions were considered, you would have approximately 54 seconds per question. Obviously, some questions may go more quickly and balance out the ones that take longer. To keep track, you need a pacing strategy. A good strategy is to establish checkpoints at 30-minute intervals. When you overview the booklet, circle the numerals corresponding to where you should be at 30 minutes, 60, 90, 120, and so on. For example, if you have 200 questions on a 3-hour exam, you should be at question number 33 at 30 minutes. As you complete the exam, check your time at the circled items. This technique keeps you from watching the clock too much, yet permits multiple opportunities to adjust your pacing.

If you find yourself spending too much time on any one question, select your best choice at that time, mark an answer, and "R" it for later review. The point is to keep going. Laboring too long on one question limits you from responding to other items you may know well. Remember, controlling your time helps you maximize your points.

ANSWERING THE QUESTIONS

- **Read and *understand* the stems and alternatives.**
  The most frequent error made on exams is misreading or misinterpreting the various aspects of a question. The **stem** is the introductory question or statement. The **alternatives** are the options from which you select the one best response. To encourage reading and understanding, use a process.
- **Follow a process to answer questions.**
  1. Quickly read the stem.
  2. Quickly read the options. (Combined, the first two steps create a preview of the item.)
  3. Carefully read, underline, and mark the stem in a timely fashion.
     - Selectively underline key words and phrases.
     - Pay attention to nouns, verbs, and modifiers.

- Circle age and gender.
- Note data in telescopic form (e.g., ↑ BP).
- Graphically represent material if it helps you to understand (e.g., diagram the renal tubule to answer a question about reabsorption).
  4. Carefully read each alternative. Mark as appropriate.
- **Consider each alternative as one in a series of true, false, or not sure (?) statements.**
  Read each alternative. Rather than slashing out the ones you eliminate, work with each one and designate it as **true, false,** or varying degrees of **true/false/?.** This marking strategy requires you to make judicious decisions about alternatives relative to the stem. It also provides a record of your original thinking, which will save you rethinking time if you need to reconsider a question. Practice this strategy on preparation questions so it becomes second nature.
- **Avoid premature closure.**
  Sometimes you may read a question and anticipate a response. Such a reaction helps focus your attention. However, be sure to read *all* the options so that you are selecting the *best* response. In one-best-answer multiple choice questions, there is one *best* and several *likely* responses. Avoid being misled; consider all the alternatives.
- **Be leery of negative stems.**
  Negative stems require shifting to a negative thinking mode to determine which alternatives are not correct. You can avoid this shift by using this strategy:
  - Circle such words as *except, least, false, incorrect, not true* to raise your awareness of them.
  - Cross out the negative and read the stem as though it were a positive.
  - Mark each option as T/F/?. The F option will then be the appropriate choice.
- **Keep your original answers.**
  To change or not to change answers is a difficult decision. The answer depends on a person's previous history. If you are the kind of student who, if you change answers, changes them from wrong to right, then selectively changing answers may be worthwhile. If, on the other hand, your past experience has been to change right answers to wrong answers, selectively changing answers is probably not a good idea. Good performers change answers, but only if they have reason, such as acquired insight or discovery of misreading or misinterpretation.

- **Maintain an even emotional keel.**
  If a question upsets you, calm yourself. Take several deep breaths. Tell yourself, "I can do this!" Give yourself a mental or physical break. Pay special attention to the next two or three questions after a bout of emotional uneasiness. It is possible to miss items when attention is diffused.

THINKING THROUGH QUESTIONS

- **Use logical reasoning and sound thinking.**
  - Read the item carefully. After careful reading, ask "What is this question really asking?" Restate it so that you know what is being asked.
  - Engage in a mental dialogue with the question. Talk to yourself about what you do know. Always start with what **you** know. Verbalize your thinking.
  - If a diagram or graphic representation is included, orient yourself to it **first** so that the options do not lead your thinking.
- **Use information found within the questions themselves to help you answer others.**
  There will not be "gimmes" on a nationally standardized exam. However, there may be items or graphics that trigger remembrances.
- **Create a diagram, chart, map, or graphic representation of given information.**
  Material that is visually presented usually helps clarify thinking. Use selective, quick sketching as warranted.
- **Reason through information like a detective.**
  - Sift through the details (preview).
  - Determine the relevant information (selectively mark).
  - Put the clues together as in solving a puzzle (reason).
- **Read carefully and note key descriptors.**
  - Note words such as *chronic, acute, greater than, less than, adult, child.*
  - Attend to prefixes such as *hyper-, hypo-, non-, un-, pre-, post-.*
- **Analyze base words and affixes.**
  Studying a question at the word level may help you remember salient information. Look for base words or related words. Determine Latin or Greek word parts and use their meanings to assist you.
- **Consider similar options equally.**
  If you mark one alternative as "false" for a particular reason and another option is qualified for the same reason, it's probably "false" as well.
- **Trust the questions.**
  The questions are designed to determine if you have a working knowledge of the material. They are not written to trick you. You need to believe that your medical school curriculum and your study efforts prepared you for most of the questions.
- **Meet the challenge of clinical vignettes.**
  Longer, vignette items challenge you to discern the relevant from the irrelevant material. In doing so, you are given multiple clues to consider. To effectively handle the vignette item, follow this strategy:
  - Scan the stem and read the first several lines.
  - Skip to the end of the stem and read the last several lines.
  - Check the alternatives to narrow your focus.
  - Now that you know what the question is about, go back to the stem; read and mark what's important to your informed decision making.
  - Make good T/F/? decisions.
- **Reread your underlines and markings when you are down to two choices, at 50/50.**
  By the time you work through a stem and numerous alternatives, it is easy to lose the gist of the question. Checking your focus by rereading only the underlines ensures that you are answering the question being posed.

ANSWERING MATCHING ITEM SETS

Matching items are used to measure your ability to distinguish among closely related items. They require knowledge of specific sets of information. As you study, be alert to potential material that could be tested in this way.

Matching items can be formatted in two ways. **Short leading list matching** items include a set of five, lettered options followed by a lead-in statement and then several numbered stems. **Long leading list matching** items include a set of up to 26 lettered options, followed by a lead-in statement and then several numbered stems.

To efficiently deal with a short leading list item, consider it as an upside-down multiple choice item with the same repeated options. To handle it effectively, do the following:

- Scan the list; determine the topic.
- Read the lead-in statement; determine the focus.
- Quickly read the stem; then read and mark key words.
- In the left margin, create a grid with A, B, C, D, E at the top.

- Make good T/F/? decisions about each stem, marking them in the grid. In this way you can see the pattern of your responses. Similarly, a grid with the item numbers can be drawn beside the leading list and responses marked there.

Handling long leading list matching items effectively requires some modifications in the process. It is not efficient to make T/F/? decisions about each option, so follow this strategy:

- Scan the list; determine the topic.
- Read the lead-in; determine the focus.
- Read a stem and generate your own response.
- Narrow the focus. Put a check mark by those related options in the long list.
- Read and mark specifics in the stem to differentiate among those alternatives you marked.
- Make good T/F/? decisions.

For each stem, mark the narrowed-list options with a different symbol (star, dash, etc.). Items are listed in logical order, alphabetically or numerically. When looking for an option such as "xanthinuria," do not start at the beginning of the list. Looking in the appropriate place saves valuable seconds.

TEST WISENESS

How a question is worded can often influence your response to it. Most clues about "test psychology" are a function of the way in which a question is worded—test constructors cannot rename body parts, drugs, diseases, and so forth. Being aware of the psychology behind the wording can often help you answer the test question.

Using techniques of test psychology to arrive at a correct answer has limited value on standardized exams because those who construct the exams are well aware of the use of these techniques. Nonetheless, being wise to these techniques of test psychology may add another point or two to your score, and they can also enhance your sense of control. Knowing these techniques provides additional strategies to employ should the question temporarily stump you.

The best way to take any exam is to be totally prepared with a strong knowledge base and personal test confidence. The following techniques should be used only if you have exhausted your knowledge base, eliminated all distractors, and cannot come up with the answer even with logical thinking and sound reasoning. Such techniques are **not** a substitute for knowledge, nor are they foolproof.

- **Identify common ideas or themes within the options and between the stem and options.**

- Circle repeated words in the options.
- Select the option with the most repeated words or phrases.
- Circle words repeated in both stem and options.
- Select the option that contains key words or related words from the stem. This is a stem/option repetition.
- **Beware of words that narrow the focus or are too extreme because they tend to be incorrect.**
  Circle such words as *all, always, every, exclusively, never, no, not, none.*
- **Options that are look-alikes are good candidates for exclusion.**
- **Note qualifiers that broaden the focus because they may be correct.**
  Circle words such as *generally, probably, most, often, some, usually.*
- **Identify antonyms or two opposing statements as potentially correct options.**
  Test constructors may use pairs of opposites, so this tip may lose its effectiveness.
- **Select the most familiar-looking option.**
  Always go from what you know. Alternatives with unknown terms may be likely distractors.
- **Select the longest, most inclusive answer.**
  This would include "All of the above" as a strong potential response.
- **In numerical items, knock out the high and low alternatives and select one in the middle that seems most plausible.**
- **In negatively stemmed questions, categorize responses; the one that falls out of the category is a likely candidate.**
- **Mark the same alternative consistently throughout the test if you have no best guess and cannot eliminate distractors.**
  Before the test, decide which letter (A, B, C, D, E) will be your choice. In this way, if you have given a question your best effort and cannot decide, mark your favorite response and move to questions that cover more comfortable material.

AFTER THE EXAM

- **Between sessions and overnight:**
  - Take a well-deserved break. Eat nutritionally.
  - If you feel the urge to study, study material that is comfortable, from a source with which you are familiar (e.g., personally developed study cards or your annotated review book).
  - If you discovered a recurring "theme," you might desire to consult that set of information.

- ● Do something pleasurable. Relax. Get a good night's rest.
- ● **After the final booklet:**
  - ● Recognize that this exam is a measure of what you know on a given day for a given set of information at a given point in time. Keep a reasonable perspective.
  - ● **Celebrate!**

References

Bushan V, Le T, Amin C: *First aid for the USMLE Step 1,* ed 5, Norwalk, Conn, 1995, Appleton & Lange.

MONEY-BACK GUARANTEE

We are confident that ACE THE BOARDS will prepare you for passing the USMLEs. We are so sure of this, that we'll offer you a money-back guarantee should you fail the USMLE. To receive your refund, simply mail us a copy of your failed USMLE report, plus the original receipt for this product. Mail these materials to:

Marketing Manager, medical textbooks
Mosby-Year Book, Inc.
11830 Westline Industrial Drive
St. Louis, MO 63146

CONTENTS

Chapter 1

Cellular Injury and Adaptation

■ **Disturbances of Homeostasis** Homeostasis is the tendency toward stability in the internal environment of cell, tissue, or organism.

● Causes of disturbed homeostasis

— *Hypoxia and ischemia*

- Hypoxia—reduced oxygenation
- Ischemia—hypoxia caused by impaired blood flow
  - Typically caused by blockage of a blood vessel by atherosclerosis or thrombus
  - Examples: myocardial infarction (heart attack), stroke
  - Reduced oxygenation with normal blood flow can occur in pulmonary failure, anemia, carbon monoxide poisoning

— *Physical agents*

- Examples: mechanical trauma, temperature extremes, radiation, electric shock

— *Chemical agents*

- Examples: therapeutic and recreational drugs, poisons, electrolytes, hormones

— *Infectious agents*

- Examples: bacteria, fungi, viruses, protozoa

— *Inflammation and immune reactions*

- Examples: autoimmune diseases

— *Nutritional imbalances*

- Examples: deficiencies of protein, calories, vitamins; excess calories, vitamins

— *Genetic abnormalities*

- Examples: mutations in single-gene encoding enzymes or structural protein, chromosomal abnormalities

— *Aging*

- Could be unique or reflect a combination of several of the above factors

● **Responses**
  • Reversible injury
  • Irreversible injury and necrosis
  • Apoptosis
  • Adaptation (establishment of a new homeostatic state)

■ **Cell Injury and Necrosis**

● **Intracellular systems involved in cell injury**
  • Aerobic respiration (mitochondrial oxidative phosphorylation): adenosine triphosphate (ATP) production
  • Integrity of membrane of cell and membranes of subcellular organelles
    • Maintaining ionic and osmotic homeostasis
  • Protein synthesis
  • Genetic apparatus (deoxyribonucleic acid [DNA] and ribonucleic acid [RNA] synthesis)
  • These systems are interrelated

● **Morphologic changes of cell injury become apparent only after critical biochemical events**
  • Morphologic changes of necrosis take more to become evident than do those of reversible cell injury

● **Type, duration, and severity of injury affect cellular reaction**

● **Properties of cell that affect the response to a potentially injurious agent**
  • Metabolic rate
    • Cells with high metabolic rates (neurons, heart muscle cells) are more susceptible to ischemic-hypoxic injury than those with low metabolic rates
  • Specific receptors for infectious agents (e.g., lymphocytes for human immunodeficiency virus [HIV])
  • Affinity for toxic agent (e.g., hepatocytes for CCl_4)
  • Nutritional state (e.g., starvation increases experimental hepatotoxicity of CCl_4)
  • Individual susceptibility (e.g., to alcohol)

● **Mechanisms in cell injury and necrosis**
  — *ATP depletion*
    • Decreased mitochondrial production of ATP common consequence of hypoxia-ischemia injury and toxins
      • Reversible, at least for some time
      • Increased anaerobic glycolysis
        • Decreased pH produces chromatin clumping
        • Depletion of glycogen
      • Decreased Na^+/K^+ dependent adenosine triphosphatase (ATPase) leads to accumulation of Na^+ and water in cell and swelling

- Separation of ribosomes from rough endoplasmic reticulum and disaggregation of polysomes
  - Decreased membrane phospholipid synthesis
- — *Increased cytosolic calcium*
  - Normally, cytsol-free Ca^{2+} is 1/1000 concentration of extracellular Ca^{2+}
  - Much intracellular calcium sequestered in endoplasmic reticulum and mitochondria
  - Membrane damage and release of Ca^{2+} from intracellular stores can increase cytosol Ca^{2+}
  - Increased Ca^{2+} activates enzymes
    - Endonucleases
    - Phospholipases that degrade membranes
    - Proteases that degrade membranes, cytoskeleton
- — *Activated oxygen species and free radicals*
  - Examples: hydrogen peroxide, superoxide radical, hydroxy radical
  - Generated by normal oxidative metabolism, inflammatory cells, reperfusion after ischemia, ionizing radiation, metabolism of toxins, therapeutically administered oxygen
  - Effects
    - Peroxidation of membrane lipids
    - Posttranslational protein oxidation
    - Mutations in nuclear and mitochondrial DNA
  - Defenses
    - Vitamin E
    - Enzymes (superoxide dismutase, catalase, glutathione peroxidase)
    - Plasma proteins (albumin, ceruloplasmin, transferrin)
- — *Membrane damage*
  - Causes
    - Decreased phospholipid synthesis (ATP depletion)
    - Activation of phospholipases (especially PLA_2) and proteases
    - Peroxidation by free radicals
  - Effects
    - Increased calcium (from extracellular space and intracellular stores)
    - Release of lysomal enzymes
- ● Sequence of events and morphology of reversible (nonlethal) injury
  - Decreased ATP (see previous explanation)
  - Cellular swelling
    - Swelling of endoplasmic reticulum
    - Fluid accumulation in vacuoles ("vacuolar degeneration")

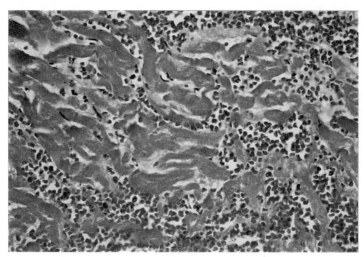

Fig. 1.1 Coagulative necrosis of cardiac myocytes in an acute myocardial infarction. The cross striations and nuclei have disappeared, but cell outlines are maintained. *(Damjanov I, Linder J:* Anderson's pathology, *ed 10, vol 1, St Louis, 1996, Mosby.)*

- Swelling of mitochondria
- Accumulation of triglycerides (fatty metamorphosis; fatty change; steatosis)
- Dilation of endoplamsic reticulum and detachment and disaggregation of polysomes
- Chromatin clumping and nucleolar abnormalities
- Cell membrane abnormalities (blebbing, loss of microvilli)

● **Transition from reversible to irreversible cell injury**

— *Irreversible mitochondrial dysfunction (even after restoration of oxygenation)*

— *Cell membrane damage*

- Progressive loss of phospholipids
- Proteolytic damage to the cytoskeleton, detaching it from the cell membrane
- Lipid peroxidation by reactive oxygen species and free radicals
- Lipid breakdown products

● **Necrosis**—the morphologic changes associated with the degradation of dead cells in living tissue

— *Nuclear changes*

- Fading of stainable chromatin (karyolysis)
- Nuclear condensation (pyknosis) and/or fragmentation (karyorrhexis)

— *Cytoplasmic changes*

- Denaturation of proteins with maintenance of cell outlines (coagulative necrosis) (Fig. 1.1)
- Enzymatic digestion of dead cells (liquefactive necrosis)

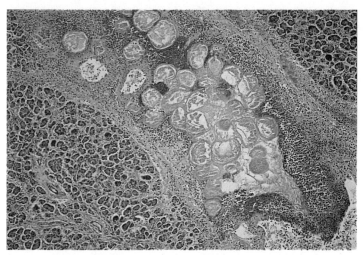

Fig. 1.2 Pancreatic fat necrosis. The interlobular fat cells are lique-fied. Acute inflammation, which frequently accompanies necrosis, is also present. *(Damjanov I, Linder J:* Anderson's pathology, *ed 10, vol 1, St Louis, 1996, Mosby.)*

— *Morphologic forms of necrosis often correlate with mechanism of injury*

Coagulative necrosis—typical of cell death caused by ischemia-hypoxia (infarction)

Liquefactive necrosis—typical of bacterial infection, central nervous system (CNS) infarction

Caseous necrosis

- Type of coagulative necrosis that typically occurs in infection with *Mycobacterium tuberculosis*
- Cheesy macroscopic appearance

Fat necrosis—liquefactive necrosis of adipose tissue adjacent to injured exocrine glands (acute pancreatitis) (Fig. 1.2)

Gangrene—infarction of extremities

- Dry gangrene

  - Sterile
  - Predominantly coagulative necrosis

- Wet gangrene

  - Secondarily infected
  - Shows liquefactive necrosis

■ Apoptosis ("Programmed Cell Death" or "Cell Suicide")

- ● A form of cell death distinct from necrosis
- ● Often dependent on RNA and/or protein synthesis
- ● Regulated by products of specific genes

  - Inhibited by bcl-2
  - Stimulated by p53

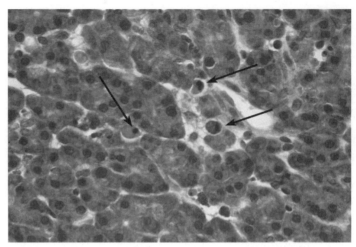

Fig. 1.3 Apoptosis in the pancreas. Note apoptotic bodies *(arrows)*: single cells with condensed nuclei. *(Damjanov I, Linder J: Anderson's pathology, ed 10, vol 1, St Louis, 1996, Mosby.)*

● Occurs in
  • Normal development (embryogenesis, clonal T cell deletion)
  • Normal cell turnover
  • Hormone-dependent involution
  • Regression of neoplasms
  • Some viral diseases (e.g., hepatitis B)
  • Ultraviolet radiation damage to skin
● Biochemical feature—endonuclease-dependent degradation of DNA into nucleosome-sized fragments
● Morphologic features (Fig. 1.3; Table 1.1)
  • Cell shrinkage
  • Chromatin condensation
  • Cytoplasmic blebs
  • Formation of apoptotic bodies
    • Membrane-bound cytoplasmic constituents +/- nucleus
  • Phagocytosis of apoptotic bodies by macrophages or neighboring parenchymal cells
  • No inflammation

■ **Intracellular Accumulations**
● Inability to metabolize certain endogenous (normal or abnormal) substances or exogenous materials can lead to their accumulation in cells
● Fatty change (steatosis)
  • Accumulation of triglycerides within parenchymal cells
  • Reversible and, by itself, not harmful
  • Mechanisms
    • Increased free fatty acid production (diabetes mellitus, decreased caloric intake)

Table 1.1 *Features of Apoptosis and Necrosis*	
APOPTOSIS	NECROSIS
Morphologic	
Death of single cells	Death of many contiguous cells
Cytoplasmic blebbing	Plasma membrane disruption
Chromatin condensation	Nuclear swelling and lysis
Cell shrinkage	Cell swelling
Lysosomes and other cytoplasmic organelles intact	Lysosomal breakdown with release of acid
Fragmentation of nucleus and cytoplasm	Cell lysis and disintegration
Phagocytosis of apoptotic bodies by adjacent cells and macrophages	Phagocytosis by macrophages
No inflammatory response	Inflammatory response frequent
Functional and Molecular	
Requires protein synthesis in early stages	Cessation of protein synthesis
Energy dependent	Energy not required
De novo transcription	Cessation of transcription
Nonrandom oligonucleosomal length DNA fragmentation "ladder"	Random DNA degradation

From Damjanov I, Linder J: *Anderson's pathology,* ed 10, vol 1, St Louis, 1996, Mosby.

- Decreased free fatty acid oxidation (anoxia)
- Decreased synthesis of lipoproteins (protein malnutrition, CCl_4)
  - Example: fatty change in liver caused by alcohol consumption
    - Probably involves several of the mechanisms mentioned immediately above
    - Can cause massive liver enlargement
- Cholesterol and cholesterol esters
  - Accumulate in macrophages and smooth muscle cells in atherosclerotic plaques
- Pigments
  - *Lipofuscin*
    - Composed of polymers of lipids and phospholipids complexed with protein
    - Thought to be derived from peroxidation of membrane phospholipids
      - Probably indicates free radical damage
    - Found in hepatocytes, cardiac myocytes in aged individuals
      - Probably does not impair cell function
  - *Iron*
    - Hemosiderin storage form of iron
    - Hemosiderosis—hemosiderin in macrophages—insignificant by itself
    - Hemochromatosis

- Iron deposited in parenchymal cells (hepatocytes, cardiac myocytes), leading to dysfunction
- Primary—genetic disorder of iron metabolism
- Secondary—acquired severe iron overload

— *Bilirubin*

- Can be seen in tissues of severely jaundiced patients
- Example: obstructive jaundice caused by carcinoma of the head of the pancreas

  - In hepatic sinusoids, Kupffer's cells, and hepatocytes

— *Carbon*

- Ubiquitous air pollutant
- Deposited in alveolar macrophages, lymph nodes (anthracosis)
- Sometimes associated with severe pulmonary fibrosis in coal miners (coal worker's pneumoconiosis)

■ **Abnormal Calcification**

● Dystrophic calcification

- Occurs in damaged or dead tissues in individuals with normal calcium homeostasis
- Found in necrotic tissues, atherosclerotic plaques, damaged heart valves

● Metastatic calcification

- Occurs in normal tissues in individuals with hypercalcemia
- Examples: primary hyperparathyroidism, malignancies involving bone

■ **Hyaline**

● Material with amorphous eosinophilic appearance in hematoxylin and eosin stained sections

● Examples

- Collagen in scar tissue
- Hyaline arteriolosclerosis

  - Hyalinization of wall of arterioles
  - Seen in aging, diabetes mellitus, systemic hypertension

- Amyloid

  - Abnormal, amorphic eosinophilic extracellular material composed of insoluble fibrils derived from normal soluble proteins
  - Many causes, including genetic disorders, chronic inflammation, certain neoplasms, Alzheimer's disease

■ **Adaptation—Establishment of a New Homeostatic State**

● Hypertrophy—increase in cell size

- Can increase the size and functional capacity of the affected tissue or organ
- Example: increased workload causes increase in the size of skeletal and cardiac muscle cells

- Increased protein synthesis, increased myofilaments, and sometimes change in protein isoforms
- In the heart, severe hypertrophy can be associated with diminished functional capacity (heart failure)
- Common causes of cardiac myocyte hypertrophy—hypertension, valvular disease

- **Hyperplasia—increase in cell number**
  - *Can increase the size and sometimes functional capacity of the affected tissue or organ*
    - Often accompanied by cellular hypertrophy, but hyperplasia more important in increasing size and functional capacity
  - *Example: stimulation of target tissue by hormones or growth factors*
    - Normal in endocrine responsive tissues during puberty, menstrual cycles, pregnancy
    - Normal response to prolonged disturbances of homeostasis
      - Example: parathyroid hyperplasia secondary to prolonged hypocalcemia (secondary hyperparathyroidism)
    - If prolonged, can be a precursor of cancer (unopposed estrogen stimulation of endometrium)
  - *Example: compensatory hyperplasia*
    - Liver regeneration after partial hepatectomy

- **Atrophy—decreased cell size**
  - Cells can have diminished functional capacity but are not dead
  - Can decrease the size and functional capacity of the affected tissue or organ
  - Example: muscle atrophy caused by decreased workload, immobilization, or denervation

- **Involution—reduction in cell number**
  - Occurs by apoptosis
  - Decreases size and functional capacity of affected organ or tissue
  - Remaining cells can be atrophic
  - Examples: hormone withdrawal
    - Normal (often cyclic) (e.g., in breast or endometrium during menstrual cycle)
    - Postmenopausal changes in endometrium and breast
    - Hypopituitarism (changes in adrenal cortex and thyroid follicular epithelium)
  - Example: development (e.g., thymic involution)

- **Metaplasia—replacement of one normal, differentiated cell type by another**
  - Example: squamous metaplasia
    - Respiratory tract columnar epithelium replaced by squamous epithelium in response to chronic irritation

● **Dysplasia—loss of individual cell uniformity and loss of arrangement within tissue**
- Often accompanies metaplasia or hyperplasia
- Characteristics of dysplastic cells
  - Hyperchromasia—increased nuclear staining in comparison to normal
  - Pleomorphism—variation in size and shape within a tissue
- Example: dysplasia of uterine cervix
  - Caused by infection with human papillomavirus
  - Can regress, persist, or progress to cancer

● **Cellular proliferative capacity and relationship to adaptive responses and repair of injury**
— *Labile cells*
- Normally proliferate continuously
  - Epithelium of skin and mucous membranes and hematopoietic stem cells
- Capable of undergoing hyperplasia and hypertrophy

— *Stable cells*
- Do not normally proliferate but can do so with the proper stimulus
  - Epithelium of endocrine and exocrine glands, cartilage
- Capable of undergoing hyperplasia and hypertrophy

— *Permanent cells*
- Incapable of proliferation
  - Neurons, cardiac muscle, skeletal muscle fibers
- Hypertrophy is sole possible growth response

— *Repair responses*
- Tissues or organs with parenchyma of labile or stable cells can repair themselves by regeneration
  - Examples: liver, bone marrow, epithelium of skin
- Tissues or organs with parenchyma of permanent cells repair by scarring
  - Often results in loss of function
  - Example: fibrous scarring in heart after myocardial infarction
  - Example: gliosis in brain after stroke

MULTIPLE CHOICE REVIEW QUESTIONS

1. In which of the following tissues is caseous necrosis most likely to occur?
    a. Those that are infected with *Pseudomonas aeruginosa*
    b. Those that are infected with *Staphylococcus aureus*
    c. Those that are infected with *Mycobacterium tuberculosis*
    d. Those that have had their arterial blood supply interrupted by thrombus
    e. Those that have lost their innervation

2. Enlargement of the left ventricle in a patient with system hypertension is most likely caused by which of the following?
    a. Amyloidosis of the left ventricle
    b. Hemosiderosis of the left ventricle
    c. Fatty change of cardiac myocytes
    d. Hypertrophy of cardiac myocytes
    e. Hyperplasia of the cardiac myocytes

3. Degradation of DNA to nucleosome-sized fragments is characteristic of which of the following?
    a. Apoptosis
    b. Dysplasia
    c. Metaplasia
    d. Coagulative necrosis
    e. Liquefactive necrosis

4. The enzyme that promotes degradation of cell membranes is which of the following?
    a. Catalase
    b. Superoxide dismutase
    c. Sodium/potassium dependent ATPase
    d. Glutathione peroxidase
    e. Phospholipase A_2

5. Which of the following is a stable cell?
    a. Cardiac myocyte
    b. Central nervous system neuron
    c. Hematopoietic stem cell
    d. Hepatocyte

Chapter 2

Inflammation and Repair

■ **Overview**

● Inflammation

— *Response of living, vascularized tissue to injury*

— *Destroys or isolates injurious agents*

— *Acute inflammation*

- Characterized by

    - Changes in blood flow
    - Increased vascular permeability
    - Infiltration of tissues by neutrophils

- Inciting agents

    - Bacteria
    - Infarction
    - Physical injury

- Time course

    - Initial response to some agents that incite inflammation
    - Lasts for no more than a few days, unless the inciting agent persists or recurs

- Outcomes

    - Resolution
    - Chronic inflammation
    - Repair

— *Chronic inflammation*

- Characterized by tissue infiltration with macrophages, lymphocytes and plasma cells, or eosinophils (all derived from blood)
- Often follows acute inflammation
- Can be the initial or only detected response to some agents or in certain diseases

    - Viral infections
    - Hypersensitivity reactions

- Granulomatous inflammation

    - A special type of chronic inflammation
    - Characterized by the presence of collections of activated macrophages (epithelioid cells)
    - Seen in delayed hypersensitivity, indigestible foreign material

- **Repair**
    - Replacement of injured tissue
    - Often begins while inflammation still present, but tends to be completed after inflammation has terminated
    - Characterized by new blood vessel formation (neovascularization) and fibrosis
- Although essential for life, inflammation and repair can be harmful in some circumstances

■ Patterns of Inflammation

- **Factors determining pattern**
    - Inciting agent
    - Time of observation
    - Immune status of host
- **Acute patterns**
    - *Transudates and exudates*
        - Transudate has low protein content
            - Specific gravity less than 1.015
            - Protein is mostly albumin
            - Reflects hemodynamic forces
        - Exudate has high protein content
            - Contains other plasma proteins in addition to albumin
            - Reflects increased vascular permeability
    - *Neutrophilic infiltration (suppuration) (Fig. 2.1)*
        Follows exudation
        Inciting agents
        - Bacteria
        - Infarction (ischemic necrosis)
        - Physical injury
        Outcomes
        - Resolution
        - Chronic inflammation
        - Abscess formation
            - Localized collection of neutrophils and dead parenchymal cells, sometimes surrounded fibrovascular tissue (indicating repair) (Fig. 2.2)
    - *Chronic inflammatory patterns*
        Eosinophilic responses (Fig. 2.3)
        - Induced by parasites or allergic reactions
        Lymphocytic and plasma cell responses
        - Found in
            - Hypersensitivity reactions
            - Viral infections
            - Neoplasms

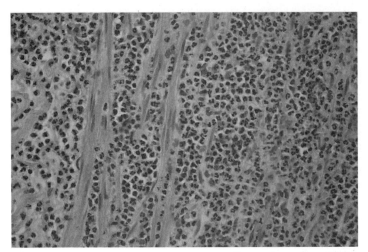

Fig. 2.1 Acute appendicitis. Neutrophils infiltrate the wall and disrupt the tissue. (*Damjanov I, Linder J:* Anderson's pathology, *ed 10, vol 1, St Louis, 1996, Mosby.*)

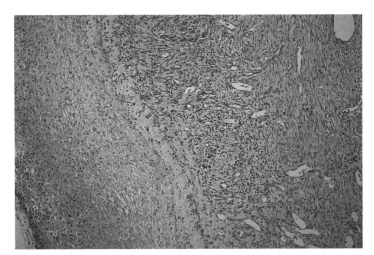

Fig. 2.2 Abscess. Note the zones of suppuration (left), neovascularization (middle), and fibrosis (right). (*Damjanov I, Linder J:* Anderson's pathology, *ed 10, vol 1, St Louis, 1996, Mosby.*)

Macrophage responses
- Often mixed with other acute or chronic inflammatory cells (Fig. 2.4)

Granulomatous response
- Granuloma—collection of activated macrophages (epithelioid cells)
  - Often surrounded by lymphocytes, fibroblasts
  - Occurs in many conditions (Box 2.1)
- Hypersensitivity type involves lymphocyte mediated response to specific antigens
  - Some apparent hypersensitivity type without identifiable antigens (e.g., sarcodosis)

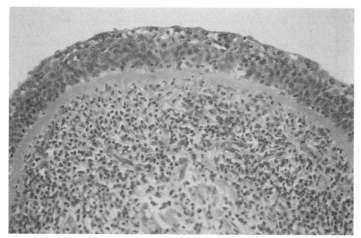

Fig. 2.3 Eosinophilic reaction. Note infiltration of bronchiole wall in an asthma patient. (*Damjanov I, Linder J:* Anderson's pathology, *ed 10, vol 1, St Louis, 1996, Mosby.*)

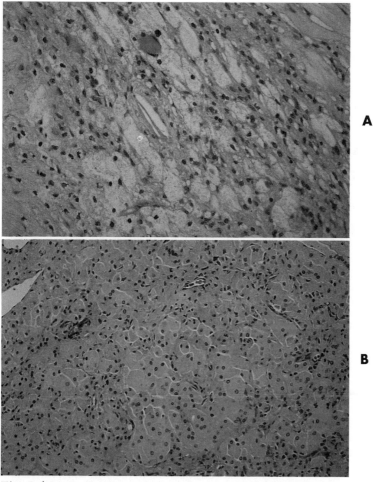

Fig. 2.4 Macrophage reactions. **A,** Foamy, lipid-containing macrophages in atherosclerotic plaque. **B,** Sheets of macrophages in a lymph node. (*Damjanov I, Linder J:* Anderson's pathology, *ed 10, vol 1, St Louis, 1996, Mosby.*)

Box 2.1

GRANULOMATOUS DISEASES

Bacterial
Tuberculosis
Leprosy
Brucellosis
Salmonellosis
Listeriosis
Syphyllis
Q fever

Metal Induced
Berylliosis
Zirconium granulomatosis

Fungal
Histoplasmosis
Blastomycosis
Coccidiomycosis
Hypersensitivity pneumonitis

Viral, Chlamydial
Cat-scratch fever
Lymphogranuloma venerum

Helminthic
Schistosomiasis
Trichiniasis
Filariasis
Capillariasis

Foreign Body Types
Foreign body pneumonitis
Silica granulomatosis

Unknown Cause
Sarcoidosis
Crohn's disease
Wegener's granulomatosis
Giant cell arteritis
Primary biliary cirrhosis
Granuloma annulare
Rheumatoid arthritis

- Persons with impaired T-cell mediated immunity will have small disseminated granulomas (miliary tuberculosis, lepromatous leprosy, human immunodeficiency virus infection)

- Nonhypersensitivity type form in response to poorly digestible materials

- Morphology affected by inciting agents (Fig. 2.5)

  - Central caseous necrosis in *Mycobacterium tuberculosis* infections

  - Eosinophils in granulomas with parasites or ova

  - Central abscesses in cat-scratch fever

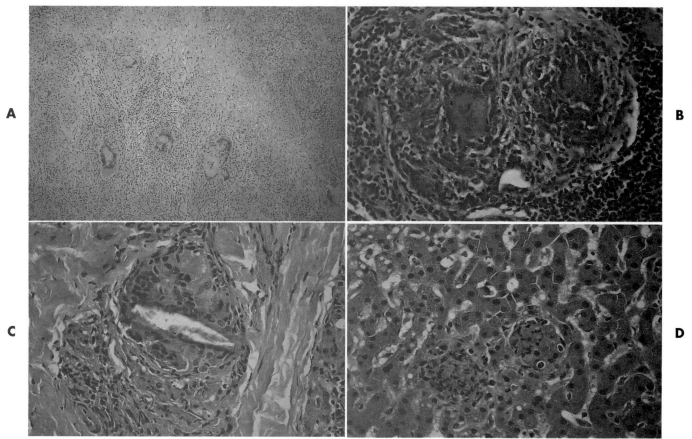

Fig. 2.5 Examples of granulomatous inflammation. **A,** Granulomas in *Mycobacterium tuberculosis.* Note caseous necrosis (upper right) and occasional multinucleated giant cells. **B,** Sarcoid granulomas. Note the tightly packed granuloma with epithelioid and giant cells. **C,** Foreign body granuloma. Note the giant cells and foreign body. **D,** *Mycobacterium avium-intracellulare* granulomas. Small granulomas in patient with HIV infection. (*Damjanov I, Linder J:* Anderson's pathology, *ed 10, vol 1, St Louis, 1996, Mosby.*)

■ **Molecules, Cells, and Stromal Elements Involved in Inflammation**

   ● Plasma proteins regulating inflammation

      — *Coagulation and fibrinolytic factors (see Bleeding Disorders chapter)*

         • Activation of a series of proenzymes ultimately generates thrombin, which cleaves fibrinogen to form fibrin and fibrinopeptides

            • Thrombin promotes leukocyte adhesion and fibroblast proliferation

            • Fibrinopeptides increase vascular permeability and attract leukocytes

         • Fibrinolytic system that breaks down blood clots generates plasmin and fibrin split products

            • Plasmin activates complement system component C3

            • Fibrin split products increase vascular permeability

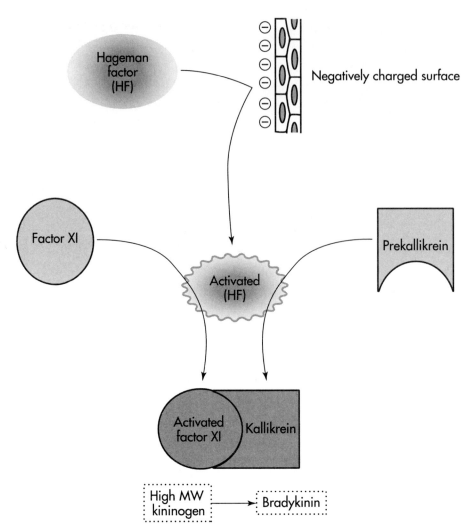

Fig. 2.6 Kinin pathway. The interaction of HF with a negatively charged surface activates coagulation factor XI and converts prekallikrein to kallikrein. The complex of the last two cleaves high molecular weight kininogen to bradykinin. (*Damjanov I, Linder J:* Anderson's pathology, *ed 10, vol 1, St Louis, 1996, Mosby.*)

— *Kinins*

• Series of proteins activated by contact (Fig. 2.6)

• Increase vascular permeability, smooth muscle contraction, and leukocyte margination

— *Complement system*

• Series of proteases activated in self-amplifying cascade

• Classic path initiated by complement fixing IgG and IgM

• Alternative path initiated by aggregated IgA, negatively charged surfaces, microorganisms (Fig. 2.7)

• Membrane active complex (C5b-C9) lyses cell membranes

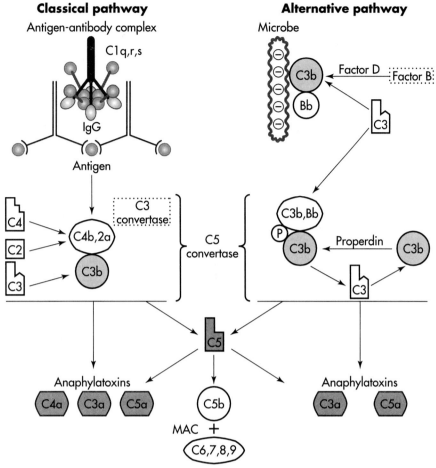

Fig. 2.7 Complement pathways. (*Damjanov I, Linder J:* Anderson's pathology, *ed 10, vol 1, St Louis, 1996, Mosby.*)

- C3a, C4a, C5a increase vascular permeability, smooth muscle contraction, histamine release

  - C5a most potent

- C5a also directs migration (chemotaxis) of leukocytes and fibroblasts

— *Immunoglobulins*

  - IgG1, IgG2, IgG3, and IgM activate classical complement cascade
  - IgA activates alternative complement pathway
  - IgG1 and IgG3 interact with leukocyte Fc receptors (see following)
  - IgE binding triggers histamine release by basophils

● Blood-borne cells in inflammation

— *Neutrophils*

  - Development

    - Mature in bone marrow

- Large storage pool in marrow
- Survive 10 hours in circulation
- About 55% of released cells marginated

- Granules

  - Primary granules appear in promyelocytes
  - Secondary granules appear in myelocytes
  - Contain enzymes that degrade bacteria and host cell components
  - Can empty into phagocytic vacuoles within neutrophils or can be released outside the cell

- Membrane receptors regulate function

  - C3b and immunoglobulin Fc receptors increase efficiency of phagocytosis
  - Receptors for chemotactic molecules (e.g., C5a)
  - Receptors (integrins) for endothelial cell addressins and extracellular matrix proteins promote adhesion

— *Mononuclear phagocytes*

Circulating monocytes and fixed tissue macrophages derived from bone marrow precursors

Tissue macrophages turnover time—4 to 15 days

Numerous secretory products (Box 2.2)

Functions

- Initiation of inflammation
- Phagocytosis
- Antigen processing and presentation

Granulomas

- Epithelioid cells (activated macrophages)

  - Activation by interferon-γ
  - Poorly phagocytic
  - Sequester ingestible materials
  - Secrete enzymes that can degrade materials

- Multinucleated giant cells formed by macrophage fusion

— *Lymphocytes*

- Found lymphoid organs (lymph nodes, spleen, thymus), submucosal lymph aggregates, in circulation
- Involved in autoimmune diseases, viral infections, and chronic inflammatory response following acute inflammation
- See Immunity chapter

— *Eosinophils*

- Derived from bone marrow precursors

  - Make up less than 5% circulating leukocytes

- Involved in allergic reactions and response to helminths
- Weakly phagocytic, at least in comparison to neutrophils

Box 2.2

SECRETORY PRODUCTS OF MONONUCLEAR PHAGOCYTES

Plasma-related Proteins

Coagulation factors
  Factors II, III, V, VII, IX, X
  Thrombospondin
  Prothrombinase
Complement components
  C1-C5
  Factors B and D
  Properdin
  C3b inactivator
Serum amyloids A and P
Apolipoprotein E
Haptoglobin and transcobalamin II

Cytokines and Growth Factors

Interleukins (IL-1a, IL-1b, IL-6)
IL-1 receptor antagonist
Tumor necrosis factor-alpha
Chemokines (IL-8, MCP-I, *gro*, IP-10)
Growth- and colony stimulating factors
  Transforming growth factor-β
  Platelet-derived growth factor
  Fibroblast growth factor
  Angiogenesis factor
  G-CSF and GM-CSF
  Erythropoietin
  Lactoferrin

Oxygen and Nitrogen Metabolites

O_2^-, H_2O_2, OH^-
Hypohalous acids
NO, NO_2, NO_3

Active lipid products

Arachidonate metabolites
  Prostaglandins
  Prostacyclin
Leukotrienes

Hydroxyeicosaenoic acids
Platelet activating factor
  and lysophospholipids

Matrix Proteins

Fibronectin
Thrombospondin
Proteoglycans

Enzymes

Proteases
Collagenases
Elastase
Plasminogen activator
Cathepsins B, L, H, N
Angiotensin convert
Phospholipase A_2
Hyaluronidase
β-Galactosidase
β-Glucuronidase
Nucleases
Ribonucleases
Sulfatases
Lysozyme
Acid phosphatases
Amylase

Enzyme Inhibitors

α_2-Macroglobulin
α_1-Antiprotease
α_1-Antichymotrypsin
Lipomodulin
Fibrinolysis inhibitor

Other Active Molecules

Vitamin D_3
Glutathione
Nucleic acid derivative

- Exert effects by degranulation (Table 2.1)

— *Basophils and mast cells*
  Both derived from bone marrow precursors

  - Basophils circulate

    - Usually less than or equal to 1% circulating leukocytes

  - Mast cells found in tissue

  Secretory granules contain histamine, carboxypeptidase A, serine proteases, glycosidases, sulfatases

  Surface IgE receptor binding IgE cross-linked with antigen leads to degranulation

  Other stimuli for degranulation—C5a, eosinophil-derived cationic protein, certain bacterial products, platelet-activating factor

Table 2.1 *Eosinophil Granule Proteins*		
PROTEIN	**MOLECULAR WEIGHT (KILODALTONS)**	**ACTION**
Major basic protein	14	Helminthotoxin, histamine-releasing factor, bactericidal
Eosinophil cationic protein	20	Helminthotoxin, histamine-releasing factor, bactericidal, neurotoxin
Eosinophil-derived neurotoxin	18	Neurotoxin, inhibits lymphocyte proliferation
Eosinophil peroxidase	66	Generates microbicidal hypohalous acids, histamine-releasing factor

— *Platelets*
- Activated on contact with exposed matrix elements (Box 2.3)
- Surface receptors for IgG and IgE permit antigen recognition with subsequent activation

● Stromal elements in inflammation

— *Endothelium*
Produce
PROSTACYCLIN (PGI$_2$)
- Antithrombotic
- Vasodilator

NITRIC OXIDE RADICAL
- Synthesized by nitric oxide synthase (NOS)
  - Using L-arginine, oxygen and reduced form of nicotinamide-adenine dinucleotide phosphate (NADPH)
  - NOS constitutively expressed in endothelium
- Antithrombotic (inhibits platelet aggregation)
- Vasodilator

ENDOTHELIN
- Peptide vasoconstrictor
Activated by inflammatory stimuli
EXPRESS ADDRESSINS THAT ALLOW FOR LEUKOCYTE ADHESION
PRODUCE CHEMOTACTIC AGENTS (E.G., PLATELET ACTIVATING FACTOR)

— *Smooth muscle cells, fibroblasts, myofibroblasts produce inflammatory mediators*

— *Matrix proteins*
- Neutrophils and some lymphocytes matrix components
- Many proinflammatory proteins bind matrix elements

Box 2.3

```
PLATELET-DERIVED INFLAMMATORY PRODUCTS

Alpha Granule Components
Adherence promoting
    Fibronectin
    Fibrinogen
    von Willebrand factor
    Thrombospondin
    Lysosome associated membrane protein
    Granular membrane protein 140
Chemotactic
    Platelet-derived growth factor
    Platelet factor 4
Growth factors
    Transforming growth factors α and β
    Basic fibroblast growth factor
    Platelet-derived growth factor
Coagulation and complement modulators
    Factors D and H
    Plasminogen
    Alpha₂ plasmin inhibitor

Dense Granule Components
Aggregation promoting
    Adenosine diphosphate
    Serotonin and calcium

Arachidonate Metabolites
Aggregation promoting
    Thromboxane A₂
Chemotactic
    12-HETE
```

HETE, Hydroxyeicosatetraeinoic acid.

● **Mediators generated by inflammatory cells**

— *Membrane lipid-derived mediators*

Generated by action of phospholipase A

• Inhibited by glucocorticoids in vitro (Fig. 2.8)

Arachadonic acid derivatives

CYCLOOXYGENASE PATHWAY ACTIVE IN MOST CELLS

• Prostaglandins active in inflammation

• Prostaglandin E_2 (PGE_2) has proinflammatory (increased blood flow, increased vascular permeability) and antiinflammatory (inhibits effector cells) actions

• Inhibited by aspirin, indomethacin

LIPOOXYGENASE ACTIVE IN LEUKOCYTES

• Leukotriene B_4 induces neutrophil chemotaxis, degranulation, and adherence to endothelium

• Other leukotrienes (LTC_4, LTD_4, LTE_4) induce histamine-independent bronchial smooth muscle contraction, vasopermeability, and mucous production

• Hydroxyeicosatetraeinoic acid (HETE) chemotactic for neutrophils and eosinophils

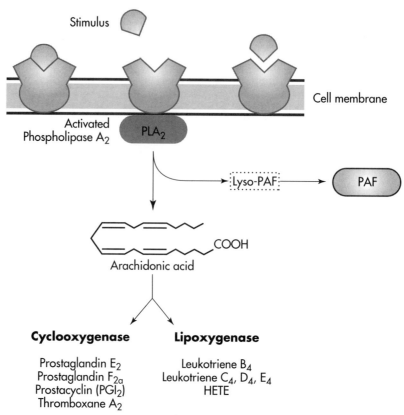

Fig. 2.8 Arachadonic acid metabolism. Activated phospholipase A_2 (PLA_2) generates platelet activating factor (PAF) and cleaves arachadonic acid (AA) from the cell membrane. AA is metabolized through either the cyclooxygenase or lipooxygenase pathway, depending upon the cell and the stimulus. *HETE,* Hydroxyeicosatetreinoic acid. (*Damjanov I, Linder J:* Anderson's pathology, *ed 10, vol 1, St Louis, 1996, Mosby.*)

Platelet-activating factor
RELEASED WITH ARACHIDONATE DERIVATIVES
PROMOTES ACTIVITY OF MOST INFLAMMATORY CELLS

— *Polypeptide mediators*

- Cytokines (Table 2.2)

  - Interferons

  - Interleukins (IL)
  - Colony stimulating factors
  - Cytotoxins

- Chemotactic cytokines (Table 2.3)

  - Belong to family of homologous genes
  - CXC type chemotactic for neutrophils
  - CC type chemotactic for mononuclear cells

- Cytokine receptors and signal transduction (Table 2.4)

Table 2.2 *Polypeptide Cytokines*

Cytokine	Molecular Weight (Kilodaltons)	Major Sources	Major Activities
Interferons			
IFN-α and IFN-β	16-20	Myeloid and stromal cells	Antiviral, activates phagocytes
IFN-γ	20-24	Lymphoid cells	Antiviral, activates phagocytes, induces class I and class II MHC antigens and IgG2α
Interleukins			
IL-1	17-18	Mostly MP but also many other cells	Promotes lymphocyte growth, cytokine adhesion molecules, fever, acute-phase protein synthesis
IL-2	15-18	Lymphocytes	Promotes lymphocyte growth, NK-cell activity, and phagocyte activation
IL-4	15-19	Lymphocytes	Promotes lymphocyte growth, IgE and IgGI synthesis, Fcε, adhesion molecules
IL-5	20	Lymphocytes	Promotes B-cell differentiation, eosinophil growth, IgE synthesis
IL-6	21-28	Leukocytes, stromal and epithelial cells	Promotes lymphocyte growth, Ig synthesis, acute-phase protein synthesis, thrombopoiesis
IL-7	25	Stromal and epithelial cells	Promotes B-cell precursor growth, T-cell growth and hematopoiesis
IL-9	32-39	Lymphocytes	Promotes T-cell growth
IL-10	35-40	Lymphocytes and MP	Promotes B-cell and mast-cell growth, inhibits IFN-γ, TNF, and IL-1 synthesis
IL-11	23	Stromal cells	Promotes lymphocyte growth and hematopoiesis
IL-12	65-75 dimer	Lymphocytes and MP	Promotes NK cell and cytotoxic T-cells; opposes IL-10 actions
IL-13	16-19	Lymphocytes	Promotes lymphocyte growth, IgE synthesis
Colony-stimulation Factors			
IL-3	14-15	Lymphocytes	Stimulates myeloid and erythroid differentiation
GM-CSF	13-14	MP, stromal cells, and endothelium	Stimulates PMN, monocyte and eosinophil growth, phagocyte activation
G-CSF	19-20	Leukocytes, stromal, endothelial and epithelial cells	Stimulates PMN differentiation
M-CSF	70-90 dimer	Leukocytes, stromal, endothelial and epithelial cells	Stimulates monocyte growth
Cytotoxins			
TNF-α	17	Mostly macrophages	Cytotoxic for some tumor cells; promotes adhesion molecules, fibroblast growth, fever, cachexia, and acute-phase protein
TNF-β	17	Lymphocytes	Activities similar to those of alpha form

Fcε, Fc receptor for IgE; *G*, granulocyte; *GM*, granulocyte-macrophage (or monocyte); *Ig*, immunoglobulin; *M*, monocyte or macrophage; *MP*, macrophage; *NK*, natural killer; *PMN*, polymorphonuclear leukocyte; *TNF*, tumor necrosis factor.

Table 2.3	*Supergene Family of Human Chemokines (Cytokines)*

CXC GROUP	CC GROUP
Interleukin-8	Monocyte chemotatic protein
gro/MGSA	RANTES
Macrophage inflam- matory protein-2	LD78
Platelet factor 4	ACT-2
IP-10	I-309

Table 2.4	*Human Cytokine Receptor Families*

FAMILY AND RECEPTOR	MOLECULAR WEIGHT (KILODALTONS)	KINASE ACCEPTOR
Immunoglobulin-like family		
IL-1	80	Yes
IL-6	80	?
Hematopoietin receptor family		
IL-2b	80	Yes
GM-CSF	85	?
IL-4	140	No
IL-7	75	?
Nerve growth factor receptor family		
TNF(p55)	55	?
TNF(p75)	75	?

GM-CSF, Granulocyte and monocyte-colony stimulating factor; *IL,* interleukin;
TNF, tumor necrosis factor.

■ Cellular and Molecular Events of Inflammation

● Changes in blood flow

— *Transient arteriolar constriction results in short-lived decrease in blood flow to affected area*

— *Followed by dilation of arterioles and opening of capillary beds results in increased blood flow (hyperemia)*

• Contributes to edema formation

• Clinical correlation—redness and warmth

— *Slowing of blood flow (stasis)*

• Increased vascular permeability (see following) causes loss of fluid and concentration of formed elements of the blood (hemoconcentration)

• Histologically, congestion (dilated small vessels packed with red blood cells)

• Allows leukocytes (especially neutrophils) to stick to vessel wall, step necessary for their infiltration of tissues

- Increased vascular permeability
  - *Permits formation of protein-rich accumulation of fluid (exudate) in the adjacent tissues*
  - *With increased blood flow, results in edema (swelling)*
  - *Mechanisms*

    Endothelial contraction in venules
    - Most common
    - Short-lived (less than 30 minutes; immediate transient response)
    - Mediated by histamine, bradykinin, leukotrienes

    Endothelial retraction
    - Delayed, transient response
    - Reorganization of cytoskeleton
    - Induced by IL-1, interferon-γ, tumor necrosis factor

    Direct endothelial injury by inciting agent
    - Immediate sustained response
      - Occurs immediately after severe injury
      - Affects arterioles, capillaries, or venules
      - Lasts until vessel blocked by thrombus or repaired
    - Delayed sustained response
      - Occurs a few hours after moderate injury (some bacterial products, thermal injury, ultraviolet [UV] radiation)
      - Involves venules and/or capillaries

    Leukocyte-mediated endothelial injury
    - Caused by release of oxygen derived free radicals and proteolytic enzymes

    Leakage from newly formed capillaries in early stages of repair
    - Persists until endothelium fully differentiated and forms intercellular junctions

- Leukocyte margination and adhesion
  - *Slowing of blood flow promotes leukocyte margination*
  - *Adhesion involves reaction between leukocyte adhesion molecules and counter receptors on endothelium*
  - *Selectins*
    - L-selectins on all leukocytes
    - E-selectins
      - Induced on endothelium by cytokines
      - Promote adhesion in acute inflammation
    - P-selectins
      - Released from alpha granules of platelet and Weibel-Palade bodies of endothelium by histamine
      - Promote adhesion in acute inflammation
    - Selectins bind carbohydrate ligands on target cells

Table 2.5 *Selectins and Integrins*

Molecule	Cells Expressing	Counterreceptor and Target Cells
Selectins		
L-selectin (LAM-1 or LECAM-1)	PMNs, eosinophils, monocytes, lymphocytes	Sialyl-fucosyl-sulfated glycoproteins (endothelium)
E-selectin (ELAM-1)	Activated endothelial cells	Sialyl Lewis X (PMNs, monocytes)
P-selectin (GMP-140)	Activted platelets and endothelial cells	Sialyl Lewis X-like (PMNs, monocytes)
Integrins		
VLA-4 ($\alpha 4\beta 1$)	Lymphocytes, monocytes, eosinophils	VCAM-1 (activated endothelium)
LFA (CDI Ia/CD18)	PMNs, monocytes, lymphocytes	ICAM-1, 2, and 3 (activated and unstimulated endothelium and other cells)
Mac-1 (CDI Ib/CD18)	PMNs, eosinophils, monocytes	ICAM-1 (activated and unstimulated endothelium and other cells)
P150,95 (CDI Ic/CD18)	PMNs, monocytes	Unknown

CD, Cluster designation; *ELAM*, endothelial leukocyte adhesion molecule; *GMP*, granule membrane protein; *ICAM*, intercellular adhesion molecule; *LAM*, leukocyte adhesion molecule; *LECAM*, lectin-cellular adhesion molecule; *LFA*, lymphocyte function-associated antigen; *Mac*, macrophage associated antigen-I; *PMN*, polymorphonuclear leukocytes; *VCAM*, vascular cell adhesion molecule; *VLA*, very late activation antigen.

— *Integrins*

   • Consist of noncovalent bound heterodimers of alpha and beta subunits

      • Named by beta subunit

   • Betaone integrins

      • Very late activation antigen (VLA) subfamily primarily bind to extracellular matrix

      • VLA-4 also binds vascular cell adhesion molecule (VCAM-1)

   • Lymphocyte function-associated antigen (LFA; CD11a/CD18), macrophage associated antigen-1 (Mac-1; CD11b/CD18), P150,95 (CD11c/CD18) are beta2 integrins

      • Alpha chain = CD11

      • Beta chain = CD18

      • Impaired CD18 leads to adhesion defect and life-threatening infections

   • Integrins bind proteins on target cells (addressins), in plasma, or in extracellular matrix (Table 2.5)

— *Steps in leukocyte adhesion (Table 2.6) (Fig. 2.9)*
   Chemotaxins

      • Directed migration of leukocyte towards chemical stimulus

      • Studied in vitro using porous membrane or gel

      • Chemotactic agents

         • Leukotriene B4

         • Platelet activating factor

Table 2.6 *Immunoglobulin Superfamily of Addressins*

MOLECULE	CELLS EXPRESSING	COUNTERRECEPTOR AND TARGET CELLS
ICAM-1	Endothelium and some epithelial cells	Mac-1 and LFA-1 (leukocytes)
ICAM-2	Endothelium	LFA-1 (leukocytes)
ICAM-3	Leukocytes	LFA-1 (leukocytes)
VCAM-1	Activated endothelium	VLA-4 (lymphocytes, monocytes, eosinophils)
PECAM-1	Endothelial junctional areas	Undefined ligand on endothelium, leukocytes, platelets

ICAM, Intercellular adhesion molecule; *LFA,* lymphocyte function-associated antigen or CDI Ia/CD18; *Mac-1,* macrophage associated antigen-1 or CDI Ib/CD18; *PECAM,* platelet-endothelial cell adhesion molecule; *VCAM,* vascular cell adhesion molecule; *VLA,* very late activation antigen.

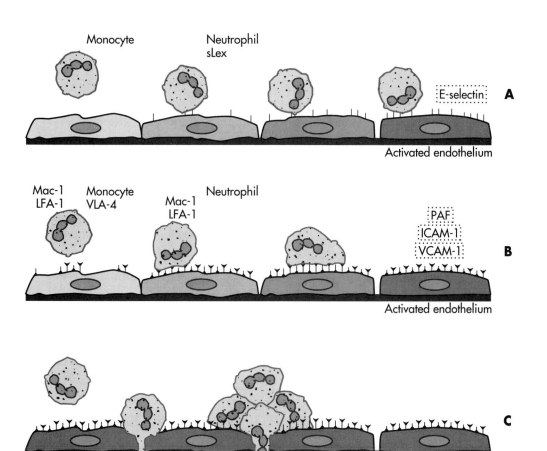

Fig. 2.9 Stages in leukocyte adherence and aggregation during inflammation. **A,** Initial interaction between sialyl Lewis X (sLex) on leukocytes and L-selectin on activated endothelium. **B,** Next, increased expression of and interactions between integrins on leukocytes and platelet activating factor (PAF) and addressins on endothelium. **C,** Increased adhesion with leukocyte aggregation and transendothelial migration. (*Damjanov I, Linder J: Anderson's pathology, ed 10, vol 1, St Louis, 1996, Mosby.*)

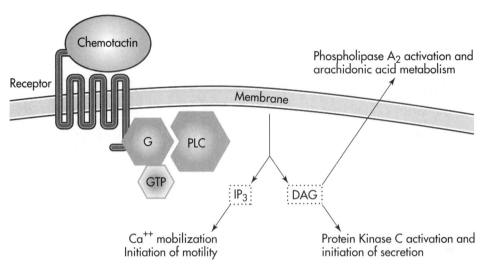

Fig. 2.10 Stimulus-response coupling after binding of chemotactic agent to its receptor. Ligand binding results in activation of the membrane-associated G protein, activation of phospholipase C (PLC) and the production of inositol triphosphate (IP$_3$) and diacylglycerol (DAG). (*Damjanov I, Linder J:* Anderson's pathology, *ed 10, vol 1, St Louis, 1996, Mosby.*)

- Complement C5a
- Interleukin-8
- Bacterial derived N-formyl peptides (e.g., N-formyl-methionyl-leucyl phenylalanin [N-FMP])
- Many of these act through G-protein receptors (Fig. 2.10)

- Move by forward projection of cytoplasm (lamellipodia)
- Requires assembly and disassembly of actin subunits
- Also involves betaone integrin mediated attachment to extracellular matrix proteins (types 1 and 4 collagen, fibronectin, laminin)

● **Leukocyte effector functions**

  — *Mechanism and cells involved depend upon the causative agent*

  - Bacteria, fungi, and parasites killed by phagocytosis and/or extracellular secretion
    - By neutrophils, eosinophils, mononuclear phagocytes
  - Virally infected cells and neoplastic cells killed by cell-mediated cytotoxicity
    - By macrophages or lymphocytes

  — *Phagocytosis*
    Attachment
    Energy independent
    Enhanced by opsonins
    Principal opsonins
    - IgG1
    - IgG3
    - C3b
    - iC3b (fragment of C3b)
    - C4b

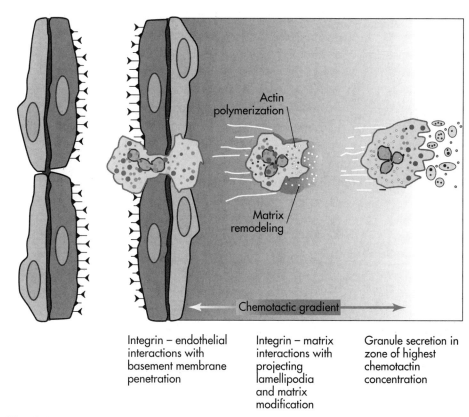

Fig. 2.11 Stages of leukocyte chemotaxis and secretion. (*Damjanov I, Linder J:* Anderson's pathology, *ed 10, vol 1, St Louis, 1996, Mosby.*)

OPSONIN RECEPTORS

- Fc receptors for immunoglobulins

  - Fc gamma R1 on mononuclear phagocytes binds IgG1 and IgG3 with high affinity
  - Other Fc receptors expressed on several cell types have lower affinity

- CR1 and CR3 (Mac-1) complement receptors found on most phagocytic cells

  - CR1 has high affinity for C3b
  - CR3 has high affinity for iC3b

WITHOUT OPSONINS, MACROPHAGES CAN BIND MANNOSE-FUCOSYL RESIDUES IN BACTERIA AND FUNGI

— *Engulfment*

- Energy dependent
- Phagocyte extends actin-rich pseudopods around particle, forming intracellular phagosome containing particle (Fig. 2.11)

— *Secretion*

Preformed granules

FUSE WITH PHAGOSOME AND PLASMA MEMBRANE, DISCHARGING CONTENTS INTO PHAGOSOME OR EXTRACELLULAR SPACE, RESPECTIVELY

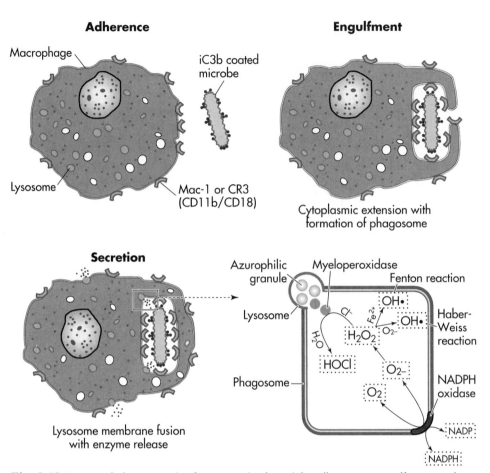

Fig. 2.12 Stages of phagocytosis of an opsonized particle-adherence, engulfment and secretion. Chemical reactions of secretion (occurring in the boxed area) are shown in the lower right. (*Damjanov I, Linder J:* Anderson's pathology, *ed 10, vol 1, St Louis, 1996, Mosby.*)

De novo synthesis of mediators
Membrane lipid derived mediators (arachidonate derivatives)
Cytokines
Enzymes
Oxygen-derived free radicals most important in microbial killing (Fig. 2.12)

- Based on NADPH oxidase (Fig. 2.13)
- Defects in NADPH oxidase result in chronic granulomatous disease
  - Repeated and often fatal bacterial infections

Nitric oxide (Fig. 2.14)

- NOS induced in macrophages, as opposed to constitutive expression in endothelium

— *Cell-mediated cytotoxicity*

- For elimination of virally infected or neoplastic cells
- Macrophages
  - Antibody-dependent cytotoxicity (ADCC)

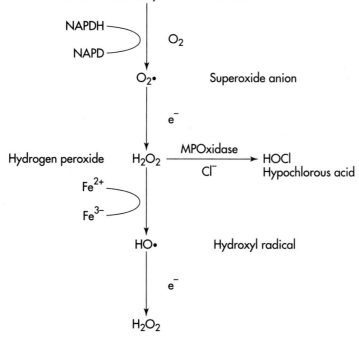

Activation and assembly of NAPDH oxidase

NAPDH
NAPD

O_2

$O_2\bullet$ Superoxide anion

e^-

Hydrogen peroxide H_2O_2 $\xrightarrow[Cl^-]{MPOxidase}$ HOCl
                        Hypochlorous acid

Fe^{2+}
Fe^{3-}

$HO\bullet$ Hydroxyl radical

e^-

H_2O_2

Fig. 2.13 Toxic oxygen species generated by phagocytes after NADPH oxidase assembly. (*Damjanov I, Linder J:* Anderson's pathology, *ed 10, vol 1, St Louis, 1996, Mosby.*)

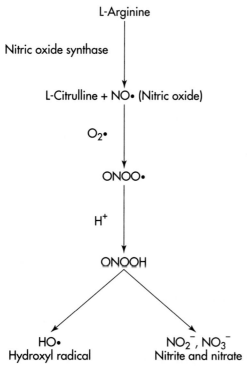

L-Arginine

Nitric oxide synthase

L-Citrulline + NO• (Nitric oxide)

$O_2\bullet$

$ONOO\bullet$

H^+

ONOOH

$HO\bullet$ NO_2^-, NO_3^-
Hydroxyl radical   Nitrite and nitrate

Fig. 2.14 Toxic nitrogen products of macrophages generated from nitric oxide. (*Damjanov I, Linder J:* Anderson's pathology, *ed 10, vol 1, St Louis, 1996, Mosby.*)

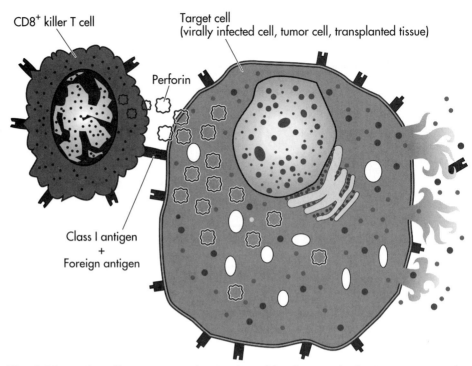

Fig. 2.15 CD8+ T-cell cytotoxicity. The CD8+ T cell binds target by foreign antigen and class I histocompatibility antigen and releases perforin, which permeabilizes the target cell membrane and kills it. (*Damjanov I, Linder J:* Anderson's pathology, *ed 10, vol 1, St Louis, 1996, Mosby.*)

- Requires target cell to be coated by antibodies recognized by Fc receptor
- Cytotoxic T cells (CD8+)
  - Antibody-independent killing using perforin (Fig. 2.15)
- Natural killer cells (NK cells; large granular lymphyocytes)
  - ADCC
  - Antibody-independent killing using cytolysin (apparently the same as perforin)

■ **Systemic Manifestations of Inflammation (Acute Phase Reaction)**
  ● Fever
    — *Mediated by effects of TNF, IL-1, and/or IL-6 on hypothalamus*
      - Direct or indirect (by induction of prostaglandins)
    — *Decreased appetite*
  ● Changes in synthesis of plasma proteins
    — *Acute phase proteins (Table 2.7)*
      - Synthesis and plasma level increases during acute phase reaction
      - SAA and CRP show greatest increase
      - Some are effectors of inflammation
      - Others (α_1-antitrypsin, cystein proteinase inhibitor, ceruplasmin) down regulate inflammation

Table 2.7 *Acute-phase Proteins*	
PROTEIN	**FUNCTION**
α_1-Antitrypsin	Antiproteinase
α_1-Acid glycoprotein	Transport protein
Cysteine protease inhibitor	Antiproteinase
Haptoglobin	Binds hemoglobin
Fibrinogen	Coagulation factor
C-reactive protein	Activates complement
Complement factor 3	Opsonin
Mannose binding protein	Opsonin
LPS binding protein	Opsonin
Ceruloplasmin	O_2 metabolite scavenger
Hemopexin	Heme binding protein
Serum amyloid A	Apolipoprotein
Serum amyloid P	Unknown

— *Negative acute phase proteins*

  • Synthesis and plasma levels decrease in acute phase reaction

    • Albumin, transthyretin

— *Regulated by IL-6 and IL-1*

● Increased white blood cell count (leukocytosis)

  • Accelerated release of postmitotic cells mediated by IL-1 and TNF

  • With prolonged stimulation, CSFs induce proliferation of precursors

  • Most bacterial infections induce neutrophilia

  • Some viral infections induce lymphocytosis

  • Parasites, allergic reactions induce eosinophilia

  • A few infections and severe debilitation can induce leukopenia (decreased white blood cell count)

■ **Repair**

● Extracellular matrix

— *Macromolecular network that surrounds stromal cells and underlies most endothelium and epithelium*

— *Collagens*

  • Structure

    • Three alpha peptide chains rich Glycine-X-Y (X and Y often proline and hydroxyproline)

    • Glycine gives right handed helical structure

    • Three alpha chains form left-handed triple helix (collagenous domain)

    • Nontriple helical domains at carboxy and amino termini

  • Fibrillar

    • Types I, II, III, V, XI

    • Provide tensile strength to tissues

- Network forming
  - Type IV (basement membrane)
— *Elastin and peripheral microfibrils*
  - Elastin is hydrophobic, insoluble, nonglycated protein core of elastic fibrils
  - Elastic fibrils surrounded by network of peripheral microfibrils
    - Fibrillin is component
— *Glycoproteins*
  Fibronectins
  - Glycoproteins
    - Two peptide subunits
  - Plasma (soluble) and cellular (insoluble) forms
    - Generated by alternative splicing of RNA and posttranslation protein modification
  - Forms deposits throughout the extracellular matrix
  - Interacts with plasma and other extracellular matrix components, cells, bacteria
  - Forms primitive matrix later replaced by scar
    - Glutamine in fibronectins allows cross linking by transglutaminases
  Tenascin
  - Glycoprotein that mediates cell-matrix interactions
  - Binds cells, fibronectin, some proteoglycans
  - Associated with fibroblasts
  Thrombospondin
  - Binds cells and extracellular matrix (ECM) components
  - Stimulates or inhibits cell migration (depending on cell type)
  - Can stimulate or inhibit formation of new blood vessels
— *Glycosaminoglycans and proteoglycans*
  - Glycosaminoglycans
    - Linear heteropolysaccharides with disaccharide repeats
    - Most are associated with proteoglycans
  - Proteoglycan—protein core plus covalently bound glycosaminoglycan side chains
  - Can be associated with other ECM components, on cell surfaces or intracellular
— *Basement membranes*
  - Specialized form of extracellular matrix at boundary between cell and stroma
    - Separate epithelia from adjacent connective tissue
    - Separate endothelia from epithelia
    - Surround individual mesenchymal cells

- Laminins
  - Glycoproteins composed of three subunits
  - Bind cells and increase cell motility
  - Interact with other extracellular matrix components
- Enactin (Nidogen)
  - Sulfated glycoprotein
- Osteonectin (SPARC)
  - Glycoprotein that interacts with type I collagen
- Type IV collagen
- Perlecan
  - Proteoglycan (core protein plus glycosaminoglycan chain)
  - Interacts with itself and with type IV collagen and laminin to form complex structures
  - Partly responsible for negative charge of basement membranes

— *Degradation*
  - Most important are metalloproteinases
    - Collagenases
    - Stromelysins
    - Gelatinases
    - Some elastases

— *Interaction with cells*
  - ECM components (fibronectin, others) contain arginine-lysine-1 asparagine (RGD) sequence that binds integrins (see previous)

- **Cells involved in repair**
  — *Endothelial cells*
    - Proliferate and form new blood vessels
      - Essential for granulation tissue and wound healing
    - Synthesize
      - Extracellular matrix components (fibronectin, elastin, collagens)
      - Vasoactive substances (affect caliber, permeability)
      - Cytokines
  — *Smooth muscle cells*
    - Secrete ECM components and growth factors
  — *Platelets*
    - Platelet plug at site of injury
    - Release mitogens, chemotactic agents, ECM components
  — *Fibroblasts*
    - Synthesize ECM
    - Myofibroblasts

- Fibroblast-like cell that has muscle contractile proteins (actin, myosin)
— *Mononuclear phagocytes*
  - Remove dead cells and damaged ECM components
— *Cell-cell interactions*
  - Cell adhesion molecules

● **Repair reactions**

— *Phases*

Inflammatory

- Repair and inflammation often coexist for first week after injury
- Fibrin clot and cross-linking of plasma protein with ECM components
- Chemotactic and mitogenic factors released by macrophages promote angiogenesis

Proliferative phase

- Development of immature, vascularized connective tissue called *granulation tissue* (Fig. 2.16)
- Cytokines and growth factors from macrophages and platelets promote chemotaxis and proliferation of endothelium, fibroblasts, myofibroblasts
- Development of ECM in granulation tissue
  - Initially ECM rich in fibronectin and proteoglycans
  - Type III collagen appears after one week
  - Type I collagen begins to appear after second week
- Angiogenesis—formation of new blood vessels from existing ones
  - Capillaries leaky initially

Maturation phase

- Decreasing cellularity
- Increasing type I collagen

● **Abnormalities of repair processes**

— *Factors that can inhibit normal repair*

- Local
  - Infections or foreign material in wound can delay healing
- Systemic factors
  - Protein malnutrition
  - Vitamin C deficiency (scurvy)
  - Synthetic glucocorticoid therapy

— *Excessive scar formation*

Keloid

- Mass composed of protuberant accumulation of connective extending beyond initial wound (Fig. 2.17)

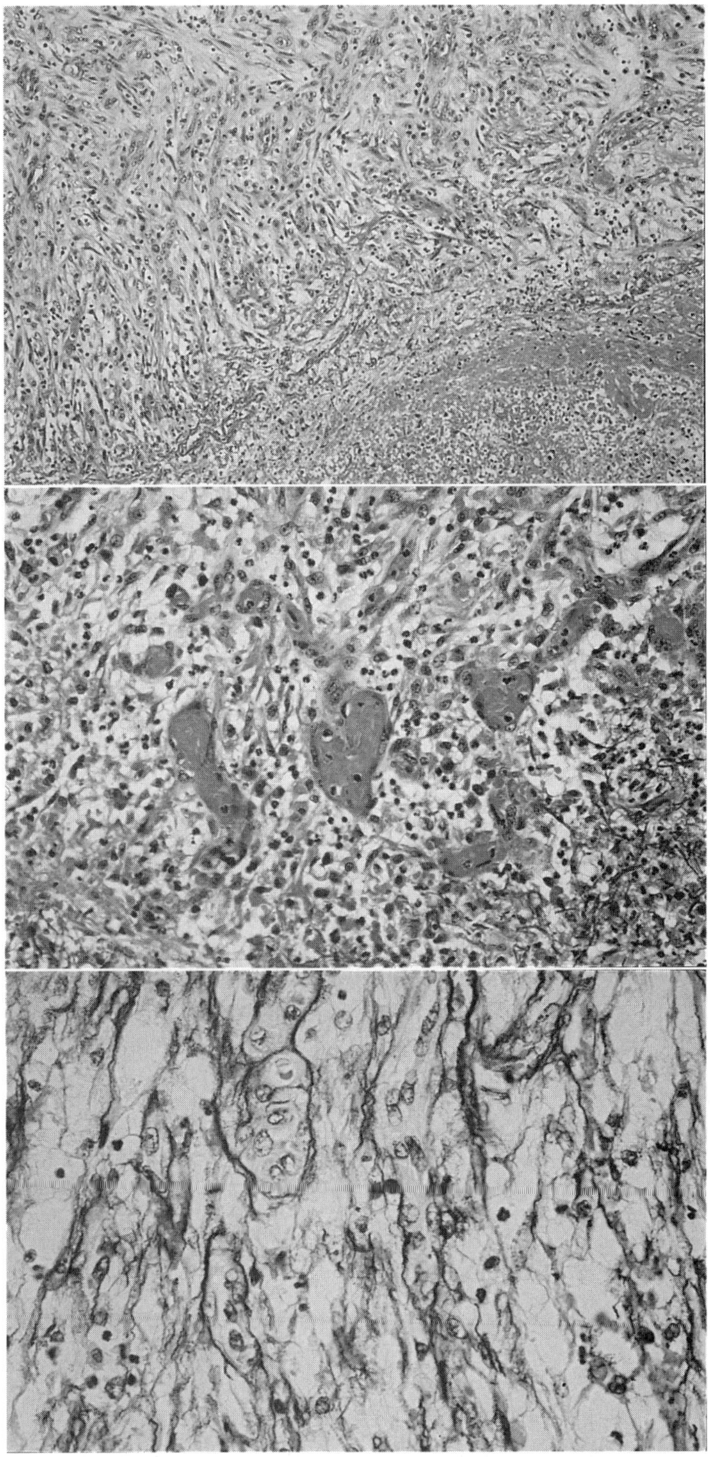

Fig. 2.16 Granulation tissue. **A** and **B,** Note the fibroblasts, capillaries, and inflammatory cells. **C,** Reticulin stain shows the fiber network. *(Damjanov I, Linder J:* Anderson's pathology, *ed 10, vol 1, St Louis, 1996, Mosby.)*

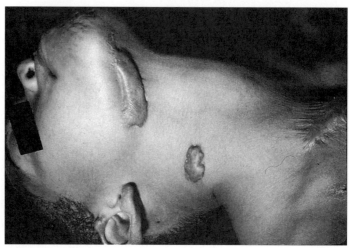

Fig. 2.17 Keloids. (*Damjanov I, Linder J:* Anderson's pathology, *ed 10, vol 1, St Louis, 1996, Mosby.*)

- Similar to hypertrophic scar, which does not extend beyond initial wound

Fibromatoses

- Proliferation of fibroblasts and other repair elements resembling neoplasm

● **Healing in specific organs**

— *Regeneration*

- Replacement of lost cells or tissue by elements of identical structure and function

— *Scarring versus regeneration*

- Chronic or massive injury, destruction of ECM framework, and low proliferative capacity of parenchymal cells favor scarring
- Acute or mild injury, preservation of ECM framework, high proliferative capacity of parenchymal cells favors regeneration

— *Example—skin*

Primary intention

- Involves wound with minimal tissue loss, no infection, and good approximation of its edges
- Initial fibrin clot
- Inflammation

  - Neutrophils enter within 24 hours
  - Macrophages within a few days

- Regeneration of epithelium

  - Stem cells migrate over wound surface
  - Maturation (differentiation) of epithelium

- Formation of granulation tissue within wound site

  - Follows macrophages

- Scarring follows granulation tissue

  - Loss of dermal appendages

Secondary intention

- Caused by larger defect than in wounds healed by primary intention

- Considerable inflammation and necrosis

- Capacity to reepithelialize lesion is exceeded

- Much more granulation tissue than with primary intention, accompanied by extensive wound contraction

  - Myofibroblasts predominant after several days

MULTIPLE CHOICE
REVIEW QUESTIONS

1. Initiation of granulation tissue formation is most closely related to the presence of which of the following?

   a. Fibronectin
   b. Tenascin
   c. Type I collagen
   d. Type III collagen
   e. Type IV collagen

2. The most important stimulus to the increase in synthesis of acute phase proteins is which of following?

   a. Interleukin-3
   b. Interleukin-6
   c. Interferon alpha
   d. Interferon gamma
   e. Prostaglandin E_2

3. Which of the following molecules is directly involved in intracellular killing of bacteria by neutrophils?

   a. Hypochlorous acid
   b. Nitric oxide
   c. Perforin
   d. Prostaglandin E_2
   e. Serotonin

4. Inflammatory response characterized by granulomas containing numerous eosinophils suggests which of the following?

   a. An allergic reaction
   b. Cat scratch disease
   c. Chlamydial infection
   d. Mycobacterial infection
   e. Parasitic infestation

5. Which of the following is most likely to be responsible for initial activation of the classical complement pathway?

   a. IgA
   b. IgE
   c. IgG
   d. Plasmin
   e. Plasminogen activator

Chapter 3

Hemodynamic Disturbances

Disorders of Perfusion

■ **Hemorrhage**

- "Bleeding" or loss of blood from the closed circulatory system
- May occur at the level of arteries, capillary beds, or veins and be either internal (into a tissue, a cavity, and organ spaces) or external
- Petechia—1 to 2 mm-sized areas of blood loss in o the subcutaneous tissue, mucous membranes, and peritoneal surfaces
- Purpura—1 to 2 cm-sized areas
- Ecchymosis—larger areas of hemorrhage, typical bruise
- Hematoma—hemorrhage into tissue forming a blood clot mass
- Hemothorax—hemorrhage into pleural cavity
- Hemoperitoneum—hemorrhage into the peritoneal cavity
- Hemopericardium—hemorrhage into the pericardium
- Hemarthrosis—hemorrhage into the joint space
- A consequence of rapid hemorrhage of over 15% of blood volume—hypovolemia and hypotension that lead to hypoperfusion of tissue
- Shock—the pathophysiologic state and all of the changes that result from an acute reduction of perfusion to the point that it is inadequate to meet the body's metabolic demands

■ **Shock**

● **Causes of shock (Fig. 3.1)**

— *Hypovolemic shock*

- External volume loss vs. internal volume loss
- Internal volume loss—sequestration of circulating fluid into various internal compartments
  - Neurogenic shock—hypovolemia caused by vasodilation, diverting blood volume to the periphery and the capacitance venous system, as may occur with induction of anesthesia or spinal cord injury
  - Anaphylactic shock—fluid loss into the interstitium accompanied by vasodilation and other inflammation-repair elements caused by type I immune-mediated injury
  - Other acute interstitial fluid losses, such as crush injuries

— *Pump failure (cardiogenic shock)*

- Decreased cardiac output from any cause

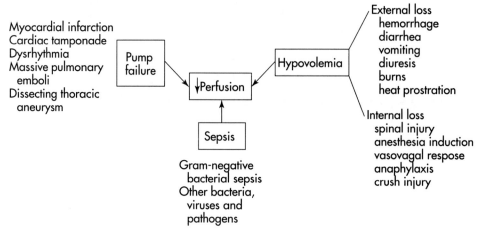

Myocardial infarction
Cardiac tamponade
Dysrhythmia
Massive pulmonary
  emboli
Dissecting thoracic
  aneurysm

Pump failure

↓Perfusion

Hypovolemia

External loss
  hemorrhage
  diarrhea
  vomiting
  diuresis
  burns
  heat prostration

Internal loss
  spinal injury
  anesthesia induction
  vasovagal respose
  anaphylaxis
  crush injury

Sepsis

Gram-negative
  bacterial sepsis
Other bacteria,
  viruses and
  pathogens

Fig. 3.1 Causes of shock.

— *Septic shock*

• The pathophysiologic changes caused by lipopolysaccharide or other toxins from infectious agents that initiate massive activation the repair and coagulation systems and release of the mediators of inflammation through the toxins' interactions with and injury to monocytes, endothelial cells, neutrophils, platelets, and other cells. The current postulated sequence of events is

   • Septicemia with a gram-negative organism
   • Lipopolysaccharide (LPS) from the bacterial cell wall interacts with the CD14 receptor of monocytes, with endothelial and other cells
   • Monocytes synthesize and release large amounts of tissue necrosis factor-α (TNF) and other mediators
   • TNF causes cardiovascular collapse and in conjunction with LPS injures endothelial cells and recruits participation of other cells and cytokines—interleukin-1, -2, -6, -8, platelet activating factor, nitric oxide, complement cascade, coagulation cascade through kinin and contact factors, leukotrienes, catecholamines, prostaglandins, endorphins, and others.
   • Toxins can also cause direct cellular injury and dysfunction

  • The result is

   • Vasodilation, myocardial dysfunction and increased vascular permeability
   • Neutrophil-endothelial adhesion and aggregation causing vascular injury, coagulation activation, thrombosis, and disseminated intravascular coagulation
   • Generalized cellular injury

  • This is manifest by

   • Hypotension and shock
   • Multiorgan dysfunction

- Diffuse alveolar lung damage and hypoxia
- Hepatic and renal failure
- Comma and death

- All the features of septic shock can be induced by injection of LPS or TNF.

— *Evolution of Shock*

- Common to all forms of shock is cellular hypoxia.
- Depending on the duration and intensity of shock, there is an increasing risk of anoxic cellular death.

Uninterrupted shock passes through phases of

- Compensation and correction

  - No irreversible tissue injury has been sustained.
  - Compensation includes volume conservation (activation of antidiuretic hormone [ADH], renin-angiotensin-aldosterone pathway) by kidneys and conservation of vital organ perfusion (baroreceptor reflexes, adrenal catecholamine output) through tachycardia and peripheral vasoconstriction.
  - Patients appear cool and clammy with a rapid weak pulse.

- Reversible progression

  - Persisting tissue hypoxia causes further cell injury and acidosis.
  - Acidosis results in secondary peripheral vasodilation worsening perfusion of essential organs.
  - Endothelial cell damage and death allows capillary leakage, neutrophil-monocyte activation, and disseminated intravascular coagulation (DIC) reducing circulating volume and oxygen delivery.
  - Renal output falls.
  - Some cells die from anoxia, releasing their cellular content, which further contributes to shock by many mechanisms including depression of cellular metabolism.

- Irreversible progression

  - Enough cell death has occurred in various organs that recovery of function is not possible.

— *Pathologic changes of shock*

- Heart

  - Epicardial and endocardial petechia
  - Contraction band myonecrosis
  - Subendocardial myocardial infarction

- Lung

  - "Shock lung" or diffuse alveolar damage
  - Capillary congestion, platelet and neutrophil capillary accumulation, interstitial edema, capillary damage and leakage, alveolar hyaline membrane formation

- Kidney

  - Cortical pallor and hyperemia of the medulla caused by vascular shunting
  - Acute tubular necrosis
  - Diffuse cortical necrosis

- Gastrointestinal tract

  - Erosions of the gastric and the intestinal mucosa produce a diffuse hemorrhagic enteropathy

- Liver

  - Centrilobular fatty change, congestion, and hepatocyte necrosis

- Central nervous system

  - Infarction in the "watershed" regions, especially with preexisting cerebrovascular disease

- Adrenal glands

  - Loss of lipid and cortical hemorrhage (characteristic of septic shock with meningococcal sepsis, known as Waterhouse-Friderichsen syndrome)

- Shock can recover with aggressive restoration of perfusion
- This is most difficult with cardiac shock (cannot replace the pump) and septic shock which accounts for their high mortality

■ Hyperemia

- Increased blood in tissues and organs
- Active

  - Occurs with arterial dilation from a variety of stimuli including neurogenic and vasoactive substances
  - The classic signs of inflammation (rubor, calor, and tumor) are caused by hyperemia

- Passive

  - Caused by obstruction of venous blood drainage
  - Commonly referred to as congestion
  - Can be generalized, usually from heart failure (nutmeg liver from chronic venous congestion) or localized because of local venous obstruction, as in cirrhosis and portal hypertension, producing splanchnic bed congestion and congestive splenomegaly
  - Passive congestion—accompanied by edema of the affected organs

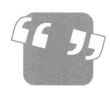

■ Thrombosis

- Thrombosis is the formation of a thrombus within the intact vascular system.
- A thrombus is an actively formed conglomerate consisting of aggregated platelets in a cross-linked fibrin meshwork that entraps red cells and leukocytes.
- Thrombi form in vessels or the heart and adhere to endothelial walls.

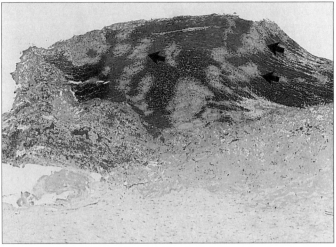

Fig. 3.2 Arterial thrombus. The pale white lines *(arrows)* composed of platelets and fibrin alternate with the dark red cell-fibrin zones to form the lines of Zahn. *(Damjanov I, Linder J: Anderson's pathology, ed 10, vol 1, St Louis, 1996, Mosby.)*

- A blood clot refers to blood coagulation occurring either postmortem in the vasculature or occurring outside the vasculature.
- Thrombosis is the result of (Virchow's triad)

  - Alterations in blood flow—stasis or turbulence
  - Endothelial damage
  - Increased blood coagulability

- Thrombi may undergo the following:

  - Lysis and dissolution through the action of the fibrinolytic system (most common outcome occurring within 24 to 48 hours)
  - Extension or propagation
  - Organization
  - Recanalization—partial reestablishment of the original lumen
  - Embolization (see following)

● **Arterial thrombosis**

  - Most common cause of death in Western world

  — *Pathology*

      - Arterial thrombi are adherent clots composed of a band of platelets and fibrin alternating with a band of fibrin and entrapped red cells.
      - The platelet-fibrin band forms a linear white-yellow zone and the fibrin-red cells a dark red zone called the lines of Zahn (Fig. 3.2).
      - The consequence of arterial thrombosis is ischemic infarction.

● **Venous thrombosis**

  - Venous thrombosis is also called phlebothrombosis, deep venous thrombosis (DVT), and, somewhat incorrectly, thrombophlebitis.

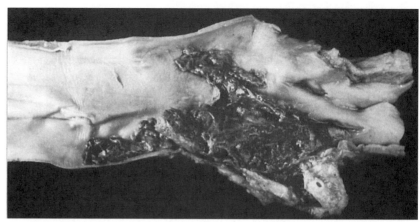

Fig. 3.3 Venous thrombus. An adherent mass of red cell and fibrin occludes a large vein. (*Damjanov I, Linder J:* Anderson's pathology, *ed 10, vol 1, St Louis, 1996, Mosby.*)

- Rather than an injury or inflammation of a vessel causing thrombosis, it is the thrombotic event that initiates the inflammation.
- Deep veins of the leg are the most common sites, followed by femoral, popliteal, and iliac veins.
- In the lower limb, the site of initiation is usually a valvular sinus.
- Proximal propagation into the thigh and iliac veins can occur and is associated with an increased risk of embolization (Fig. 3.3).
- Factors favoring DVT include

  - Inherited deficiencies of fibrinolytic and anticoagulant proteins
  - Prolonged bed rest
  - Surgery—especially lower limb orthopedic procedures
  - Old age
  - Heart failure
  - Immobilization
  - Vessel trauma
  - Pregnancy-childbirth
  - Malignancy
  - Oral contraceptives

- Most DVT are asymptomatic and clinical detection is unreliable.
- DVT and subsequent pulmonary embolization are frequent complications of hospitalization to the extent that prophylactic measures for their prevention saves lives.

— *Pathology*

- Venous thrombi appear as firm casts, focally adherent to the walls.
- Lack distinct lines of Zahn, but have fine fibrin strands that are visible traversing the thrombus on cross-section.
- Postmortem clots differ by being rubbery, unattached to the vessel wall, and, as they occur after some sedimentation of the blood has occurred, show a zonal appearance with dark red dependent ar-

eas (red currant jelly) and yellowish translucent (chicken fat) overlying areas.

■ Embolism

- Occlusion of a vascular lumen by any material that has been carried though the arterial or venous system
- Thromboembolism
  - A thrombus that has detached and been carried to a new intravascular site where it lodges and obstructs blood flow
  - The most common embolism
- Other embolic materials can be
  - Gases—nitrogen in decompression sickness or air introduced directly into the veins
  - Foreign bodies—bullets, catheter fragments
  - Fat—after hip fractures
  - Tumor—a mechanism of metastasis
  - Amniotic fluid—with childbirth

- **Venous pulmonary thromboembolism**
  - Most common source is from the leg veins, and 50% of patients have no symptoms of the primary thrombosis.
  — *Pulmonary emboli may result in*
    1. Sudden death
       - Frequent in hospitalized patients
       - Caused by acute right sided heart failure from sudden obstruction of over half of the pulmonary vascular bed
       - A saddle embolus—a large thromboembolus that lodges at the bifurcation of the pulmonary artery

    2. Pulmonary infarction
    - Emboli must lodge in an end artery, and the secondary blood supply from the bronchial arteries must be compromised (usually caused by preexisting cardiopulmonary disease)
      - Occurs about once in every five pulmonary emboli
      - Pathology

        - Grossly—dark red hemorrhagic, wedge-shaped lesions with base on the pleural surface
        - Microscopically—coagulative necrosis

    3. No symptoms
    - Most common result of pulmonary thromboembolism (¾ of patients)
    - Does not have infarction because of the dual pulmonary blood supply
      - Thrombus usually undergoes lysis and resolution
      - Rarely with recurrent small emboli, pulmonary hypertension and cor pulmonale develop from gradual reduction of the pulmonary arterial bed

- ● Paradoxical embolus

  - • An arterial embolus that arises in the venous system and gains access to systemic circulation via a right-to-left cardiac shunt to become an arterial embolus.

- ● Arterial or systemic emboli

  - • Most commonly arise from the heart after infarction with mural thrombosis, less frequently from atherosclerotic plaques or aneurysms
  - • Emboli lodge at arterial bifurcations and almost always result in infarction unless collateral blood supply is good
    - • Sites of emboli are

      - • Lower extremities
      - • Brain—causing a stroke
      - • Viscera—renal, mesenteric, and splenic
      - • Upper extremities

- ● Fat embolus

  - • Occurs after trauma involving fractures to the long bones
  - • May be immediate or more commonly delayed in onset up to a few days
  - • Produces neurologic symptoms, respiratory insufficiency, petechia, and thrombocytopenia
  - • Widespread microvasculature deposition of neutral fat can be readily identified in lungs, kidneys, and other organs in many patients with trauma, but only a very small number develop fat embolism syndrome
  - • Source of fat—both direct entry from fatty tissue and likely de novo metabolic production of some triglycerides

- ● Air embolus

  - • Release of gases from solution as in decompression sickness or barotrauma with small gas bubbles obstructing the microcirculation

    - • Acutely—in the bones causing pain ("the bends") and in the lungs causing "the chokes"
    - • Chronically—producing avascular necrosis of bones

  - • Direct introduction of gas

    - • Usually air through trauma to the great veins of the neck or chest
    - • Cardiac problems require a large air bolus (100 ml or more)

- ■ **Infarction**

  - • Reduction in blood supply to a tissue or organ is called *ischemia.*
  - • An area of coagulative necrosis in an organ or tissue caused by ischemia is called an *infarct.*
  - • Infarcts are almost always caused by arterial occlusion.
  - • Vascular occlusion may be from thrombosis (most common), embolus, torsion atherosclerosis, and other mechanisms causing ischemia or infarction.

  - ● Pathology—two gross morphologic types

    - • Pale or anemic infarcts

      - • In solid tissue especially kidney, brain, spleen, and heart

- Initially appear slightly darker, wedge-shaped areas (pointing towards the site of occlusion), becoming soft, pale, tan-yellow, and surrounded by a peripheral hyperemic zone by about 24 to 48 hrs
- Microscopically—coagulative necrosis

- Red or hemorrhagic infarct

  - From hemorrhage into an infarcted area
  - More common in loose expansile tissue, tissue with dual blood supply, infarction caused by venous occlusion, and infarcts that become reperfused (i.e., lysis of a thromboembolus)
  - Gross: deep red, firm and sharply demarcated areas
  - Microscopic—interstitial hemorrhage, vascular dilation and congestion with coagulative necrosis

■ Edema

- Condition of excess fluid in the interstitial space
- Local—inflammation, regional venous or lymphatic obstruction
- Generalized—severe, called anasarca
- Collection of edema fluid in body cavities known as—hydrothorax, hydropericardium, and ascites (peritoneal cavity)
- Caused by an imbalance in factors moving fluid out of vascular fluid space and those moving fluid back into the circulation
- Increased hydrostatic pressure

  - Localized venous obstruction—venous thrombosis, portal hypertension
  - Generalized increased venous pressure—cardiac failure

- Decreased plasma oncotic pressure (decreased return of fluid to vessels)

  - Low serum albumin from decreased synthesis (liver disease, malnutrition) or increased loss (burns, nephrotic syndrome)

- Lymphatic obstruction from scarring or tumor
- Increased sodium and water retention

  - Renal disease or as a secondary response to some of above causes through renin-angiotensin-aldosterone mechanism
  - Disruption of the capillary endothelial integrity can also cause fluid and plasma leakage

- ● **Pulmonary edema**

  - Usually cardiac disease producing increased venous pressure and decreased lymphatic return
  - Early increased venous pressure causes an increase in lymphatic flow and shunting of pulmonary blood flow from lower lung fields to upper
  - Detected on x-ray film as Kerley B lines in the lower lungs (dilation and edema around the pulmonary lymphatics that run in the septa) and increased prominence of upper lung vasculature
  - As fluid accumulates in the alveoli it is visible on x-ray film or audible on auscultation

  - *Pathology*

    - Gross—lungs weight is increased, and they ooze fluid when cut
    - Microscopic—dilation and congestion of capillaries, expanded

lymphatic and perilymphatic tissue along the bronchovascular bundles and lobular septa, pale pink fluid in the alveoli

- Chronic edema can lead to intraalveolar hemorrhage and hemosiderin deposition (in pulmonary macrophages equal heart failure cells) and fibrosis

Multiple Choice Review Questions

1. Common causes of shock include all *except* which of the following?
   a. Collapse after rapid return to the upright position after blood donation
   b. *E. coli* sepsis following ureteral obstruction with a calculus
   c. Saddle pulmonary embolus
   d. Massive hematemesis from esophageal varices
   e. Myocardial infarction

2. Virchow's triad (factors favoring thrombosis) includes which of the following?
   a. Leukocytosis, thrombocytosis, and erythrocytosis
   b. Increased plasminogen, increased protein C, and increased protein S
   c. Occult cancer, heart failure, and jaundice
   d. Hyperglycemia, hyperlipidemia, and hypertension
   e. Stasis, vascular injury, and hypercoagulability

3. For severe hepatic disease, edema results primarily from which of the following?
   a. Hyponatremia
   b. Hypergammaglobulinemia
   c. Hypoproteinemia
   d. Anemia
   e. Hypocalcemia

4. From which of the following sites do the most clinically significant systemic emboli arise?
   a. Mural thrombi within the heart after myocardial infarction
   b. Thrombi within the atrial appendages with atrial fibrillation
   c. Heart valve vegetations
   d. Pulmonary venous thrombi
   e. Ulcerated atherosclerotic plaques

5. A young female suffers multiple, bilateral fractures of the femur after being struck by a car while crossing an intersection. Two days after admission she develops dyspnea, confusion, and conjunctival petechia and dies. The most likely finding at autopsy is which of the following?
   a. Multiple pulmonary embolus
   b. Widespread fat emboli of lung, brain, and kidney
   c. Aspiration pneumonia and microvascular thrombi from disseminated intravascular coagulation
   d. Myocardial infarction with mural thrombus and multiple systemic arterial emboli
   e. Occult endocarditis with widespread septic embolization from vegetations

Chapter 4

Immunity

All pathologic immune reactions represent a normal protective immune function against pathogens that become destructive and cause disease.

■ **Anaphylaxis and Atopy (Type I Immune Injury) (Fig. 4.1)**

- Allergic reactions refer, in common terms, to altered immune responses dependent on the binding of antigens to mast cells and basophils through their passively acquired membrane-bound IgE.

- Clinical anaphylaxis consists of acute (usually termed *anaphylactic*) or chronic and recurrent (usually termed *atopic*) reactions.

- Normal immune function of this process is thought to be an initiation of a local inflammatory reaction to aid in toxin neutralization and in the expulsion of intestinal parasites.

- Allergy prone individuals are known as *atopic.*

- Antigens causing allergic reactions are called *allergens.*

- Mast cell or basophil degranulation and release of histamine, heparin, and serotonin account for the acute reactions and recruitment of T cells and eosinophils for the persistent features.

- Histamine causes

    - Arteriolar vasodilation (H2 receptors) producing local hyperemia or systemic shock

    - Smooth muscle and endothelial cell constriction (H1 receptors) producing edema, bronchospasm, diarrhea, and micturition

- Synthesis and gradual secretion of prostaglandins and leukotrienes produce the chronic phase of a more sustained inflammatory reaction with infiltration by neutrophils and eosinophils.

- Local anaphylaxis presents as urticaria or wheal and flare reaction and hives.

    - There is a regional histamine effect with itchy, raised pale area (wheal) and surrounding erythema (flare) that resolves in 15 to 20 minutes.

- Generalized anaphylaxis presents as anaphylactic shock with cardiovascular collapse caused by arteriolar dilation and increased vascular permeability.

- Other disorders caused by this immune reaction are allergic rhinitis (hay fever), food allergy, insect bite allergy, and asthma.

■ **Cytolytic Reactions (Type II Antibody-mediated Toxicity) (Fig. 4.2)**

- Direct binding of antibody to antigens on the cell surface

    - Complement (C) cascade activation and cell lysis

    - Phagocytosis of cells with bound Ig's and C (opsonization)

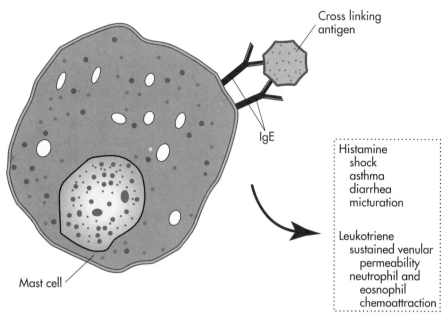

Fig. 4.1 Anaphylaxis. An antigen cross links surface-bound IgE on mast cells, releasing the granule-stored mediators.

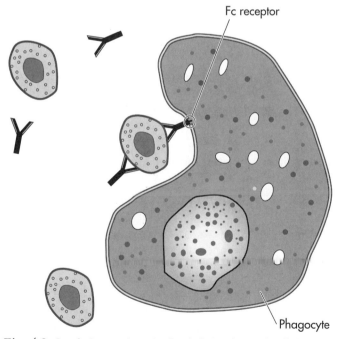

Fig. 4.2 Cytolytic reaction. Antibody bound to red cells binds to phagocytes through the phagocyte Fc receptors.

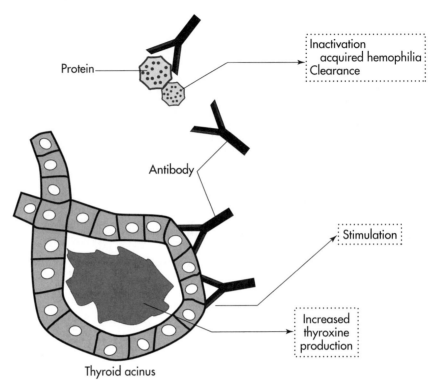

Fig. 4.3 Antibody-mediated activation and inactivation. The binding of antibodies can result in neutralization of proteins or stimulation of cells.

- The normal immune function—direct lysis and phagocytosis of bacteria and other susceptible pathogens
- Phagocytes—recognize cells labeled with complement and/or immunoglobulin by their C3b or Fc receptors
- Disease states include—hemolytic transfusion reactions, immune neutropenia, immune thrombocytopenia, autoimmune hemolytic anemia, some drug-induced reactions (especially thrombocytopenia and hemolytic anemia) and Rh disease of the newborn, alloimmune neonatal neutropenia, and thrombocytopenia

■ **Antibody-mediated Activation and Inactivation (Type II Antibody-mediated Toxicity) (Fig. 4.3)**

- Antibodies to functionally important molecules cause their inactivation or antibodies to important receptors cause their activation or inactivation resulting in disease states.
- The normal immune function for this reaction is the neutralization of toxins or blockage of viral receptors.
- Examples:
  - Acquired hemophilia—antibody inactivates normal factor VIII
  - Graves' disease—antibodies to thyroid-stimulating hormone (TSH) receptor produce hyperthyroidism
  - Myasthenia gravis—antibodies to the acetylcholine receptor cause persistent stimulation and muscle weakness
- Many other diseases result from this mechanism.

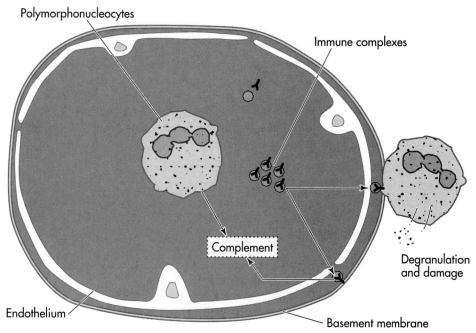

Fig. 4.4 Immune complex disease. Antibodies bind to tissue antigens, or soluble antigen-antibody complexes are deposited in tissues activating an inflammatory reaction.

▪ Immune Complex Disease (Type III Immune Injury) (Fig. 4.4)

• Antibodies bind to tissue antigens (i.e., basement membrane) to form antigen-antibody (ag-ab) complexes or soluble circulating ag-ab complexes are deposited in the tissue.

• Ag-ab complexes are capable of activating complement evoking an acute inflammatory reaction.

• Antibodies directed towards fixed tissue antigens often included in type II injuries (antibody-mediated injury), but result in injury similar to immune complex disease.

• Normal immune function of this reaction is to elicit an acute inflammatory response at the site of pathogens.

• Attracted neutrophils cause destruction by granule release.

• The sites of the immune complex deposition characterize some disorders.

• Serum sickness

  • 10 to 14 days after administration of nonhuman sera
  • During the antigen excess phase, immune complexes are not cleared by the fixed phagocyte system efficiently and deposit in vessels and glomeruli
  • Neutrophils infiltrate and acute inflammation results
  • Clinical—fever, arthritis, vasculitis, and glomerulonephritis

• Vasculitis

  • Deposition of immune complexes in the vessel walls
  • Pathology—neutrophilic inflammation, vessel thrombosis, fibrinoid ne-

crosis, leakage of red cells, and neutrophil degeneration, leaving nuclear debris called *leukocytoclastic vasculitis*

- Pattern seen with vasculitis occurring in other disorders, including systemic lupus erythematosus (SLE)

- Glomerulonephritis

  - Immune complexes—the most common cause of glomerulonephritis
  - Glomerular basement membrane—exposed to antibodies binding to the membrane or to the deposition of circulating complexes

- Goodpasture's syndrome is caused by antiglomerular basement membranes antibodies affecting predominantly the lungs and the kidneys.

- Bullous pemphigus is caused by antiepidermal basement membrane antibodies.

■ Delayed Hypersensitivity (Type IV Immune Injury)

- Immune injury resulting from sensitized T helper (CD4$^+$) cells (T-DTH) that recognize antigens presented in the context of major histocompatibility complex (MHC) class II become activated and attract nonspecific inflammatory cells, and result in chronic inflammation and tissue destruction.

- Activated monocytes cause most of the tissue destruction and, by producing cytokines, help establish the chronic inflammation.

- The intradermal injection of *Mycobacterium tuberculosis* derived purified protein derivative (PPD) in a sensitized individual (a TB skin test) is the paradigm of this response.

  - Pathology

    - Sensitized lymphocytes infiltrate around small veins and venules, followed by monocytes, nonspecific lymphocytes, basophils, and other cells.
    - Proliferation of T-DTH produces blast transformation of some cells.

- This immunologic response is critical to controlling various infections, including mycobacteria, syphilis, other bacteria, fungi, viruses, and parasites as evidenced by the susceptibility of acquired immunodeficiency syndrome (AIDS) patients.

- Disorders thought to arise through this mechanism include postvaccinial encephalomyelitis, multiple sclerosis, and transplant rejection.

- Direct activation of T-DTH cells by superantigens results in some types of food poisoning, toxic shock syndrome, rheumatic fever, scarlet fever, and scalded skin syndrome from *Staphylococcus aureus* and *Staphylococcus pyogenes* toxins.

■ T Cell-mediated Cytotoxicity (Type IV Hypersensitivity) (Fig. 4.5)

- Specifically sensitized T cells (CD8) recognize antigens (in the context of MHC class I) and destroy the cells directly.

- These cytotoxic T cells (T-CTL) kill the target cells utilizing their granule components, especially perforin and granzymes.

- Natural killer (NK) cells can also kill by a similar mechanism.

- The normal function of this immune reaction is thought to be protection against intracellular organisms, especially killing of virus infected cells and possibly tumor responses.

  - Contact dermatitis

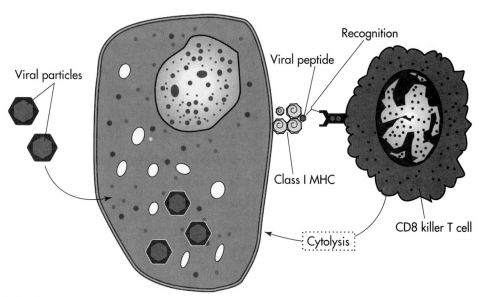

Fig. 4.5 Cell-mediated cytotoxicity. Sensitized T cells recognize antigens destroying cells directly.

- Antigens, usually lipid-soluble, are reactive chemicals or metals that penetrate the epidermis and bind to local proteins in a haptenlike fashion.
- Prior sensitization is required.
- Pathology consists of perivenous accumulation of lymphocytes and monocytes with edema. The lymphocytes infiltrate the epidermis, causing edema (spongiosis), death of epidermal cells, and development of intraepidermal vesicles (small fluid-filled, blisterlike lesions).
- Poison ivy reaction is an example of this response.

- Graft rejection—T-CTL is the major mechanism involved in graft rejection, along with T-DTH.

Granulomatous Reactions

- Granuloma are focal inflammatory collections of macrophages, typically multicellular with histiocytes, epithelioid macrophages, giant cells, lymphocytes, and plasma cells as components.
- Epithelioid histiocytes are transformed macrophages characterized by abundant eosinophilic cytoplasm (resembling squamous epithelium) and pale vesicular nuclei with a central nucleolus.
- They form as the result of prolonged delayed type hypersensitivity (DTH) and cytotoxic lymphocytes (CTL) responses to persistent organisms or antigens that are poorly degradable.
- Granulomatous hypersensitivity is a type of type IV, cell-mediated immune response.
- Normal function is directed to certain pathogens, notably leprosy, tuberculosis, some fungi, and helminths.

Table 4.1 *Common* Autoantibodies in Systemic Autoimmune Disease*

Antinuclear antibodies (various staining patterns)	SLE, undifferentiated connective tissue disease (UCTD), drug-induced SLE, Sjögren's syndrome, scleroderma/CREST, polymyositis, dermatomyositis, overlap syndrome
Rheumatoid factor	Rheumatoid arthritis, scleroderma, MCTD, Sjögren's syndrome
Anti-double-stranded DNA	SLE
Sm (Smith)	SLE
SS-A/Ro	SLE, Sjögren's syndrome
Histone	Drug-induced SLE, SLE
SS-B/La	Sjögren's syndrome
Ribonucleoprotein (RNP)	SLE, Sjögren's syndrome, scleroderma, polymyositis, UCTD
Scl-70 (DNA topoisomerase 1)	Scleroderma
Centromere	CREST
Jo-1 (histidyl-tRNA synthetase)	Dermatomyositis/polymyositis

*Gives the disease best characterized by a positive finding and those diseases with over 25% of cases positive.
SLE, Systemic lupus erythematosus; *MCTD,* mixed connective tissue disease; *CREST,* *c*alcinosis, *R*eynaud's phenomenon, *e*sophageal motility disorders, *s*clerodactyly, and *t*elangiectasia.

- Pathologic reactions involving granuloma include berylliosis, Crohn's disease, sarcoidosis, granulomatous vasculitis, primary biliary cirrhosis, and Wegener's granulomatosis.

■ **Autoimmunity and Autoimmune Diseases**

- Dysfunction of the immune system is caused by failure to recognize self and the development of a humoral and/or cellular immune response directed at one's own tissue that results in autoimmune disease.

- Autoantibody detection and monitoring is useful in diagnosis of diseases and their follow-up (Table 4.1).

- Presence of an autoantibody is not sufficient for a diagnosis because low-titer autoantibodies are common in normal people, and the absence of a high-titer autoantibody can be seen in an autoimmune disorder.

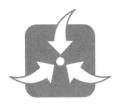

- Failure of self-tolerance (clonal deletion, clonal anergy, and clonal ignorance) and immune regulation (antiidiotypes and specific suppressor T cells) are postulated etiologies for autoimmunity.

- Genetic factors

  - Closely linked to the major histocompatibility (MHC) locus haplotypes and female sex, but also include the T cell receptor and B cell immunoglobulin gene repertoires
  - Human leukocyte antigens (HLA) DR3—insulin-dependent diabetes mellitus (IDDM), SLE, Sjögren's syndrome, Graves' disease, myasthenia gravis, dermatitis herpetiformis
  - HLA DR4—rheumatoid arthritis, IDDM, and pemphigus vulgaris
  - HLA B27—spondylitic arthropathies

- Environmental factors

  - Most frequently infectious pathogens

- Less often drugs and chemicals
- May function as molecular mimics, result in formation of new self-determinants, or release sequestered antigens by tissue damage
- Coxsackievirus B—IDDM, gastrointestinal
- Urinary tract infections—spondyloarthropathies

- Basic mechanisms of autoimmunity are abnormal presentation of autoreactive antigens and abnormal regulation of the immune system
- Autoimmune disease may be classified as systemic or organ specific.
- Diagnosis is based on the combination of clinical finding and results of laboratory tests for marker autoantibodies as proposed by the American Rheumatism Association.

Systemic Lupus Erythematosus

- A chronic, idiopathic, multiorgan autoimmune inflammatory disease with widespread tissue damage and characteristic autoantibodies
- Common (1/700 prevalance in females of reproductive age)
- Familial predisposition and association with inherited complement deficiency and HLA B8, DR2, and DR3
- Immune complex mechanism of tissue injury

- Pathology

  - Skin—may be part of systemic lupus or the skin-limited discoid lupus

    - Hyperkeratosis, basal layer liquefactive degeneration, follicular plugging, telangiectasis, and superficial and deep perivascular lymphohistiocytic infiltration
    - Basement membrane thickened on periodic acid-Schiff (PAS) stains and dermal hyaluronic acid increase by alcian blue staining
    - Leukocytoclastic vasculitis (clinically palpable purpura)
    - Lupus band test—immunofluorescent along the basement membrane of skin for immunoglobulins and complement

  - Kidney—immune complex nephritis, poor prognosis, varing degrees of glomerular inflammation; heavy subendothelial deposits can result in "wire loop" thickening of the capillary wall
  - Cardiovascular system

    - Pericarditis—common
    - Libman-Sacks endocarditis—see cardiovascular disease

  - Pulmonary system

    - Pleuritis and a variety of changes including acute pneumonitis, acute alveolar hemorrhage, diffuse alveolar damage, and chronic interstitial disease

  - Brain—seizures and cerebritis, poor prognostic sign
  - Musculoskeletal system—symmetrical, nondestructive, polyarthritis
  - Lymph nodes and spleen—follicular hyperplasia, plasmacytosis, focal necrosis with hematoxylin bodies (purple bodies formed of fragmented nuclei)
    - Hematologic

- Autoimmune hemolytic anemia, thrombocytopenia, and neutropenia
- Lupus anticoagulant and antiphospholipid antibodies

■ Scleroderma

- Idiopathic disorder characterized by increased collagen deposition, vascular endothelial injury and vessel obliteration associated with perivascular lymphoid infiltrates and epidermal atrophy
- Progressive systemic sclerosis (PSS) is the generalized form
- CREST—calcinosis, Raynaud's phenomenon, esophageal motility disorder, sclerodactyly, and telangiectasia is the more organ-limited form

  - Skin involvement is usually hands and face
  - More indolent than PSS

- Women of reproductive age, but less common than SLE

● Pathology

- Skin—tightening, atrophy, and loss of mobility give rise to the stiff, clawlike hands and masklike facies, focal ulceration of the finger tips, and calcification can occur

  - Dense dermal fibrosis with epithelial thinning, atrophy, and loss of adnexal structures except for hypertrophy of erector pili muscle, vascular obliteration

- Lungs—interstitial fibrosis, pulmonary hypertension common in CREST
- Heart—restrictive cardiomyopathy
- Gastrointestinal tract—muscularis propria and submucosa fibrosis, epithelial atrophy and focal ulceration causes dysphagia, abdominal pain, and obstruction
  - Kidneys—renal failure is the most common cause of death

    - Obliterative vasculopathy of the interlobular arteries
    - Malignant hypertension may eventuate

  - Musculoskeletal—synovitis similar to rheumatoid arthritis but without joint destruction, less commonly myositis

■ Sjögren's Syndrome

- Idiopathic autoimmune disorder characterized by destruction of lacrimal and salivary glands producing keratoconjunctivitis sicca (dry eyes) and xerostomia (dry mouth)
- May be primary (sicca syndrome) or associated with rheumatoid arthritis and other autoimmune disorders
- Female predominance with mean age of 50 years
- HLA-B8, DR3 association

● Pathology

- Infiltration and destruction of salivary and lacrimal glands with formation of myoepithelial islands also called *benign lymphoepithelial lesions* (commonly biopsy minor labial salivary glands) (Fig. 4.6)
- An indolent, malignant, B cell lymphoma of the monocytoid or marginal zone type may arise from this background

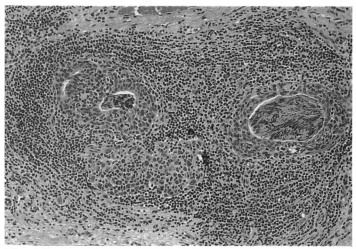

Fig. 4.6 Myoepithelial sialoadenitis. Dense lymphocytic infiltration and proliferation of epithelial and myoepithelial cells results in epimyoepithelial islands. (*Damjanov I, Linder J:* Anderson's pathology, *ed 10, vol 2, St Louis, 1996, Mosby.*)

- May develop peripheral vasculitis with cryoglobulinemia, Raynaud's phenomenon, and tubulointerstitial nephritis

■ **Immunodeficiency**

● Primary

— *Severe combined immunodeficiency (SCID)*

- Immunodeficiency characterized by lack of both T and B cell function
- Many genetic etiologies
- Usually manifest by 3 months with failure to thrive and evidence of persistent viral, fungal, or other infection and lymphopenia with lymphoid depletion of lymphoid tissue
- Survival—depends on immune reconstitution with bone marrow transplant

X-linked

- Most common type of SCID (60%)
- Mutation of the interleukin-2 receptor gamma chain gene on Xq13
- Severe T cell deficiency but may have B cells that resemble neonatal B cells with expression of CD5 and CD11c
- The immunoglobulins are not produced in response to specific challenge

Other SCIDs

- Autosomal recessive
- Deficiencies of the purine degradation enzymes adenosine deaminase and nucleoside phosphorylase are common
- Failure to express MHC class I and II antigens results in SCID like immunodeficiency
- Other defects are not yet characterized

— *X-linked agammaglobulinemia (Bruton's)*
  - Recurrent pyogenic infections in males after age 6 months
  - Low levels of all classes of immunoglobulin and depletion of normal mature B cells from blood and lymphoid tissue
  - Defect in the cytoplasmic signal-transducing molecule btk or the *B* cell *ty*rosine *k*inase gene at Xq22
  - Treated by immunoglobulin replacement

— *IgA deficiency*
  - Common with about 1 in 700 incidence
  - Most asymptomatic, but some have gastrointestinal and respiratory disorders or autoimmune diseases
  - May have antibodies to IgA; blood product transfusions can cause anaphylaxis

— *Common variable immunodeficiency*
  - Onset in second and third decades with hypogammaglobulinemia and impaired specific antibody response
  - Heterogeneous inheritance and defects of B and T cell interaction
  - Recurrent sinopulmonary or gastrointestinal tract infections and sometimes autoimmune peripheral blood cytopenias, collagen vascular disease, generalized lymphoid hyperplasia, inflammatory bowel disease, and widespread, nonspecific granuloma
  - Predisposition to lymphoid malignancies and gastric carcinomas

— *Other immunodeficiencies*
DiGeorge syndrome
  - Small facies, truncus arteriosus, thymic and parathyroid aplasia or hypoplasia
  - Abnormal development of the third and fourth pharyngeal pouches and heart occurring at 4- to 6-week gestation
  - Most sporadic with death caused by tetany or heart failure

Ataxia-telangiectasia
  - Cerebellar ataxia, oculocutaneous telangiectasia with recurrent infections presenting at about 1 year of age
  - Autosomal recessive
  - *ATM* gene at 11q22, possible cell cycle regulating kinase
  - Appear to have a DNA repair problem with spontaneous translocation involving the T cell receptor genes and susceptibility to ionizing radiation and a predisposition to development of lymphoid malignancies

Wiskott-Aldrich syndrome
  - Eczema, thrombocytopenia, and recurrent infection
  - X-linked with survival into teens
  - Gene identified on Xp11 and cloned, but is a unique protein of unknown function

X-linked lymphoproliferative syndrome (Duncan's syndrome)
  - Inability to handle infection by the Epstein-Barr virus

— *Chemotaxis disorders*
Leukocyte adhesion defect

- Caused by mutation in the CD18 beta chain common to a number of surface adhesion molecules on leukocytes
- Poor scar formation, recurrent respiratory infections, and diarrhea with peripheral blood leukocytosis

— *Defective bacterial killing*
Chronic granulomatous disease

- Inability of the phagocytes to produce superoxide and other reactive oxygen forms essential in bacterial killing
- Caused by a deficiency in respiratory burst pathway involving the membrane-bound NADPH (reduced form of nicotinamide-adenine dinucleotide phosphate) oxidase
  - Nitroblue tetrazolium test reveals this defect in the neutrophils
  - X-linked for the deficiency of membrane cytochrome b at Xp21
  - Other autosomal forms with defects in other burst pathway proteins
  - Inability to kill catalase-positive organisms, such as *S. aureus,* results in formation of abscess characterized by central necrosis and a surrounding granulomatous response

■ Acquired Immunodeficiency Syndrome

- Caused by infection by the human immunodeficiency virus (HIV) (commonly type 1 in North America, but type 2 may be seen in Africa and India)
- Cytopathic nontransforming type C retrovirus resembling the lentivirus family that primarily infects and destroys T cells
- Spread through exchange of body fluids by intravenous or sexual routes
- CD4 is the receptor molecule for the HIV
- CD4 expressing cells include T cell subsets, macrophages, monocytes, and microglial cells of the central nervous system
- Primary infection (1 to 12 wks)

  - Flulike symptoms, dissemination of virus
  - Drop in CD4 T cells

- Clinical latency (mean of 10 years)

  - Immune response to virus with reduction in the viral replication
  - Gradual decline in helper T cells

- Symptomatic AIDS

  - Development of infections and malignancies characteristic of severe T cell depletion secondary to HIV
  - 2 to 3 years until death

- ● Pathology

  - Lymphoid tissue

    - Persistent generalized lymphadenopathy
    - Nonspecific changes in lymph nodes includes—follicular hyperpla-

sia, clusters of monocytoid B cells in sinusoids, and multinucleate giant cells from T helper cell fusion induced by the virus

- Eventually nodes show generalized lymphoid depletion
- Salivary gland—changes resembling Sjögren's syndrome
- Hematologic manifestations
- Anemia of chronic disease, thrombocytopenia (often immune based)
- Common infections
    - *Pneumocystis carinii,* cytomegalovirus, *Cryptosporidium parvum, Toxoplasma gondii, Mycobacterium avium-intercellulare* complex, *Mycobacterium tuberculosis, Candida* organisms, Epstein-Barr virus (EBV)
- Neoplasms
    - Non–Hodgkin lymphoma—often disseminated and extranodal; usually aggressive B cell types with EBV present in 40%
    - Kaposi's sarcoma—most frequent in homosexual males, a herpes virus recently isolated
    - Carcinoma—usually lung, larynx, and uterine cervix; higher incidence of human papillomavirus (HPV) associated carcinoma
- Nervous system
    - Frequent site of abnormalities
    - Encephalitis, AIDS-related dementia, progressive multifocal leukoencephalopathy, JC virus (papovavirus), myelopathy, peripheral neuropathy, and myopathy

■ Transplantation Pathology

● Transplantation genetics

- Blood-group and tissue-type (MHC) matching is important for graft survival.
- The closer to identical matches, the better the organ survival or the less chance of graft-versus-host (GVH) disease in bone marrow transplantation.
- With full matching, graft failure and GVH disease is presumed to be caused by other "histocompatibility" antigens.
- Allogeneic refers to genetically different individuals.
- Syngeneic refers to genetically identical individuals.
- Autograft refers to a graft of one's own tissue.

— *Allograft rejection*

- Recipient's immune system recognizes the HLA difference between itself and the graft and mounts a cellular (T cell) and antibody response

Classification

- Relates to time course, histologic composition, and mechanism of rejection
- Hyperacute—implies preformed antibodies binding to the graft with complement-mediated cell damage
- Acute—implies a T cell-mediated graft rejection

- Chronic—implies a humoral-mediated mechanism, targeting the vascular endothelium occurring over greater periods of time

● **Renal transplantation**

— *Hyperacute rejection*

- Preformed antibodies to ABO blood group, HLA class I, and graft endothelium antigens fix complement-causing vascular injury, inflammation, and necrosis
  - Occurs within minutes to days of revascularization
  - Immunoflourescense demonstrates immunoglobulins and complement in the vessels and glomeruli resulting in acute inflammation, neutrophil infiltration, vascular thrombosis, and ischemic necrosis

— *Acute rejection*

- Occurs weeks to years after grafting
- Most common type is cellular tubular rejection
- Pathology—lymphocytes, transformed lymphocytes, plasma cells, and macrophages infiltrate around vessels, interstitium, and into the tubules (tubulitis); lymphocytes are mostly CD8 positive T cells

— *Chronic rejection*

- Progressive decline in renal function months to years after engraftment
- Pathology—atrophic lesions consisting of interstitial fibrosis, glomerular and tubular shrinkage with damage to the vessels and chronic ischemia
  - Vascular changes consist of fibrosis and narrowing
  - May be the result of accumulated episodes of acute rejection

MULTIPLE CHOICE
REVIEW QUESTIONS

1. Which of the following is the most common form of immunodeficiency?

    a. Severe combined immunodeficiency
    b. Chronic granulomatous disease
    c. Common variable immunodeficiency
    d. Ataxia-Telangiectasia
    e. X-linked agammaglobulinemia

2. X-linked severe combined immunodeficiency is caused by an inherited defect in which of the following?

    a. Adenosine deaminase
    b. Interleukin-2 gamma chain
    c. MHC class I gene expression
    d. B cell tyrosine kinase (btk gene)
    e. Nucleoside phosphorylase

3. Pathologic skin changes of SLE may include all *except* which of the following?

    a. Dense dermal fibrosis
    b. A positive immunofluorescent band test
    c. Follicular plugging
    d. Thickening of the epidermal basement membrane
    e. Leukocytoclastic vasculitis

4. HLA DR4 is more prevalent in which of the following autoimmune disorders?

    a. SLE
    b. Rheumatoid arthritis
    c. CREST
    d. Ankylosing spondylosis
    e. Sjögren's syndrome

Chapter 5

Overview of Infectious Diseases

■ **Agents of Infectious Disease**

- Bacteria (including spirochetes, chlamydiae, rickettsiae)
- Fungi
- Viruses
- Protozoans
- Helminths
- Prions

■ **Disease-causing Agents Vary in Complexity**

- Free-living microorganisms, which contain all the necessary equipment to sustain themselves outside host cells (e.g., bacteria)
- Incomplete organisms (saprophytes), which require preformed organic matter for food (e.g., fungi)
- Organisms that require more of the processes of host cells to survive (e.g., rickettsiae, chlamydiae)
- Organisms totally dependent on host cell metabolic processes (e.g., viruses)
- Large, complex, multicellular parasites (e.g., helminth worms)
- Infectious agents that cause fatal disease and apparently are able to capture cellular mechanisms so that more of the agent is made, but function without the aid of nucleic acids (e.g., prion ["slow virus"] agents)

■ **Microorganisms (Particularly Bacteria) Can Be Divided into Three Categories**

- Pathogenic (cause disease)
- Nonpathogenic (do not cause disease)
- Either—dependent upon host

  - *Note:* These are relative terms, and a microorganism's ability to cause disease (pathogenicity) depends on many factors, including many external to the organism itself.

■ **Some Pathogens Are Aided in Their Ability to Cause Disease by Certain Unique Properties**

- Toxin production (e.g., *Clostridium tetani*)
- A structure that protects it from attack by the host's defenses (e.g., the polysaccharide capsule of *Streptococcus pneumoniae* inhibits attack [phagocytosis] by macrophages)

- Elaboration of enzymes that aid spread through tissues (e.g., "flesh eating" streptococci)

  - These special properties, however, are exceptional.
  - *Note:* The capacity to produce disease by *any* agent is more dependent on host **defense mechanisms (or lack thereof)** than any characteristic of the agent itself. The distinction between pathogen and nonpathogen is blurred and may vary with the age of the patient, the patient's previous experience with the organism, the state of the host's immune system, coexisting diseases or microorganisms, and many other factors.

Some organisms can cause disease only *if* and *when* they multiply in the human under specific circumstances such as location, pH, oxygen tension (e.g., *C. tetani* can proliferate and produce toxin only in deep wounds protected from oxygen)

■ Human

- Is inhabited by large numbers of microbial organisms (normal endogenous microbial flora) normally nonpathogenic, some actually beneficial, which may, nevertheless, produce disease under the right circumstances
- Is exposed to large numbers of exogenous microorganisms in the environment, such as in soil, water, air

  - Most are nonpathogenic but may become so under the right circumstances.
  - Some are inherently pathogenic *if* they gain entry.
  - Some produce products (toxins) that are dangerous if they are ingested (e.g., in food) even though the microorganisms themselves are not present (e.g., botulism and staphylococcal food poisoning).
  - Some produce toxins as they grow within the host that have detrimental effect on the host (e.g., gram-negative Enterobacteriaceae).
  - Some produce their major consequences for the host solely by way of a toxin produced as they grow within the host (e.g., *C. tetani*).

- Is exposed to animals, which harbor different families of microorganisms that sometimes can be transmitted to humans and cause disease, directly or through vectors (e.g., insects); these diseases are known as *zoonoses*

■ Of All Sources of Human Microbial Infection, the Most Important Source of the Organisms Is the Human Being

- Normally present endogenous microbial flora, if conditions are suitable (diminished host defenses), may cause disease (e.g., as a complication of acquired immunodeficiency syndrome [AIDS]).
- Some humans ("carriers") may harbor more virulent, disease-causing organisms (with or without themselves being ill) and may transmit these organisms, and the diseases, to others.

  - An example of a disease that can be transmitted when the individual is overtly ill is the common cold (caused by a variety of different viruses).
  - Examples of diseases that may be transmitted to others without the carrier being overtly ill are typhoid fever and diphtheria.

■ Transmission of Microorganisms

- Is favored by close contact with humans or animals harboring the disease-causing microorganisms; these may be transmitted to others by respiratory droplet infection, direct contact with infected sites, contamination of physician's hands, contact with mucosal surfaces during sexual intercourse (e.g., tuberculosis, leprosy, all of the sexually transmitted diseases)

• May occur through contaminated food or water (cholera, salmonella infections, *Escherichia coli* 0157:H7)

• May take place by contamination of wounds or other breaks in the skin (e.g., tetanus, rabies)

• By insects, human or animal bites, or contaminated needles (e.g., rabies, encephalitis-producing viruses, human immunodeficiency virus [HIV])

• Transplacental or perinatal transmission, from mother to child (e.g., HIV, syphilis, herpes, hepatitis B)

■ **Common Terms**

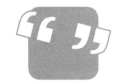

• Pathogen—a microorganism that causes clinically significant disease

• Virulence—"poisonous," sometimes used to refer to the degree of pathogenicity

• Communicability—the ability of a microorganism to pass from the source and infect others; some factors influencing communicability may have nothing to do with the organism itself (e.g., the percentage of the population that is immune; the more immune members in a population, the less likely a nonimmune member of that population will be infected [herd immunity])

• Invasiveness—the ability of a microorganism to multiply in or on the tissues of the host; invasiveness depends on the properties of the microorganism, the host, and host-organism interactions

• Opportunistic pathogen—an organism that does *not* cause disease in a normal host but can do so when host defenses are impaired (e.g., in AIDS); *Candida albicans* and *Pseudomonas aeruginosa* (a fungus and a bacterium, respectively) are two common organisms seen mainly in hosts with impaired immunity

LESIONS OF INFECTIOUS DISEASE

The host can mount many defenses against disease-causing microorganisms. Once having gained entry to the host, if the invaders are not contained by these host defenses, the disease-causing infectious agents can damage cells and tissues by a wide variety of different mechanisms, some highly characteristic for particular organisms or groups of organisms, some quite nonspecific. The changes in organs and tissues caused by the infectious agents of disease therefore form a broad spectrum of damage. This portion of the discussion will illustrate some of the kinds of damage caused by microorganisms and relate them to the groups of microorganisms with which they are often associated.

■ **Infection (and Tissue Damage) without Inflammation (or with Very Minimal Degrees of Inflammation)**

● Prion ("slow virus") disease

• A relatively new class of infectious agent, discovered only within the past 25 years

• Causes invariably fatal central nervous disease without cellular inflammatory infiltrates or detectable humoral antibody responses

• Is *not* a virus in the usual sense—apparently contains no DNA or RNA and represents an altered form of an endogenous protein; it affects the central nervous system only (although it can be isolated from almost any tissue or body fluid) and can only be detected by biologic assay (i.e., by injection into experimental animals)

  • Prion-caused diseases—bovine spongiform encephalitis, scapie (sheep), kuru, and Creutzfeld-Jakob disease

  • Characteristic tissue changes—vacuoles within the processes of nervous system cells, giving the tissue, by light microscopy, the appearance of a sponge with many small holes; hence, these diseases are known as the "spongiform encephalopathies" (more detail in the Neuropathology chapter)

● Fungi

— *Cryptococcus neoformans* A budding yeast, normally causes severe chronic or granulomatous inflammation. *Occasionally,* however, it may cause severe damage to the nervous system over a long period of time, but with only a very low grade chronic (mononuclear) inflammatory cell response. This rare type of reaction is included to point out that, even if inflammation is absent or minimal, the etiology for this process may still be an infectious agent.

  • *Note:* The term *chronic* is used in two different ways (one temporal and the other related to the predominant type[s] of inflammatory cells)

    • To indicate that the disease process has been present for a considerable period of time

    • To indicate that the inflammatory response is mononuclear (lymphocytes and/or plasma cells and/or macrophages), even though the inflammation may have been present for only a few hours

■ **Exudative Inflammation without Tissue Damage**

● Exudative inflammation

  • Increased vascular permeability and leukotaxis, predominantly of neutrophils.

  • Many neutrophils, protein-rich fluid, and fibrin present in the lesions

— *Pneumococcal pneumonia (Streptococcus pneumoniae)*

  • Severe acute inflammation (increased vascular permeability and outpouring of inflammatory cells—in the acute phase predominantly neutrophils) usually involves an entire lobe of the lung, limited to the alveolar air spaces.

  • In adequately treated cases or where spontaneous resolution occurs (without treatment, patients either recover or die), the lung may return to baseline normal without residua because the walls of the alveoli have not been significantly damaged.

■ **Inflammation on the Surface of Organs, with or without Inflammation of Underlying Tissues**

● Empyema

  • Suppuration (exudative inflammation and pus formation) within a natural tissue space or organ cavity, often appears as a layer of purulent exudate covering the surface of an organ.

    • *Suppuration* means pus formation; *purulent* means consisting of pus; *pus* means viscous, liquefied exudate, the product of liquefactive necrosis, rich in neutrophils, tissue debris, serum, and, often, microorganisms

- Empyema is commonly seen within the pleural cavity, gallbladder, subdural space and nasal sinuses.

    - A wide variety of organisms including bacteria and fungi may be associated with this type of lesion; *viruses are not.*

● **Acute or chronic inflammation within the cerebral and/or spinal subarachnoid space is a subtype of the above but is generally called** *meningitis*

    - Its full name is *cerebrospinal* (since the subarachnoid space is in continuity over the brain and spinal cord) *leptomeningitis* (inflammation of the pia and arachnoid).

    - Inflammation involving the dura mater is *pachymeningitis.* Many different organisms, including bacteria and fungi, may be responsible.

    - A very severe acute virus infection of neural parenchyma may kill nervous system cells at such a rapid rate that the products of the dead cells may be chemotactic for neutrophils (i.e., acute meningeal inflammation may be present).

● **Pseudomembrane formation**

    - Some infections that involve mucosal surfaces of organs have severe inflammation limited to the mucosa, with exudate that appears to lie on the surface of the mucosa forming a membranelike covering.

    - Inflammation spreads across the surface rather than into the depths of the tissue.

    - If the pseudomembrane is stripped off, the superficial damage becomes apparent with ulcerations of the underlying tissue. This type of inflammation is seen in the gastrointestinal tract with overgrowth of certain enteric opportunists after antibiotic therapy or in immunosuppressed patients (e.g., *Clostridium difficile*).

    - Diphtheria is also characterized by a membrane that forms on the mucosa of the upper respiratory tract.

        - This membrane contains the bacteria and inflammatory cells.
        - A toxin, secreted by the bacteria *Corynebacterium diphtheriae* is absorbed into the blood stream and causes severe damage to other organs, especially heart and nerves.

■ **Diffuse Inflammation of the Parenchyma of an Organ (Usually Accompanied by Some Degree of Diffuse Parenchymal Damage)**

    - This type of reaction, with either acute or chronic inflammation, may be interstitial inflammation

    - It may also be the result of autoimmune phenomena directed against normal bodily constituents (myelin, muscle, thyroid hormone, DNA, etc.), directed against the antigens of a transplanted organ, or as a reaction to drugs, and may present an extremely vexing diagnostic dilemma to clinician and pathologist alike

    - As a morphologic entity, this type of lesion is often named for the involved organ with the suffix-*itis* appended, indicating inflammation; often *acute* or *chronic* is also added to further describe the appearance (e.g., *chronic interstitial nephritis* means chronic interstitial inflammation of the renal parenchyma; *acute myocarditis* means acute inflammation of the muscle of the heart; *chronic interstitial pneumonitis* means chronic inflammation involving the walls of the alveolar air spaces, often with little or no inflammation within the air spaces themselves and is a common reaction in lungs infected with a virus).

■ **Inflammation of the Parenchyma with Focal Tissue Damage**

● Necrotizing inflammation

• Acute or chronic inflammation resulting in significant damage to the cells and tissues of the organ—necrosis of lung parenchyma (e.g., "necrotizing pneumonia") is inflammation within the alveolar air spaces with damage to the alveolar walls themselves

• Necrotizing pneumonia—common with almost any type of infectious pneumonia with the exception of pneumococcal pneumonia

● Abscess

• A focus of total liquefactive necrosis of the parenchyma of an organ, usually filled with pus (cellular debris, acute and/or chronic inflammatory cells, protein-rich fluid and fibrin, and the microorganisms, alive and dead)

• *Staphylococcus aureus*—the bacterium most commonly associated with abscesses but there are many others that may form abscesses (so may fungi and protozoans)

■ **Cytopathic-Cytoproliferative Inflammation**

• With certain microorganisms, *especially viruses,* cellular proliferation and/or the formation of multinucleated giant cells may be the initial response to the infection and be much more striking than other facets of the inflammatory response.

• An example of this type of response occurs with measles virus infection, especially in children, especially in the appendix and in the lung, where the alveolar air spaces may be lined by bizarre, multinucleated giant cells (Warthin-Finkeldey giant cells).

• Epithelial proliferation also occurs in the skin in response to infection with papilloma viruses; the growth is commonly called a wart.

■ **Granulomatous Inflammation**

• Granuloma is a specific inflammatory lesion.

• Tuberculosis, leprosy, parasitic (worm) infestations, syphilis, certain viral infections are all common infectious causes of granuloma formation.

• A foreign-body granuloma is an example of a noninfectious granuloma.

• Other diverse diseases, such as granulomatous enteritis (Crohn's disease), and sarcoidosis, are diseases not proven to be infectious in nature but are characterized by the formation of granulomas.

• Granulomatous inflammation also may be seen in patients with autoimmune disease and in drug reactions.

• Granuloma is a circumscribed inflammatory lesion characterized by the presence of altered *histiocytes (epithelioid cells),* which are themselves derived from monocytes.

• When a granuloma resides within the parenchyma of an organ, it usually destroys and replaces the normal parenchyma in that location.

• Chronic mononuclear inflammation and multinucleated giant cells do not form a necessary part of the definition of the lesion, although they are often present.

● Although recognizing these patterns of inflammation leads the pathologist to certain pathways of diagnostic investigation, there are many pitfalls to be avoided

1. *None of the reactions described above are specific for a particular organism.* Many organisms can elicit one or more of these inflammatory reactions, de-

pending upon a variety of factors related to the time course of the illness, such as the degree and quality of host resistance, or therapy that may have been applied.

2. *None of the reactions described above is specific for an infection with a microorganism at all*—these reactions to infective microorganisms and all of the various inflammatory reactions can be mimicked by other disease processes not caused by infection.

- Examples: Edema may mimic the "spongiform" degeneration associated with a prion ("slow virus") agent.

  - Diffuse acute inflammation is usually present around acute infarctions.
  - A foreign body, such as a piece of glass, may elicit the formation of a granuloma.
  - The analgesic, phenacetin, if taken to excess, causes severe, chronic, interstitial inflammation in the kidneys.
  - Multiple sclerosis, a disease of unknown etiology but probably mediated by a delayed hypersensitivity autoimmune reaction directed against central nervous system (CNS) myelin, is associated with perivascular mononuclear inflammation similar to that seen with viral infections of the nervous system.

3. *Inflammation caused by infection is rarely pure but is often of mixed character.* This is because of the time course of the disease, the patient's previous experience with the organism, the drugs that may have been used to treat the patient, and a variety of other factors.

- The physician, to be successful, must learn to apply the *art,* as well as the *science,* of medicine to decipher these diagnostic riddles; the life of each patient hinges on the proper solution of the mystery.

MYCOBACTERIAL INFECTIONS

■ Tuberculosis (TB)

- A widespread, chronic, highly contagious disease caused by *Mycobacterium tuberculosis* (an "acid-fast" organism)

  - Poor socioeconomic conditions (crowding, poor hygiene, poor nutrition) and underlying immunosuppression are responsible for a dramatic increase in TB.
  - One third (⅓) of the world's population is infected with the bacterium but most of these are asymptomatic and do not even know they have been infected at some time in their lives.

- May affect any organ or tissue; the lungs are the most common site

- Lesions are typically granulomatous, with necrosis resembling curds of cheese; hence, "caseous" necrosis

  - Adjacent small lesions coalesce to form larger lesions.
  - Chronic inflammatory cells, fibroblasts, and multinucleated giant cells of the Langhans' type, with their nuclei deployed about the periphery of the cells like a necklace of beads, are also commonly present (Fig 5.1).

- Virulence of the bacterium is related to complex lipids and carbohydrates in the cell wall; these are also involved in the delayed hyper-

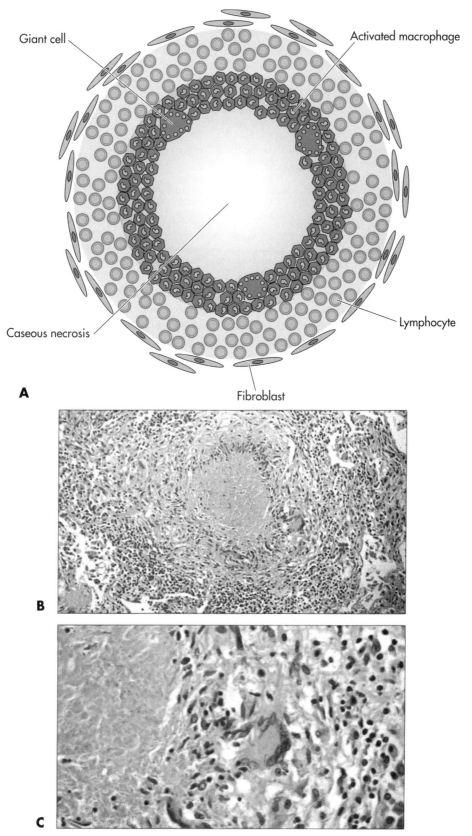

Fig. 5.1 Tuberculosis. **A,** Diagrammatic representation of a tuberculous granuloma. Central caseous necrosis is surrounded by activated macrophages (histiocytes) and occasional Langhans' giant cells. **B,** Photomicrograph of pulmonary granuloma (tubercle) with features corresponding to diagram in **A. C,** Higher power view of **B,** demonstrating a Langhans' giant cell. (*From Stevens A, Lowe J:* Pathology, *London, 1995, Times Mirror International.*)

sensitivity state that develops in tuberculosis and plays an important role in the course of the disease and in the containment of the infection

- Primary tuberculosis is an infection in someone who has not been previously exposed *or* who cannot react immunologically.

- The primary lung lesion—the most common type—is a single, necrotic, subpleural focus that becomes granulomatous in an upper segment of the lower lobe or a lower segment of the upper lobe of one lung. By the second week after infection, the lesion develops a necrotic, caseous center. This lesion is known as the *Ghon focus.*

- Tubercle bacilli drain to the regional (tracheobronchial) lymph nodes causing caseating granulomas there. The lung lesion plus the lymph node lesions are known as the *Ghon complex.*

- Usually the disease does not progress beyond this stage; one sees gradual shrinkage, fibrosis, and calcification of the lesions, but the bacilli within may remain viable indefinitely. The organism is contained (imprisoned) at this site.

- The skin test for TB becomes positive in 2 to 4 weeks after initial infection. The delayed hypersensitivity state develops about the same time the granulomas become necrotic (10 to 14 days).

- Progressive primary tuberculosis appears in some patients when the lesions do not regress, but grow large, forming large granulomatous masses in matted hilar lymph nodes; in the lung, the primary focus may erode into a bronchus, spreading bacilli throughout the bronchial tree and causing multiple additional granulomas. Bacilli may also enter the blood stream and become disseminated throughout the body including the brain, where tuberculous meningitis is a common complication. When the granulomas are disseminated and small, the term *miliary* tuberculosis applies, with millet-seed (canary seed) sized granulomas scattered throughout the parenchyma of the affected organs (Fig. 5.2).

- Secondary tuberculosis is reexposure to tubercle bacilli in a previously exposed and sensitized individual. The reexposure to the bacilli may be exogenous (from the outside) or endogenous (release of bacilli from previously quiescent primary lesions in the same host).

- Secondary lesions are typically in the *apical or posterior segments* of the lungs, resulting from hematogenous (blood-borne) seeding of bacilli; these areas probably reflect a favorable environment for growth because of their higher oxygen tension. Lesions (granulomas) may progress and spread (progressive secondary tuberculosis) or regress to fibrocalcific nodules (arrested tuberculosis).

- Secondary lesions may erode into bronchi (the patients may cough up necrotic material containing many tubercle bacilli), erode into an artery spreading bacilli to other organs, or erode into the pleural space giving rise to tuberculous empyema.

- Continuous reticuloendothelial system stimulation may result in "secondary" amyloidosis in the liver, spleen, and kidneys.

- *Note:* In primary infection, local tissue damage is usually insignificant and clinically silent. In secondary tuberculosis, tissue damage is more intense because of the full effects of the delayed hypersensitivity state. However, the delayed hypersensitivity aids in the con-

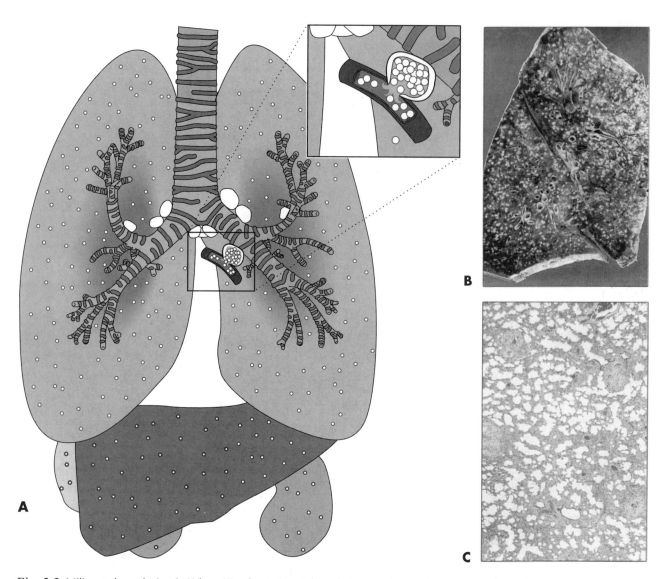

Fig. 5.2 Miliary tuberculosis. **A,** When *Mycobacterium tuberculosis* organisms gain access to the pulmonary venous system, systemic dissemination of the disease occurs (e.g., liver, spleen, kidneys). When these organisms gain access to the pulmonary arterial system, dissemination throughout the lungs occurs. **B,** Photograph depicts a child's lung featuring numerous small yellow-white tuberculous granulomas. **C,** Low-power photograph of tuberculous granulomas (tubercles); note the giant cells featured in many of these space occupying lesions.

tainment of the disease, preventing (possibly fatal) spread throughout the body. Miliary dissemination is much more likely, therefore, to occur in primary TB. Inoculation with a strain of bacillus (Bacille Calmette-Guérin ([BCG] or the vole TB bacillus) not pathogenic for humans but able to produce cross-reacting delayed hypersensitivity, has been used as a form of protective immunization for people in danger of exposure to TB, such as workers in TB sanitoria.

● Key points

- *Mycobacterium tuberculosis* (M.t.b.) cases have been on the increase (even *without* the AIDS epidemic); TB in the United States increased each year from 1985 to 1992; since 1992 the number of new cases has stabilized.

- Multiple drug resistant M.t.b. cases are on the increase (as many as 20% of isolates in some communities).
- M.t.b. is a *major* infection in the AIDS population.

■ Nontuberculosis Mycobacteria

- Also known as mycobacteria other than tuberculosis (MOTT, or atypical mycobacteria)

● *Mycobacterium avium-intracellulare complex*

- A number of MOTT organisms are capable of causing human disease, but the most clinically relevant culprits here have been within the *Mycobacterium avium-intracellulare* grouping (MAI).
- Historically, MAI organisms (which are essentially ubiquitous in nature) have caused medically significant disease in middle- to older-aged men, many of whom had underlying pulmonary disease (especially chronic obstructive pulmonary disease [COPD], usually associated with cigarette smoking).
- Infections of MAI are *not* highly contagious (in contradistinction to M.t.b.) but rather appear to be acquired from the environment by hosts who are at least somewhat predisposed to lung infection.
- The infection has historically involved, and been more or less limited to, previously diseased lung (virtually exclusively) and may be difficult to eradicate, often requiring 3 to 5 antimicrobial drugs for treatment.
- This scenario changed rather dramatically after 1981, at which time we recognized the first cases of what would become known as the AIDS epidemic.
- Since this time, we have come to realize that MAI infections in AIDS patients are notorious for becoming *disseminated* beyond the pulmonary portal of entry.
- Favorite sites in AIDS patients include the gastrointestinal tract, bone, liver, lymph nodes, and CNS, but virtually any other body site may be infected. Eradicating this organism in AIDS patients is often essentially impossible.
- Key point: In *non-AIDS* patients, the inflammatory response to MAI is usually the expected type (granuloma formation). *But in AIDS patients, the inflammatory response to MAI is usually not that of discrete granuloma formation but rather diffuse sheets of histiocytes literally stuffed with organisms.*

● Non-MAI MOTT

- *Mycobacterium fortuitum-chelonei complex*—infections usually involve skin or eye (cornea) as well as lung; may also contaminate medical prostheses (e.g., cardiac valves, mammary augmentation devices); *M. fortuitum-chelonei is now the second most common MOTT grouping associated with human disease*
- *M. kansasii*—causes pulmonary infection resembling classical M.t.b.; most cases in southern, western, and midwestern United States; rarely disseminates, except for AIDS patients
- *M. ulcerans*—causes chronic skin ulcers in patients living in tropical locales
- *M. marinum*—associated with chronic ulcerating skin granulomas ("swimming-pool granulomas")

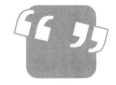

- *M. szulgai*—may cause granulomatous infection in lung, lymph nodes, joint tissues

- *M. scrofulaceum*—a common cause of infectious cervical lymphadenitis in children; rarely causes pulmonary disease

- *M. xenopi*—may cause pulmonary disease; may be seen in immuno-suppressed hosts

- *M. malmoense*—associated with pulmonary disease (rarely seen, however)

- *M. haemophilium*—causes skin infections, mainly in immunosuppressed lymphoma as well as renal transplant patients

- *M. simiae*—sometimes seen in handlers of monkeys; can cause pulmonary disease in humans

- *M. genovense*—recently identified in pulmonary and extra pulmonary sites

AIDS (Acquired Immunodeficiency Syndrome)

In 1981, five young male homosexuals contracted *Pneumocystis carinii* pneumonia, a disease previously virtually unknown except for children with protein-calorie malnutrition or in severely immunodeficient adults. At about the same time, an outbreak of a rare malignancy (Kaposi's sarcoma) was reported in a group of previously healthy, young gay males. Thus began an epidemic that has spread worldwide. As of late 1995, over 476,000 AIDS cases have been diagnosed in the United States; nearly 300,000 of these persons have died already. Globally, the World Health Organization estimates that 20 million are *infected* and that there are over 1 million HIV-positive persons in North America alone. Most, if not all, will eventually die of complications of this disease unless there are major advances in diagnosis, prevention, and treatment.

Although this epidemic traces its roots to the homosexual-bisexual population, it has effectively been spread into the heterosexual population, mainly by injection drug users.

Therefore, the disease is now rapidly spreading into the heterosexual, non-drug-using population through promiscuity, prostitution, and contaminated blood (although this is now a minor factor in the United States) and has been introduced into the lives of the famous and wealthy along with the average and poor: Arthur Ashe and Magic Johnson are recent examples.

■ **Epidemiology** Our understanding of the distribution of AIDS has constantly evolved since 1981 and is still evolving. Major populations at risk:

- Homosexual or bisexual males historically constituted the largest single group infected

- *Injection drug users and their sexual contacts now account for an ever-increasing number of cases at risk*

- Heterosexual contacts of members of the above groups or other heterosexuals already infected

- Hemophiliacs, especially those who received factor VIII concentrates prior to 1985

- Other recipients of blood or blood products

- A small percentage of cases in which the mode of transmission is unknown

- Occasional health-care workers accidentally infected from patients or from laboratory accidents

■ AIDS Virus

- Previously known as HTLV-III (Human T-cell leukemia virus type 3) and by other names, the virus is now known as HIV-1 (human immunodeficiency virus type 1). There is also an HIV-2 described that may be even more virulent than type 1, but this is seen almost exclusively in West Africa.

- A *retrovirus*—a member of the family that includes human T-cell leukemia virus type 1, a transforming virus that causes neoplastic transformation of its target cells, in this case CD4$^+$ helper T lymphocytes, gives rise to T-cell leukemia, a relatively rare variety of white blood cell neoplasia. HIV, in contrast, is cytolytic for helper T cells and thus produces profound immunodeficiency rather than T-cell neoplasms.

- The HIV-1 virion has an icosahedral structure (a regular polyhedron with 20 plane faces) 72 projecting external spikes that are formed by the two major viral envelope proteins, gp120 and gp41. The core contains four nucleocapsid proteins and two copies of the single-stranded, HIV-1 genomic RNA that is associated with various preformed viral enzymes, including reverse transcriptase.

- Human CD4$^+$ T lymphocytes are the specific targets for this virus because the CD4 antigen on their surfaces represents the major, if not the sole, high-affinity receptor for the virus. These cells are regulators and effectors of normal immune response, and the killing of these cells results in profound immunodeficiency.

- The virus also infects monocytes and macrophages but has much less cytopathic effect on these cells, which probably serve as a reservoir for the virus and disseminate the virus throughout the body, including to the brain. The virus may also infect glial cells, gut epithelium, and bone marrow precursors of the normal circulating blood cells.

- The virus gains entry to the target cells by attaching at a CD4 receptor site and fusing with the cell membrane. After internalization, the outer portions of the virion are stripped off (uncoating), and viral replication begins by the generation of a first-strand DNA copy of the viral RNA mediated by the viral reverse transcriptase enzyme. Second-strand DNA is also generated, yielding a double-stranded DNA replica of the original RNA viral genome. This replica enters the nucleus of the cell and is inserted into the host genome by another viral enzyme, viral integrase.

- After entry into the cell the virus may establish a latent or persistent form of the infection. It is estimated that for every T cell that actively produces virus, nine others contain latent virus. The reasons for this are not completely understood.

- Expression of the HIV-1 genes is characterized by cytoplasmic expression of viral mRNAs uniquely encoding the HIV-1 regulatory proteins, structural and enzymatic proteins, which are mediated by specific viral regulatory proteins including Tat, Nef, Rev, and others, and the complete virus is eventually assembled.

  - *Note:* One viral enzyme, protease, cleaves precursor viral proteins and is the target of a new class of anti-AIDS viral agents which holds some promise.

- The exact mechanism(s) by which the virus kills infected cells is (are) not completely understood, but is (are) probably multifactorial. One possible mechanism involves cell fusion leading to multinucleated syncytia (giant cells) that ultimately die.

■ Transmission

- Sexual contact (including vaginal and anal-receptive intercourse)

  - Possibility of transmission by kissing unproven and uncertain (but probably very low or negligible)

- Parenteral inoculation

  - Injection drug users sharing needles
  - Administration of contaminated blood or blood products

- Perinatal transmission from infected mother to child during pregnancy or in the immediate postpartum period

  - Risk approximately 15% to 30% if mother is infected

- AIDS—*not* transmitted by casual (nonsexual) contact, even close family contacts

  - Health-care workers who have contracted the disease—usually by way of accidental parenteral inoculation by needle stick or contamination of non-intact skin or mucous membranes by blood (0.3% risk at each percutaneous exposure)

■ Clinical Features (Spectrum Ranging from Asymptomatic Infection to Full-blown AIDS)

- 30% to 50% of infected patients—develop an acute illness resembling influenza or infectious mononucleosis (Epstein-Barr virus); sore throat, muscle aches, fever, rash, sterile leptomeningitis are common
  - Persistent generalized lymphadenopathy; modest depletion of CD4$^+$ cells
  - AIDS-related complex (ARC)—intermittent or continuous long-lasting fever (3 months or longer), weight loss, and diarrhea; CD4$^+$ cell count is reduced, and the CD4:CD8 (helper to suppressor) ratio is reversed (normal 2:1); anemia, leukopenia, thrombocytopenia, and elevation of serum gamma globulins often present
  - Full blown AIDS—opportunistic infection and/or opportunistic cancer in setting of marked decline in the immune system, especially helper T lymphocytes; typically occurs when CD4$^+$ T lymphocytes are less than 200/mm^3 of blood

■ Morbidity

● Opportunistic infections

- *Pneumocystis carinii* pneumonia (65% of AIDS patients get this at some time)
- Candidiasis (mouth, esophagus, bronchopulmonary); at least 50% of AIDS patients get some sort of candida infection
- Cytomegalovirus infection—most common of the opportunistic viral infections to afflict AIDS patients
- Other viral infections, including other members of the herpesvirus group (herpes simplex virus 1, [HSV1], HSV2, herpes zoster [HZ], EBV).
- Polyoma virus infection of the brain, causing progressive multifocal leukoencephalopathy

- Other fungal infections—*Cryptococcus* and *Aspergillus* organisms, *Histoplasma capsulatum* and *Coccidioides immitis*
- HIV-1 encephalopathy, caused by intrinsic deleterious effect of HIV itself on neural cells
- Vacuolar myelopathy (vacuolated degeneration of the spinal cord)
- Mycobacterial infections, including tuberculosis and nontuberculosis (especially MAI, *M. kansasii*)
- *Toxoplasma gondii*
- Cryptosporidial and giardial infections of the bowel mucosa
- Legionella pneumonia
- Salmonella sepsis
- Bacillary angiomatosis—a blood vessel proliferation resembling angioma
  - Caused by infection with *Bartonella henselae* and *Bartonella quintana*
- Shigella infection
- Oral hairy leukoplakia (related to EBV and/or human papillovirus [HPV] infection)
- Other opportunistic infections (the possibilities are almost limitless)

- **Neoplasms**
  - Kaposi's sarcoma—a malignant blood vessel neoplasm
  - Lymphomas, mainly B-cell non-Hodgkin's (including CNS B cell lymphomas [microgliomas])
  - Squamous cell carcinoma of the uterine cervix

— *Diagnosis*
  - *ELISA* (enzyme-linked immunosorbent assay) serum antibody detection (for screening) and Western blot ("gold standard confirmatory test")
  - *Detection of viral antigen in serum* (especially p24)
  - *Detection of viral nucleic acid* (nucleic acid hybridization after polymerase chain reaction amplification)
  - *Direct viral culture* (done essentially in research labs only)

— *Time course (usual) (Fig. 5.3)*
  - Exposure to seroconversion—6 to 8 weeks typically, *but* may be months to 1 year
  - Seroconversion to clinical AIDS—months to years (up to 10 years)
  - Clinical AIDS to death—months to years, often with a superimposed cancer, typically lymphoma and/or Kaposi's sarcoma

- **Sexually Transmitted Diseases (STDs)** A rampant problem, STDs affects millions of Americans. Women may develop pelvic inflammatory disease (PID), which can cause **infertility** and is a predisposing factor for **ectopic pregnancy**, an important cause of maternal death.

  - **Human papilloma virus**
    - A DNA virus (with over 70 known types) associated with peculiar histologic changes in squamous cells (koilocytic atypia); causes raised, wart-

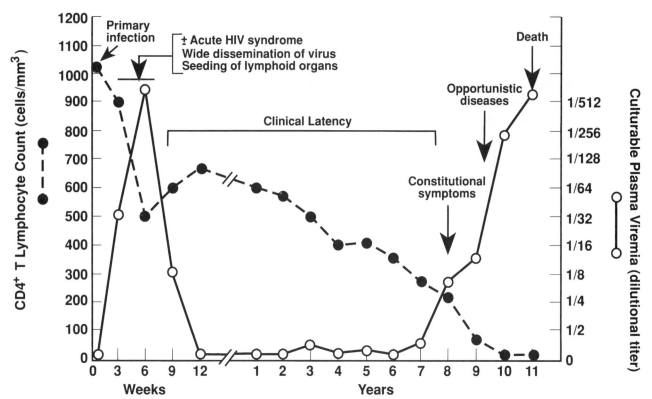

Fig. 5.3 HIV infection time course. This figure presents the usual time course of events involved with HIV infection. (*From Pantaleo G, Graziosis C, Fauci AS: N Engl J Med 328:327, 1993.*)

like lesions on the perianal area, vulva, vagina, and cervix (condyloma acuminatum or venereal warts).

• Lesions in the cervix are usually flat and associated with squamous dysplasia; *HPV 6 and 11 are the serotypes most often associated with condyloma, whereas HPV 16, 18, 31, 33, 35, and 45 are most often identified in cases of dysplasia and squamous cell carcinoma (in situ and invasive) of the lower genital tract.*

● Gonorrhea—*Neisseria gonorrheae*

• A gram-negative diplococcus that causes urethritis, cervicitis, and inflammation of vulvovaginal glands in the acute phase. *50% of women are asymptomatic.*

• Without treatment, the organism may ascend to the fallopian tubes thereby causing PID.

• *Gonorrhea is a common cause of PID in young women* (an estimated *3 million* cases of gonorrhea occur annually in the United States and an increasing number of cases are penicillin resistant).

● Chlamydia—*Chlamydia trachomatis*

• A bacterial organism that is an obligate intracellular parasite, causes symptomatic "nongonococcal urethritis" in the male but frequently causes asymptomatic urethritis and cervicitis in the female.

• *Untreated, this organism may also cause PID.*

• Much less commonly, different serotypes of this organism cause *lymphogranuloma venereum,* a disease associated with a progression from ulcerative genital lesions to swollen inguinal lymph nodes with spontaneous drainage and, ultimately, scarring accompanied by lymphatic obstruction and resultant genital elephantiasis.

- Syphilis—*Treponema pallidum*

    • This spirochete causes a primary chancre followed by a secondary phase (rash, lymphadenopathy, condyloma latum).

    • Untreated, the organisms remain latent, causing a tertiary phase years later (cerebral and cardiovascular lesions, localized gummas). Treatment availability has made tertiary syphilis rare.

    • Transmission to fetus (in utero) can result in congenital syphilis (abnormalities in the bones, teeth, eyes, and meningitis, deafness, thrombocytopenia, and even fetal death).

- *Trichomonas vaginalis*

    • This protozoan causes *severe cervicitis and vaginitis.*

    • Infection is *self-limited,* but the inflammation it produces may complicate interpretation of the cervical Pap smear.

- Herpes simplex virus, type II (HSV-2)

    • Transmitted by sexual contact or during childbirth, this DNA virus causes *recurrent* painful vesicles usually involving the vulva but also the vagina and cervix. The virus remains dormant within nerve tissue.

    • Transmission to infants during delivery may lead to fatal herpetic infection of the neonate.

- Granuloma inguinale—*Calymmatobacterium granulomatis*

    • A gram-negative intracellular coccobacillus, causes a chronic ulcerating and granulating disease of the genital area that may result in extensive disfigurement; uncommon in the United States.

- Chancroid—Haemophilus ducreyi

    • A gram-negative coccobacillus, causes a soft chancrelike lesion that appears on the genitals followed by enlargement of draining regional lymph nodes; uncommon in the United States.

MULTIPLE CHOICE
REVIEW QUESTIONS

1. Which of the following pathogens most often causes abscess formation?

    a. Cytomegalovirus (CMV)
    b. Prions
    c. *Treponema pallidum*
    d. *Staphylococcus aureus*

2. Of the following agents, which is the most common cause of pelvic inflammatory disease?

    a. *Trichomonas vaginalis*
    b. *Treponema pallidum*
    c. *Neisseria gonorrhoeae*
    d. Herpes simplex virus Type 1
    e. Herpes simplex virus Type 2

3. You are a resident drawing blood from a patient known to be infected by the HIV-1 and you accidentally stick yourself with a needle contaminated by this patient's blood. What is your risk of acquiring HIV infection via this single percutaneous exposure?

    a. 0%
    b. 0.3%
    c. 5%
    d. 50%
    e. 95%

4. Bacillary angiomatosis is a histologically benign blood vessel proliferation (resembling an angioma) caused by infection with which of the following agents?

    a. *Bartonella henselae*
    b. *Pneumocystis carinii*
    c. *Mycobacterium avium-intracellulare*
    d. *Toxoplasma gondii*
    e. *Aspergillus fumigatus*

5. The most common location for involvement by secondary tuberculosis is which of the following?

    a. Spleen
    b. Pleural space
    c. Apical or posterior lung segments
    d. Brain
    e. Gastrointestinal tract

Chapter 6

Neoplasia

- ■ **Definitions**
  - ● Neoplasm (new growth)
    - • "A neoplasm is an abnormal mass of tissue, the growth of which exceeds and is uncoordinated with that of the normal tissues and persists in the same excessive manner after cessation of the stimuli which evoked the change."—Sir Rupert Willis
  - ● Other definitions
    - • Tumor—commonly used as a synonym for neoplasm
    - • Cancer—malignant neoplasm
    - • Parenchymal cells—proliferating neoplastic cells
      - • Neoplasms classified by their parenchymal cells
    - • Stroma—connective tissue support framework and blood supply of the neoplasm
  - ● Nonneoplastic masses sometimes confused with neoplasms
    - — *Hamartoma*
      - • Malformation composed of disorganized cells or tissues native to the site
      - • Example: pulmonary hamartoma composed of cartilage, respiratory epithelium, sometimes other elements
    - — *Choristoma (heterotopic rest; heterotopia)*
      - • Normal tissue in the wrong location
      - • Example: pancreatic tissue in stomach or small intestine
    - — *Hematoma—localized collection of blood in tissue or body cavity*
    - — *Inflammatory masses*
      - • Abscesses
      - • Granulomas
- ■ **Nomenclature of Neoplasms (Table 6.1)**
  - ● Nomenclature based on two distinctions
    - • Benign or malignant
    - • Mesenchymal or epithelial
  - ● Benign neoplasms—root + -oma
  - ● Malignant neoplasms
    - • Mesenchymal—root + -sarcoma
      - • Sarcoma is the general term for malignant mesenchymal neoplasm

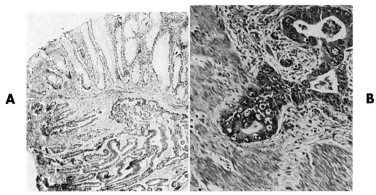

Fig. 6.1 Adenocarcinoma of the colon. **A,** Note the abnormal glandlike structures invading the submucosa and muscularis; some normal mucosa is preserved. **B,** Invasion of the muscularis is shown at a higher power than **A.**   (*Damjanov I, Linder J:* Anderson's pathology, *ed 10, vol 1, St Louis, 1996, Mosby.*)

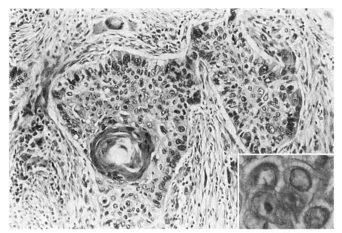

Fig. 6.2 Squamous cell carcinoma. This well-differentiated example shows keratin pearls and intercellular bridges (inset).   (*Damjanov I, Linder J:* Anderson's pathology, *ed 10, vol 1, St Louis, 1996, Mosby.*)

- Epithelial—root + -carcinoma (Figs. 6.1 and 6.2)
  - Carcinoma is the generic term for malignant epithelial neoplasm
- Several important exceptions
  - Leukemia and lymphoma are malignant

■ **Characteristics of Neoplasms**
  ● Differentiation
  - Neoplasms are differentiated by the degree to which parenchymal cells resemble comparable normal cells in appearance and function.
  - Benign neoplasms tend to be well differentiated.
  - Malignant neoplasms can be well differentiated or poorly differentiated.
    - Anaplasia—lack of histologic differentiation

Table 6.1   *Nomenclature of Tumors*

CELL OR TISSUE OF ORIGIN	BENIGN	MALIGNANT
Tumors of Epithelial Origin		
Squamous cells	Squamous cell papilloma	Squamous cell carcinoma
Basal cells		Basal cell carcinoma
Glandular or ductal epithelium	Adenoma	Adenocarcinoma
	Papillary adenoma	Papillary adenocarcinoma
	Cystadenoma	Cystadenocarcinoma
Transitional cells	Transitional cell papilloma	Transitional cell carcinoma
Bile duct	Bile duct adenoma	Bile duct carcinoma (cholangiocarcinoma)
Islets of Langerhans	Islet cell adenoma	Islet cell carcinoma
Liver cells	Liver cell adenoma	Hepatocellular carcinoma (hepatoma)
Neuroectoderm	Melanocytic nevus	Malignant melanoma
Placental epithelium		Choriocarcinoma, hydatidiform mole
Renal epithelium	Renal tubular adenoma	Renal cell carcinoma (hypernephroma)
Respiratory tract		Bronchogenic carcinoma
Skin adnexal glands:		
Sweat glands	Syringoadenoma, sweat gland adenoma	Syringocarcinoma, sweat gland carcinoma
Sebaceous glands	Sebaceous gland adenoma	Sebaceous gland carcinoma
Germ cells (testis and ovary)		Seminoma (dysgerminoma)
		Embryonal carcinoma, yolk sac tumor
Tumors of Mesenchymal Origin		
Hematopoietic and lymphoid tissues		Leukemias
		Lymphomas
		Hodgkin's disease
		Multiple myeloma
Neural and retinal tissue		
Nerve sheath	Neurilemoma, neurofibroma	Malignant peripheral nerve sheath tumor
Nerve cells	Ganglioneuroma	Neuroblastoma
Retinal cells (cones)		Retinoblastoma
Connective tissue		
Fibrous tissue	Fibroma	Fibrosarcoma
Fat	Lipoma	Liposarcoma
Bone	Osteoma	Osteogenic sarcoma
Cartilage	Chondroma	Chondrosarcoma
Muscle		
Smooth muscle	Leiomyoma	Leiomyosarcoma
Striated muscle	Rhabdomyoma	Rhabdomyosarcoma
Endothelial and related tissues		
Blood vessels	Hemangioma	Angiosarcoma
		Kaposi's sarcoma
Lymph vessels	Lymphangioma	Lymphangiosarcoma
Mesothelium	Benign mesothelioma	Malignant mesothelioma
Meninges	Meningioma	Malignant meningioma
Uncertain origin		Ewing's tumor
Other Origins		
Renal anlage		Wilms' tumor
Trophoblast		Choriocarcinoma, hydatidiform mole
Totipotential cells	Benign teratoma	Malignant teratoma

From Damjanov I, Linder J: *Anderson's pathology,* ed 10, vol 1, St Louis, 1996, Mosby.

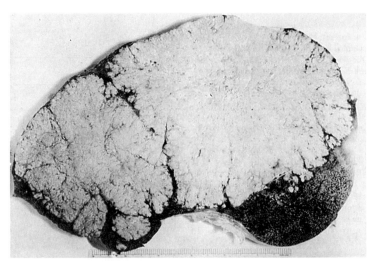

Fig. 6.3 Liver metastasis. Most of the liver in this section is replaced by metastasis from a colon carcinoma. *(Damjanov I, Linder J:* Anderson's pathology, *ed 10, vol 1, St Louis, 1996, Mosby.)*

● **Growth rate**
  • Benign neoplasms tend to grow slowly.
  • Malignant neoplasms tend to grow rapidly and sometimes erratically.

● **Local growth patterns**
  — *Benign neoplasms*
      • Cohesive, expansile masses
      • Localized—do not invade or metastasize
  — *Malignant neoplasms*
      • Progressively invade and destroy adjacent tissues
      • In situ cancer—preinvasive form of cancer

● **Metastasis (plural, metastases)**
  • Neoplastic implants not continuous with the primary site
  • The definitive proof of malignancy
  • All malignant neoplasms can metastasize but a few types almost never do (e.g., basal cell carcinoma of the skin)
  — *Pathways*
      • Seeding of body cavities and surfaces
      • Lymphatic
        • Many cancers first spread to regional lymph nodes
      • Hematogenous (venous)
        • Tend to follow venous drainage
        • Liver (via portal venous system) or lungs (via systemic veins and right side of the heart) tend to be involved initially and most prominently (Figs. 6.3 and 6.4)

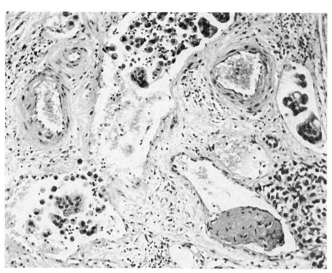

Fig. 6.4 Vascular invasion. Note malignant cells within several small veins in this example of a carcinoma of the pancreas.
(*Damjanov I, Linder J:* Anderson's pathology, *ed 10, vol 1, St Louis, 1996, Mosby.*)

■ Cancer Epidemiology and Etiology

- ● United States cancer statistics (1996 estimates from Parker SL et al., *CA,* 46:5-27, 1996)

  — *1,359,000 new cases*

    • Males, 764,000; females, 595,000

    • Excluded

      • In situ cancers (>50,000 cases/year)
      • Nonlethal skin cancers (800,000 cases/year)

  — *555,000 cancer deaths (23% of all deaths)*

    • Males, 292,000; females, 263,000

  — *Leading sites of origin of cancer cases*

    • Males—prostate, 41%; lung, 13%; colon and rectum, 9%; urinary tract, 7%; lymphoma and leukemia, 6%; oral cavity, 3%; skin (melanoma), 3%; pancreas, 2%

    • Females—breast (invasive), 31%; lung, 13%; colon and rectum, 11%; lymphoma and leukemia, 8%; uterus (corpus and unspecified sites), 6%; ovary, 6%; urinary tract, 4%; uterine cervix, 3%; skin (melanoma), 3%

  — *Leading sites of origin of cancers that cause death*

    • Males—lung, 32%; prostate, 14%; colon and rectum, 9%; lymphoma and leukemia, 9%; urinary tract, 5%; pancreas, 5%; skin (melanoma), 2%; oral cavity, 2%

    • Females—lung, 25%; breast, 17%; colon and rectum, 10%; lymphoma and leukemia, 8%; ovary, 6%; pancreas, 5%; urinary tract, 3%; uterus (corpus and unspecified sites), 2%; uterine cervix, 2%

- ● Changes in cancer mortality in the United States since 1930

    • Cancer death rate increased in males, decreased slightly in females
    • Marked increase in deaths from lung carcinoma (both sexes)

- Increased incidence because of cigarette smoking
- Marked decrease in deaths from stomach carcinoma and hepato-cellular carcinoma (both sexes)
  - Decreased incidence caused by unknown reasons (possibly diet in the case of stomach cancer)
- Marked decreased in deaths from carcinoma of uterine cervix
  - Early detection from screening (Pap smear) and treatment

- **Factors that affect the likelihood of developing cancer or of developing specific cancers**
  - *Geography*
    - Worldwide—the incidence of specific cancers varies greatly with location
    - Probably reflects both environmental and genetic factors
      - In most cases, environmental factors are more important
  - *Age*
    - Cancers become much more common with aging.
    - In the United States, most cancer mortality occurs in persons 55 to 75 years old.
    - Children and adults tend to develop different types of cancers.
  - *Sex*
    - In the United States, males have a greater lifetime risk of developing invasive cancer than do females (47.12% vs. 38.41%).
    - In the United States, females have a greater risk of developing invasive cancer early in life than do males.
      - Up to age 39 years, 1.94% of females and 1.73% of males develop invasive cancer.
      - Ages 40 to 59 years, 9.19% of females and 7.99% of males are affected.
  - *Race*
    - African Americans have greater cancer incidence and mortality than do Caucasians.
      - Incidence—439 vs. 406/100,000 population
      - Mortality—228 vs. 170/100,000 population

- **Types of environmental factors involved in cancer development**
  - *Diet*
    - Carcinogens in diet
      - Polycyclic hydrocarbons from smoked fish, meat
      - Aflatoxin B1 (from *Aspergillus flavus*)
    - Metabolism of dietary nitrites, amines, and amides to nitrosamines and nitrosamides
    - Lack of protective factors
      - Fiber
      - Vitamins A, C, and E
      - Selenium

  — *Tobacco*

- Carcinogens in cigarette smoke

  - Polycyclic hydrocarbons (e.g., benzo[a]pyrene)
  - Nitrosamines

- Cigarette smoking and lung cancer

  - About 80% of lung carcinomas occur in cigarette smokers
  - Smokers have tenfold greater risk of developing lung carcinoma than nonsmokers

- Other tobacco-related carcinomas—oral cavity, pharynx, larynx, esophagus, urinary bladder

  — *Alcohol*

- Increased risk of cancer of the liver (via increased cirrhosis)
- Increases risk of cancers of oral cavity, pharynx, larynx, esophagus (synergistic with tobacco)

  — *Industrial chemicals*

- Asbestos—malignant mesothelioma and lung carcinoma
- β-naphythalamine and bladder carcinoma in dye workers
- Many others

  — *Infectious agents*

- Oncogenic viruses

  - Papillomaviruses—genital tract and oral cavity carcinoma
  - See following

- *Helicobacter pylori*

  - Bacteria that causes many cases of gastritis and peptic ulcers
  - Related to carcinoma and lymphoma of stomach

  — *Natural and therapeutic radiation*

- Sunlight (ultraviolet B) and skin cancers
- Ionizing radiation—leukemias, thyroid carcinoma, others

● **Heredity and cancer**

  — *Cancer family syndromes*

- Increased risk of common type of cancer(s)

  - Often apparent autosomal dominant inheritance and incomplete penetrance
  - Sometimes earlier onset than in sporadic types of same cancer

- Hereditary nonpolyposis colorectal cancer (Lynch syndrome)

  - Autosomal dominant increased risk of colorectal carcinoma
  - Three or more members affected in two or more generations with at least one with onset by age 50 years
  - In some families, increased risk of other malignancies
  - Could account for 5% of all colorectal carcinoma cases
  - Most caused by inherited mutation in one of four genes encoding deoxyribonucleic acid (DNA) mismatch repair enzymes

- Familial breast cancer
- About 80% caused by mutations in BRCA1 or BRCA2

— *Autosomal dominant inherited cancer syndromes*

- Strong family history of uncommon cancer and/or marker phenotype
- Familial retinoblastoma
- Multiple endocrine neoplasia, type 1, type 2A, type 2B
- Familial adenomatous polyposis of colon

  - Hundreds of colon adenomas, with cancer developing in one or more
  - Mutations in APC (adenomatous polyposis coli) gene

- Neurofibromatosis 1 and 2

— *DNA repair defects (autosomal recessive)*

— *Immune deficiency syndromes (mostly X-linked recessive)*

● Acquired premalignant conditions

— *Some benign neoplasms can become malignant*

- Example: villous adenoma of the colon
- Generally, benign neoplams do not become malignant

— *Dysplasia*

- Disorderly proliferation of cells (usually epithelium)

  - Loss of normal orientation
  - Loss of cellular uniformity

- Example: cervical dysplasia
- Most examples of dysplasia do not become malignant

— *Several nonneoplastic conditions involving persistent regeneration or chronic inflammation occasionally give rise to malignancies*

- Cirrhosis
- Chronic inflammatory bowel disease
- Atrophic gastritis (pernicious anemia)
- Solar keratosis of skin

■ **Molecular Basis of Cancer Development**

● Nonlethal genetic damage underlies carcinogenesis

- More than one mutation involved

● Protooncogenes

— *Cellular genes that can become activated to become cancer causing oncogenes*

- Names derived from names of retroviruses that contain homologous oncogenes responsible for their transforming abilities

  - Protooncogenes: c-onc
  - Viral oncogenes: v-onc

— *Encode proteins involved in normal cell differentiation or proliferation*

- Growth factors: c-sis (platelet derived growth factor subunit; PDGF-B)
- Growth factor receptors: c-erbB family (epidermal growth factor receptor family), c-fms (colony stimulating factor-1 receptor)
- Signal transduction proteins: ras family
- Transcription factors: c-myc family, c-jun, c-fos

— *Activation of protooncogenes*

- Point mutation: changes function
- Translocation
  - Increased expression
  - Production of fusion proteins with different functions
- Amplification: increased expression

— *Example: ras*

- Several ras genes (c-Ha-ras, c-Ki-ras, others) each encode different protein, p21.
- p21 is active when it binds GTP, and inactive when it binds GDP.
  - Binding of peptide growth factors to their receptors indirectly (via grb2-sos) promotes nucleotide exchange and activation.
  - Associated GTPase inactivates p21.
- Activate p21, in turn, activates a series of cytoplasmic protein kinases, which in turn activate transcription factors (c-fos, c-jun).
- Point mutations make ras oncogenic by decreasing GTPase activity.
- 20% to 30% of human neoplasms contain ras gene with oncogenic mutations (including many examples of carcinoma of lung, bladder, colon).

● **Tumor suppressor genes (anti-oncogenes)**

— *Encode proteins that normally inhibit cell proliferation*

- Cell surface protein: DCC (cell adhesion)
- Signal transduction protein: NF-1 (GTPase activator)
- Proteins that regulate transcription: p53, pRb

— *Loss (deletion) or inactivation of both copies can cause cancer.*

- Germline mutations in anti-oncogenes can result in familial cancers.

— *Example: Rb*
Encodes a nuclear protein, pRb

- Activity is decreased by phosphorlyation.
- When active (hypophosphorylated), Rb binds and sequesters certain transcription factors (E2F family), whose activities are needed for DNA synthesis.

- Phosphorylation state (activity) of pRb correlates with cell cycle.

  - Growth factors stimulate cyclin dependent kinases that phosphorylate (inactivate) pRb.
  - After mitosis, phosphates desphosphorylate (activate) pRb.

Familial retinoblastoma

- Accounts for about 40% of cases of this rare ocular neoplasm
- Autosomal dominant
- Two separate events inactivating both copies of Rb gene ("2 hits")

  - First, germline mutation (deletion usually)
  - Second, acquired mutation in retinoblast

- Often multiple
- Often have another malignancy in childhood (osteosarcoma)

Sporadic retinoblastoma

- Accounts for 60% of cases
- Loss or inactivation of both Rb alleles in same retinal cell
- Single

Rb mutated in many common neoplasms

— **Example: p53**

Nuclear protein (active as tetramer)

- Binds DNA, activates transcription

Functions

- Inhibits cell proliferation

  - Induces protein (cip1/sdi/WAF1) that inactivates cyclin associated kinases needed for intitiation of DNA synthesis

- Necessary for apoptosis in some situations (after DNA damage)

p53 gene most commonly mutated gene in human cancers

- Inactivation of both copies
- Occurs in at least 50 different types
- 70% colon carcinomas, 50% lung carcinomas, and 40% breast cancer

Most mutations missense near DNA binding site

- Mutations change DNA binding and increase stability (increase detectability in clinical samples).

Germline p53 mutations: Li-Fraumeni syndrome

- Autosomal dominant tendency to develop one or more cancers at early age

● **Genes involved in apoptosis (programmed cell death)**

- Decreased amount or activity of agent promoting apoptosis (e.g., p53) or activation of inhibitor of apoptosis
- bc1-2, an inhibitor of apoptosis

- First identified in B cell lymphoma—overexpressed because of translocation

- ● DNA repair genes
  - — *Mismatch repair genes*
    - Familial nonpolyposis colorectal carcinoma
      - In >90% of cases, tumors exhibit microsatellite instability (replication error phenotype).
      - In 70% of cases, germline mutation in one of four DNA mismatch repair genes has been found; tumor shows mutation of other allele.
    - Replication error phenotype and/or acquired mutation of mismatch repair gene in tumor occasionally seen in sporadic colorectal or endometrial cancers
  - — *Mutations in other DNA repair genes*
    - Responsible for autosomal recessive syndromes with increased likelihood of skin cancers

- ● Molecular basis of multistep carcinogenesis
  - Transformation of cultured human cells requires expression of more than one oncogene
  - Human neoplasms show more than one (often several) genetic alterations
  - Colorectal carcinoma model (based on carcinomas developing in patients with familial adenomatous polyposis, but applicable to apparently noninherited colorectal carcinoma)
    - Progressive development of morphologic abnormalities: hyperproliferative epithelium→ adenoma (various stages)→ carcinoma
    - Progressive acquisition of genetic abnormalities—loss-inactivation of APC, loss DNA methylation, Ki-ras activation, loss DCC, inactivation p53

- ● Chromosomal (karyotypic) changes
  - Genetic abnormalities of cancer—first identified by studying preparations of chromosomes with the light microscope (karyotype)
  - Many neoplasms commonly exhibit nonrandom chromosomal abnormalities
  - — *Types*
    - Balanced translocations
    - Deletions
    - Amplifications
      - Double minutes (dms)—small chromosome-like structures
      - Homongeneous staining regions (HSRs)—abnormal regions within chromosomes
  - — *Examples*
    Philadelphia chromosome in chronic myelogenous leukemia
    - Reciprocal translocation involving chromosomes 9 and 22

- Philadelphia chromosome is abnormal chromosome 22
- Involves protooncogene c-abl on chromosome 9 and bcr on chromosome 22
- Results in production of an abnormal fusion protein, p210 bcr/abl, which is likely to contribute to the development of the disease

Amplification of N-myc in neuroblastoma and of c-erb2 in breast cancer

- Indicates poor prognosis

■ Growth of Neoplastic Cells

● Neoplasms are clonal; they arise from a single cell

● Kinetics

— *The original cell must divide many times before it can produce a clinically detectable mass*

- By this time the neoplasm has completed most of its life cycle.
- Thirty population doublings would produce 10^9 cells.
  - This is equivalent to 1 g mass (clinically detectable in some circumstances).

— *Factors determining doubling time*

- Length of cell cycle
- Percent of dividing cells (growth fraction)
  - Cancers with high growth fraction are more susceptible to many types of chemotherapy than those with a low growth fraction
- Cell loss

● Progression and heterogeneity

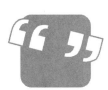

- Progression—"acquisition of permanent, irreversible qualitative changes in one or more characteristics of a neoplasm"—L. Foulds
- While a neoplasm originates from a single cell, eventually it is composed of subsets of descendants differing in various properties.
  - Properties include physiologic, morphologic, chemical, karyotypic, and genetic.
  - Since 30 or more cell divisions have occurred by the time most neoplasms are clinically detectable, they can be quite heterogeneous.
  - Neoplasm can develop new characteristics after clinical detection.

● Angiogenesis

- Neoplasms must be vascularized in order to grow

— *Peptide angiogenic factors*

- Derived from neoplastic cells (e.g., angiogenin)
- Derived from inflammatory cells infiltrating the neoplasm

● Invasion and metastasis

- Malignancies contain subsets of cells with varying abilities to invade and metastasize

— *Steps in invasion and metastasis*

- Detachment from primary
- Invasion through basement membrane and interstitial connective tissue
- Intravasation (includes passage through endothelial basement membrane)
- Circulation
- Attachment to endothelial basement membrane
- Extravasation (adhesion to and penetration of endothelial basement membrane)
- Proliferation at the distant site

— *Necessary for invasion of extracellular matrix (ECM)*

ECM—basement membrane and interstitial connective tissue

- Collagen

    - Fibrillar (type I)
    - Nonfibrillar (type IV, basement membrane)

- Glycoproteins

    - Laminin (most abundant basement membrane glycoprotein) binds cell surfaces and other ECM components
    - Fibronectin binds to ECM components and to cells (via integrins)

- Proteoglycans—glycosaminoglycan + protein core

Attachment to basement membrane laminin and fibronectin

- Increased binding of these by carcinoma cells in comparison to normal epithelium

Activation of proteolytic enzymes that degrade ECM components

- Secreted by neoplastic cells or by fibroblasts and macrophages (induced by neoplastic cells)
- Type IV collagenase (a metalloproteinase) degrades basement membrane collagen
- Cathepsin D (cysteine protease), urokinase-like plasminogen activator (serine protease) that degrade laminin, fibronectin, protein cores of proteoglycans
- Protease inhibitors

Motility factors

- Autocrine (i.e., made by the neoplasm)
- Local growth factors
- ECM degradation products

— *Genetic control*

- Increased expression of proteins whose activities promote invasion and metastasis

    - Example: metalloproteinases
    - Detection in primary could be useful in predicting likelihood of metastasis

- Decreased expression of proteins that suppress metastasis

— *Patterns of metastasis*

- Some malignancies metastasize to particular sites.

  - Adhesion molecules on neoplastic cells
  - Chemoattractants secreted by tissue

- Some tissues are very resistant to metastases (heart, skeletal muscle).

■ Carcinogenesis

● Chemical

— *Initiation and promotion*

- Initiation—rapid, irreversible, caused by DNA damage
- Promotion—affects initiated cells
- Complete carcinogen—both an initiating and promoting agent
- Incomplete carcinogen (more common)—initiating agent only

— *Initiating agents*

- Direct acting agents do not require metabolic activation

  - Example: alkylating agents used for cancer chemotherapy

- Indirect acting agents require metabolic activation

  - Original agent, procarcinogen; activated metabolite, ultimate carcinogen
  - Activation by cytochrome P-450-dependent monooxygenases
  - Examples: polycyclic hydrocarbons (e.g., benzo[a]pyrene), aromatic amines and azo dyes (e.g., β-naphythylamine), natural products (aflatoxin B1)

- Direct acting and ultimate carcinogens usually highly electrophilic

— *Promoters*

- Augment tumorogenicity of some carcinogens
- Not by themselves carcinogenic or mutagenic

  - Increase proliferation of initiated cells

- Examples: phorbol ester TPA (activator of protein kinase C)

● Radiation

— *Ultraviolet (UV) radiation*

- Exposure to sunlight can induce cancers in exposed skin
- UV causes pyrimidine dimer formation

  - Marked increase in skin cancer susceptibility in persons with inherited DNA repair defects (e.g., xeroderma pigmentosum)

— *Ionizing radiation*

- Direct or indirect (via free radicals) damage to macromolecules
- DNA damage most important in carcinogenesis

  - Double strand breaks, activation of oncogenes or inactivation of antioncogenes

- **Viral**
  - — *Oncogenic DNA viruses*

    Transforming ability

    - Stable integration of viral DNA into host genome prevents viral replication
    - Expression of viral early genes in transformed cells

    Human papilloma viruses (HPV)

    - There are ≥ 60 genetically distinct types.
    - It is a suspected sexually-transmitted agent responsible for squamous cell carcinoma, of the uterine cervix, its precursors, and low risk genital warts.
      - "High-risk" types (16 and 18 most common) are involved in a majority of these cancers and are presumed precursors.
      - "Low-risk" types (6 and 11) are involved in genital warts.
    - HPV is also involved in other genital tract, anal, oral cavity, laryngeal carcinomas.
    - In invasive cancers, virus is integrated, and integration sites are clonal.
    - In precursor lesions and warts, virus is episomal (not integrated).
    - Integration disrupts early region genes that repress expression of proteins that bind and inactivate antioncogenes.
      - E6 binds and destabilizes p53 (via ubiqutin).
      - E7 binds and sequesters underphosphoylated pRb.

    Epstein-Barr virus (EBV)

    INFECTS B LYMPHOCYTES, OROPHARYNGEAL EPITHELIUM

    BURKITT'S LYMPHOMA

    - B cell origin
    - Most common childhood neoplasm in central Africa
    - Also found outside of Africa
    - EBV implicated in pathogenesis of Burkitt's lymphoma in Africa

    EBV AND BURKITT'S LYMPHOMA IN AFRICA

    - EBV genome occurs in > 90% of neoplasms.
      - Antibodies fight against viral capsid antigens in 100% of patients.
      - Antibody titers correlate with risk of developing the disease.
    - EBV is not the sole factor.
      - EBV infection occurs outside of Africa.
      - EBV causes infectious mononucleosis.
      - Most non-African Burkitt's lymphomas do not contain EBV.
      - Both African and non-African Burkitt's lymphoma contain overexpressed c-myc related to translocation.
      - EBV immortalized B lymphocytes are not tumorogenic in vitro and do not overexpress c-myc.

Also implicated in B cell lymphomas and smooth muscle neoplasms in immunosuppressed (AIDS, transplantation), nasopharyngeal carcinoma in southern China, a few cases of Hodgkin's disease

Hepatitis B virus (HBV)

- There are strong epidemiologic associations between HBV infection and risk of developing hepatocellular carcinoma.
- HBV DNA is integrated into host genome (clonal within tumor).
- Mechanisms of action are unclear.

— *Oncogenic ribonucleic acid (RNA) viruses*

- Animal oncogenic retroviruses
  - Acutely transforming—encode v-onc
  - Slowly transforming—integrate adjacent to c-onc
- Human T cell leukemia virus type 1 differs from animal retroviruses
  - Lacks v-onc, consistent integration site
  - Encodes tax activates transcription of host genes (including growth factor and receptors) and induces T cell proliferation
- Hepatitis C virus

■ **Tumor Immunology**

● Tumor antigens

— *Tumor-specific antigens occur in some experimental models*

— *Tumor-associated antigens*

- Oncofetal antigens are found in embryonic tissues and neoplasms, not in normal adult tissues.
  - Carcinoembryonic antigen (CEA), α-fetoprotein
- Onconeural antigens are expressed in relatively immunologically privileged nervous system and some neoplasms.

● Mechanisms

- Cytotoxic T cells
- Natural killer cells
- Macrophages
- Antibodies

● Immunosurveillance

- High risk of malignancy in immunosuppressed individuals
  - Often B cell lymphomas, sometimes related to EBV infection
- Postulated that in immunocompetent hosts malignancies evade immunosurveillance
  - Loss of antigens during progression
  - Production of immunosuppressants (e.g., transforming growth factor-β)

- Immunotherapy
  - *Antibodies—target toxin to neoplasm*
  - *Cytokines*
  - *Adaptive cellular therapy*
    - Tumor-infiltrating lymphocytes
    - Patient peripheral blood lymphocytes treated with interleukin-2
  - *Vaccines*

Clinical Aspects of Neoplasia

- Effects of neoplasms on the host
  - *Local and hormonal effects*
    - Destruction of an endocrine gland by primary or metastatic neoplasm: decreased hormone secretion
    - Excess hormone secretion by neoplasm of an endocrine gland
    - Erosion of mucosal surfaces (causing bleeding or secondary infection)
    - Compression or destruction of areas of brain
  - *Cachexia*
    - Loss of lean body mass and fat, accompanied by anorexia, weakness, anemia
    - Occurs in malignancies
    - Possibly humorally mediated (tumor necrosis factor-α, other cytokines)
  - *Paraneoplastic syndromes*
    - Not explained by local effects of neoplasm or by secretion of hormone normally found in the tissue with the neoplasm
    - Occur in 10% of patients with malignancy
    - Importance
      - Can be presenting sign or symptom
      - Can cause significant morbidity and even mortality
      - Can cause diagnostic dilemmas
    - Endocrine—ectopic hormone
      - Neoplastic production of hormone not usually produced in that tissue
      - Example: ectopic production of adrenocorticotropic hormone (ACTH)
    - Neuromuscular
      - Some caused by antibodies to onconeural antigens
      - Example: degeneration of sensory, visual system, cerebellar neurons
      - Example: axonal neuropathies
    - Others
      - Dermatologic—acanthosis nigricans, dermatomyositis
      - Hypercoaguable states

- Hypertrophic osteoarthropathy, clubbing of digits
    — *Example: hypercalcemia*
        - Primary hyperparathyroidism
        - Osteolytic metastases
        - Humorally mediated, associated with malignancies (parathyroid hormone related peptide, cytokines)
        - Nonneoplastic causes

● **Grading and staging of cancer**
    — *Histologic grading—grades I to III (or IV)*
        - Subjective assessment of degree of differentiation
        - Mitotic counts (hard to standardize and reproduce)
    — *Staging*
        - Commonly used for predicting prognosis and determining therapy
        - For many cancers, staging is the most important prognostic feature
            - The higher the stage, the shorter the survival

● **Laboratory evaluation of neoplasms**
    — *Screening, diagnosis, staging, monitoring response to therapy*
    — *Morphologic diagnosis and classification*
        - Cytologic
            - Smears, body fluids, fine needle aspiration biopsies
        - Histologic (more common)
            - Incisional or excisional biopsies and resection specimens
        - Supplementary techniques
            - Immunohistochemistry for tumor antigens, differentiation markers
            - Electron microscopy
        - Example: classification of bronchogenic carcinoma of lung
            - Small cell carcinoma and nonsmall cell carcinoma (adenocarcinoma, squamous cell carcinoma, large cell carcinoma)
            - Small cell carcinoma proliferates more rapidly, has a worse prognosis, and is treated differently than nonsmall carcinoma
    — *Chemical*
        - Measurement of hormones, tumor markers in blood for diagnosis or monitoring
            - Hormone (example): calcitonin for medullary thyroid carcinoma
            - Tumor markers—carcinoembryonic antigen, α-fetoprotein
        - Assay receptor content in neoplasms
            - Example: estrogen receptors in breast carcinoma for predicting response to antiestrogen therapy

— *Karyotypic*

- Chromosomal abnormalities found in specific neoplasms
- Example: Philadelphia chromosome in chronic myelogenous leukemia

— *Molecular*

- Genetic markers for neoplasia or cell type
- Example: immunoglobulin gene rearrangements in B cell lymphoma
- Example: increased sensitivity for detection of malignant cells by detection of oncogenic mutations

MULTIPLE CHOICE REVIEW QUESTIONS

1. Exposure to ultraviolet light is most important in the development of which of the following?

    a. Basal cell carcinoma of the skin
    b. Squamous cell carcinoma of the lung
    c. Hepatocellular carcinoma
    d. Papillary carcinoma of the thyroid
    e. Acute myelogenous leukemia

2. The agent or category of agents most clearly associated with carcinoma of the uterine cervix is which of the following?

    a. *Apergillus flavus*
    b. *Helicobacter pylori*
    c. *Schistosomiasis hematobium*
    d. Epstein-Barr virus
    e. Papillomaviruses

3. In females in the United States, the greatest number of deaths results from cancers arising in which of the following?

    a. Breast
    b. Colon and rectum
    c. Lung
    d. Skin
    e. Uterus

4. The gene that encodes a protein that binds to and inhibits the activity of transcription factors is which of the following?

    a. p53
    b. Rb
    c. bCl-2
    d. Ki-ras
    e. c-sis

5. Which of the following enzymes or class of enzymes is responsible for metabolic activation of procarcinogens?

    a. Myeloperoxidase
    b. Tyrosine kinases
    c. Cytochrome P450 cyclooxygenases
    d. Superoxide dismutases
    e. Cathepsin D

Chapter 7
Genetic Diseases

MENDELIAN DISORDERS

■ **Patterns of Mendelian Inheritance**

● Autosomal dominant

- Account for about half of mendelian disorders
- Typically vertical transmission from one generation to the next
- 50% of children of an affected parent are also affected
- Exceptions
  - New mutations
  - Variable penetrance

● Autosomal recessive

- About one third of mendelian disorders
- Often shows horizontal pattern of inheritance (affected children of heterozygous, unaffected parents)
- In a family with affected child—probability of each subsequent child being affected is 25%

● X-linked

- Mutation on X chromosome
- Affected father passes trait to 50% of daughters (obligate carriers)
- Obligate carrier mother
  - 50% of daughters also obligate carriers
  - 50% of sons affected

■ **Specific Mendelian Disorders**

● Marfan syndrome

- Autosomal dominant disorder of connective tissue, involving skeleton, eyes, cardiovascular system
- Almost all cases caused by mutations in gene encoding fibrillin (15q21.1)

— *Morphology*
  Skeleton

  - Tall, long extremities (long legs account for increased height) and digits

- Kyphosis or scoliosis
- Deformed chest (pigeon breast or pectus excavatum)

Eye

- Bilateral ectopia lentis (subluxation or dislocation)
  - Very characteristic of Marfan syndrome

Cardiovascular

- Cystic medionecrosis involving aorta
  - Severe dilation of aortic root, potentially causing aortic valvular insufficiency
  - Tears of aortic intima can produce intramural hematoma and dissection
- Mitral valve prolapse can produce mitral insufficiency

Clinical features

- Variable
- 30% to 45% die from aortic dissection

● Familial hypercholesterolemia

— *Mutation in gene encoding low-density lipoprotein (LDL) receptor affects about 1/500*

— *LDL receptor function*

- High-affinity receptors found on many cell types, but hepatic receptors functionally most important (liver clears 70% LDL)
- Responsible for clearance of plasma intermediate density lipoprotein (IDL) and LDL
- Hepatocytes responsible for clearance of 70% of plasma LDL

— *Mutations in LDL receptor*

- Type I
  - Most common
  - At the 5′ end of the gene
  - Affect transcription
  - No receptors produced (null allele)
- Type II
  - Receptors accumulate in endoplastic reticulum and cannot be transported to Golgi (transport deficient)
- Type III
  - In LDL-binding region
  - Defective in binding
- Type IV
  - In cytoplasmic region
  - Receptors not internalized

— *Effects of mutations*

- Increased LDL level caused by
  - Decreased clearance of LDL and IDL

- Increased synthesis (from increased LDL)
- Homozygotes have no functioning receptors; heterozygotes have 50% normal functioning receptors

— *Clinical features*

- Homozygotes affected earlier and more severely
- Elevated plasma cholesterol
- Xanthomas
- Accelerated atherosclerosis
  - Homozygotes can have myocardial infarction before age 20 years

● Cystic fibrosis

- Most common autosomal-recessive disorder in persons of European ancestry (1:2000 affected)
- Involves lung, pancreas, gastrointestinal tract, reproductive tract

— *Cystic fibrosis gene and protein*

- Located on 7q31
- Encodes CFTR (cystic fibrosis transmembrane conductance regulator)
  - Transmembrane chloride ion channel at apical membrane of epithelium
  - Contains two transmembrane domains, two intracellular nucleotide binding domains, and one intracellular regulatory region

— *CF gene mutations*

- ΔF508 accounts for 70% of mutant alleles
  - Deletion of three nucleotides encoding amino acid 508 in one of the nucleotide-binding regions
  - Results in defect in intracellular transport and glycosylation and premature degradation of protein
- More than one hundred other mutations
  - Can affect nucleotide binding or regulatory regions
  - 5 account for about half of the non-ΔF508 mutations
- ΔF508 mutations tend to confer the most severely affected phenotype

— *Pathogenesis*

- Underlying abnormality is defective chloride transport
- Sweat glands
  - Decreased resorption of sodium and chloride from lumen
  - Increased sweat chloride
- Airways
  - Decreased chloride resorption from airway lumen
  - Increased sodium and water resorption
  - Probability of infection increased

- *Pseudomonas aeruginosa*—elaboration of alginate protects organism from antibodies and antibiotics

— *Morphology*

- Organs involved and severity varies
- Lungs

    - Distension of bronchioles, with thick mucus and hyperplasia and hypertrophy of mucous-secreting cells
    - Chronic bronchitis
    - Bronchiectasis

- Pancreas

    - Less severe cases, only mucous plugs and dilation of ducts
    - Obstruction of ducts
    - Atrophy of glands
    - Progressive fibrosis
    - Most severe cases, fibrous or fatty replacement of acini with only residual ducts and islets

- Epididymis and vas deferens

    - Obstructed or absent

— *Clinical features*

- Extremely variable, in part depending upon mutations involved
- About 5% of cases present at birth with intestinal obstruction (meconium ileus)
- Malabsorption caused by exocrine pancreatic insufficiency
- Chronic obstructive pulmonary disease and right sided heart failure
- Chronic lung infections

    - *Pseudomonas aeruginosa, Pseudomonas capacia,* and *Staphylococcus aureus*
    - Most common cause of death

- Infertility

    - In almost all affected males who survive
    - In some males, infertility is only manifestation

- Elevated sweat chloride used as diagnostic test

    - Sweat chloride >60 mEq/L on two separate tests, using adequate volume of sweat (>50 mg)

- Alpha$_1$-antitrypsin deficiency

    — *Alpha$_1$-antitrypsin*

    - Hepatocytes are the major source of plasma alpha$_1$-antitrypsin
    - Potent inhibitor of the enzyme neutrophil elastase (NE)
    - Protects extracellular structures from degradation by NE released from activated or disintegrated neutrophils

— *Genetics of alpha₁-antitrypsin*

- Gene is extremely polymorphic—about 75 alleles
- Alleles given a letter designation, based on electrophoretic mobility of the protein, often preceded by Pi (for protease inhibitor)
- Null alleles cause complete absence of alpha₁-antitrypsin
- Alleles can be simply classified as "normal" or "at risk"
- Four common normal alleles (M) and several rare ones
- Known at-risk alleles most common in persons of Northern European ancestry

  - S (frequency—2% to 4% in Northern Europeans)
  - Z (frequency—1% to 2% in Northern Europeans; estimated 20,000 to 40,000 ZZ homozygotes in the United States)
  - Null alleles are rare

— *Genetics of alpha₁-antitrypsin deficiency*

Null alleles—complete absence of alpha₁-antitrypsin

- Gene deletion
- Absence of transcripts
- Premature termination

Z allele

- Point mutation
- Normal alpha₁-antitrypsin messenger ribonucleic acid (mRNA) amount
- Secretion is about 10% of normal

  - Protein has abnormal 3D structure
  - Accumulates in rough endoplastic reticulum

S allele

- Point mutation
- mRNA normal in amount
- Protein has an abnormal 3D structure, causing intracellular degradation

Other alleles (all rare)

- Can cause decreased secretion and intrahepatocyte accumulation, intracellular degradation, or decreased activity

— *Emphysema and alpha₁-antitrypsin*

Etiology

- Environmental—smoking increases risk in susceptible individuals

Genetic risk of emphysema

- MM, MZ, SS have no increased risk
- SZ has mildly increased risk (alpha₁-antitrypsin sometimes below critical level)
- ZZ (alpha₁-antitrypsin below critical level) and null/null (alpha₁-antitrypsin absent) have high risk

Pathogenesis

- When serum alpha$_1$-antitrypsin is less than the critical level of 11 μM, the lower respiratory tract is prone to damage by NE released from neutrophils normally in the lung

  - Effects of cigarette smoking

    - Attracts neutrophils to the lung
    - Increases the amount of NE released per neutrophil
    - Oxidatively damages alpha$_1$-antitrypsin, decreasing its activity
    - Imbalance between NE (excess) and alpha$_1$-antitrypsin (deficient) destroys alveolar walls, causing air space enlargement

Morphologic manifestation

- Panacinar emphysema involving lower lung fields

  - Enlargement of the acini from the respiratory bronchiole to the terminal alveoli

Clinical course

- Signs and symptoms—forced expiration, barrel chest, difficulty in breathing on exertion
- Lungs hyperinflated on chest x-ray film
- Prognosis—poor

— *Liver disease and alpha$_1$-antitrypsin*

- Etiology—genetic

  - Occurs in patients with Z and certain rare alleles

- Pathogenesis

  - Caused by accumulation of alpha$_1$-antitrypsin in hepatocytes
  - Other factors must be involved—neonatal hepatitis (see following) occurs in <20% of persons with ZZ

- Morphologic manifestations

  - Intrahepatocyte accumulation of alpha$_1$-antitrypsin
  - Cholestasis (impaired bilirubin excretion), inflammation, hepatocyte necrosis
  - Sometimes, cirrhosis

- Clinical course

  - Neonatal hepatitis that usually resolves, but can progress to cirrhosis
  - Hepatitis, cirrhosis, hepatocellular carcinoma later in life

CYTOGENETIC DISORDERS

■ Normal Karyotype

- Somatic chromosomal complement of 46 chromosomes aligned in standard sequence based on size, centromere location, and banding pattern
- Preparation of karyotype

  - Requires cells capable of proliferation in culture
  - Giemsa staining (G banding) most commonly used (Fig. 7.1)

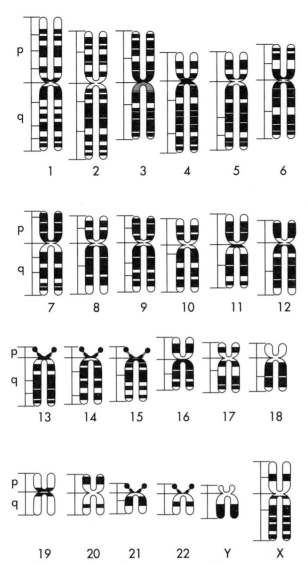

Fig. 7.1 Schema of chromosomes (G banded) according to the Paris Conference (ISCN 1985). *(Adapted from Damjanov I, Linder J:* Anderson's pathology, *ed 10, vol 1, St Louis, 1996, Mosby.*

■ Abnormal Karyotype

● Nomenclature (Table 7.1)

● Numerical abnormalities

- Normal haploid gamete (N), 23 chromosomes; normal diploid (2N), 46 chromosomes
- Euploid, exact multiple of N (e.g., triploid 3N, 69 chromosomes)
- Aneuploid, noneuploid state
  - Monosomy, single copy of one chromosome
  - Trisomy, three copies of one chromosome
  - Usually caused by failure to separate during division (nondisjunction)

Table 7.1 *Cytogenetics Nomenclature*

del	Deletion, or loss, of a chromosome segment. EXAMPLE: del(13)(q14) = deletion of band 14 located on the long arm of chromosome 13.
der	Structurally abnormal chromosome created by the rearrangement of two or more chromosomes or more than one rearrangement in the same chromosome.
dup	Duplication, a replicated or duplicated chromosome segment next to itself; if in the same orientation = *direct* duplication *(dir dup);* if inverted = *inverted* duplication *(inv dup).*
i	Isochromosome, a symmetric chromosome composed of duplicated long or short arms formed after misdivision of the centromere in a transverse plane. EXAMPLE: i(5)(p10), duplication of the short arm of chromosome 5 with loss of the long arm.
ins	Insertion, a chromosomal segment from one chromosome is inserted into a nonhomologous chromosome; similar to a duplication, an insertion can be direct or inverted. EXAMPLE: dir ins(10;3)(q22;p14p24) = a direct insertion of the chromosomal segment of a short arm of chromosome 3 (p14-p24) into chromosome 10 at q22.
inv	Inversion, a segment of a chromosome is reversed 180 degrees; a *paracentric* inversion does not involve the centromere in the inversion, a *pericentric* inversion does (a break in each chromosomal arm is necessary). EXAMPLE: inv(2)(p14q22) is a pericentric inversion involving the centromere of chromosome 2.
p	Short arm of a chromosome (from French *petit*).
q	Long arm of a chromosome (letter following *p*).
t	Translocation, a *reciprocal* translocation is an exchange of chromosomal material between two or more nonhomologous chromosomes (may be balanced or unbalanced); a *Robertsonian* translocation involves acrocentric chromosomes with fusion at the centromere and loss of the short arms and satellites. EXAMPLE: t(9;11)(q31;q21.1) denotes a reciprocal translocation involving breaks at band 31 on the long arm of chromosome 9 and at band 21.1 on the long arm chromosome 11 with exchange of the segments distal to those breakpoints.
+ (plus sign)	Added chromosome (+8) or chromosomal segment (8q+).
– (minus sign)	Lost (deleted) chromosome (–7) or chromosomal segment (5q–).

From Damjanov I, Linder J: *Anderson's pathology,* ed 10, vol 1, St Louis, 1996, Mosby.

- **Structural abnormalities**
  - Breakage and rejoining of broken ends to form new combinations
  - Balanced (no change in genetic information) or unbalanced (gain or loss of genetic information)

Clinical Abnormalities

- Spontaneous abortions
  - *50% have chromosomal abnormalities (Table 7.2)*
    - 95% of chromosomally abnormal conceptuses abort spontaneously
    - Mostly, aneuploid
      - 45,X most common

Table 7.2 *Chromosomal Abnormalities Occurring in Recognized Human Abortuses*

Type of Abnormality	Percentage of Chromosomally Abnormal Abortuses	Percentage Survival to Term
Trisomies of autosomes		
16	15	0
13, 18, and 21	9	15
All others	27	~0
Sex chromosomal abnormalities XXY, XYY, XXX	1	75
45,X	18	1
Triploidy	17	~0
Tetraploidy	6	0
Structural abnormalities (such as translocations, balanced and unbalanced)	7	~55

From Damjanov I, Linder J: *Anderson's pathology*, ed 10, vol 1, St Louis, 1996, Mosby.

- Percent of newborns with chromosomal abnormality—0.5%
- Autosomal disorders (Table 7.3)

  — *Most common features—mental retardation, growth retardation, somatic abnormalities*

  — *Maternal age >35 years increases risk for many*

  — *Down syndrome*

    - 1/800 births
    - 95% have trisomy 21 (47,XX, +21)
    - 4% unbalanced translocation of long arm of 21 to another chromosome, usually 22 or 14, e.g., m 46,XY, -14, +t(14q21q)

      - Usually have parent with balanced translocation

    - 1% mosaics
    - Region responsible 21q22
    - Manifestations—mental retardation, flat face, upward slanting palpebral fissures, epicanthic folds, simian crease in hands, cardiac septal defects, tenfold to twentyfold increased incidence of acute leukemia, immune deficiency and infections, premature Alzheimer's disease in long-term survivors

  — *Other trisomies less common (each less than 1/6000 births)*

    - Usually fatal in first year
    - Trisomy 13 (Patau's syndrome)

      - About 1/6000 births
      - Cleft lip and palate, cardiac anomalies, microcephaly

    - Trisomy 18 (Edwards' syndrome)

      - About 1/8000 births
      - Growth retardation, overlapping fingers, cardiac anomalies

Table 7.3 *Dectection of Chromosome Abnormalities at Amniocentesis in Pregnancies of Women Over 35 Years of Age Compared with Rates Determined from Surveys of the Newborns*

Type of Chromosome Abnormality	Prenatal Diagnoses (%)	Newborn Surveys Including All Maternal Ages	
		%	Fraction
Autosomal Abnormalities			
Trisomy 21	1.16	0.12	1 in 700
Trisomy 18	0.23	0.01	1 in 3000
Trisomy 13	0.07	0.01	1 in 5000
t(13q14q)	0.05	0.07	
Other balanced structural rearrangements	0.18	0.12	
Extra marker chromosome	0.06	0.02	
Other unbalanced structural rearrangements	0.08	0.06	
Sex Chromosome Abnormalities			
47,XXX	0.25f	0.10f	1 in 800f
47,XXY	0.33m	0.09m	1 in 700m
47,XYY	0.07m	0.09m	1 in 800m
45,X	0.09f	0.01f	1 in 2500f
Other unbalanced	0.05	0.06	

From Damjanov I, Linder J: *Anderson's pathology*, ed 10, vol 1, St Louis, 1996, Mosby.
f, Rates for females; *m*, rates for males.

— *Cri du chat syndrome*

- Deletion of short arm of chromosome 5 (5p-)

  - Critical resion 5p15

- Cat cry during first year of life, mental retardation, microcephaly, round facies
- Compatible with survival into adulthood

● Sex chromosome disorders

— *X chromosome inactivation*

- Usually random process by which genes on one X chromosome not transcribed in a particular cell
- Abnormal X chromosomes can be preferentially inactivated
- Equalizes expression of X-encoded genes in males and females
- Condensed, inactive X chromosome seen as sex chromatin (Barr) body

  - Dense granule adjacent to nuclear membrane in interphase cells
  - Altered numbers of Barr bodies present in females with abnormalities of X chromosome number (e.g., XXX will have 2 Barr bodies)

— *Turner syndrome*

- Female hypogonadism with X monosomy
- 45,X most common but several other numerical or structural abnormalities possible (Table 7.4 lists other abnormalities)

Table 7.4	*Types and Relative Percentages of Chromosomal Abnormalities in Turner's Syndrome*
45,X	53%
45,X/46,XX mosaics	15%
46,X,i(Xq)	10%
45,X/46,X,i(Xq) mosaics	8%
46,XXq– or 46,XXp– deletions	6%
Other 45,X/? mosaics	8%

From Damjanov I, Linder J: *Anderson's pathology*, ed 10, vol 1, St Louis, 1996, Mosby.

- Loss of Xp determines short stature and somatic abnormalities
- Loss of Xq determines abnormal gonadal function
- Clinical features (variable)
  - Most 45,XO conceptuses do not survive to birth
  - Manifestations in those who are born are quite variable, including short stature, lymphedema, web neck, shield chest and wide-spaced nipples, aortic coarctation, primary amenorrhea, fibrous and atrophic ovaries, infantile genitalia, and failure of breast development

— *Klinefelter's syndrome*
  - Male with more than one X chromosome
  - 80% 47,XXY; most others mosaics (e.g., 46,XY/47,XXY)
  - Clinical features include eunichoid body habitus, infertility, atrophic testes with Leydig cell hyperplasia, failure of male secondary sex characteristics, gynecomastia, elevated follicle-stimulating hormone (FSH) and estrogens; decreased androgens, minimal or no intellectual impairment

— *XYY*
  - Tall, behavioral difficulties (controversial)

NON-MENDELIAN INHERITANCE

■ Mutations in Mitochondrial DNA

- ● Mitochondrial genome distinct from nuclear chromosomes
  - 16kb circular deoxyribonucleic acid (DNA)
  - Encodes transfer RNA (tRNA), ribosomal RNA (rRNA), 22 proteins
  - Inherited from mother
- ● Mitochondrial diseases from mutations in mitochondrial DNA
  - Passed from mother to children of either sex (different from X-linked)
  - Variable phenotypic expression caused by random distribution of normal and abnormal mitochondria in different tissues
  - Tend to affect tissues most dependent on oxidative phosphorylation (central nervous system, skeletal muscle, heart muscle)

- Diseases from point mutations in mitochondrial DNA
  - Leber's hereditary optic neuropathy
  - MELAS (mitochondrial myopathy, encephalopathy, lactic acidosis, stroke)
  - MERRF (myoclonus epilepsy with ragged red fibers)
- Disease from deletion of mitochondrial DNA
  - Kearns-Sayre syndrome (chronic external ophthalmoplegia, retinal degeneration, heart block)
- Mutations in mitochondrial DNA (especially in brain and heart) accumulate with aging
- Most mitochondrial proteins encoded by genomic DNA and most genetic mitochondrial diseases are mendelian

Genomic Imprinting

- Functional differences between maternal and paternal genes (e.g., so that only one is expressed)
  - *Might be mediated by methylation*
- Prader-Willi and Angelman's syndromes
  - *Chromosomal region involved*
    - About 1000 kb on 15q11-13
    - Prader-Willi syndrome locus is active on paternal chromosome
    - Angelman's syndrome locus is active on maternal chromosome
    - Within this region there is a locus that controls its imprinting
    - Inactive DNA is hypermethylated
  - *Prader-Willi syndrome*
    - About 70% have interstitial deletion involving 15q11-13 in paternal chromosome
    - Most of the rest exhibit uniparental disomy (both chromosomes of maternal origin)
    - Clinical features—small hands and feet, developmental delay, hyperphagia and obesity, short stature, hypogonadism, and hypopigmentation
  - *Angelman syndrome*
    - About 70% have 15q11-13 deletion in maternal chromosome
    - Some of the remaining 30% have uniparental disomy (both chromosomes of paternal origin)
    - Clinical features—mental retardation, seizures, inappropriate laughter

Unstable Number of Trinucleotide Repeats

- Fragile X syndrome
  - *Most common form of inherited mental retardation in males (1:1000 to 1:1500 affected)*
  - *Karyotypic abnormality*
    - Discontinuity or constriction on the distal long arm of X (Xq27.3)

- Chromatid breaks when cell cultured in folate-deficient medium
— *Differences from normal X-linked disorders*
  - Carrier males
    - About 20% of males who carry mutation are phenotypically and cytogentically normal
    - Can transmit disease through unaffected daughters to grandchildren
  - About 30% of carrier females are phenotypically affected (mentally retarded)
  - Sherman's paradox
    - Position in pedigree affects risk of being phenotypically affected
    - Daughter of carrier male has 75% risk of having affected son in comparison to about 18% chance of transmission by other heterozygotes
  - Anticipation
    - Clinical features worsen with passage to successive generations
— *Role of tandem CGG repeats*
  - Normal individuals have 10 to 50 repeats
  - Normal transmitting males and carrier females have 52 to 200 repeats (premutation)
  - Affected individuals have 200 to 500 repeats (full mutation)
  - Amplification of repeats converts premutations to full mutations
    - Process much more likely to occur during oogenesis than spermatogenesis
— *Clinical features*
  - Mental retardation
  - Long face, large mandible, everted ears
  - Large testicles
  - Diagnosis
    - Cytogenetic
    - Southern blot can distinguish premutations from full mutations
- **Other trinucleotide repeat disorders involve nervous system**
  - Huntington's disease
  - Myotonic dystrophy

MULTIPLE CHOICE
REVIEW QUESTIONS

1. The most probable karyotype of a male infant with a flat face, epicanthic folds, a simian crease, and an atrial septal defect is which of the following?

    a. 46,XY, −14, +t(14q21q)
    b. 47,XY, +21
    c. 45,XO
    d. 46,XXY
    e. 46,5q−

2. Which of the following is an individual homozygous for null alleles of alpha$_1$-antitrypsin most likely to manifest?

    a. Meconium ileus and chronic bronchitis
    b. Chronic bronchitis only
    c. Meconium ileus and panacinar emphysema
    d. Neonatal hepatitis and panacinar emphysema
    e. Panacinar emphysema only

3. Alzheimer's disease is most characteristic of patients with which of the following?

    a. Down syndrome
    b. Edwards syndrome
    c. Familial hypercholesterolemia
    d. Marfan syndrome
    e. Patou syndrome

4. Genomic imprinting most likely involves which of the following?

    a. Expansion of trinucleotide repeats in nuclear DNA
    b. Expansion of trinucleotide repeated sequences in mitochondrial DNA
    c. Deletion of specific chromosomes
    d. Methylation of nuclear DNA
    e. Methylation of mitochondrial DNA

Chapter 8

Environmental and Nutritional Diseases

DISEASES CAUSED BY STARVATION OR MALNUTRITION

Inadequate nutrition or starvation is a major cause of human disease, both in this country and abroad.

- Forms of malnutrition

  - Inadequate caloric intake
  - Inadequate protein intake
  - Inadequate vitamin/mineral intake
  - Mixed forms (combinations of the above)
  - Adequate caloric intake, but inadequate protein or vitamin-mineral intake (e.g., kwashiorkor; overindulgence in "empty calories," such as refined sugars or alcohol; protein-vitamin-mineral deficiencies may be present even though obesity may be severe)

- Malnutrition may occur in spite of adequate available nutrients.

  - Psychiatric disturbances (e.g., anorexia nervosa)
  - Physical disease preventing adequate food intake (e.g., poor teeth; oral, esophageal, or gastric carcinoma)
  - Loss of ingested nutrients because of disease (e.g., nausea or vomiting associated with medical treatment, such as chemotherapy for neoplasia; vomiting of pregnancy; iron loss from chronic gastrointestinal bleeding or excessive menstruation)
  - Malabsorption or inadequate utilization of ingested nutrients (e.g., liver, gallbladder or pancreatic disease; malabsorption syndromes; chronic diarrhea associated with intestinal parasites; inadequate absorption of vitamin B_{12} in pernicious anemia or with infestation of the freshwater fish tapeworm *Diphyllobothrium latum;* drug-induced malabsorption; malabsorption from excessive intake of foods containing artificial fat; genetic disorders)
  - Relative malnutrition from increased nutritional requirements (e.g., during a rapid growth phase in childhood or adolescence; during pregnancy; in the course of protein-losing diseases; during healing after massive trauma or burns)
  - Inadequate protein-vitamin-mineral content of preparations in total parenteral feeding

- Functional deficits (e.g., apathy, poor concentration, loss of memory, poor stamina) may precede structural lesions by a considerable period.

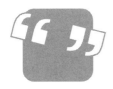

- Malnutrition contributes to immune deficiency, infection by contagious diseases or parasites that, in turn, intensify the malnutrition.

■ **Protein and Calorie Malnutrition**

- Common in this country and abroad
- Children, adults, and elderly are all affected
- Maternal malnutrition predisposes to prematurity and low infant birth weight

● Severe malnutrition states

— *Kwashiorkor—"disease of displaced children"*

- Caused by protein insufficiency (often with adequate caloric intake, usually from carbohydrates)
- Also affects children weaned to an inadequate or high carbohydrate diet

- There is low serum albumin, hepatomegaly, fatty liver, peripheral or generalized edema, anemia.
- Subcutaneous fat may be abundant.
- Dermatoses with flaking of skin and depigmentation or hyperpigmentation occurs.
- Moon facies may be present; hair is fine, poorly rooted, pale, and often banded, reflecting periods of better nutrition alternating with periods of starvation.
- Atrophy of bowel mucosa, loss of microvilli, and absence of normal mitotic activity in mucosal crypts may be caused by intestinal parasites that are commonly present (*Ascaris, Strongyloides, Trichuris* organisms, amoebas).
- Bone marrow atrophy and iron deficiency anemia commonly present.
- Listlessness, apathy, and lethargy are characteristic.

- If adequate diet restored, fat is mobilized and health can be restored, often with little or no permanent damage; reports of mental or growth retardation in children following kwashiorkor are difficult to confirm

— *Marasmus*

- Wasting, from lack of all nutrients (i.e., starvation)

- Stunted growth, lack of body fat, atrophy of muscles, redundant skin, bone marrow atrophy, iron deficiency microcytic or mixed microcytic-/macrocytic (from folate deficiency) anemia all result from starvation.
- No hepatomegaly or edema is present; however, starvation states intermediate between kwashiorkor and marasmus occur, with some features of both.

- Children are hungry, eat voraciously if fed
- If adequate nutrition restored, and parasitic and bacterial infections controlled, most physical deficits can be reversed, including stunted growth; permanent intellectual deficits may remain because of lack of brain development with loss of neurons in children, but difficult to measure

■ **Obesity** The obverse of marasmus, obesity is a common problem in the United States. While obesity occurs when caloric intake exceeds caloric requirements, many other factors are often involved.

- Genetic factors may contribute, as suggested from studies of twins separated at birth.
- Familial dietary customs and food preferences exert powerful influences on the amount and type of food intake.
- Possible individual differences in the efficiency of digestion and utilization of nutrients are reported.

● **Obesity may result in**

- Social ostracism, sometimes leading to psychiatric disturbance, including depression
- Shortened life span
- Non–insulin-dependent diabetes mellitus
- Hypertension, atherosclerosis, and heart disease, including coronary artery disease
- Cholesterol gallstone formation

■ **Vitamin Deficiencies and Toxicities** Vitamins are required as cofactors or as prosthetic groups on enzymes involved in metabolic reactions. Most vitamins require exogenous sources, although some can be synthesized endogenously; endogenous synthesis is usually inadequate during periods of starvation.

● **Fat-soluble vitamins (A, D, E, K)—may be stored and mobilized during starvation, delaying deficiency states**

— *Vitamin A*

- Retinoids (compounds with vitamin A properties) and many of their derivatives, found in animal products, including eggs, butter, meat, milk, fish, liver; retinol is the most potent retinoid.

- Carotenoids (vitamin A precursors, including beta-carotene) naturally occur in green and yellow vegetables.
- Absorption requires the digestive enzymes and salts needed to absorb fats.
- During periods of adequate nutrition, sufficient vitamin A is stored to prevent deficiency states during long periods of starvation; hydrolysate esters with vitamin A activity are bound to transthyretin (retinol-binding protein, prealbumin); all cells have specific binding sites, where the vitamin is taken in and transported to the nucleus by other specific proteins.
- Deficiency results in

  - Keratinization of the ocular conjunctivae (xerophthalmia)
  - Corneal ulcerations (keratomalacia) and scarring, eventually leading to blindness
  - Depletion of retinal visual pigments causes night blindness
  - Epithelial metaplasia, especially of mucous-secreting and transitional epithelia
  - Depletion of antioxidant capacity in cells
  - Impaired immunity and high infection rate, especially in children

- Reduction of cell-growth regulation, possibly leading to increased incidence of neoplasms (now questionable in the light of recently released research studies); increased incidence of lung and skin tumors and reduced growth and reproductive capacity in laboratory animals

- Desquamation of epithelial cells may lead to stone formation in the urinary tract and block the lumina of glandular ducts

- Follicular keratosis caused by squamous metaplasia of sebaceous and sweat glands causes or intensifies acne

- Excessive intake of vitamin A may result in nausea, vomiting or diarrhea, headache (possibly related to inadequate or overabundant production of cerebrospinal fluid), depressed levels of consciousness or excitation and hyperactivity, alopecia; chronic toxicity may cause premature closure of fontanelles in children or lymphadenopathy and hyperostoses in adults; yellowing of skin may be confused with true jaundice.

— *Vitamin D*

- Normally formed in skin from 7-dehydrocholesterol acted upon by ultraviolet light and converted to vitamin D_3; also abundant in foods such as fortified milk, saltwater fish and grains, which contain ergosterol, converted to vitamin D_2 after ingestion.

- The vitamin must be converted to its biologically active form in the kidney after being carried there by a transporting alpha globulin protein produced in the liver.

- Metabolites of vitamin D act to maintain adequate serum levels of calcium and phosphate for proper mineralization of bone.

- Deficiencies result from

  - Poor maternal nutrition with adverse consequences to fetus and young infant and, following birth, to inadequate diet and inadequate exposure to sunlight; in the elderly, osteomalacia results from restricted diets and inadequate exposure to sunlight

  - Conditions that impair absorption of fat (e.g., pancreatic disease, biliary disease, sprue, regional enteritis)

  - Extensive liver disease, interfering with blood transport protein production

  - Extensive renal disease, which inhibits formation of active metabolites of vitamin D; in renal failure, acidosis and azotemia inhibit absorption of calcium from gastrointestinal tract; secondary hypoparathyroidism from renal failure results in "renal osteodystrophy"

  - In protein-losing renal disease (nephrotic syndrome)—depletion of the transport globulin

  - Drugs (phenobarbital, phenytoin) accelerate degradation of vitamin D via induction of P-450 enzymes

  - Genetic diseases that restrict conversion of vitamin D to its active metabolites (vitamin D-dependent rickets, type I)

  - Genetic diseases with deranged end-organ receptors and in-

adequate calcium absorption from the gastrointestinal tract (vitamin D-dependent rickets, type II)
- Rare paraneoplastic syndromes that cause phosphorus wasting
- Excessive use of antacids, such as Mylanta, which contain aluminum hydroxide that binds phosphate and interferes with absorption

- Deficiency in adults results in osteomalacia with impaired mineralization of osteoid during bone remodeling.

- Loss of skeletal mass predisposes to fractures and vertebral column deformities
- Looser's zones or Milkman's fractures—narrow radiolucent lines in long bones or pelvis; may be poorly healed, spontaneous stress fractures or erosions by penetrating arteries; diagnostic when present radiographically
- Bone pain and proximal limb weakness—common clinical signs

- Deficiency in children results in rickets caused by inadequate mineralization, especially of epiphyseal cartilage that does not mature and then overgrows.

- Osteoid matrix, deposited onto the masses of immature cartilage, causes osteochondral junctions to become irregularly enlarged; capillaries overgrow, marrow becomes fibrotic
- Irregular bone growth results in poor rigidity of the bones and distortion of the skeleton by the pull of the muscles
- There is protrusion ("bossing") of the frontal area of the skull from excessive osteoid formation; the chest becomes deformed with enlargement of the costochondral junctions ("rachitic rosary"); improperly mineralized ribs pulled inward, resulting in anterior bulging of the sternum ("pigeon-breast"); legs become bowed, spine may be deformed

- Restoration of proper diet and vitamin D supplementation promote proper mineralization of the skeleton, but major skeletal deformities remain.

- Hypervitaminosis D is rare, but may predispose to renal stones and metastatic calcifications because of hypercalcemia.

— *Vitamin E*

- 4 related tocopherols, all antioxidants, have vitamin E activity; the principle and most potent compound is alpha-tocopherol.
- Vitamin E protects polyunsaturated fatty acids in biologic membranes from peroxidation; diets containing abundant polyunsaturated fatty acids increase vitamin E and other antioxidant requirements.
- Vitamin E is found most abundantly in fish, grains, and vegetables; after ingestion, chylomicrons transport the vitamin in the blood for storage, mainly in adipose tissue, muscle, and in the liver; a specific transport protein is not required.

- Dietary deficiency is rare; deficiency states usually occur with

  - Premature and term low birth-weight infants because of immaturity of the liver and gastrointestinal tract and feedings often high in polyunsaturated fats
  - Small bowel diseases, including regional enteritis, celiac disease, or any other condition predisposing to steatorrhea and malabsorption of fats, including pancreatic diseases, especially cystic fibrosis
  - Cholestasis from any cause with resulting decreased fat absorption
  - Rare genetic disorders that impede absorption of vitamin E or its transport in the blood (e.g., abetalipoproteinemia)

- Deficiency is associated with

  - Posterior column spinal cord degeneration, in vitamin E malabsorption syndromes in adults and children; numerous dystrophic axons and demyelination present within the degenerated posterior columns; peripheral neuropathies and pigmentary retinal degeneration also reported, as well as myopathies and depositions of lipoid pigments within the cytoplasm of muscles fibers; lesions seem more significant in patients who have not received replacement vitamin E therapy; direct correlation with vitamin E deficiency often difficult to prove, however
  - Massive overdoses of vitamin E are associated with difficulties in absorbing the other fat-soluble vitamins and enteritis, especially in infants

— *Vitamin K*

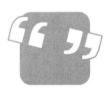

- Vitamin K is a cofactor for liver carboxylase conversion of glutamyl residues in some proteins (especially in clotting factors VII, IX, and X and prothrombin) to gammacarboxyglutamates; these proteins require carboxylation to provide calcium-binding sites for binding to phospholipid surfaces in the formation of thrombin.

- Vitamin K is abundant in dairy products, green vegetables, and liver.

- As with all fat-soluble vitamins, absorption is impeded by pancreatic, biliary, and gastrointestinal diseases; normal intestinal flora synthesize small amounts of vitamin K.

- Little vitamin K is stored; however, efficient reconstitution after its carboxylation reactions makes ingestion of only minimal amounts of exogenous vitamin K necessary in healthy individuals.

- Vitamin K deficiency may result, in addition to malabsorption conditions, from use of some antibiotics that inhibit vitamin K recycling; from liver disease, which reduces the synthesis of vitamin K precursors; and from therapeutic or unintentional intake of vitamin K antagonists, including dicumarol and warfarin (often used in rat poisons).

- Vitamin K deficiency may occur in neonates because of poor transport of the vitamin across the maternal circulation and lack of intestinal flora in the newborn to synthesize the vitamin; breast-fed babies are more likely to develop vitamin K deficiency than fortified formula-fed babies.

• Vitamin K deficiency results in inadequate clotting response and hemorrhage; in deficient newborn infants, intracerebral hemorrhage, gastrointestinal bleeding, and umbilical hemorrhage are often serious problems.

• Dietary overconsumption of vitamin K with toxicity does not occur.

● **Water-soluble vitamins**—The vitamin B-complex that includes thiamine (vitamin B_1), riboflavin (vitamin B_2), niacin, pyridoxine (vitamins B_6), ascorbic acid (vitamin C), and cyanocobalamin (vitamin B_{12})

• B-complex vitamins are ubiquitous and easily absorbed; adequate amounts can usually be obtained from diets containing green leafy vegetables, milk, eggs, meat, fish, and cereals; citrus fruits and vegetables, especially tomatoes, are rich in vitamin C.

— *Thiamine (B_1)*

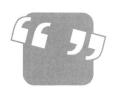

• Although the vitamin is widely available, refined foods (white flour, refined white sugar, polished white rice) contain inadequate amounts of vitamin B_1.

• Coffee, tea, and raw freshwater fish have **anti**thiamine activity.

• Absorption involves passive diffusion when there are high concentrations in the gastrointestinal tract (especially the small intestine) and energy-dependent absorption when concentrations are low.

• Phosphorylation is required to produce the active form (thiamine pyrophosphate), which is important in maintenance of nerve membrane integrity and conduction (especially in peripheral nerves), in oxidative decarboxylation of alpha-ketoacids in adenosine triphosphate (ATP) synthesis, and in pentose phosphate pathway.

• Thiamine deficiency damages peripheral nerves ("dry" beriberi), producing polyneuropathy of both motor and sensory nerves, usually beginning distally in legs and feet, progressing proximally, and later involving trunk and arms; myelin degenerates, then axons; anterior horn cells and posterior columns may be secondarily involved in severe prolonged deficiencies.

• In the central nervous system (CNS), Wernicke's encephalopathy most often affects alcoholics, with petechial hemorrhages in the mamillary bodies, walls of the third ventricle, periaqueductal gray matter, floor of the fourth ventricle, thalamus, and cerebellum; death may result if condition is not recognized and promptly treated with replacement therapy. Symptoms include ophthalmoplegias, ataxia, and mental confusion; Korsakoff's psychosis often follows Wernicke's encephalopathy and is characterized by loss of recent memory and confabulation (tendency of victims to fill in memory gaps with well-constructed fictions). Mamillary bodies are brown and small, neuronal loss and gliosis are present.

• Heart (in "wet" beriberi) may be minimally or severely enlarged with dilation of all chambers and thinning of the ventricular walls; changes are not unique to thiamine deficiency. Consequences of the heart failure include peripheral vasodilation and high-output cardiac failure, decreased renal blood flow, water retention, and peripheral edema.

• Thiamine in large doses produces flushing of skin and dizziness, but effects of administration of even large doses of thiamine are not serious or permanent.

— *Riboflavin (B₂)*

• Abundant in cereals, eggs, milk, fruit, and liver

• Acts as cofactor for many enzymes after conversion to flavin mononucleotide and flavin-adenine dinucleotide

• Deficiency causes mucosal fissuring, with inflammation of the lips, mouth, and tongue, dermatitis, and vascularization of the cornea

— *Niacin*

• Involved in many biochemical reactions as part of nicotinamide adenine dinucleotide (NAD) and NAD phosphate (NADP)

• Deficiency results in pellagra, with its classic triad of dementia, dermatitis, and diarrhea (the "3 Ds")

— *Pyridoxine (B₆)*

• Abundant in cereals, milk, meat, and fish

• Deficiency causes confusions or dementia, inflammation of lips, mouth and tongue, and peripheral neuropathy

• Isoniazid therapy for tuberculosis, L-dopa treatment for Parkinson's disease, antihypertensive drug therapy, and use of oral contraceptives associated with pyridoxine deficiency

• Pyridoxine dependency syndromes reported, including homocystinuria, requiring very large doses of the vitamin

— *Cyanocobalamin (B₁₂)*

• Ubiquitous in foods, but requires gastrointestinal intrinsic factor for absorption

• Deficiency causes megaloblastic (pernicious) anemia and subacute combined degeneration of spinal cord (also known as posterolateral degeneration)—bilateral, edematous, spongy demyelination, and axonal degeneration of both the posterior columns (afferent sensory tracts carrying proprioception and two-point discriminative touch sensations) *and* the posterolateral columns ("lateral columns") carrying corticospinal (pyramidal) motor tracts

— *Ascorbic acid (vitamin C)*

• Deficiency often affects the elderly and chronic alcoholics; both groups frequently have inadequate diets

• Cannot be synthesized in the body

• Necessary for many oxidation-reduction reactions, protecting lipids from peroxidation, and for collagen, chondroitin sulfate, and osteoid matrix synthesis; also important in synthesis of neurotransmitters and carnitine

• Mild deficiency associated with lethargy, weakness, and tendency to bruise easily

• Severe deficiency—causes scurvy, with bleeding gums, hyperkeratosis of hair follicles with a perifollicular skin rash, and petechial, subperiosteal, and intracranial hemorrhages; condition often affected seamen on long voyages until it was finally recognized that citrus

fruits corrected the problem; hence, the term for British sailors—
"Limeys"

   • Some have advocated very large doses of vitamin C for protection against common cold and in treatment of cancer; most studies have shown little or no effect on either condition; consequences of ingestion of megadoses of vitamin C—increased iron absorption, possible iron overload, acidosis, especially when chronic renal disease is present, uricosuria, and the formation of renal stones

■ **The Influence of the Diet on Cancer**

   • Exogenous carcinogens, ingested with food, may promote carcinogenesis.

   • Aflatoxin produced by *Aspergillus flavus* contamination of grains has been linked to hepatocellular carcinoma in Africa.

   • Saccharin and other artificial sweeteners have been linked to neoplasms (at least in experimental animals).

   • Barbecuing (producing aromatic hydrocarbons) has been suggested as a contributing factor in gastrointestinal carcinogenesis.

   • Endogenous carcinogens, synthesized from ingested foods have been suggested as contributing factors in production of some neoplasms (e.g., eating smoked meats containing nitrites that are converted in the body to nitrosamines, have been linked to an increased incidence of carcinoma of the stomach).

   • Protective factors in food (or a lack thereof) might influence the incidence of cancer (vitamin A's value as a protective factor against carcinoma of the colon has recently been disproved in a study of 26,000 physicians). A high-fiber diet, by speeding transit of feces through the colon and thereby lowering the colonic exposure to carcinogens from food or metabolites of bile acids, or by diluting these carcinogens by increasing the bulk of the stool, is thought to be valuable in reducing the incidence of colonic carcinoma, diverticulosis, and diverticulitis.

ENVIRONMENTAL AND OCCUPATIONAL DISEASE

The detrimental impact of the environment on human health is enormous. *Homo sapiens,* according to some pessimists, has despoiled its nest virtually to the point of no redemption. Air, soil, and water pollution, depletion of the ozone layer, man-made and naturally occurring radioactive material (NORM) pollution of soil, ground water, and air, therapeutic and "recreational" drug use and abuse, occupational psychological and physical stress (e.g., carpal tunnel syndrome in computer operators), and trauma all take their toll on health.

■ **Climate, Atmosphere, and the Ozone Layer**

   ● Global warming

   • Certain gases ("greenhouse gases") trap infrared radiant energy; these gasses—water vapor, CO_2, methane, O_2, and chlorofluorocarbon compounds—contribute significantly to earth surface warming.

   • Humans have significantly increased atmospheric content of these gases in the last 250 years.

   • Large increases in CO_2 content in the atmosphere are partly from expanding human population, from decreasing forest and grasslands vegetation that take in CO_2 (and produce O_2), and from industrial emissions.

• Earth surface temperature has warmed measurably (approximately 0.5° C since 1900), largely from increases in greenhouse gases. Predicted continued increases, as much as 5° to 10° C in the next few centuries if efforts are not made to reverse this trend, will have devastating effects on plants and animals, causing flooding from melting of the polar ice caps, contaminating of fresh water sources, and, at the same time, causing increased evaporation of surface water (adding further to the greenhouse effect). Increased atmospheric temperature will increase mortality from heatstroke; dehydration of flora and fauna alike will escalate, respiratory disease incidence will increase, and disruption of ecosystems and changing microbiologic populations may possibly cause disease epidemics.

• Current technologies, if properly applied, can delay or reverse this trend.

● Depletion of the ozone layer

• Chlorofluorocarbon compounds, used as aerosol propellants and as refrigerants, and other atmospheric pollutants, by providing free radicals that convert ozone to oxygen, destroy the ozone layer, which is produced in the upper atmosphere by the action of solar radiation on oxygen and sparse nitrogen dioxide molecules. Gases used in fire extinguishers, containing bromine ions, are equally destructive to ozone.

• Atmospheric layer of ozone acts as a screen against penetration of ultraviolet (UV) radiation into our environment.

• Significant losses of ozone over both polar regions, which has already occurred, correlates with

• Marked increases in nonmelanotic skin cancers in whites
• Doubling of the rate of skin melanoma in the United States; even greater increases elsewhere
• Increases in the incidence of ocular cataracts
• Impact on the food chain, including possible destruction of phytoplankton, food for many sea dwellers, with eventual depletion of important human food sources higher in the food chain

■ **Outdoor Air Pollution**

• Inhaled air may contain a variety of organic and inorganic particulate substances, gases, and microbiologic agents, some injurious to all and some to sensitive individuals in varying degrees. Important outdoor air pollutants are listed in Table 8.1.

• Atmospheric temperature inversions increase the concentration of pollutants near the ground.

• Most affected by outdoor pollution are asthmatics, those with chronic obstructive pulmonary disease and cardiovascular disease, children (outdoors when ozone levels are highest), joggers, runners, and outdoor exercisers.

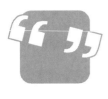

■ **Indoor Air Pollution**

• Numerous gases, volatile and semivolatile organic compounds, insect and animal products, bacteria, fungi and spores, noxious particulate materials (e.g., asbestos and particulates from smoke), and the radioactive gas radon pollute indoor air. Some are listed in Table 8.2.

■ **Tobacco and Smoking**

• Cigarette smoking is responsible for greater morbidity and mortality in the United States than all other pollutants combined. Pipe and cigar smoking,

Table 8.1 *Common Outdoor Air Pollutants*

POLLUTANT	SOURCES	FORMATION	EFFECTS
Particulates (especially those less than 10 microns in diameter) containing organic carbon, aluminum, calcium, silicon, and sulfates, nitrates, and ammonium ions	Coal burning, engine exhausts, wood smoke Aerosol sulfates	Generated by industry, automobiles, heating of homes, forest fires Ammonia neutralization of H_2SO_4 aerosols	Asthma, emphysema, other respiratory diseases; increased cardiovascular disease
Ozone (O_3)	Nitric oxide (NO) from automobile exhaust plus sunlight	NO, in car exhaust, is oxidized to NO_2. O_3 forms in the presence of NO_2 plus sunlight and hydrocarbons	Ozone-sensitive crop damage. Reduction in expiratory flow rate; asthma worsened, especially when mixed with acid (sulfate) aerosols
Hydrogen sulfide Chlorine Ammonia	Industry, industrial accidents	Manufacturing; accidental release from storage; release from large deposits of organic matter	Nausea, eye irritation, respiratory irritation, decreased lung function, expecially with repeated chlorine exposure

NO_2, Nitric dioxide.

Table 8.2 *Common Indoor Air Pollutants*

POLLUTANT	SOURCES	EFFECTS
Animal dander, saliva, feces, urine	Pets, rodents	Allergic reaction, asthma attacks
Rug mites	Mite feces, body parts	Allergic reaction, asthma attacks
Bacteria, fungi, viruses	Animals and humans; outside air; molds and spores	Infections, allergic reactions, asthma attacks
Combustion products, including particulate SO_2 and NO, NO_2 CO, tobacco smoke (primary and "secondhand")	Fireplaces, gas stoves and pilot lights, outside air, cigarettes and matches, space heaters	Irritants to respiratory tract; CO competes for O_2 in hemoglobin
Formaldehyde	Insulation, plywood, particle board	Respiratory tract irritation, allergic reactions, possible respiratory cancer
Other volatile and semivolatile organic compounds (e.g., benzene, tetrachloroethylene, polychlorobiphenyls (PCBs)	Paint, dry-cleaning fluids, solvents, polishes, pesticides, electrical transformers, ceiling tiles, glues, cigarette smoke	Respiratory tract irritation, cancer
Radon	Seepage into houses from soil	Lung cancer
Asbestos	Insulation, fire proofing	Mesothelioma

SO_2, Sulfur dioxide; *NO*, nitric oxide; *NO_2*, nitric dioxide; *CO*, carbon monoxide; *O_2*, oxygen.

chewing tobacco, and snuff ("smokeless tobacco") contribute additionally to morbidity and mortality, especially to deaths from cancer of the oral cavity and upper airway and digestive tracts.

• Tobacco smoke contains numerous carcinogens including polycyclic hydrocarbons and nitrosamines, irritants including formaldehyde (possibly also a carcinogen), nitrous and nitric oxides, amines, carbon monoxide, and nicotine. Recent reports suggest that nicotine levels have been carefully controlled by the manufacturers to keep smokers addicted.

• Nicotine addiction is comparable in all respects to alcohol, heroin, and cocaine addiction, including relapse rates. Nicotine easily enters the nervous system across the blood-brain barrier and binds to receptors, most numerous in the thalamus and hypothalamus, hippocampus, cerebral cortex, and dopaminergic nuclei. There it facilitates release of acetylcholine and other neurotransmitters in the brain, sympathetic nervous system, and autonomic ganglia and potentiates increases in beta-endorphin, growth hormone, and adrenocorticotropic hormone (ACTH). Nicotine use promotes weight loss in adults and also in the unborn fetus, directly resulting in low birth-weight babies in mothers who smoke.

• Pregnant women who smoke increase the risk of fetal death, early neonatal mortality, and mortality sudden infant death syndrome (SIDS).

• Smoking-related myocardial infarction causes about 20% of deaths from heart disease; deaths from lung cancer are almost as numerous. The rate of lung cancer deaths in females is steadily approaching that of males, as female pack/year numbers increase. Chronic obstructive pulmonary disease and some cases of bladder carcinoma, myelogenous leukemia, multiple myeloma, lymphoma, and anal, penile, and vulval malignancies can be linked to smoking. "Secondhand smoke" (smoke inhaled by nonsmokers from the environment) has been shown to increase atherosclerosis and respiratory diseases.

• Smoking is statically related to increased incidence and delayed healing of peptic ulcers, granulomatous enteritis (Crohn's disease), early onset of menopause, osteoporosis, and Graves' disease.

• The adverse effects of tobacco smoking can reduced or reversed, albeit slowly, by cessation of smoking. Many positive effects begin as early as one year of total abstinence, but rates of morbidity and mortality, especially in rates of myocardial infarction and lung carcinoma, do not equal those of nonsmokers for about 20 years. Structural lung damage, (e.g., emphysema, fibrosis), however, cannot be reversed.

■ **Alcohol Abuse**

• Various estimates indicate that 10% to 33% of the population of the United States are heavy users or addicted abusers of ethyl alcohol (ETOH).

• Drinking more than 1g/kg of body weight per day of ETOH puts the drinker at risk for damage (e.g., a six-pack of 12 oz bottles of beer for a 70 kg man). The exact mechanisms by which ETOH induces damage are still debated. Malnutrition, often associated with heavy ETOH consumption is probably *not* responsible for most damaging effects of heavy consumption, except for vitamin deficiency-induced CNS disease.

• ETOH is readily absorbed through the stomach and metabolized mainly by the action of liver alcohol dehydrogenase; the resulting acetaldehyde, which itself may be toxic, is metabolized to acetate by aldehyde dehydrogenase. In this reaction, nicotinamide adenine dinucleotide (NAD) is reduced to NADH; the increased NADH/NAD ratio may underlie some forms of alcoholic organ damage.

• Hepatic microsomal P-450 oxidases acting on ETOH, also yielding acetaldehyde, is a secondary metabolic pathway.

● **Central nervous system diseases associated with ETOH usage (also see Breast chapter)**

• Acute effects—euphoria, incoordination, dizziness, headache, ataxia (depending upon blood levels and tolerance); increasing blood concentrations result in confusion, coma, and death, often from aspiration, airway obstruction and respiratory depression

- Effects of chronic ETOH use

  - Wernicke's syndrome (an acute syndrome affecting chronic drinkers with hemorrhages, neuronal loss, and gliosis of the mamillary bodies, walls of third ventricle, cerebral aqueduct, quadrigeminal plate, floor of fourth ventricle, cerebellum, thalamus)—patients show eye movement disturbances and other cranial nerve abnormalities, ataxia, depressed sensorium, and disturbed cognition; syndrome is largely caused by thiamine deficiency, reversible with prompt thiamine administration, but may be fatal if not treated.

  - Korsakoff's psychosis (atrophic, brown mamillary bodies, probably also related to thiamine deficiency—a late effect of sublethal Wernicke's syndrome) involves there is severe, permanent loss of recent memory and confabulation.

  - Cerebral cortical atrophy occurs in most heavy drinkers to some degree—with lowered brain weight, cerebral cortical neuronal loss, cerebellar atrophy, and cerebellar Purkinje cell loss, more severe in the vermis than in the lateral cerebellar hemispheres, causing ataxic gait, tremor, and incoordination.

  - Central pontine myelinolysis, a softened, demyelinated area in the central basis pontis causing spastic paralysis and quadriplegia is often fatal; not restricted to alcoholics; caused by rapid shifts in sodium (Na) concentration in the blood.

  - Marchiafava-Bignami disease, with softening and degeneration of the central portion of the corpus callosum, is possibly related to ingestion of Italian red wine containing naturally occurring cyanide.

- **Liver disease associated with alcoholism**

  - The most common complication of heavy, chronic ingestion of ETOH
  - Liver abnormalities are progressive

    - Fatty liver (which may be present after relatively little ETOH intake), with liver enlargement and softening as triglycerides accumulate within hepatocytes; reversible if ETOH ingestion stops

    - Alcoholic hepatitis occurs with increased and prolonged intake; fever, leukocytosis, liver pain, and jaundice may be present as well as fat accumulation in hepatocytes, centrilobular hepatic necrosis, accumulation of Mallory's alcoholic hyalin in liver cells, and acute and chronic (mononuclear) inflammatory cell infiltration; partial or complete regression can occur if ETOH intake is discontinued, but continued ingestion leads to development of cirrhosis

    - Alcoholic micronodular cirrhosis (Laennec's cirrhosis)—characterized by interlacing fibrous collagenous bands, distortion of hepatic architecture, and eventual shrinkage and uniform nodularity of the parenchyma; regenerating nodules usually present with increased risk of developing hepatocellular carcinoma; scarring causes increased resistance to venous blood flow through the liver, portal hypertension, esophageal varices, often resulting in fatal hemorrhage, hemorrhoids, caput medusae, jaundice, liver failure, and death

● **Alcoholic cardiomyopathy (myocardial disease in the absence of coronary artery disease)** Probably more common than any other form of cardiomyopathy (including those associated with vitamin deficiencies, viral infections or diphtheria)

  • Cardiac dilation and/or congestive heart failure results.

  • ETOH is toxic to all striated muscle; in addition to cardiomyopathy, alcoholic skeletal myopathy may also occur.

  • Moderate alcohol ingestion is associated with *increased* levels of serum high density lipoprotein (HDL) and *decreased* coronary artery disease.

  • Heavier intake of ETOH, however, damages the liver and lowers HDL, increasing the incidence of atherosclerotic coronary artery disease.

● **Pancreatic disease and ETOH**

  • Pancreatitis, acute and chronic, is common in alcoholics; alcoholism is probably the most common risk factor for pancreatitis in men.

    • The exact mechanism(s) by which alcoholism is related to the pathogenesis of pancreatitis is still undetermined. Reflux of bile into the pancreatic duct during vomiting, spasm of the sphincter of Oddi, or gallstones causing pancreatic duct obstruction have all been proposed.

    • Pancreatitis, regardless of etiologic mechanisms, is characterized by activation of pancreatic secretions within the pancreas, with lipid and protein digestion of pancreatic parenchyma, including the islets.

    • Severe abdominal pain radiating to the back, often with shock, occurs. Blood pancreatic enzymes are elevated. Mortality is high.

● **Fetal alcohol syndrome**

  • Maternal alcohol ingestion directly affects the unborn fetus, and heavy intake results in retardation of fetal growth, microcephaly, other nervous system malformations, and mental retardation of affected children. Cardiac, urologic, and skeletal defects and facial abnormalities also occur.

■ **Other Injurious Toxic Substances**

  • Injury from toxic chemicals or drugs may result from accidental exposure (e.g., industrial accidents; children who swallow paint chips, cleaning fluids, solvents, or medications in the course of play), inadvertent overdoses of therapeutic drugs, idiosyncratic drug reactions, deliberate poisoning (suicide attempts or murder), or use of illegal "recreational drugs" (intrinsically potentially dangerous, but often and unexpectedly mixed with other toxic drugs or chemicals).

● **Illicit or licit drug abuse**

  • Illicit (illegal) or legal drugs with psychoactive and addicting properties or side effects may be used inappropriately (abused) to achieve an altered mental state.

  • Addiction is the craving for, or compulsive use of a drug, despite the known potential for adverse medical, social, economic or legal consequences.

  • Physical and mental damage may stem from the long-term use of a drug or from other diseases contracted during the administration of a drug (e.g., AIDS and hepatitis acquired through shared needles).

- Social and legal consequences of drug addiction stem from the constant need of the drug, often resulting in antisocial acts (robbery, blackmail, extortion, prostitution, murder) to obtain the drug or funds to buy the drug.

  - Diacetylmorphine (heroin) is illegal in the United States but still legal in other countries for medical use. Tolerance develops with use, and ever higher doses are required to provide the "high." An acute overdose (an unusually large dose in a tolerant individual or a "normal" dose, previously tolerated, in an individual who has gone through withdrawal) frequently causes acute pulmonary edema. Other complications of use include tetanus (from contaminated material used to "cut" [dilute] concentrated drug), acquired immunodeficiency syndrome [AIDS], hepatitis, and malaria (from blood contamination of shared needles). Scarring of, and around, veins used for injection may form subcutaneous "ropes." Hepatic triaditis, lymphoid hyperplasia of the spleen, and mild-to-moderate hepatosplenomegaly are common. Granulomas may form at injection sites from fillers (starch, talc, dust balls) or filter material (cotton fibers) used to "cut" and prepare concentrated drug for street sale. Similar particles or granulomas may be found in the lungs, often polarizable in microscopic sections. Bacterial endocarditis, especially of the tricuspid valve, results from trauma to the valve induced by foreign particulates in the injected drug, contaminated with bacteria or fungi (heroin itself is also commonly contaminated, as is the "cutting" material). *Staphylococcus aureus* valvular infection is the most common, but gram-negative rods and *Aspergillus flavus* infections also occur. Heroin-associated nephropathy, a progressive nephrotic syndrome, also affects heroin addicts.

  - Cocaine is a surface anesthetic and vasoconstrictor, used legally by physicians, and a central nervous system and cardiovascular stimulant. However, cocaine is highly addicting and may cause bizarre behavior, psychoses, seizures, hypertension, cerebral vasculitis, cerebral hemorrhage, ischemic strokes, cardiovascular hyperstimulation, and arrhythmias, all potentially lethal. Use predisposes to cerebral fungal infections. In pregnant women, cocaine can cause placental abruption and spontaneous abortion, and cocaine is sometimes illegally used as a deliberate abortifactant. "Sniffing" (nasal ingestion) is probably the most common route of administration. Chronic sniffing leads to nasal septal perforations. It may also be smoked or injected intravenously, and it is readily absorbed from the gastrointestinal tract or vagina. It has caused the demise of users, smugglers, or dealers who have swallowed or hidden plastic packets of the drug internally to thwart arrest for possession, when the packets burst. "Freebase" cocaine is created by dissolving cocaine hydrochloride in alkaline water, extracting with ether, and then evaporating the ether with heat (a spoon held over a match), a dangerous procedure because of fire-explosion hazard (which nearly caused the death of the entertainer Richard Pryor). Heating cocaine HCl, dissolved in water with baking soda, precipitates the insoluble base ("crack cocaine"). Tolerance tends to *decrease* with use, predisposing to overdose.

- Amphetamines, because of cardiovascular stimulation, often mimic cocaine effects.

- Marijuana is a respiratory irritant when smoked. Use alters perceptions, especially when used with ETOH, which poses a significant driving hazard. Cannabinoids (the active ingredients) have powerful antinausea effects and would be potentially useful to control vomiting associated with cancer chemotherapy, if legal objections could be overcome.

- Numerous other hallucinogenic drugs are "on the street," including phencyclidine hydrochloride (PCP) ("angel dust"), lysergic acid diethylamide (LSD), psilocybin, and mescaline. "Designer" drugs (illegal compounds slightly altered chemically to avoid prosecution for possession of specifically prohibited substances) may have unexpected and severe side effects (e.g., a severe parkinsonian syndrome induced by the use of N-Methyl-4-phenyl-1,2,3,6-tetrahydrophridine [MPTP]).

- Therapeutic psychoactive drugs (e.g., Valium, phenobarbital, antidepressants, etc.) are commonly abused or mixed with illegal drugs to potentiate their effect, sometimes with unexpected or lethal consequences, and may also be addicting when used alone.

● Lead

- Lead slowly accumulates with continued exposure and, particularly in children, may cause irreversible damage before the cause is recognized.

- Sources of lead intoxication include lead paint in older housing, a major hazard, especially for children who find the flakes "tasty." Newsprint, contaminated soil, edibles grown in that soil, and lead plumbing in old houses are other sources of exposure. For adults, industrial exposure (lead mining, smelting, and fabricating industries, lead-acid battery manufacturing and salvaging) is the most common source. General contamination of the environment from lead compounds in gasoline, used until recently to control engine "knocking," exposes everyone (some of the compounds now used instead of lead may be even more toxic, especially for children).

- Lead is absorbed through the gastrointestinal tract or lungs, posing a risk for electronics workers and stained-glass artisans because of inhalation of hot gasses during soldering (solder usually contains lead and tin). Deficiencies of normal dietary metals (iron, zinc, calcium) facilitates absorption.

- In children, most of the absorbed lead accumulates in the bones and teeth, about 10% remains in the blood, and a small fraction remains in the soft tissues transiently. The bony deposits remain until the bone salts are recycled, a slow process that keeps blood levels of lead high for extended periods.

- Blood, nervous system, gastrointestinal tract, and kidneys are the principle sites of lead action, usually through the denaturing of proteins and interference with enzymes by binding to sulfhydryl groups.

- In the blood, lead interferes with iron binding to the hemoglobin molecule, zinc protoporphyrin being formed instead; basophilic stippling of red blood cells is characteristic, and a hypochromic, microcytic, or hemolytic anemia is common.

- Central nervous system damage, particularly in children, may be severe, with death of neurons in the cerebral hemispheres and cerebellum, demyelination, gliosis, and edema. In mild poisoning, only mild-to-moderate cognitive dysfunction may be present. In adults, the peripheral nervous system is preferentially involved. A demyelinating motor neuropathy, particularly of the nerves supplying the extensors of the wrist and foot, results in wrist or foot "drop."

• Abdominal pain and rigidity of the abdomen from muscle spasm ("lead colic") occurs in adults and may be mistaken for a surgically correctable condition. A dark "lead line" of precipitated lead sulfide may be present along the gingival margin.

• Chronic renal interstitial tubulonephritis is less common than other manifestations of lead poisoning but eventually leads to decreased glomerular filtration rate and renal failure. Uric acid excretion falls ("saturnine gout").

● **Mercury**

• Most contamination is natural, from the earth's crust. However, significant additional contamination of the environment has occurred through the activities of man, via industry, mining, burning of coal and oil, incinerators, mercury compounds in germicides and pesticides, and through improper disposal of batteries.

• Elemental mercury vapor is toxic, travels through the air for great distances, contributes to acid rain, and contaminates ground water. Thus plants, including some grains, and fish become contaminated, poisoning the food chain.

• All forms of mercury (elemental, inorganic, and organic compounds) are toxic.

• Metallic mercury damages the gastrointestinal system, cardiovascular, hepatic and hematopoietic systems, and the unborn fetus. Mercury and inorganic mercury compounds from gastrointestinal ingestion are particularly toxic to kidneys (membranous glomerulonephritis, proteinuria, proximal renal tubular necrosis). Chronic inhalation of mercury in gaseous form and ingested organic mercurial compounds damage the nervous system (tremors, memory loss, blindness, and spasticity, caused by neuronal loss, gliosis, cerebral and cerebellar atrophy, and peripheral nerve damage). Mercurial compounds used in the hat industry were responsible for the bizarre behavior of the "mad hatter" in *Alice in Wonderland.* Organic mercurial salts, especially the most toxic methyl mercury, in contaminated sea water, are absorbed and concentrated by fish and, when the fish are eaten, cause severe paralysis, spasticity, and death. An enormous tragedy with much morbidity and loss of life occurred in Japan via industrial dumping of methyl mercury-contaminated waste (Minamata Bay disease); cerebellar destruction with severe loss of internal granular neurons was characteristic.

● **Arsenic**

• Industrial poisoning is most commonly related to herbicide, pesticide, and fertilizer (phosphate fertilizers are often contaminated with arsenicals) manufacturing and use, and in workers and nearby residents of smelting industries.

• Trivalent arsenicals are known pulmonary and skin carcinogens.

● **Cyanide**

• Cyanide is often present in smoke, especially in the burning of silk, wool, and some plastics.

• Cyanide inhibits cellular respiration by binding to cytochrome oxidase and causes severe anoxic injury to the brain, liver, kidney.

■ Reactions to Legal and Therapeutic Drugs

• Any legal, prescription, or over-the-counter drug, in overdose or misuse, may cause damage to tissues or organs or even death. However, numerous unusual, unwanted, damaging, or lethal reactions may occur when drugs are used for their intended purposes in normal doses. These range from tinnitus (e.g., aspirin) to anaphylaxis (e.g., penicillin).

• Some drugs (e.g., thalidomide) cause severe birth defects if taken during pregnancy.

• Some drugs (e.g., estrogens) have associations with cancer of the breast or endometrium.

■ Physical Injury

• Tissue damage results from mechanical forces, abnormal temperatures, or abnormal atmospheric pressure or electromagnetic radiation.

• Mechanical forces may produce scrapes (abrasions), tears (lacerations), cuts (incisions), bruises (contusions), hemorrhages, fractures (including compound fractures where the bone ends or fragments lacerate tissues), crush injuries, or unconsciousness, or temporary or permanent amnesia without detectable structural damage (concussion).

• Localized, highly elevated temperature produces tissue damage (usually cutaneous burns). The seriousness of these burns depends upon the extent of body surface damaged and depth of the burn. Shock, hypovolemia, plasma protein loss, secondary infection, and gastrointestinal ulceration and bleeding from stress complicate recovery. Excessive heat may also damage internal structures or organs, and associated noxious fumes (carbon monoxide, sulfur dioxide, and many other noxious gasses) may cause additional damage.

• Heat stroke (with physical effort—"exertional heat stroke") usually features a cessation of sweating and dry skin. Respiratory alkalosis occurs because of hyperventilation. Dilation of skin vessels sometimes causes low blood pressure, decreased cerebral blood flow, fainting, or unconsciousness.

• Hypothermia may be generalized or localized. Generalized hypothermia slows body processes, including brain functions, and may cause death without necrosis of tissues. Slowing of the metabolic rate, however, may permit resuscitation after prolonged exposure. Localized chilling or freezing causes freezing with ice crystal formation in intracellular and extracellular body fluids, increasing electrolyte concentrations and causing death of cells. Vascular constriction during slowly developing localized hyperthermia is associated with increased vascular permeability and edema. Rapid, localized cooling, when prolonged, causes vasoconstriction and anoxic-ischemic injury; if warming then occurs, increased blood flow in cold-damaged blood vessels causes edema.

• Caisson disease ("the bends") affects divers and workers in tunnels exposed to long periods of increased atmospheric pressure. During decompression, excess gases (oxygen, nitrogen, and, if used, helium) dissolved in the blood are released forming bubbles, and gaseous emboli cause respiratory difficulty, chest pain, and joint pain (which gives the condition its name). Emboli occluding small osseous blood vessels may cause delayed necrosis. Recompression and very slow decompression is the treatment of choice.

• Gaseous emboli may form during hyperbaric oxygen therapy, scuba diving and positive-pressure ventilation. Increased intraalveolar pressure tears alveolar walls, with the air or oxygen gaining access to blood vessels and dissecting through tissue planes. Gas in blood vessels impedes blood flow, causes ischemic changes in brain and heart, and may cause sudden death. Gaseous emboli may also be introduced during intravenous administration of fluids, if the drip chamber is not full, and foam, forming in the heart, restricts blood inflow and outflow.

- Electrical currents passing through the body may cause localized surface or internal heating with destruction of tissue or may disrupt the electrical regulation of brain and heart. Heating increases with electrical resistance, causing localized burning of tissues (e.g., an electrical current passing through dry skin). However, current easily passes through wet tissues (e.g., electrocution while emersed in a bath), disrupting cardiac and neural electrical regulation, often with death, but without burning tissues. The electrodes used in execution by an electric chair are kept moistened with saline-soaked sponges. Survivors of lightning strikes often exhibit bizarre psychiatric disturbances which may be permanent, presumably from electrical changes within the brain.

■ Radiation Injury

- The electromagnetic radio spectrum—wave propagated energy including electrical and radio waves, infrared, visible and ultraviolet light, microwaves, x-rays, cosmic rays, and gamma radiation; all of these are suspected or proven causes of biologic change.

- Electrons (beta particles), alpha particles, protons, deuterons, mesons, and neutrons are particles with specific mass, size, and charge that are emitted by radioactive materials and constitute *particulate radiation.*

  - Ionizing radiation—when electromagnetic or particulate radiation of sufficient energy hits a biologic target, it displaces electrons orbiting around nuclei (producing ions).

● **Target effect** Energy directly hitting atoms, proteins, membranes, or enzymes (DNA is the most vulnerable target) within a cell causes structural changes; single- or double-stranded breaks of chromosomal DNA, if not promptly repaired, result in DNA mutations impairing DNA function.

● **Indirect effect** Radiation may produce intracellular free radials (especially from ionization of cellular water) that react with other cellular atoms and molecules, including DNA, producing alterations with potentially serious consequences.

  - Although ionization occurs instantaneously, the observed effects occur after a *latent period;* tumor formation or mutations may only become apparent years later.

  - If the dose of radiation is low, and the cells have the necessary repair mechanisms, recovery can occur.

● **With increasing doses of radiation, progressively more severe damage occurs**

  - Cell swelling and nuclear chromatin damage occur after low dosage radiation; both are reversible.

  - With higher doses, cell swelling, pyknosis or fragmentation of nuclei, cell disruption, and cell death occur.

  - Other disturbances, including inhibition of cellular mitotic division, particularly in actively dividing cells, lead to cell death; nuclear division without cytoplasmic division results in the formation of multinucleated giant cells.

• Chromosomal translocations and deletions occur from DNA alterations.

• Repeated exposure to radiation causes cumulative damage, if repair is incomplete between doses.

• Cells may also become radiation resistant during repeated exposure to low-dosage radiation.

● **The effects of ionizing radiation depend upon**

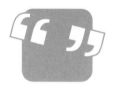

• The type of radiation, the time period over which the radiation occurs, and the total dose

• *Linear energy transfer (LET)*—a measure of energy loss per unit of distance travelled and a function of the velocity, mass, and charge of the radiation; it therefore indicates the probability of the radiation effect in a given area. High mass-low velocity particles (e.g., alpha particles) expend their energy within a short distance of travel and have a high *LET* value; high velocity-low mass radiation (e.g., gamma rays) penetrate deeply, but because of their low mass, strike fewer targets along their path and have a low *LET* value

• *Relative biologic effectiveness (RBE)*—a measure of the ability (effectiveness) of different forms of radiation to produce a biologic effect

   • Different types of cells have different sensitivities to ionizing radiation. Lymphoid, hematopoietic, and germ (gonadal) cells are the most sensitive. Gastrointestinal mucosal cells, endothelial cells, and hair follicles are moderately sensitive. Glandular epithelium, especially of pancreas and breast, bladder epithelium, brain, and growing bone and cartilage are less sensitive or exhibit delayed effects. Mature bone and cartilage, muscles, and peripheral nerves have low radiation sensitivity.

   • Sensitivity of cells depends upon their *mitotic* rate (rapidly dividing cell populations are sensitive; hence the effectiveness of radiation on cancer), *phase of the cell cycle at the time of radiation* (cells are most sensitive during G_2 [immediately prior to mitosis] and during mitosis, less sensitive during G_1, and the least sensitive during S phase), *the ability of the cells to repair radiation damage* (e.g., in xeroderma pigmentosum, inability to repair sunlight-induced DNA damage results in a high rate of skin malignancies), and *the degree of local oxygenation* (the greater the amount of available oxygen, the greater the local formation of damaging free radicals). Poorly vascularized tissues are therefore less sensitive to radiation damage than highly vascularized tissues.

● **Cellular, tissue, and organ alterations induced by radiation**

• To a greater or lesser extent, all cells are vulnerable to radiation. For a given dose of radiation, not all cells of the same type in the irradiated area react equally.

• The nucleus is the principle target (pyknosis, karyorrhexis, karyolysis, abnormal mitoses, abnormal nuclear morphology).

• Cytoplasmic changes also occur (swelling, mitochondrial abnormalities, endoplasmic reticulum disruption, cell membrane breaks).

- Vascular changes are common, especially at high radiation doses (dilation, swelling of vascular endothelium, thromboses, hemorrhage).

- Skin changes occur with externally delivered radiation and partially depend upon the area of skin exposed, dose, and type of radiation (erythema, edema, blistering, desquamation, chronic dermatitis, hyperpigmentation or depigmentation, loss of hair, ulceration, fibrosis, cancer, vascular damage in the underlying dermis).

- Lymphoid tissues and hematopoietic cells are extremely sensitive, changes often appearing within hours (lymphopenia, shrinkage of lymph nodes and spleen). If the patient survives, still-viable stem cells restore the lymphocyte population within a few weeks or months. The granulocyte population falls more slowly (during the first and second weeks after high-dose exposure) partly because a supply of mature, radiation-resistant granulocytes is always held in reserve within the marrow and gradually released, even if stem cells are rapidly destroyed. Granulocytes may be restored within a few months. The platelet population falls even more slowly, and restoration is also more delayed. Red cell precursors are radiation sensitive, but mature red cells are not. Destruction of erythrocyte precursors results in anemia.

- Radiation also increases the incidence of leukemia.

- Germinal epithelium and germ cells are radiation sensitive; sterility results. Mature sperm cells are relatively resistant, as are the body of the uterus and cervix. Local implantation of radioactive pellets may therefore be used for the treatment of cervical and endometrial carcinoma.

- The lungs are sensitive to radiation damage. Acute radiation change causes increased vascular permeability, with congestion, pulmonary edema, protein (including fibrin) exudation into the alveolar air spaces and hyaline membrane formation, restricting oxygen interchange across alveolar walls. Vascular and alveolar wall fibrosis occur later with alveolar obliteration ("radiation pneumonitis"). Inhalation of radioactive dust by miners or radon contamination of housing may be involed in the pathogenesis of bronchogenic carcinogenesis.

- Radiation affects the midgastrointestinal tract, particularly the small intestines and colon (esophagus and rectum are relatively resistant). Epithelium, especially the crypt cells with their rapid turnover rate, are most affected and show mitotic abnormalities and cellular pleomorphism and necrosis. Clinically, victims develop nausea, vomiting, and diarrhea, often bloody. Vascular thickening, submucosal atrophy, gut wall fibrosis, and strictures follow.

- The central nervous system of the embryo and fetus is radiosensitive; the adult central nervous system is amazingly radioresistant. Vascular changes, however, induce secondary changes (ischemia, necrosis, demyelination, gliosis).

- **Whole body radiation** Even relatively low doses (100 to 1000 rad) induces acute radiation syndrome (acute nausea, vomiting, and diarrhea, with destruction of gastrointestinal mucosa, hematopoietic cell destruction, pancytopenia, anemia and death); symptoms and signs become progressively more severe with increasing radiation dose, as does mortality.

- **Late effects of radiation** Reports include increased rate of still-births, fetal anomalies and mutations with in utero radiation, and congenital anomalies, mental retardation, and the early development of cancer in children and young adults, but definitive epidemiologic confirmation is lacking, in spite of careful study of atom bomb victims in Japan. Radiation to shrink tonsils and adenoids in children (an old form of therapy) is associated with increased risk of development of thyroid carcinoma during adulthood. Also controversial are reports of increased rates of cancer in people residing near high tension lines or users of portable and cellular telephones and in amateur radio operators. Increased risk of fetal anomalies and stillbirths has also been reported with the use of electric blankets or waterbeds with electric heaters during pregnancy (low-frequency electromagnetic radiation).

MULTIPLE CHOICE
REVIEW QUESTIONS

1. An obese child with severe nutritional protein deficiency probably has which of the following?

    a. Marasmus
    b. Lead poisoning
    c. Kwashiorkor
    d. Fetal alcohol syndrome
    e. Rickets

2. Non-enriched white bread, polished white rice, and refined white sugar are extremely deficient in which vitamin?

    a. A
    b. B_1
    c. C
    d. D
    e. E

3. Isoniazid therapy for tuberculosis should be accompanied by which of the following supplements?

    a. Vitamin A
    b. Thiamin
    c. Pyridoxine
    d. Ascorbic acid
    e. Niacin

4. Further depletion of the ozone layer in the upper atmosphere may lead to which of the following?

    a. A general increase in earth surface temperature
    b. Destruction of microscopic sea creatures (phytoplankton) important in the food chain
    c. An increased rate of lung cancer
    d. Further destruction of rain forest areas
    e. An increase in chlorofluorocarbon compounds in the atmosphere

5. Consequences of alcohol abuse include all *except* which of the following?

    a. Wernicke's encephalopathy
    b. Posterolateral degeneration of the spinal cord (subacute combined degeneration)
    c. Central pontine myelinolysis
    d. Marchiafava-Bignami syndrome
    e. Korsakoff's psychosis

Chapter 9

Diseases of Childhood

OVERVIEW

■ **Different Age Groups with Different Diseases and Risks of Mortality**

- Highest mortality in first year of life—700-1000/100,000

  - Perinatal conditions (low birthweight, respiratory distress syndrome, intrauterine hypoxia/birth asphyxia, birth trauma) most important
  - Congenital anomalies
  - Sudden infant death syndrome

- Ages one to four—40/100,000
- Ages four to fifteen—18/100,000
- Injuries—most common cause of death in children greater than 1 year

■ **Birth Weight and Gestational Age**

● Classification

- Appropriate for gestational age (AGA; 10th to 90th percentile), large for gestational age (LGA), small for gestational age (SGA)
- Term (thirty-eighth to forty-first week), postterm, preterm
- Increased risk of mortality in low-birth-weight infants

● Intrauterine growth retardation (IUGR)

- At least ⅓ of infants born less than 2500 g are term
- Causes—fetal, placental, or maternal factors (most common)
- Growth retardation can be symmetric (proportionate; type I) or asymmetric (disproportionate; type II) with relative sparing of brain
- Fetal factors

  - Chromosomal abnormalities (trisomies 21, 13, 18; XO; triploidy)
  - Congenital anomalies
  - Infections
  - Results in symmetric growth retardation

- Placental factors

  - Placental lesions (infarction, infection, abruption, placenta previa)
  - Multiple gestation
  - Confined placental mosaicism (mutation occurring in dividing trophoblast or inner cell mass, therefore affecting placenta only)
  - Results in asymmetric growth retardation

- Maternal factors

  - Toxemia

- Chronic hypertension
- Alcohol and narcotics
- Heavy cigarette smoking
- Therapeutic drugs (dilantin, antimetabolites)

● **Prematurity**

— *Immature organ systems can be direct cause of death in early preterm infants and affect survival of late preterm ones*

— *Lung*

- Alveolar differentiation does not begin until about seventh month of gestation and is not complete until midchildhood
- The less mature the lung, the more impaired the gas exchange

Morphology of immature lung

- Grossly unexpanded
- Incomplete alveolar expansion
- Amniotic material (squames, lanugo hairs, mucous) within alveoli indicates respiratory distress

Other organs

- Kidneys

  - Incomplete glomerular development
  - Renal function usually adequate to maintain viability

- Brain

  - Smooth surface caused by delayed development of convolutions
  - Poor myelination
  - Vital brain centers developed enough to maintain viability, but some functions impaired (temperature regulation, vasomotor control, respiratory rate, muscle activity)

● **Apgar score**

- Measured at 1 or 5 minutes
- Evaluates heart rate, respiratory effort, muscle tone, response to nasal catheter, color—each on scale of 0 (worst) to 2 (best)
- Correlates with survival at 28 days, not long-term neurologic prognosis

● **Birth Injuries**

— *LGA infants at greatest risk*

— *Most common*

- Fractures (clavicle, humerus)
- Facial nerve or brachial plexus injuries
- Intracranial

— *Morbidity—immediate (fractures) or delayed (nervous system injuries)*

— *Intracranial hemorrhage—most common serious injury*

Predisposing factors

- Prolonged labor
- Hypoxia

- Bleeding disorders
- Vascular anomalies

Consequences

- Disruption of brain substance
- Increased intracranial pressure
    - Can cause herniation of medulla through foramen magnum with respiratory depression

CONGENITAL ANOMALIES

■ Morphologic Abnormalities

- Some present at birth
- Some not apparent until later

● **Functionally or cosmetically significant ones present in estimated 3% of live births**

- Most frequent congenital anomalies in the United States
    - Hypospadias (urethral orifice on ventral side of penis)—0.28%
    - Clubfoot—0.25%
    - Ventricular septal defect—0.15%

● Definitions

— *Malformations*

- Intrinsic abnormalities occurring during development
- Can involve one or several organs

— *Deformations*

- Mechanical alteration in form usually arising in late fetal life
- Usually caused by fetal growth outpacing uterine growth in late gestation
- Contributory factors
    - Maternal (first pregnancy, small uterus, bicornuate uterus, leiomyomas)
    - Fetal-placental (oligohydramnios, multiple fetuses, abnormal fetal presentation)
    - Common example: clubfoot

— *Disruptions*

- Destruction or interference with originally normal body part or region
    - Acquired
    - Example: amniotic band

— *Sequence*

- Single anomaly affects multiple organs
- Example: oligohydramnios (Potter's sequence)
    - Causes of oligohydramnios—rupture of amnion, placental insufficiency, renal agenesis
    - Oligohydramnios leads to fetal compression

- Flattened face, deformed hands and feet, chest compression with lung hypoplasia

— *Syndrome*

- Several apparently pathogenically related defects not explained by a single initiating anomaly

— *Agenesis*

- Complete absence of organ and its primordium

— *Aplasia*

- Absence of organ caused by failure of anlage to development

— *Hypoplasia*

- Underdevelopment of an organ

— *Atresia*

- Absence of opening of a hollow organ, such as the intestine

● **Causes of malformations**

— *Genetic—30% to 50%*

- Chromosomal abnormalities—10% to 15%

- Most common—Down syndrome
- Most not familial

- Single gene inheritance—2% to 10%
- Multifactoral inheritance—20% to 25%

— *Environmental—10% to 15%*

- Maternal or placental infections—2% to 3%

- Rubella before 16 weeks causes cataracts, heart defects, deafness
- Cytomegalovirus—second trimester infection affects central nervous system (retardation, microcephaly, deafness)
- Herpes simplex

- Maternal diseases—6% to 8%
- Drugs and chemicals—1%
- Radiation—1%

— *Unknown—40% to 60%*

● **Pathogenesis**

— *Effects of timing of injury*

- Early embryonic period (weeks 1 to 2)

- Zygote division, implantation
- Little susceptibility to teratogens
- Injury followed by death or recovery

- Later embryonic period (weeks 3 to 9)

- Formation of organs
- High susceptibility to teratogens
- Major organ malformations

- Fetal period (after week 9)

  - Growth and maturation of organs
  - Low susceptibility
  - Growth retardation, minor organ malformations

PERINATAL INFECTIONS

■ Routes of Infection

- ● Transcervical infection

  - Most bacteria, a few viruses (e.g., herpes simplex type 2)
  - Aspiration of infected amniotic fluid usually shortly before or at birth
  - Mechanisms

    - Premature rupture of membranes caused by inflammation
    - Premature labor caused by prostaglandins from inflammatory cells or microorganisms

  - Morphology of placenta

    - Chorioamnionitis—inflammation of fetal membranes
    - Funisitis—inflammation of umbilical cord

  - Fetal manifestations

    - Pneumonia, sepsis, meningitis

- ● Transplacental infections

  - Most parasites, most viruses, a few bacteria *(Listeria)*
  - During gestation or, less commonly, during delivery
  - Placenta shows villitis (inflammation of villi)

- ● TORCH infections (*t*oxoplasmosis, *o*ther agents, *r*ubella, *c*ytomegalovirus, *h*erpes simplex)

  - — *Similar signs and symptoms from infection with one of several organisms*

    - Occur in 1% to 5% of liveborn infants in United States

  - — *Toxoplasma*

    - 25% of women of childbearing age asymptomatically infected
    - Intrauterine infection in less than 0.1% of pregnancies

  - — *Other*

    - Syphilis

      - Results from infection of mother during pregnancy
      - About ⅓ cases result in intrauterine death
      - Congenital syphilis in about 0.05% liveborns

    - Tuberculosis
    - *Listeria*
    - *Leptospira*
    - Epstein-Barr virus

- Human immunodeficiency virus
- Parvovirus B19
- Varicella-zoster virus

— *Rubella*

- Extremely rare in United States because of vaccination

— *Cytomegalovirus*

- About 65% of women of childbearing age infected
- About 2% of newborns congenitally infected (most common fetal viral syndrome)

— *Herpes simplex*

- Infection usually occurs during birth to actively infected mother

  - Transmission to newborn avoided by cesarean section

— *Manifestations of TORCH infections*

- General—fever, prematurity, SGA
- Central nervous system

  - Microcephaly
  - Hydrocephalus
  - Encephalitis

- Eyes

  - Visual impairment
  - Chorioretinitis

- Hepatosplenomegaly
- Hemolytic anemia
- Pneumonitis
- Myocarditis

DISORDERS OF THE PREMATURE INFANT

■ Respiratory Distress Syndrome of the Newborn (Hyaline Membrane Disease)

- ● Etiologic factors

  - Prematurity most important

    - Less than 28 weeks, greater than 50% risk
    - 32 to 36 weeks, 20% risk
    - After 36 weeks, risk less than 5%

  - Other factors

    - Maternal diabetes mellitus
    - Delivery by cesarean section
    - Neonatal asphyxia
    - Twin pregnancies

- **Pathogenesis**
  - *Fundamental defect—surfactant deficient in amount and quality*
  - *Surfactant synthesis*

    Synthesized by type II pneumocytes, which become maximally active after 35 weeks' gestation

    Consists of
    - 90% lipids
      - Dipalmitoyl phophatidylcholine (lecithin) predominant
      - Amniotic fluid lecithin:sphingomyelin ratio less than 2:1 indicates fetal lung immaturity and risk of respiratory distress
    - Surfactant proteins

    Synthesis stimulated by corticosteroids, inhibited by insulin
  - *Reduced alveolar surfactant → atalectasis → under ventilation of collapsed areas → reduced oxygen and acidosis → damaged type II pneumocytes → further reduction in surfactant and hyaline membrane formation*

- **Morphology**
  - Gross—dark red and airless
  - Collapsed alveoli, dilated alveolar ducts and respiratory bronchioles
  - Hyaline membranes line alveolar ducts
    - Amorphous eosinophilic material
    - Composed of fibrin and debris from necrotic epithelium

- **Clinical features**
  - Increased inspiratory effort and respiratory rate within an hour of birth followed by cyanosis
  - Severe cases unresponsive to oxygen therapy
  - Mortality 30% (50% in infants under 30 weeks)
  - Infants survive 4 days—tend to recover

- ■ **Other Pulmonary Complications**
  - **Pulmonary interstitial emphysema**
    - Develops in 30% of infants born under 1500 g who have respiratory distress syndrome
    - Caused by barotrauma in immature airways
  - **Massive pulmonary hemorrhage**
  - **Bronchopulmonary dysplasia**
    - Continuing requirement for mechanical ventilation and oxygen therapy in patient with respiratory distress syndrome for more than 1 month after birth
    - Pathogenic factors—prematurity (40% incidence in infants less than 1000 g), mechanical ventilation, oxygen toxicity
    - In those dying of respiratory distress syndrome, histologic manifestations of bronchopulmonary dysplasia seen after about 1 month
    - Cardiovascular and pulmonary manifestations (Table 9.1)

Table 9.1 *Pathologic Changes in Bronchopulmonary Dysplasia*

STAGE	PULMONARY FINDINGS	CARDIAC FINDINGS

Exudative, and early reparative (1 to 2 weeks)	Hyaline membranes
	  Bronchial necrosis
	  Bronchiolitis obliterans
	  Bronchiolectasis
	Early septal fibrosis
	Mucosal dysplasia and necrosis of trachea and bronchi
	Interstitial edema, with or without emphysema
		Patent ductus arteriosus

Subacute, fibroproliferative	Bronchiolitis obliterans Bronchiolectasis	
Chronic fibroproliferative (months)	Gross appearance like cobblestones Interstitial fibrosis Smooth muscle proliferation Honeycomb lung Vascular wall thickening No bronchiolitis obliterans or bronchiolectasis Mucosal metaplasia, trachea, bronchi, bronchioles Muscular hyperplasia, trachea, bronchi	With or without left ventricular hypertrophy With or without cor pulmonale
Longstanding "healed" (months to years)	Alveolar septal fibrosis Pulmonary vascular hypertensive changes, low grade Pleural fibrosis	Biventricular hypertrophy with or without myocardial or endocardial fibrosis

Based on Stocker JT, Dehner LP: Acquired pulmonary disease in the pediatric age group. In Dail DH, Hammer SP, editors: *Pulmonary pathology,* New York, 1987, Springer-Verlag.

■ Cardiovascular Manifestations

- Patent ductus arteriosus

  - Remains patent after normal time of closure (4 days)
  - Occurs in one third
  - Recovery from lung disease—lowers pulmonary pressure, causing persistent left-to-right shunt

- Persistent pulmonary hypertension of the newborn (persistent fetal circulation)

  - Continued high pulmonary vascular resistance with impaired gas exchange

■ Central Nervous System Manifestations

- Kernicterus

  - Grossly visible yellow staining with histologic damage of specific nuclei caused by hyperbilirubinemia

- Germinal matrix and intraventricular hemorrhage

  - Occurs in 30% born before 35 weeks and up to 70% less than 1000 g
  - Rupture of thin-walled veins in periventricular matrix
  - Sometimes ruptues into ventricles

- Periventricular leukomalacia

  - Often coexists with intraventricular hemorrhage
  - Necrosis and gliosis in subependymal white matter

■ Necrotizing Enterocolitis

- Results from ischemia, bacterial colonization, excess protein in lumen

  - Primarily affects terminal ileum and ascending colon, but can be more extensive
  - Hemorrhage, inflammation and necrosis confined to mucosa or extending through wall, in more severe cases

- Clinical features—abdominal distension, ileus, diarrhea, possible perforation with sepsis

SUDDEN INFANT DEATH SYNDROME (SIDS)

■ Definition

- Sudden death of infant not expected from history and not explained by a thorough autopsy

■ Epidemiology and Etiology

- Incidence—2/1000 live births
- Most occur within first 6 months of life
- Usually occurs at night or while sleeping
- Maternal risk factors

  - Low socioeconomic status
  - First pregnancy before age 20 years
  - Cigarette smoking during pregnancy
  - Use of drugs during pregnancy

- Infant risk factors

  - Low birth weight
  - Prematurity
  - Sibling of SIDS victim
  - Prone sleeping position
  - Illness (usually gastrointestinal) in preceding 2 weeks

TUMORS

■ Sometimes Difficult to Distinguish True Neoplasms from Nonneoplastic Masses

- Heterotopia (choriostroma)

  - Microscopically normal cells or tissue in abnormal site

- Hamartoma

  - Growth composed of mature elements native to organ in which it is found but not showing the normal architecture of the organ

■ Benign Neoplasms and Neoplastic-like Conditions

- ● Hemangioma
  - Authorities disagree whether they are true neoplasms or hamartomas
  - Most often located in skin, especially on face and scalp
  - Irregular, blue-red mass that can be flat or elevated
  - Can enlarge with growth of child or spontaneously regress
  - Rarely, manifestation of von Hippel-Lindau disease

- ● Teratoma
  - — *Two incidence peaks*
    - About age two
    - Late childhood-early adulthood
  - — *Sacrococcygeal teratomas*
    - Most teratomas in infants and young children
    - Found in 1/20,000 live births
    - About 10% associated with congenital anomalies
    - About 75% histologically mature and have benign course
    - About 12% clearly malignant (e.g., containing endodermal sinus elements) with lethal course
    - About 12% have some immature elements
      - Malignant potential correlates with amount of immature elements

■ Malignant Neoplasms

- ● Differences between childhood and adult malignancies
  - Much less common in children than in adults
  - Adults and children—generally different types of malignancies
  - Pediatric malignancies often closely related to developmental abnormalities
  - Neonatal neoplasms sometimes regress spontaneously

- ● Acute leukemia causes majority of cancer deaths in pediatric age group
  - Most are acute lymphoblastic leukemia

- ● Small, round, blue-cell tumors of childhood
  - Solid tumors that can be confused histologically
  - Includes
    - Lymphoma (see White Blood Cell Diseases chapter)
    - Neuroblastoma (see Endocrine Diseases chapter)
    - Retinoblastoma (see Eye chapter)
    - Rhabdomyosarcoma (see Bone, Joint, and Soft Tissue Disorders chapter)
    - Ewing's tumor (see Bone, Joint, and Soft Tissue Disorders chapter)
    - Wilms' tumor (see Kidney and Urinary Tract chapter)

Multiple Choice Review Questions

1. The greatest vulnerability to agents causing major organ malformations occurs during which of the following?

   a. Weeks 1-2 of gestation
   b. Weeks 3-9 of gestation
   c. Weeks 10-20 of gestation
   d. Weeks 21-36 of gestation
   e. After week 36 of gestation

2. Increasing levels of which of the following are responsible for increased synthesis of surfactant beginning at about the eighth month of gestation?

   a. Aldosterone
   b. Chorionic gonadotropin
   c. Cortisol
   d. Insulin
   e. Somatostatin

3. Bronchopulmonary dysplasia and necrotizing enterocolitis are most likely to be seen in a patient with which of the following diseases?

   a. Cystic fibrosis
   b. Down syndrome
   c. Infant respiratory distress syndrome (hyaline membrane disease)
   d. Renal agenesis
   e. Sudden infant death syndrome (SIDS)

Chapter 10
Amyloidosis

■ **Overview**

● Amyloidosis—a heterogeneous group of diseases characterized by deposition of amyloid in various tissues and organs

● Amyloid—an abnormal, insoluble material composed primarily of protein fibrils derived from normal, soluble proteins

• Chemical composition of the amyloid fibrils—varies among different clinical forms of amyloidosis

• Other components of amyloid

• P component

• Proteoglycans

● Amyloidosis—can be systemic or localized to one organ or tissue

• Localized mass of amyloid—amyloid tumor (amyloidoma)

■ **Morphology and Physical Nature**

● Diagnosis depends upon recognition in tissue

● Amorphous, eosinophilic, extracellular material (Fig. 10.1)

• Sometimes associated with pressure atrophy of adjacent cells

● Distinctive histochemical properties that aid in identification of amyloid

• Metachromatic

• Certain dyes (e.g., crystal violet) will turn amyloid purple in tissue sections.

• Congophilic

• In tissue sections stained with Congo red amyloid will turn pink (Fig. 10.2, A).

• When viewed with a polarizing microscope amyloid in Congo red-stained sections has green birefringence (Fig. 10.2, B).

● Ultrastructure

• Composed of nonbranching fibrils of indefinite length and width of 7.5 to 10 nm (Fig. 10.3)

• Can form aggregates, bundles, or meshwork

• Extracted amyloid—pentagonal structures, called the P component

● X-ray crystallography

• Shows that amyloid fibrils have a cross β-pleated sheet structure responsible for the various morphologic properties described above

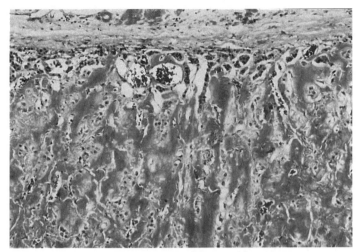

Fig. 10.1 Histology of amyloid in adrenal cortex. Note the amorphous material replacing most of the cortex, except for some compressed cortical cells under the capsule. (*Damjanov I, Linder J:* Anderson's pathology, *ed 10, vol 1, St Louis, 1996, Mosby.*)

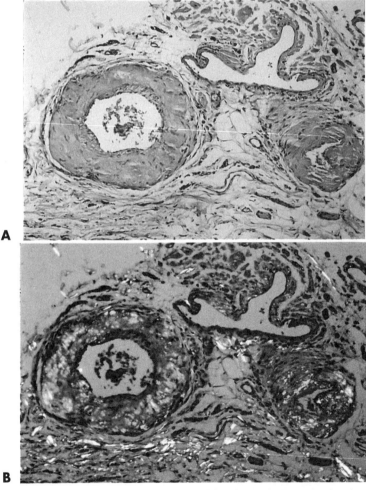

Fig. 10.2 Histology of amyloid in a blood vessel, Congo red stain. **A,** Note the amorphous material in the vessel wall. **B,** Note the birefringence in the same section viewed with polarized light. (*Damjanov I, Linder J:* Anderson's pathology, *ed 10, vol 1, St Louis, 1996, Mosby.*)

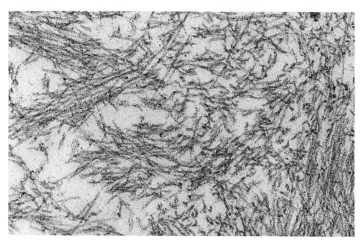

Fig. 10.3 Ultrastructure of amyloid. Note the fibrils with the characteristic 7 to 10 nm diameter of nonbranching structure and occasional parallel bundles. (*Damjanov I, Linder J:* Anderson's pathology, *ed 10, vol 1, St Louis, 1996, Mosby.*)

■ Amyloid P Component

- Makes up about 15% of the mass of amyloid deposits
- Composed of glycoprotein AP, which is identical to plasma protein SAP
- Found in all forms of amyloid
- Bound to amyloid fibrils in a calcium-dependent fashion
- Might protect the amyloid fibrils from proteolysis, contributing to persistence of amyloid

■ Chemical Nature of Amyloid Fibril Proteins

● Amyloid fibril proteins

- Vary among different clinical forms of amyloidosis
- Classification of amyloidosis based on the chemical nature of the amyloid fibrils

● AL

- Derived from immunoglobulin light chains or their amino terminal fragments
  - Probably specific amino acid sequences within some light chains make them liable to be deposited in the tissue as amyloid fibrils
- Source of light chain   paraprotein
  - Abnormal monoclonal immunoglobulin or free light chain
  - Almost all patients with AL amyloid have paraprotein detectable in serum or urine or both
  - Only a minority of persons with paraprotein develop amyloidosis
  - Seen in persons with multiple myeloma or benign monoclonal gammopathy

- **AA**
  - Derived from amino terminus of plasma protein serum amyloid A (SAA)
    - Synthesized by hepatocytes
    - Circulates associated with high-density lipoprotein (HDL_3)
    - Concentration—increases markedly as a consequence of injury or inflammation (i.e., is an acute phase reactant)
  - Fibril in secondary (reactive) amyloidosis and familial Mediterranean fever

- **ATTR**
  - Derived from the plasma protein transthyretin (TTR; also called pre-albumin)
    - Synthesized by hepatocytes
    - Binds thyroxine and retinol binding protein, carrier for vitamin A
    - Concentration—decreases with injury or inflammation (negative acute phase reactant)
  - 30 different amino acid substitutions in TTR that can cause familial amyloidosis
    - Most typical clinical manifestation is polyneuropathy, sometimes associated with other neurologic disorders.
    - Familial amyloid cardiomyopathy also occurs.
    - ATTR can be treated by liver transplantation (remove source of the abnormal normal TTR).
  - Amyloid fibrils in senile amyloidosis derived from apparently normal TTR

- **Aβ**
  - Amyloid β and (or β-amyloid) protein is 39–42 amino acid peptide derived from a larger protein called amyloid β precursor protein (βAPP).
    - Normal precursor processing (constitutive pathway) generates a nonamyloidogenic peptides that can be secreted.
    - Processing by lyosomal-endosomal pathway generates potentially amyloidogenic peptides.
  - Aβ induces apoptosis in cultured central nervous system neurons.
  - Amyloid derived from Aβ is found in
    - Senile plaques and blood vessels in brains of Alzheimer's disease patients, adults with Down syndrome, and normal older individuals
    - Cerebral blood vessels in congophilic angiopathy
    - Inclusions in muscle in inclusion body myositis
  - Point mutations in the AβPP gene (on chromosome 21) account for a small percentage of examples of familial early onset Alzheimer's disease.
    - Most cases of familial Alzheimer's disease are caused by mutations in other genes.

- **Peptide hormone-derived amyloid**
  - *ACal*
    - Derived from procalcitonin, precursor of calcitonin, a peptide hormone produced by the C cells of the thyroid and by medullary thyroid carcinomas
    - About 80% of medullary thyroid carcinomas—contain amyloid derived from procalcitonin
  - *AIAPP*
    - Derived from islet amyloid protein (IAPP; also called amylin)
      - Hormone secreted by β cells of endocrine pancreas
      - Opposes insulin action on skeletal muscle
      - Affects secretion of other islet cell hormones
    - Makes up the fibrils of amyloid present in the islets of most patients with type II diabetes mellitus and in some islet cell neoplasms
  - *AANF*
    - Derived from hormone atrial natriuretic peptide (ANP; also called atrial natriuretic factor, ANF)
    - Makes up the amyloid fibrils in isolated atrial amyloidosis that commonly occurs in the elderly
- **Others**
  - *Aβ₂M*
    - Derived from $β_2$-microglobulin, plasma protein that associates with class I histocompatibility antigens on cell surfaces
    - Amyloid fibril protein in amyloidosis in chronic hemodialysis patients
      - Chronic renal failure patients can have markedly elevated plasma $β_2$-microglobulin, not all of which is removed by dialysis
    - Amyloid involves synovium, joints, tendon sheaths; sometimes amyloid tumors are present
  - *ACys*
    - Derived from cystatin C (gamma trace protein), a proteinase inhibitor produced by neurons and endocrine cells
      - Concentration higher in cerebrospinal fluid than in plasma
    - Mutant (amino acid substitution) can form cerebral vascular amyloid in autosomal dominant cerebral hemorrhage (Iceland)
  - *AKer*
    - Derived from keratin, the intermediate filament protein of epithelium
    - Amyloid fibrils in the rare skin condition called lichen amyloidosis
  - *AApoAI*
    - Derived from apolipoprotein AI, major protein component of HDL

- Mutant (amino acid substitution) can produce familial polyneuropathy

— *AGel*

- Derived from gelsolin, an actin-binding protein present in the cytoskeleton
- Mutant (amino acid substitution) can produce familial polyneuropathy

— *ALys*

- Derived from lysozyme, an antibacterial enzyme found in secretions, neutrophils, and macrophages
- Mutant (amino acid substitution) can produce familal systemic amyloidosis

— *APrP*

- Derived from prion protein (PrP^C), expressed in most neurons
- In prion diseases—posttranslational processing of PrP^C converts it to a 33-35 kDa sialoglycoprotein, PrP^{Sc}, which is infectious
  - Partial proteolysis of PrP^{Sc} generates PrP-27-30, which forms amyloid
- Prion diseases
  - Scrapie (sheep)
  - Kuru
  - Creutzfeld-Jakob disease (CJD)
  - Gerstmann-Sträussler-Scheinker (GSS) disease
  - Fatal familial insomnia
  - In some examples of familial prion diseases (familial CJD, GSS disease, fatal familial insomnia) point mutations in PrP^C found

■ **Clinicopathologic Correlations**

● **Primary and myeloma-associated amyloid**

- AL amyloid derived from immunoglobulin light chain of paraprotein
  - About 10% have multiple myeloma (myeloma-associated amyloidosis); less commonly, other types of lymphoid malignancies.
  - Most have no associated malignant disease (primary amyloidosis).
- Multiple myeloma
  - A malignant neoplasm of plasma cells is characterized by multiple osteolytic lesions and paraprotein.
  - Approximately 10% of patients with multiple myeloma have amyloidosis.
  - Usually these patients present with amyloidosis and have a poor prognosis.
- Primary amyloidosis
  - Almost all of these patients have paraprotein with no underlying malignancies (benign monoclonal gammopathy).

- Many have a modest increase in the number of plasma cells in the bone marrow.

- Almost always systemic amyloidosis, most prominently involving peripheral nerves, tongue, skin, heart, and gastrointestinal tract

  - Left ventricular involvement can cause fatal disturbance of cardiac rhythm or congestive heart failure.

- **Secondary amyloidosis**

  - Major fibril protein—AA is derived from acute phase reactant SAA.
  - Secondary to some other condition

    - As many 15% to 25% of rheumatoid arithritis patients develop secondary amyloidosis.
    - Other predisposing inflammatory conditions are dermatomyositis, scleroderma, and chronic inflammatory bowel disease.
    - Chronic infections include tuberculosis, bronchiectasis, chronic osteomyelitis.
    - Some neoplasms occur, such as renal cell carcinoma and Hodgkin's disease.

  - Amyloidosis is usually systemic, most prominently involving spleen, liver, kidneys, and adrenals.
  - Amyloidosis can be clinically significant, causing proteinuria and renal failure.
  - Treatment of the underlying disorder might arrest the development of amyloidosis.
  - Familial Mediterranean fever is sometimes associated with systemic amyloidosis similar to secondary amyloidosis.

    - Autosomal recessive disorder is most common in Armenians, non-Ashkenazi Jews, Turks, Arabs.
    - Characteristics are attacks of fever accompanied by inflammation of serosal surfaces, with amyloid in some families.

- **Senile systemic amyloidosis**

  - ATTR amyloid fibrils derived from apparently normal TTR
  - Involves heart, blood vessels, and lung
  - Cardiac left ventricular amyloid—can cause arrhythmias or heart failure

MULTIPLE CHOICE REVIEW QUESTIONS

1. A 49-year-old woman with rheumatoid arthritis for about twenty years develops protein in the urine that becomes progressively more severe. A renal biopsy shows amyloid replacement of many glomeruli. It is most likely that the amyloid fibrils are which of the following?

   a. AA
   b. AL
   c. AGel
   d. Aβ
   e. Aβ2M

2. An 87-year-old woman dies of heart failure that is unresponsive to usual medical therapy. At autopsy the left ventricle is enlarged, primarily by amyloidosis. Amyloid is also present in many blood vessels. It is most likely that the amyloid fibrils are a derivative of which of the following?

   a. Amyloid P component
   b. Amylin
   c. Atrial natriuretic peptide
   d. Transthyretin
   e. Retinol binding protein

Chapter 11

Blood Vessels

BASIC "GAME PLAN" FOR BLOOD VESSELS

■ **Arteries: Three Major Types**

- Large elastic (e.g., aorta)
- Medium sized, muscular (e.g., temporal artery)
- Arterioles (0.3 mm or less internal diameter)
- *Note:* The divisions among these three types are not completely distinct.

● **Histology**

- All arteries have three layers.

    - *Tunica intima,* the inner one, consists of a single layer of endothelial cells lining the lumenal surface as well as a basement membrane, beyond which are varying amounts of connective tissue stroma (mostly collagen); beyond this is a discrete band of elastic fibers that separates the tunica intima from the tunica media (internal elastic lamina).

    - *Tunica media,* the middle one, comprises most of the thickness of the arterial wall; it is composed mainly of smooth muscle, elastic fibers and connective tissue ground substance (proteoglycan); outermost elastic fibers form a discrete band known as the external elastic lamina.

    - *Tunica adventitia,* the outermost arterial layer, consists of irregularly deployed collagen and elastic fibers. Also seen within the adventitia of large arteries are nutrient blood vessels that supply the large artery itself (these are known as vasa vasosa) and lymphatic channels and nerves.

    - *Note:* Elastic arteries have *prominent* internal elastic laminas and external elastic laminas as compared to the medium-sized muscular arteries, where these structures are much less pronounced; in addition, the tunica media of elastic arteries is liberally endowed with elastic fiber bands. Muscular arteries, like elastic arteries, have vasa vasora. Finally, arterioles (internal diameter of 0.3 mm or less) have all three of the above layers and a poorly formed internal elastic lamina.

■ **Capillaries**

- These small-caliber vessels have a single layer of continuous endothelial cells resting upon a basement membrane; external to this, there is no other connective tissue.

- However, located around the basement membrane are pericytes, which provide structural support and contain the contractile protein myosin.

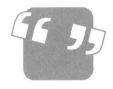

- Pericytes also probably help in the production of basement membrane material.

■ Veins

- These possess much thinner walls than arteries.

  - Endothelial luminal lining
  - Small amount of subendothelial connective tissue with small elastic fiber component
  - Smooth muscle coat
  - Variably formed adventitia

Basic Disease Processes Affecting Blood Vessels

■ Mechanical-Physiologic Disorders

- **Ruptured vessels**

  - Ruptured vessels are usually caused by traumatic injury but *may be secondary* to spontaneous rupture of a vessel already weakened by some other disease process.

    - In either case, one sees hemorrhage into various tissue locales.

  - Blood that exits from and coagulates outside of blood vessels is referred to as a *coagulum* (or clot) whereas blood that coagulates within the vascular tree is called a *thrombus.*

- **Thrombosis**

  - Thrombosis occurs when blood coagulates within the vascular tree.
  - A thrombus consists of platelets, fibrin, and entrapped blood cells (mostly red blood cells [RBCs]).
  - To a certain degree, and in many clinical circumstances, thrombosis represents a normal protective mechanism designed to staunch blood loss when vessel walls are breached.
  - Thrombosis requires a delicately choreographed "ballet" involving platelets, endothelial cells, circulating coagulant proteins, the fibrinolytic system (to remove thrombi at a later time), and the inflammatory and complement cascades.
  - Normally, excessive thrombosis is prevented by the following mechanisms.

    - *Intact endothelial cell monolayer* (endothelium) keeps platelets (which form the primary hemostatic plug when vessel walls are breached) from coming into contact with collagen and von Willebrand factor.
    - *PGI$_2$ (prostacyclin) and nitric acid,* found within endothelial cells, prevent adhesion and aggregation of platelets.
    - *Thrombomodulin* on the endothelial surface binds to any locally produced thrombin, and this complex activates an anticoagulant mechanism involving protein C and protein S.
    - Endothelial cells produce *anticoagulant, heparin-like substances.*
    - Endothelial cells produce plasminogen activators, which initiate local clot lysis (*fibrinolysis*).

● **Factors predisposing to pathologic (abnormal) thrombus**

  • Previously damaged blood vessel wall, (atheroma formation, aneurysm, inflammatory process)

  • Low blood flow (stasis) states

  • Changes in the coagulability of blood (increased coagulant proteins, decreased anticoagulant proteins, decreased activity of fibrinolytic system)

  • *Note:* Not all thrombi are 100% occlusive

    • This is especially true in the aorta and heart, where they usually do *not* totally occlude but rather form raised nodules (or plaques) attached to vessel or cardiac chamber walls (mural thrombus formation). Finally, thrombi occurring on cardiac valves have a polypoid appearance and are called *vegetations.*

● **Possible outcomes of pathologic thrombus formation (assuming patient survival)**

  • *Growth of thrombus* within vessel lumen/cardiac chamber is called propagation of thrombus.

  • *Lysis of thrombus* is accomplished by patient's own fibrinolytic system, sometimes assisted by exogenous fibrinolytic therapy.

  • Ingrowth of granulation tissue from vessel wall is the *organization of a thrombus;* eventually, new (smaller) vascular channels will be created and this is called a *recanalization of thrombus.*

  • Fragments of the thrombus may break off and be carried to some other site in the vascular tree to form a *thromboembolism.*

● **Embolus formation**

  • This is often, though not always, intimately related to prior thrombus formation.

  • Embolism refers to vascular occlusion caused by material that has been transported to the occlusion site by the bloodstream; the mass of material so deposited is an embolus and need not necessarily consist of thrombus, although this is clinically the most important source of emboli.

  • Thromboemboli are emboli resulting from fragments of a previously formed thrombus transported to the occlusion site.

  — *Clinically significant thromboembolic scenarios*

    • Pulmonary thromboemboli originating in systemic veins, usually of leg and pelvis, can cause pulmonary infarcts.

    • Thromboemboli from heart can travel via the arterial system to numerous sites, including brain, kidneys, spleen, gastrointestinal tract, and limbs.

    • Thromboemboli arising from common carotid artery thrombosis can result in brain vascular occlusions (*cerebrovascular events*).

    • Thromboemboli arising in abdominal aorta can occlude renal arteries, mesenteric arteries and their ramifications, and leg arteries.

    • *Note:* Materials other than thrombi can form emboli, although these scenarios are *much less* often encountered than are thromboembolic ones in clinical medicine.

      • Air (introduced by trauma or medical intervention)

      • Amniotic fluid (obstetrical complication)

Table 11.1   *Clinical Aspects of Shock*

TISSUE	EARLY SHOCK	LATE SHOCK
Skin	Pale and cold	Cyanosed
Kidneys	Low urine production	Necrosis of tubular epithelium
Gut	Bowel stasis	Necrosis of lining epithelium
Lung	Tachypnea	Necrosis of alveolar epithelium
Liver	Fatty change	Necrosis of centrilobular cells
Brain	Reduced conscious level	Necrosis of neurons; coma
Heart	Tachycardia	Myocardial necrosis

From Stevens A, Lowe J: *Pathology,* London, 1995, Times Mirror International.

- Nitrogen (decompression sickness)
- Cholesterol (derived from atheromas)
- Fat and bone marrow (caused by traumatic bone injury)
- Neoplastic cells
- Intentional, therapeutic (used to occlude the blood supply to inoperable vascular lesions, usually in the brain; occlusion caused by injected wire, gel foam, glue, or balloons)

● Thrombophlebitis (phlebothrombosis)

- Refers to inflammation within thrombosed veins
- Most common sites—calf, femoral, popliteal, iliac, periprostatic, and periuterine veins
- Predisposing factors

  - Prolonged bed rest
  - Cardiac failure
  - Postoperative state
  - Pregnancy-postpartum state
  - Anticoagulant protein deficiency (e.g., antithrombin III, protein C, protein S)
  - Hyperlipidemia
  - Cigarette use

● Shock

- In contradistinction to the *local* impairment of blood flow caused by thromboemboli, *shock results from a systemic reduction in the flow of blood to the body's tissues.*

— *Causes of shock*

  - "Pump" failure (cardiogenic)
  - Reduced blood volume (hypovolemia)
  - Abnormal dilation of peripheral vessels, resulting in lack of venous blood return to heart (septic shock which is endotoxin shock caused by infection; anaphylactic shock, neurogenic shock)

— *Clinical mainfestations of shock are summarized in Table 11.1*

— *Protective mechanisms operative during shock*

  1. Activation of renin-angiotensin-aldosterone axis to cause sodium and water retention and increased blood volume
  2. Increased catecholamine output, causing tachycardia and vaso-

constriction of certain vascular beds (and resultant blood shunting away from them)

3. If shock persists, however, metabolic acidemia supervenes; this results in vascular dilation, hypotension, and shunting of blood away from the kidneys and gastrointestinal tract in a valiant attempt to protect the brain and heart

4. In late shock, irreversible cell damage is seen

— *Possible clinical consequences of the above four processes (hemorrhage, thrombosis, embolism, and shock)*

• *Ischemic change* to tissues suffering from a reduction of blood supply; this implies damage and, eventually, focal scattered individual cell death *but not wholesale tissue death*

• *Infarction*—actual wholesale tissue death caused by marked reduction or total lack of blood supply; usually occurs when vascular occlusion is abrupt

— *Infarction usually results in coagulative necrosis, with the infarct's shape corresponding to the territory of the occluded vessel*

• *Arterial infarct*

• After occlusion, the affected tissue becomes pale and swollen; in 2 days, this changes to a pale yellow appearance (because of the accumulation of neutrophils).

• Subsequently, a red, hyperemic border appears along the infarct's margins.

• In about 10 days, granulation tissue grows into the infarcted area, with eventual infarct replacement by scar tissue.

• *"Hemorrhagic" (venous) infarction caused by obstruction of venous drainage*

• When blood cannot drain from a tissue because of obstructed venous outflow, arterial blood nonetheless continues to enter that tissue, thereby resulting in a rapid rise in small blood vessel pressure and eventual rupture and hemorrhage of these vessels.

• This finally results in a tissue resistance so high as to choke off the arrival of arterial blood, and one sees an infarct.

• *Hemorrhagic infarcts are dark, because of congestion by trapped, deoxygenated RBCs.*

• *Note:* The usual etiology for hemorrhagic (venous) infarction is torsion of an organ's vascular pedicle.

■ **Degenerative Disorders** These represent the most important causes of morbidity (illness) and mortality (death) in the United States today.

● **Arteriosclerosis** A general, rather all-encompassing moniker that simply refers to thickened and hardened arteries and may be of several types.

• Thickened, hardened arteries are prone to:

• Reduce blood flow to tissue, thereby potentially causing ischemia and even infarction

• Rupture (caused by structural weakening) with consequent hemorrhage

• Develop pathologic thrombosis

● **There are four major types of arteriosclerosis**

— *Atherosclerosis*

• *Atherosclerosis* is the most common form of arteriosclerosis.

• It affects large- and medium-sized arteries (almost always those with a diameter greater than 2 mm) and is predominantly seen in vessels exposed to the high pressure of the systemic circulation.

• Thus, the pulmonary arteries normally are not involved by this process unless there happens to be coexisting heart and/or lung disease.

• Also, veins are not affected (except in those used to bypass blocked arteries because only then are they exposed to systemic blood pressures [such as in coronary artery bypass grafting]).

• Key lesion of atherosclerosis is accumulation of lipid-rich material within the intima of arteries (atherosclerotic plaque or atheroma); this is often associated with at least some degree of inflammatory cell response. The genesis of atherosclerosis is depicted in Fig. 11.1.

Atherosclerosis risk factors

• Hyperlipidemia (particularly cholesterol and low density lipoproteins)

• High density lipoproteins are actually *protective* against the development of atherosclerosis.

• Hypertension
• Diabetes mellitus
• Cigarette smoking
• Old age
• Male gender
• Familial history
• Obesity

Complications of arterial atherosclerosis

• Reduction in caliber of vessel lumen with possible ischemic/infarctive complications in tissue served by affected vessels
• Thrombosis superimposed upon an atheroma
• Hemorrhage into an atheroma, with resultant reduction in vessel lumenal diameter and occlusion of that vessel
• Aneurysm formation

— *Hypertensive arteriosclerosis*

Benign hypertension

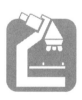

• Arterial wall thickening develops slowly over time as a result of stable hypertension.

• One sees thickening of small artery walls caused by intimal fibroelastic proliferation and media smooth muscle proliferation; arterioles show a thickened wall caused by deposition of a smudgy, red, hyaline material as seen on standard microsections.

"Malignant" hypertension

• Arterial wall thickening develops over a short time course when hypertension is severe and of more sudden onset.

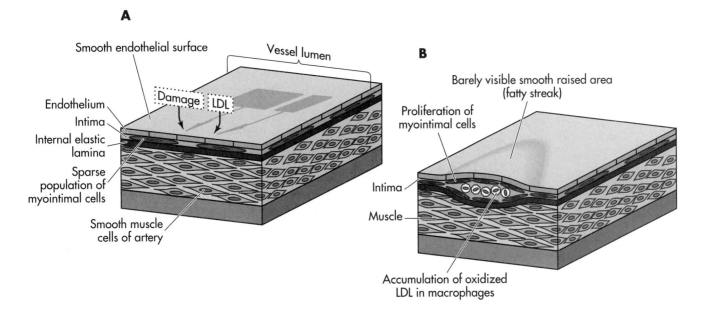

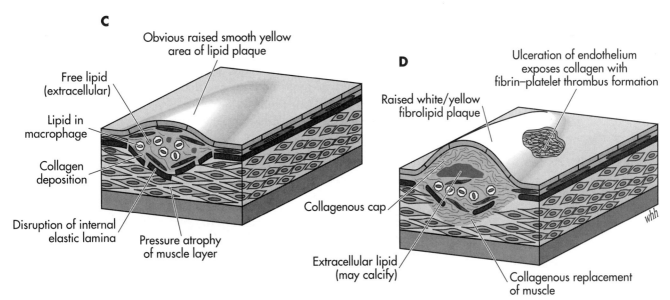

Fig. 11.1 Genesis of an atheromatous plaque. **A,** Damage to endothelial monolayer allows cholesterol-laden low density lipo-proteins *(LDL)* into intima. **B,** Intimal macrophages take up lipid material to produce a fatty streak. **C,** Macrophages produce cy-tokines that stimulate proliferation of myofibroblasts which produce collagen and initiate fibrosis of plaque. **D,** Fibrous plaque hardens; endothelium ulcerates and thrombosis typically ensues.

- In small arteries, there is intimal fibroblastic proliferation.
- Arterioles show necrosis of their walls with accumulation of fi-brin material (fibrinoid necrosis).

— *Arteriolosclerosis*

Two main types of this lesion

- *Hyaline type* is identical to the hyaline thickening seen in benign hypertension (see preceding); this type may also be seen, however, as an aging concomitant and in diabetes mellitus.

Table 11.2 *Types of Aneurysms*

Type	Site	Cause	Incidence
Atherosclerotic	Abdominal aorta	Thinning and fibrous replacement of media	Common
Syphilitic	Ascending aorta and arch	Inflammatory destruction of media and fibrous replacement	Now rare
Berry	Cerebral arteries	Congenital defect(s) in elastic lamina-media	Common
Infective (mycotic)	Any	Destruction of wall by pathogen in infected thrombus	Rare

From Stevens A, Lowe J: *Pathology,* London, 1995, Times Mirror International.

- *Proliferative type* may be seen in malignant hypertension (see preceding) but also in other conditions, including scleroderma (progressive systemic sclerosis), hemolytic-uremic syndrome, congenital rubella, and homocystineuria.

  - Microscopically, can see one of three patterns
  - "Onion skin" proliferation of intimal smooth muscle
  - Accumulation of mucinous material within tunica intima—mucinous intimal thickening
  - Fibroblastic proliferation in tunica intima, with collagen and elastic fiber deposition

— *Mönckeberg's medical calcific sclerosis*

  - An age-related, idiopathic (etiology unknown) disorder characterized by calcification (and sometimes osseous metaplasia) centered in the tunica media

● Aneurysms

- *Aneurysms* are *abnormal, focal vascular dilations,* the clinical importance of which are mostly possible complications, including rupture and a nidus for thrombus formation.

  - Most frequently they are caused by underlying atherosclerotic disease, but there are other causes, including previous syphilis, congenital vessel wall weakening; and active infection (known also as a mycotic aneurysm, which is a bit of a misnomer because any infectious agent [*not* just fungal] can cause this).
  - Aneurysm types are summarized in Table 11.2.
  - Most aneurysms arise in the aorta between the renal arteries and the aortic bifurcation into the common iliacs.

- *Dissecting (false) aneurysms* result from an arterial intimal tear, thereby allowing blood beneath the tunica intima and into the arterial wall; this blood tracks into the tunica media and splits it, thereby forming a false channel.

  - *Hypertension is the important predisposing factor and is seen in 70% of cases.*

- Other causes include medial mucoid degeneration, Marfan syndrome, Ehlers-Danlos syndrome, and atherosclerosis.
- Rare cases are iatrogenic (caused by medical instrumentation of an arterial wall with subsequent damage to it).

■ Vasculitis Disorders

- These are characterized by primary inflammation of and damage to blood vessel walls; any blood vessel may be affected.
- Depending upon the severity of this vasculitis, blood vessels may be transiently or permanently damaged.
- Box 11.1 categorizes vasculitic disorders.
- ● Three major types of vasculitis
  - — *Hypersensitivity*
    - *Hypersensitivity* is the most common type and usually presents as a skin rash; it involves capillaries and venules primarily.
      - Most commonly seen as a manifestation of a drug reaction (drug induced vasculitis), but also may be seen in bacteremia, viremia, serum sickness, cryoglobulinemia, and Henoch-Schönlein purpura
      - Genesis—immune complexes become trapped in vessel walls; this triggers complement activation and neutrophil chemotaxis
      - Histologically, destruction of affected vessel walls and infiltration by neutrophils and leakage (extravasation of RBCs) from these inflamed and damaged vessels

  - — *Autoimmune disease associated*
    - Especially seen in systemic lupus erythematosus and rheumatoid arthritis
  - — *Systemic disorders of uncertain etiology*   There are a number of such disorders but only four will be briefly addressed here.
    Polyarteritis nodosa
    - A systemic disorder characterized by vasculitis involving small- and medium-sized arteries
    - Clinically manifests as focal organ infarction caused by occlusion of inflamed or damaged vessels
      - *Target organs*
        - Kidneys
        - Heart
        - Gastrointestinal tract
        - Liver
        - Central nervous system
        - Skin
        - Skeletal muscle
        - Nerve tissue
    - Idiopathic, although some cases are associated with chronic hepatitis B antigenemia and others are associated with group A streptococcal infection

Box 11.1

TYPES OF VASCULITIS

Direct Infection of Vessels
Bacterial vasculitis (such as neisserial)
Mycobacterial vasculitis (such as tuberculous)
Spirochetal vasculitis (such as syphilitic)
Rickettsial vasculitis (such as Rocky Mountain spotted fever)
Fungal vasculitis (such as aspergillosis)
Viral vasculitis (such as herpes zoster)

Immunologic Injury
Immune complex-mediated vasculitis
   Henoch-Schönlein purpura
   Cryoglobulinemic vasculitis
   Lupus vasculitis
   Rheumatoid vasculitis
   Serum sickness vasculitis
      Induced by whole serum
      Induced by heterologous proteins
   Infection-induced immune complex vasculitis
      Viral (such as hepatitis B and C)
      Bacterial (such as group A *Streptococcus*)
   Paraneoplastic vasculitis
   Behçet's disease
   Some drug-induced vasculitides (such as sulfon-amide-1 induced vasculitis)
Direct antibody attack-mediated vasculitis
   Goodpasture's syndrome (mediated by anti-basement membrane antibodies)
   Kawasaki disease (possibly mediated by anti-endothelial antibodies)
Antineutrophil cytoplasmic autoantibody-mediated vasculitis
   Wegener's granulomatosis
   Microscopic polyangiitis (microscopic polyarteritis)
   Churg-Strauss syndrome
   Some drug-induced vasculitides (such as thiouracil-1 induced vasculitis)
Cell-mediated vasculitis
   Allograft cellular vascular rejection

Unknown
Giant cell (temporal) arteritis
Takayasu arteritis
Polyarteritis nodosa
Behçet's disease

From: Damjanov I, Linder J: *Anderson's pathology,* ed 10, vol 1, St Louis, 1996, Mosby.

• Histologically characterized by transmural blood vessel acute inflammation and necrosis.

Buerger's disease (thromboangiitis obliterans)

• Clinically this presents with inflammation-mediated occlusion of peripheral arteries in the upper and lower extremities; sometimes this progresses to gangrene.

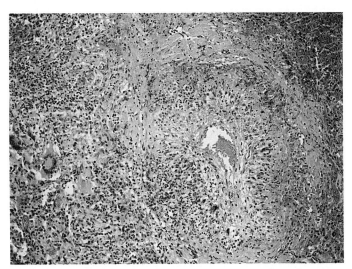

Fig. 11.2 Wegener's granulomatosis. This photomicrograph of lung tissue shows necrotizing granulomatous inflammation involving a small pulmonary artery (to the right) as well as lung parenchyma. (*From Damjanov I, Linder J:* Anderson's pathology, *ed 10, vol 1, St Louis, 1996, Mosby.*)

- *There is a strong association with heavy cigarette use and male gender.*
- Histologically, one sees segmental arterial wall infiltration by, initially, neutrophils followed by lymphocytes and monocytes (sometimes accompanied by giant cells).

Wegener's granulomatosis (WG)

- WG is a potentially multi-organ disease characterized by necrotizing, granulomatous inflammation that *may* involve the orbital region, upper respiratory tract, lungs, skin, and kidneys
- *Classic triad of WG (not all cases are "classic")* includes the following:

  - Systemic necrotizing vasculitis
  - Necrotizing granulomatous inflammation of lower or upper respiratory tract or both
  - Necrotizing glomerulonephritis

- The vasculitis of WG involves small- to medium-sized vessels (capillaries, arterioles, venules, small arteries) (Fig. 11.2).
- *Note:* More than 90% of WG have, in their serum, an antibody directed against neutrophil cytoplasm; specifically, this antibody is directed to proteinase -3 and is called antineutrophilic cytoplasmic antibody (ANCA). The antibody (which is distinct from another antibody that reacts to myeloperoxidase in the perinuclear cytoplasm of neutrophils) is only rarely seen in other vasculitis disorders.

Giant cell arteritis (temporal arteritis)

- This is a potentially systemic disease seen most commonly in females over 50 years old.
- It tends to target medium-sized muscular arteries of the head and neck, *particularly the temporal artery (but also the ophthalmic artery).*

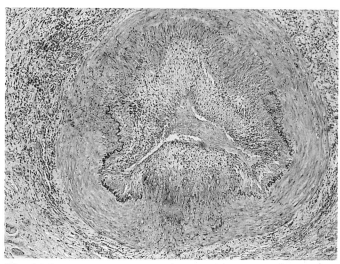

Fig. 11.3 Giant cell arteritis. This photomicrograph features a temporal artery with transmural inflammation and disruption of the internal elastic lamina. (*From Damjanov I, Linder J:* Anderson's pathology, *ed 10, vol 1, St Louis, 1996, Mosby.*)

• Patients typically have ill-defined systemic complaints (headaches, malaise, fatigue, fever); *erythrocyte sedimentation rate is usually high, and patients often have an associated polymyalgia rheumatica.*

• Lesions are segmental and often "skip" areas of involved artery.

• Histologically, one sees a full thickness vessel wall granulomatous inflammatory process featuring monocytes, lymphocytes, histiocytes, and giant cells; this process is often centered about the internal elastic lamina and/or the external elastic lamina (Fig. 11.3).

• *Note:* A frequent and devastating consequence of this vasculitis is sudden blindness caused by involvement of the ophthalmic artery.

■ **"Tumors"-Malformations**

● Venous

• Far and away the most common abnormalities of veins involve dilation and congestion with blood.

— *Varicose veins*

• Persistently distended superficial lower extremity veins (long and short saphenous) that result from incompetency of venous valves

— *Hemorrhoids (piles)*

• Distended internal and/or external hemorrhoidal veins in the anorectal region

• Pain, bleeding, protrusion, and pruritus are common symptoms

— *Varicocele*

• Persistent vein distension in pampiniform plexus of the spermatic cord within the scrotal sac

— *Esophageal varices*

• A result of portal hypertension associated with hepatic cirrhosis

- Dilated venous channels (which may thrombose and/or bleed) in the esophageal submucosa

● **Vascular malformations**

- *Hemangiomas* (angiomas)—developmental vascular malformations

  - *Capillary*—consists of numerous small, capillary-like vessels
  - *Cavernous*—consists of numerous, widely dilated vessels that have the appearance of thin-walled veins

- Arteriovenous malformations

  - Often seen in the brain, but may be seen elsewhere
  - May spontaneously bleed and compress surrounding tissue
  - Histologically, an admixture of benign arteries and veins that produce a mass lesion

● **Vascular neoplasms**

— *Glomus tumor (glomangioma)*

  - Classically presents as a tender, painful finger nodule
  - Histologically, benign small vessel channels surrounded by glomus cells (neuroendocrine cells)

— *Hemangioendothelioma*

  - A neoplasm derived from endothelial cells; some have malignant potential

— *Hemangiopericytoma*

  - A neoplasm composed of pericytes, which are specialized cells that surround blood vessels and have a "supportive" role for endothelial cells

    - Some have malignant potential

— *Angiosarcoma*

  - A malignant neoplasm composed of endothelial cells that form vascular channels

    - Highly malignant in many cases
    - Clinically often presents as a bluish red, raised lesion
    - May occur in limbs that have been subjected to long-standing lymphedema
    - May be seen in visceral organs, such as liver

— *Kaposi's syndrome (KS)*

  - Probably derived from endothelial cells but may arise from pluripotent mesenchymal cells
  - Prior to the acquired immunodeficiency syndrome (AIDS) epidemic, KS in the United States was seen almost exclusively on the skin of the legs of elderly men (often of Mediterranean descent); these lesions were relatively indolent, uncommonly metastasizing or causing death of the patient.
    - Three phases of AIDS-related KS
      - Patch phase—flat purple lesions
      - Plaque phase—slightly raised, firm, purple lesions

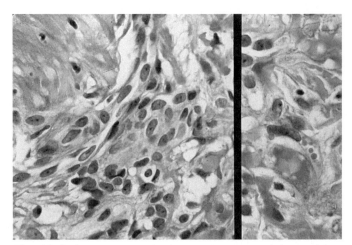

Fig. 11.4 Photomicrograph of Kaposi's sarcoma; left panel features the atypical spindle cells characteristic of this lesion while the right panel depicts the hyaline protein droplets also typically seen in this neoplasm. (*From Damjanov I, Linder J:* Anderson's pathology, *ed 10, vol 1, St Louis, 1996, Mosby.*)

- Nodular phase—dome-shaped, firm, blue lesions

- Histologically, numerous slitlike vascular channels lined by atypical spindle cells; extravasated RBCs, extravascular hemosiderin (iron containing protein), and hyaline droplets (usually within macrophages) also seen (Fig. 11.4)

- Recent evidence suggests that the genesis of Kaposi's sarcoma may involve human herpesvirus-8 infection

MULTIPLE CHOICE REVIEW QUESTIONS

1. When blood coagulates outside the vascular tree, it is referred to as which of the following?

    a. Thrombus
    b. Embolus
    c. Clot
    d. Thromboembolus
    e. Organized thrombus

2. The most common and clinically significant type of arteriosclerosis encountered in the United States is which of the following?

    a. Atherosclerosis
    b. Mönckeberg's medial calcific sclerosis
    c. Arteriolosclerosis
    d. Hypertensive arteriosclerosis
    e. Buerger's disease

3. The most common type of vasculitis observed in the United States is which of the following?

    a. Hypersensitivity
    b. Autoimmune disease associated
    c. Polyarteritis nodosa
    d. Wegener's granulomatosis
    e. Giant cell arteritis

4. An 85-year-old woman presents with sudden onset of severe headache as well as fever and malaise. An erythrocyte sedimentation rate (ESR) is markedly elevated and you order a temporal artery biopsy; the pathology report reveals the presence of full-thickness arterial granulomatous inflammation with inflammatory giant cells centered about a disrupted internal elastic lamina. This patient has which of the following?

    a. Wegener's granulomatosis
    b. Polyarteritis nodosa
    c. Hypersensitivity vasculitis
    d. Giant cell arteritis
    e. Buerger's disease

5. A 25-year-old man, who admits to long term use of injection drugs, presents to your office with fatigue and multiple raised, purplish skin and buccal mucosal lesions. You biopsy one of the skin lesions, and the pathologist reports that there is a vascular proliferation characterized by slit-like vessels lined by very atypical spindle cells; extravasated RBCs and extracellular hemosiderin deposition are also noted. Your patient has which of the following?

    a. Bacillary epithelioid angiomatosis
    b. Kaposi's sarcoma
    c. Glomus tumor
    d. Squamous cell carcinoma
    e. Melanoma

Chapter 12

Heart

■ **Valvular Disease**

● Rheumatic heart disease

• The pancarditis and symptom complex is seen in 1% to 3% of people within 6 weeks of a group A beta-hemolytic streptococcal infection (usually pharyngitis) frequently between the ages of 6 to 15 years.

• Incidence has risen in the last decade.

• Mechanism is thought to be immunologic injury evoked by cross-reactivity of tissue antigens with streptococcus.

• Diagnosis of acute rheumatic heart disease requires two major or one major and two minor Jones Criteria (Box 12.1).

• Without adequate penicillin prophylaxis, recurrent episodes of rheumatic fever may give rise to chronic rheumatic heart disease, the major cause of acquired valvular heart disease throughout the world.

— *Pathology*

• Chronic inflammation and the pathognomonic Aschoff bodies around small vessels in the connective tissue of the heart (primary target), joints, central nervous system, lungs, blood vessels, and skin

• Aschoff bodies

• **Exudative phase**—areas of edema, increased ground substance, and degeneration of collagen—fibrinoid necrosis

• **Granulomatous phase**—organization to form nodules within the interstitium and connective tissue consisting of lymphocytes, histiocytes, plasma cells, and multinucleated giant cells (Aschoff giant cells) centered on the fibrinoid necrosis

• **Healing phase**—residual scarring and fibrosis

• **Anitschkow's or Aschoff cells**—large histiocytes with central oval nuclei in which the chromatin has condensed towards the center to form an irregular linear shape that looks caterpillar-like

• Pericardium

• Fibrinous pericarditis—dense, reddened, shaggy exudate composed of fibrin and chronic inflammatory cells with fibroblasts and Aschoff cells in adjacent areas

• Myocardium

• Myocarditis with Aschoff bodies

Box 12.1

JONES CRITERIA

Major manifestations
   Carditis, polyarthritis, chorea, erythema marginatum,
     subcutaneous nodules
Minor manifestations
   Clinical—arthralgia, fever
   Laboratory—elevated erythrocyte sedimentation rate
     or C-reactive protein, prolonged P-R interval
   Supporting evidence of antecedent group A strep-
     tococcal infection
         Positive throat culture or rapid streptococcal
           antigen test
         Elevated or rising streptococcal antibody titer

Modified from Damjanov I, Linder J: *Anderson's pathology,* ed 10, vol 1,
St Louis, 1996, Mosby.

- Endocarditis
  - Most serious manifestation because of sequelae of chronic valvular disease
  - Initially edema and swelling with 1 to 2 mm fibrinous vegetations along the valve closure lines known as verrucous endocarditis
  - Healing with scarring and fibrosis, resulting in chronic valve disease (see following)
  - Always involves the mitral valve, frequently alone or with the aortic valve, less commonly the tricuspid valve, and rarely the pulmonary valve

- **Mitral stenosis**
  - Rheumatic fever is the only common cause (90%), however, Aschoff bodies almost never found at this stage
  - Long latent period of 20 years
  - Complications—thromboembolism, infective endocarditis, chronic pulmonary congestion, and dyspnea
  - *Pathology*
    - Valve leaflets thickened by collagenization and occasional calcium deposits
    - Leaflet fusion along the commisure and chord shortening results in a "fishmouth" appearance to the valve

- **Mitral insufficiency**
  - Causes—rheumatic heart disease, rupture of the chordae tendineae, ischemic papillary muscle dysfunction, mitral valve prolapse, calcification of the mitral valve ring, and infective endocarditis
  - Acute insufficiency—results in pulmonary edema and left ventricular failure
  - Chronic insufficiency—results in low cardiac output with fatigue and weakness

● Calcification of mitral valve ring

  • Common, usually asymptomatic elderly women
  • Calcifications—may form nodules behind the valve leaflets but, in contrast to chronic rheumatic valve disease, the leaflets are unaffected
  • Impairment of systolic contraction of the ring—may cause insufficiency

● Mitral valve prolapse

  • Common, usually asymptomatic
  • Estimated at 5% to 10% of population
  • Often an autosomal dominant predisposition
  • Secondary associations—inherited connective tissue disorders, such as Marfan syndrome, osteogenesis imperfecta, cardiomyopathy, polyarteritis nodosa, and others
  • Symptomatic cases frequently associated with myxomatous or mucoid degeneration of the valve, producing excess valve tissue that bulges and prolapses into the left atrium during systole
  • Increased risk for infective endocarditis and sudden death
  • Clinical—midsystolic click-murmur is classic auscultory finding, severe insufficiency may necessitate valve replacement

  — *Pathology*

    • Leaflets enlarged and chords stretched
    • A clear gelatinous appearance to the thickened leaflets on cross section
    • Microscopic—myxoid change consists of an increase of pale pink-staining proteoglycans in the valve matrix that may form focal cystic spaces

● Aortic stenosis

  • Frequent in the elderly
  • Calcific degeneration—most common cause of isolated stenosis
  • Chronic rheumatic valve disease—most common cause if there is coexisting mitral valve disease
  • Congenital bicuspid valves predisposed to calcification

    • Dystrophic calcium deposition in a "wear and tear" setting

  • Pathology

    • Large calcium masses arising in the lower portions of the cusps that protrude into the sinus of Valsalva
    • In contrast to rheumatic aortic stenosis, the free margins of the valves unaffected and not fused
    • Severe left ventricular hypertrophy results from working against the stenotic, high pressure gradient

  • Clinical—dizziness and syncope on exertion from an inability to increase cardiac output

    • Heart failure, is frequent; valve replacement effective

  • Complications—infective endocarditis

- **Carcinoid heart disease**
  - Occurs in 50% of patients with carcinoid syndrome
  - Affects predominantly the right side of the heart
  - Tricuspid and pulmonary valves, chordae, and the adjacent endocardium thickened by white plaques
  - Plaque composed of myxoid, glycosaminoglycan-rich material layered over normal valve tissue
  - Causes tricuspid regurgitation and pulmonary stenosis, resulting in right atrial dilation and right ventricular hypertrophy

- **Endocarditis**
  - Inflammation of the endocardium, including the heart valves
  - Infective and noninfective etiologies

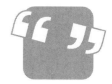

— *Rheumatic valvulitis (noninfective)*
  - Small, 1 to 2 mm, nondestructive, sterile, warty, or verrucous vegetations along the margins of cusps and leaflets

— *Libman-sacks endocarditis (noninfective)*
  - Complication of systemic lupus erythematosus (SLE)
  - Several mm-sized vegetations on the valves along the lines of closure but also elsewhere on the valve surface, valve underside, and atrial or ventricular endocardium

  - Composed of fibrinoid material often with hematoxyphil bodies and a mixed inflammatory infiltrate, overlying an area of edema or fibrinoid necrosis of the valve
  - Differentiated from rheumatic fever by the absence of Aschoff bodies
  - Vegetations seldom embolize

— *Nonbacterial thrombotic endocarditis (NBTE)*
  - Also called marantic endocarditis
  - Occurs in severe catabolic states
  - Variably sized tan vegetations ranging from 1 mm (resembling rheumatic lesions) to several mm and larger (resembling infective endocarditis)
  - Occur along the lines of valve closure, most commonly on the mitral and aortic valves
  - Composed of sterile bland thrombus
  - Can embolize systemically

— *Infective endocarditis*
  - Inflammation of the endocardium caused by an infectious agent
  - Changes in the etiologic organism over the past century reflects antibiotic treatment, IV drug abuse, and immunodeficiency
  - Classification no longer acute or subacute, but by organism
  - Pathology

    - Most commonly the mitral and aortic valves
    - With IV drug abuse affects the right side valves

- Destructive vegetations of varying size, appearance, and location
- Microscopic—fibrin-platelet thrombi with leukocytes and clumps of organisms that produce a localized, necrotizing process in the underlying tissue, sometimes with microabscess formation

- Complications

1. Cardiac

  - Acute valvular insufficiency—destruction and perforation of a valve often precipitates congestive heart failure, most frequent complication
  - Abscess formation and fistulization
  - Suppurative pericarditis

2. Septic embolization and systemic sepsis

  - Cerebral abscess, lung abscess, osteomyelitis, and other septic foci

3. Infectious arteritis and thrombosis

  - Thromboembolic infarction in various organs

4. Circulating immune complexes

  - Glomerular nephritis, some cutaneous lesions
  - Predisposing factors
  - Children—congenital heart disease
  - Adults—mitral valve prolapse and congenital heart disease
  - Congenital heart disease—patent ductus arteriosis, tetralogy of Fallot and ventricular-septal defect
  - Other factors—rheumatic heart disease; IV drug abuse; cardiac prosthesis; indwelling vascular catheters; transient bacteremic-producing manipulations, including dental (brushing teeth, dental visits), genitourinary tract (catheterization), gastrointestinal tract (endoscopy), obstetric (delivery), and other, more obvious, surgical procedures; elderly often calcific aortic stenosis and bicuspid aortic valve; diabetes; alcoholism; immunosuppresion; and neutropenia
  - No predisposition in up to 25% of patients

- Organisms

  - Varies with predisposition; virtually all microorganisms encountered
  - General community—*Streptococcus viridens* (65%) most common overall, with *Staphylococcus aureus* (25%) next
  - IV drug abuse—*S. aureus* (60%), *Streptococcus* organisms and *Pseudomonas aeruginosa*
  - Prosthetic valves—coagulase-negative methacillin-resistant *Staphylococcus* organisms (60%)
  - Immunosuppression and hospital acquired—various nosocomial and exotic organisms

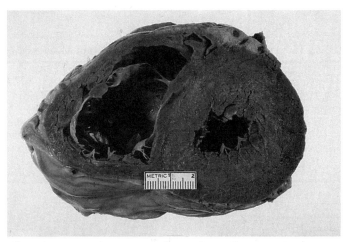

Fig. 12.1 Hypertensive heart disease. The left ventricle is uniformly thickened in a concentric fashion. (*Damjanov I, Linder J: Anderson's pathology, ed 10, vol 1, St Louis, 1996, Mosby.*)

■ Myocardial Disease

● **Hypertrophy and dilation**

• Normal heart—weight up to 350 g, but varies in proportion to body size and sex, left ventricular wall up to 1.5 cm and the right up to 0.5 cm

• Cardiomegaly—enlarged heart, may be from dilation, hypertrophy, or both

— *Cor pulmonale*

• Right-sided cardiac hypertrophy, dilation, and failure caused by primary pulmonary disease

• Most common cause—chronic obstructive lung disease

• Other causes—chronic hypoxemia (kyphoscoliosis, obesity), vascular obliteration (idiopathic [primary], recurrent thromboembolism) or the combination of hypoxemia and vascular obliteration (emphysema, pneumoconiosis)

• Pathology—thickening of the ventricular wall and hypertrophy of myocytes, often with coronary atherosclerosis

— *Hypertensive heart disease*

• Left ventricular hypertrophy caused by chronic systemic hypertension or outflow obstruction from aortic valve disease, aortic stenosis, or coarctation

• Pathology

• Relatively uniform thickening of the left ventricle and septum in a symmetrical, circular fashion described as concentric that decreases the chamber size

• Dilation occurs with heart failure

• Microscopic—marked myocyte hypertrophy with nuclear enlargement and hyperchromasia

• Often accompanied by ischemic atherosclerotic changes (Fig. 12.1)

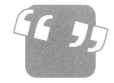

Table 12.1 *Cardiomyopathies*

Type of Cardiomyopathy	Specific Cause (Secondary)	Indirect Cause of Myocardial Dysfunction
Dilated (systolic disorder)	Infective myocarditis; hemochromatosis; chronic anemia; alcohol; adriamycin; sarcoidosis	Ischemic heart disease; valvular heart disease; hypertensive heart disease; congenital heart disease
Hypertrophic (diastolic disorder)	Friedreich's ataxia; glycogen storage disease; infants of diabetic mothers	Hypertensive heart disease, especially in older patients; aortic stenosis
Restrictive (diastolic and systolic disorder)	Amyloidosis; pancardiac radiation-induced fibrosis	Pericardial fibrosis, effusion (constriction)

From Damjanov I, Linder J: *Anderson's pathology*, ed 10, vol 1, St Louis, 1996, Mosby.

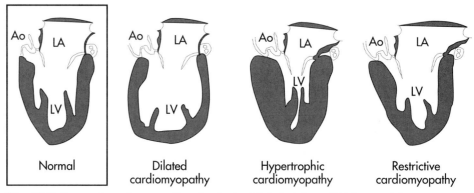

Fig. 12.2 Types of cardiomyopathy. *Ao,* Aorta; *LA,* left atrium; *LV,* left ventricle. (*Damjanov I, Linder J:* Anderson's pathology, *ed 10, vol 2, St Louis, 1996, Mosby.*)

— *Cardiomyopathy*

• Cardiac disease caused by myocardial dysfunction that excludes ischemia, hypertension, valvular disease, congenital abnormalities, and inflammatory disorders

• Functionally divided into dilated, hypertrophic, and restrictive types that may be caused by idiopathic (primary) or known (secondary) causes (Table 12.1 and Fig. 12.2)

— *Dilated cardiomyopathies*

• The most common type of cardiomyopathy, characterized by

• Large, heavy hearts; prominant dilation of the chambers, especially the ventricles; soft, "floppy" ventricular walls

• Progressive loss of cardiac output caused by systolic failure (decreased ejection fraction)

• Severe congestive heart failure

• Intraventricular mural thrombi common, producing pulmonary and systemic thromboembolism

• Microscopic—interstitial fibrosis, myocyte hypertrophy, and hyperplasia

• May represent an end stage of many pathogenic processes, including toxins (anthracyclines, ethanol, cobalt, cyclophosphamide, catecholamines), metabolic (beriberi, scurvy, vitamin E and selenium deficiency, malnutrition, hypo- and hyperkalemia), endocrine disorders (hyper- and hypothyroidism, acromegaly), infectious agents (viral myocarditis), hypertension, pregnancy, and severe persistent anemia

- Secondary causes must be excluded before a diagnosis of idiopathic dilated cardiomyopathy made and few differences between primary and most secondary causes of cardiomyopathy seen pathologically

- Idiopathic cardiomyopathy—has familial association in about 20% of cases

— *Hypertrophic cardiomyopathy*

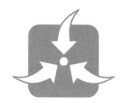

- Uncommon cardiomyopathy characterized by abnormal cardiac hypertrophy inappropriate for the hemodynamic load

- Over ½ cases—familial; numerous point mutations in the beta myosin heavy chain gene and, less commonly, in the troponin T gene identified

- Clinical—asymptomatic, dyspnea on exertion, angina and heart failure or sudden death in young adults with exertion

- Pathology

    - Enlarged heart
    - Predominantly left ventricular hypertrophy that is often asymmetrical with a septal to free wall ratio of greater than 1.5
    - Atria—may be dilated
    - Microscopic—myocytes are arranged in a random fashion with bundles at right angles rather than the normal parallel

— *Restrictive cardiomyopathy*

- Uncommon cardiomyopathy characterized by diminished diastolic filling sometimes accompanied by decreased myocardial contractility (systolic defect) caused by endocardial or myocardial abnormalities

- Interstitial infiltration—idiopathic fibrosis, amyloidosis, sarcoidosis (restrictive and dilated), carcinoma, radiation

- Endomyocardial disease—endomyocardial fibrosis, endomyocardial fibroelastosis

- Storage diseases—hemochromatosis (may be restrictive or dilated), glycogenosis, mucopolysaccharidosis, hemochromatosis

- Idiopathic or primary cases show only interstitial fibrosis

- Clinical—progressive heart failure

● **Endomyocardial fibrosis**

- Uncommon disorder characterized by restrictive thickening of the endocardium

- Etiology thought to be persistent hypereosinophilia with eosinophils damaging the endocardium

- In tropical regions, eosinophilia usually associated with parasitic infections; in Western nations, a greater variety of causes seen, including parasites, vasculitis, hypersensitivity, myeloproliferative disorders, and idiopathic (Löffler's syndrome)

- Acute—infiltration of the endocardium and subendocardium by eosinophils and myocardial necrosis and vascular damage
- Mural thrombi—may form and embolize
- Late stages—marked fibrosis and thickening of the endocardium with resulting valvular retraction-incompetence and restrictive cardiomyopathy

● Myocarditis

- An inflammation of the myocardium with leukocyte infiltration, myocyte degeneration, and necrosis in the absence of ischemia
- Clinical—sudden death and/or acute heart failure at any age

— *Viral myocarditis*

- Most cases of myocarditis presumed viral in origin, although specific identification of a virus is almost always lacking
- Symptoms—may begin days to weeks after an infection
- Most recover, very few progress to dilated cardiomyopathy
- Suspect pathogens—echo virus, coxsackievirus, influenza virus, or other viruses
- Viral cultures from heart biopsies usually negative, but polymerase chain reaction and electron microscopy may be positive
- Direct viral effects or immunologic injury most likely mechanisms of damage
- Pathology

  - Enlarged hearts with soft, flabby myocardium and dilated chambers
  - Variable infiltrate of lymphocytes (usually T cells) and monocytes with necrosis of adjacent individual myocytes

— *Other infectious myocarditis*

- Bacteria—brucellosis, diphtheria (toxin), meningococcus, borellia (Lyme disease)
- Chlamydia—psittacosis
- Chagas' disease—most common cause of myocarditis in South America caused by *Trypanosoma cruzi*

— *Hypersensitivity myocarditis*

- Drugs—methlydopa, sulfonamides, others
- Infiltrate—often includes eosinophils

— *Giant cell myocarditis*

- Rare disorder characterized by an infiltrate of lymphocytes, monocytes, plasma cells, eosinophils, and multinucleate giant cells
- Unknown etiology, but may be seen with SLE, thymoma, and thyrotoxicosis

● Cardiac tumors

- Primary tumors much less common than metastasis

— *Myxoma*

- Most common primary tumor, benign
- Sporadic in adults, but may be familial in younger patients

- Clinical—mitral valve dysfunction, embolic phenomena or elevated interleukin (IL)-6 levels producing fever, weight loss, and increased immunoglobulin levels
    - Pathology

        - Polypoid mass arising in the left atrium
        - Lobulated, glistening, and gelatenous with areas of hemorrhage
        - Microscopic—myoxma cells (delicate stellate or polygonal cells with bland nuclei) in an abundant proteoglycan-rich myxoid matrix

— *Rhabdomyoma*

    - Very rare, but the most common primary cardiac tumor of infants and children
        - May be hamartomas; up to ½ associated with tuberous sclerosis
    - Most—multifocal and microscopically composed of "spider" cells with central nuclei and abundant vacuolated cytoplasm (caused by glycogen) in which cytoplasmic strands extend to the cell margins as the spider legs

- **Ischemic heart disease**

    - Heart disease caused by inadequate blood flow to meet myocardial demands
    - Leading cause of death in North America
    - Coronary artery atherosclerosis of the epicardial arteries—overwhelmingly the most common etiology
    - Risk factors for atherosclerosis

        - Major factors—smoking, elevated plasma lipid levels, hypertension, family history, and diabetes
        - Other factors—obesity, male sex, increasing age, and lack of regular exercise

    - Clinical—angina, sudden death, myocardial infarction, and chronic ischemic heart disease

— *Angina*

    - Ischemic myocardial pain in the absence of infarction
    - Stable exertional type

        - Predictable pain after a constant amount of exertion that has remained unchanged for long periods
        - Morphology—fixed point stenosis of one or more coronary arteries that limits the increased blood flow normally seen with exercise

    - Unstable angina

        - Less predictable, episodic pain that may occur at rest and increase in frequency over time
        - High risk for myocardial infarction
        - Morphology—nonocculsive coronary artery thrombosis overlying a disrupted plaque

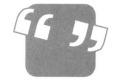

- Symptoms caused by distal embolization of platelet aggregates
- Variant or Prinzmental's angina
  - A form of unstable angina occurring at rest but stable over time
  - Morphology—a segment of usually mild coronary atherosclerosis associated with vasospasm on coronary angiography
— *Sudden death*
  - Primarily caused by ventricular fibrillation
  - Preexisting ischemic heart disease common, and may be first symptom
  - Occurs with or without thrombosis and infarction
  - ½ of patients successfully resuscitated from sudden ventricular fibrillation—do not subsequently show a myocardial infarction
— *Acute myocardial infarction*
  - An area of ischemic myocardial necrosis
— *Causes and modulators of myocardial ischemia*
  Reduction of blood flow
  - Atherosclerosis
    - Stenosis is considered significant when the diameter of the vessel is reduced more than 75%.
    - Within the first hour, 90% of patients with infarcts have complete thrombotic occlusion of the regional coronary artery by angiography (left anterior decending—anterior and septal left ventricle [LV]; circumflex—lateral LV wall and right coronary—posterior LV wall and septum).
    - At 4 to 24 hours 50% to 70% of arteries will be patent after spontaneous fibrinolysis.
  - Collateral coronary flow
    - Sudden occlusion of coronary arteries results in infarction; however, gradual occlusion allows expansion of the normal anastamosis from a nonoccluded coronary vessel to compensate for the reduced flow.
    - This explains seemingly paradoxical infarcts in the distribution of one coronary artery when the acute thrombosis is identified in another.
  Other causes of reduced coronary artery blood flow
  - Thromboembolism—rare, usually arising from thrombi in the heart
  - Coronary arteritis—polyarteritis in adults and Kawasaki Syndrome in children
  - Congenital anomalies, coronary artery dissection, aortic dissection
  General decrease in oxygen delivery
  - Anemia, carbon monoxide or carbon dioxide exposure
  - Shock—usually results in subendocardial infarction

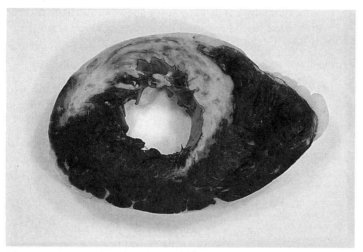

Fig. 12.3 Acute myocardial infarction. The special stains show loss of cardiac enzymes (pale areas) in the anterior and septal region, corresponding to the distribution of an occluded left anterior descending coronary artery. (*Damjanov I, Linder J:* Anderson's pathology, *ed 10, vol 2, St Louis, 1996, Mosby.*)

Increased oxygen requirements

- Tachycardia, pregnancy, valvular disease, hypertension

— *Pathology*

- Two basic types of infarcts—transmural and subendocardial
- **Transmural infarctions**—involve the full thickness of the myocardium

    - Result from acute thrombotic obstruction of a coronary artery and occur in that artery's distribution (modified by collateral flow)

- **Subendocardial infarctions**—involve the inner portion of the left ventricle in a circumferential pattern

    - Result of generalized myocardial hypoperfusion or hypoxemia and not associated with coronary thrombosis

- Patchy focal myocardial necrosis—seen in a number of conditions, including catecholamine excess, viral illness, and other toxins, but not considered part of myocardial infarction
- Ischemic necrosis—does not begin until about 20 to 40 minutes after blood flow has stopped
- If reperfusion occurs within this time, complete recovery possible, but delays result in some necrosis

— *Gross changes*

- 12 to 24 hours—infarcted area appears slightly paler (with special whole tissue staining for dehydrogenase depletion, the infarcted zone may be highlighted earlier) (Fig. 12.3)
    - 24 to 48 hours—pallor, slightly yellow
    - 3 to 10 days—soft, yellow zone with later hyperemic rimming,

becomes maximal at 10 days, may show hemorrhage if thrombolysis has occurred, weakest period for myocardial wall strength

> • Weeks to months—gradual replacement from outside in by pale tan fibrosis; age indeterminate after scarring is complete

— *Light microscopic changes*

12 to 24 hours—early neutrophilic infiltration followed by increased eosinophilia of the myocytes (early coagulative necrosis)

> • Thin "wavy" fibers—change seen in adjacent myocardium from stretching of the myocytes caused by akinesis of the infarcted area
> • Contraction band necrosis—also called *reperfusion injury*
>> • Describes the thick hypereosinophilic bands of hypercontracted sarcomeres and degenerate proteins that cross the dead myocytes at right angles
>> • Seen at the edges of infarcts, with fibrinolytic therapy of coronary thrombosis and bypass grafting

24 to 72 hours—neutrophilic infiltration peaks, progression of coagulative necrosis with loss of cross striations and nuclei by about 72 hours

3 to 7 days—neutrophils undergo karryorhexis and disappear, macrophage phagocytosis of myofibers, early repair response with neovascularization, proliferation of fibroblasts, and neocollagen deposition beginning at the infarct edges

7 to 21 days—repair process shifts to collagenization as neovascularization and inflammatory infiltrates resolve

3 weeks onward—the fibrosis becomes more dense, the cellarity diminishes, and most debris is removed

Age of the scars—indeterminate; scars may be the only finding at autopsy of previous silent infarcts that may account for ¼ of all nonfatal infarcts

— *Complications of infarcts*

> • Dysrhythmia (most frequent), cardiogenic shock, extension of infarction, myocardial wall rupture (highest risk 2 to 7 days postinfarction), papillary muscle rupture, aneurysm, mural thrombosis and embolism, and pericarditis
> • Dressler's (postmyocardial infarction) syndrome—delayed pericarditis occuring 2 weeks to 3 months after infarction or open heart surgery

■ Pericardial Disease

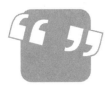

• Pericardial effusion—increased fluid in the pericardial sac greater than the usual 50 ml

> • Serous effusion—transudate with low protein and cell count
> • Chylous effusion—lymphocyte and fat rich (chylomicrons) from the thoracic duct
> • Cardiac tamponade—diminished cardiac filling caused by pressure of pericardial fluid, producing low cardiac output that may be fatal in acute cases

● Pericarditis

> • Inflammation of the pericardium

- Acute—multiple etiologies, including autoimmune, viral infection, bacterial infection, myocarditis, myocardial infarction, uremia, radiation, and asbestosis

    - May be fibrinous, purulent, or hemorrhagic

    - Constrictive—adherent, fibrotic process that restricts filling and increases venous pressure, leading to low output, systemic edema, and ascites

        - Occurs after purulent pericarditis, tuberculous pericarditis (common in underdeveloped countries), radiation, surgery, or idiopathically (probably postviral, common in Western world)

■ Congenital Heart Disease (CHD)

- Developmental abnormalities of the cardiovascular system present at birth likely caused by environmental or inherited factors
- About 1% of births (excluding the 1% to 2% of the population with bi-cuspid aortic valves)
- Mitral valve prolapse—occurs in about 5% to 10% of the population but generally not present at birth
- Hereditary

    - Multifactorial—increased risk in siblings and offspring of individuals with CHD, some single gene and chromosomal abnormalities (Down syndrome, trisomies, and Turner's syndrome)

- Environmental

    - Exposure to teratogens
    - Alcohol, amphetamines, chemotherapy, anticonvulsants, hormones, thalidomide, retinoic acid
    - Congenital infections—rubella syndrome
    - Other diseases—diabetes, SLE, phenylketonuria

- Ventricular septal defects—account for ⅓ of all lesions noted at birth
- An additional ⅓—atrial septal defects, patent ductal artery (ductus arteriosis), pulmonary stenosis, and tetralogy of Fallot

● Ventricular septal defect (VSD)

- Openings in the ventricular septum that allow blood to flow from the higher pressure left ventricle to the right
- Most common CHD
- Extracardiac malformations present in 25% of cases
- Membranous VSDs—have a valve forming one of the borders and are most common type of VSD (80%)
- Muscular VSDs—may be more common but tend to close spontaneously
- Without closure

    - Large defects—ventricular overload and heart failure
    - Smaller defects—pulmonary hypertension and plexogenic pulmonary vascular disease may develop

- Clinical—large defects need closure by surgical patching, increased risk of endocarditis

- **Atrial septal defects (ASD)**
  - Abnormal communication between left and right atrium (not including the common probe patency of the fossa ovalis found at 25% of autopsies)
  - A defect at the fossa ovalis (ostium secundum type of ASD)—the most common (90%) with sinus venosus and primum types less common
  - Clinical—pulmonary hypertension (10%) and heart failure (10%) develop less rapidly than in VSD; ASD—one of the most common congenital heart disorders to present in adults (age 30 years)
  - Complications—parodoxical embolism and endocarditis

- **Atrioventricular septal defect (AVSD)**
  - A less common defect caused by a persistent common atrioventricular canal (endocardial cushion defect)
  - Without involvement of the valve leaflets results in primum type of ASD
  - ⅓ of AVSDs have Down syndrome or about 20% of all those with Down syndrome have AVSD

- **Patent ductus arteriosus (patent ductal artery, PDA)**
  - Failure of the fetal pulmonary blood shunt to close off in response to the increased arterial oxygen content after birth
  - Common in rubella syndrome, in preterm births (usually closes spontaneously), and in hypoxemic neonates
  - After birth—shunt becomes left to right with exposure of the pulmonary vasculature to both increased flow and increased pressure
  - Large shunts—lead to early left heart hypertrophy and failure, smaller shunt to pulmonary hypertension
  - Complications—increased risk of endocarditis
  - Patency—prostaglandin dependent
    - Prostaglandin inhibitors can close a PDA in premature infants.
    - PGE_2 can keep a PDA open for infants that need the shunt to survive, such as complete transposition of the great arteries.

- **Truncus arteriosis (persistent truncal artery)**
  - Failure of the common single great artery to be divided into the aorta, the pulmonary arteries, and coronary arteries
  - Must occur with a VSD
  - May be familial or associated with DiGeorge syndrome
  - Untreated—90% die in the first year from pneumonia or heart failure, with the remainder as children or young adults from pulmonary hypertension

- **Anomalous pulmonary venous connection (drainage)**
  - Pulmonary veins—lack direct connection to the left atrium
  - May be partial, involving only some of the veins, or complete with no direct connections
  - Complete must have a patent foramen ovale or an ASD to survive

- **Tetralogy of Fallot**
  - Consists of subpulmonary stenosis, ventricular septal defect, overriding aorta, and right ventricular hypertrophy

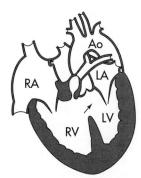

Fig. 12.4 Classic tetralogy of Fallot. There is a ventricular septal defect, an overriding aorta, right ventricular hypertrophy, and stenosis of the pulmonary outflow. *Ao,* Aorta; *RA,* right atrium; *LA,* left atrium; *RV,* right ventricle; *LV,* left ventricle. (*Damjanov I, Linder J:* Anderson's pathology, *ed 10, vol 2, St Louis, 1996, Mosby.*)

- Additional cardiac abnormalities common
- Most common type of congenital cyanotic heart disease
- Pulmonary stenosis and the VSD—produce a right-to-left shunt with peripheral cyanosis
- Clinical—about 90% long-term survival with surgical correction

  - Mortality about 95% uncorrected at 40 years

- Complications—heart failure, endocarditis, brain abscess, and cerebral thrombosis associated with secondary polycythemia (Fig. 12.4)

● **Complete transposition of the great arteries**
- Aorta connected to the right ventricle and pulomonary artery to the left ventricle with normal atrioventricular connections
- Causes cyanotic heart disease in the neonate with survival dependent on the presence of a right-to-left shunt from a PDA, ASD, or a VSD
- Clinical—90% 5-year survival with surgical correction, 90% mortality at 1 year if left uncorrected

● **Coarctation of the aorta**
- Localized constriction of the aortic arch usually opposite the site of the ductal artery
- Common in males but also seen in Turner's syndrome
- Often with bicuspid aortic valve, PDA, and other anomalies
- Clinical—produces a marked difference between arm and leg blood pressures

  - Dilation of subcostal arteries from increased collateral flow that causes the radiologic sign of notched ribs

- Concentric left ventricle hypertrophy and right ventricle hypertrophy if there is a patent ductal artery
- Complications—cystic medial necrosis of the aorta with dissection, infectious endocarditis, rupture of congenital cerebral aneurysm, and heart failure

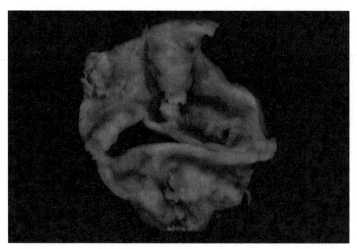

Fig. 12.5 Bicuspid aortic valve. Only two valve cusps are present, and the valve is stenotic from calcification. (*Damjanov I, Linder J: Anderson's pathology, ed 10, vol 2, St Louis, 1996, Mosby.*)

- Mortality as high as 75% by age 45 years
- **Bicuspid aortic valve**
  - 1% to 2% of population
  - Males more frequent
  - Usually an isolated anomaly
  - Clinical—long asymptomatic phase; endocarditis common before the age of 40 years
  - Complications—calcification with stenosis and/or regurgitation most common (Fig. 12.5), acute dissection because of weakened aortic arch showing dilation and cystic medial degeneration

Multiple Choice
Review Questions

1. A 20-year-old male has a brachial artery blood pressure of 200/140 mm Hg but blood pressure measured at the anterior tibial artery is 90/50. The best explanation is which of the following?

   a. Tetralogy of Fallot
   b. Ventricular septal defect
   c. Coarctation of the aorta
   d. Patent ductus arteriosus
   e. Atrial septal defect ostium secundum type

2. A common complication in this patient would include all *except* which of the following?

   a. Infective endarteritis
   b. Cerebral hemorrhage
   c. Congestive heart failure
   d. Cystic medial necrosis of the aorta
   e. Cyanosis

3. The most common complication of myocardial infarction is which of the following?

   a. Ventricular rupture
   b. Pericardial tamponade
   c. Ventricular aneurysm
   d. Pulmonary embolism
   e. Dysrhythmia

4. The organism most frequently causing endocarditis in the general community is which of the following?

   a. *Streptococcus pyogenes*
   b. *Streptococcus viridans*
   c. *Pseudomonas aeruginosa*
   d. *Klebsiella pneumoniae*
   e. *Candida albicans*

5. Tetralogy of Fallot consists of which of the following?

   a. Subpulmonary stenosis, ventricular septal defect, overriding aorta, and right ventricular hypertrophy
   b. Subpulmonary stenosis, ventricular septal defect, overriding aorta, and left ventricular hypertrophy
   c. Aortic stenosis, ventricular septal defect, overriding aorta, and right ventricular hypertrophy
   d. Subpulmonary stenosis, atrial septal defect, overriding aorta, and right ventricular hypertrophy
   e. Subpulmonary stenosis, ventricular septal defect, patent ductal artery, and right ventricular hypertrophy

Chapter 13

Lung

■ **Vascular-Hemodynamic Disorders Affecting the Lung**

● Pulmonary emboli

• *Pulmonary emboli* are important because they can occlude vessels in the pulmonary arterial system and cause pulmonary infarction.

• *The vast majority of clinically encountered pulmonary emboli are thromboemboli that arise in deep leg veins (calf, femoral, iliac, popliteal) passing through the venous circulation and right side of the heart to become lodged in the pulmonary vasculature (Fig. 13.1 and Box 13.1).*

• *Other types of embolic material* (i.e., air, amniotic fluid, fat) *may also constitute pulmonary emboli.*

• *Note:* Pulmonary infarction is seen in only about 10% of thromboemboli patients because of the lung's dual arterial blood supply (pulmonary arterial system and the bronchial arteries arising from the aorta).

- Recurrent thromboemboli may damage pulmonary arterial system and lead to pulmonary hypertension and, eventually, right sided heart failure.

- *Massive* pulmonary thromboemboli, especially those involving the pulmonary artery bifurcation point (saddle embolus), can cause acute right sided heart failure and sudden death.

— *Clinical facts*

• *Pulmonary thromboembolism constitutes the most common cause of preventable death in hospitalized patients.*

• Diagnosis is often exceedingly difficult, because of relative nonspecificity of patient's signs and symptoms.

• *Most cases of pulmonary thromboembolism are clinically asymptomatic.*

• Clinical presentation depends upon how extensive the pulmonary arterial blockage is and the time course during which this process occurred.

- If 60% or more of the pulmonary arterial blood flow is halted, the heart is no longer able to pump blood through the lungs and rapid death ensues *(massive pulmonary embolus).*

- When midsized pulmonary arteries are occluded, one has a significant pulmonary embolic event, and patients typically present with dyspnea, fever, tachycardia, chest pain and sometimes even hemoptysis *(major pulmonary embolus).*

- When small pulmonary arterial vessels are occluded by thromboemboli, one has *minor pulmonary embolism* and patients may not even have any symptoms at all.

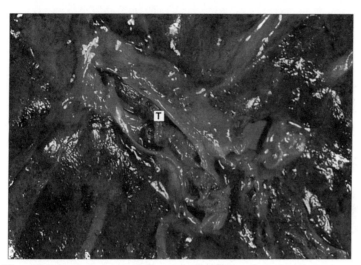

Fig. 13.1 Pulmonary thromboembolus. The main pulmonary artery is occluded by a large thromboembolus (T). *(From Stevens A, Lowe J: Pathology, London, 1995, Times Mirror International.)*

Box 13.1

CLINICAL CONDITIONS
PREDISPOSING TO LEG VEIN THROMBOSIS

Thrombosis arising in deep leg veins may be completely asymptomatic or may cause mild pain and tenderness in the muscles, sometimes with development of ankle edema.

Clinical situations predisposing to development of deep leg vein thrombosis are:
- Immobility and bed rest
- Postoperative period
- Pregnancy and postpartum period
- Oral contraceptive therapy with high-estrogen preparations
- Nephrotic syndrome
- Severe burns
- Trauma
- Cardiac failure
- Disseminated malignancy

In many of these situations it is clinical practice to give prophylactic treatment with heparin to prevent development of thrombosis, combined with physiotherapy to the legs.

From Stevens A, Lowe J: *Pathology,* London, 1995, Times Mirror International.

- Two main, long-range consequences of pulmonary thromboembolism are *increased pulmonary* arterial pressure (which taxes the right heart) and lung ischemia in ventilated (aerated) areas not being perfused with blood.

- *Treatment* is with fibrinolytic agents (tissue plasminogen activator, streptokinase) and/or heparin, depending upon clinical circumstances.

● Pulmonary edema

   • *Pulmonary edema* is defined as increased fluid within alveolar walls and, often, within the alveolar spaces themselves.

   • *Most common cause of pulmonary edema is left sided heart failure;* this is because of an increase in "back pressure" within alveolar capillaries.

   • In severe cases of pulmonary edema, alveolar capillaries rupture and spill red blood cells (RBCs) into alveolar spaces.

      • The resultant hemoglobin released is phagocytosed by macrophages, which accumulate an iron-containing, pigmented protein known as hemosiderin.

      • These hemosiderin-laden macrophages are dubbed "heart failure cells."

   • *Note:* Pulmonary edema is also a prominent feature of adult respiratory distress syndrome (ARDS); for a discussion of this entity, see restrictive lung diseases.

● Pulmonary hypertension

   • *Pulmonary hypertension* is increased pulmonary arterial pressure; this brings about irreversible pulmonary arterial vessel wall changes, thereby stressing the right side of the heart and causing *cor pulmonale* (right heart enlargement and failure).

   — *Causes of pulmonary hypertension*

      • Chronic obstructive airway disease (especially chronic bronchitis and emphysema)

      • Histologically, pulmonary arterial vessel wall medial hypertrophy and intimal proliferation

● Pulmonary vasculitis (angiitis)

   • Inflammation of pulmonary vessel walls, often with thrombosis and pulmonary necrosis (example, Wegener's granulomatosis); for a more complete review, see Blood Vessels chapter.

■ **Infective Diseases of the Lung** A commonly encountered category of disease in clinical medicine

● Infection of bronchi and bronchioles

   • *Most often caused by viruses* (especially respiratory syncytial virus, influenza virus, adenovirus)

   • Bacteria also may be culprit here

● Pneumonia

   • Defined as *infective* lung inflammation and consequent consolidation (firmness caused by filling up of alveolar spaces by inflammatory materials, especially neutrophils)

      • In *bronchopneumonia,* primary infection occurs in the *bronchi* and then spreads to adjacent alveoli; at least initially, consolidation is patchy within affected lung tissue.

      • In *lobar pneumonia,* the offending organisms gain entry to distal air spaces without a preceding bronchial colonization phase. There is a rapid spread of infection to involve the *entire pulmonary lobe.* Histologically, as in the appearance for bronchopneumonia, this le-

Table 13.1 *Viral Infections of the Lower Respiratory Tract*

Virus	Nucleic Acid	Family	Tracheo-bronchitis	Bronchi-olitis	Interstitial Pneumonia	Focal Necrosis	Intranuclear Inclusion	Cytoplasmic Inclusion
Influenza	RNA	Orthomyxoviridae	+	+	+	–	–	–
Parainfluenza	RNA	Paramyxoviridae	+	+	+	–	–	+
Measles	RNA	Paramyxoviridae	+	+	+	–	+	+
Respiratory syncytial virus	RNA	Paramyxoviridae	+	+	+	–	–	+
Adenovirus	DNA	Adenoviridae	+	+	+	–	+	–
Herpes simplex	DNA	Herpetoviridae	+	+	+	+	+	–
Varicella-zoster virus	DNA	Herpetoviridae	+	+	+	+	+	–
Cytomegalo-virus	DNA	Herpetoviridae	–	+	+	+	+	+

From Damjanov I, Linder J: *Anderson's pathology,* ed 10, vol 1, St Louis, 1996, Mosby.

sion features alveolar spaces filled with exudate material (especially neutrophils).

— *Pneumonia facts*

• *The most common cause of community-acquired pneumonia is Streptococcus pneumoniae* (accounts for 35% of all cases).

• *Haemophilus influenzae infection is a common cause of community-acquired pneumonia* (accounting for about 10% of all cases) and is particularly prevalent among children, patients over 60 years of age, and those with underlying chronic obstructive airway disease (i.e., chronic bronchitis and emphysema).

• *Atypical (walking) pneumonia,* caused by infection with *Mycoplasma pneumoniae* (Eaton agent) or *Chlamydia pneumoniae,* accounts for 10% of all community-acquired pneumonia.

  • *Note:* This type of pneumonia is histologically characterized by chronic inflammatory cell infiltrates (lymphocytes, monocytes) within alveolar walls rather than neutrophils within alveolar spaces.

• *Viral pneumonia* accounts for about 10% of community-acquired pneumonias; their further significance, however, is related to the fact that these infections are often complicated by the development of a bacterial "superinfection," commonly *Staphylococcus aureus,* which is a pyogenic (pus-producing) organism notorious for causing abscess formation.

  • *Key point:* Viral pathogens cause an interstitial pneumonia wherein the inflammatory cells are mainly lymphocytes, plasma cells, and monocytes situated in alveolar septae; furthermore, some severe viral pneumonias are associated with alveolar lining cell damage and the clinical appearance of ARDS. Table 13.1 lists pertinent viral infections of the lung.

• In stark contradistinction to the case for hospital-acquired pneumonia, non-Haemophilus gram-*negative bacilli bacteria account for approximately 5% of community-acquired pneumonia;* the organisms most commonly responsible are *Klebsiella pneumoniae* and *Legionella pneumophilia.*

- 30% of community-acquired pneumonia patients have negative microbiologic cultures, usually because of prior antibiotic administration.

- Hospital-acquired (nosocomial) pneumonia is *most commonly caused by gram-negative bacilli bacteria* (60% of nosocomial pneumonia), especially *Escherichia coli, Klebsiella pneumoniae,* and *Pseudomonas, Proteus,* and *Serratia* organisms.

- Certain hospital locales may also harbor *Legionella pneumophila* organisms (usually within standing water supplies).

- *Aspiration pneumonia* is often seen as a result of regurgitation of gastric contents during loss of consciousness (or in stroke patients).

  - *Key points:* Gastric acid causes a chemical pneumonitis that can lead to ARDS; furthermore, organisms causing pneumonia in these patients often include anaerobes (especially *Fusobacterium* and *Bacteroides* organisms). *In hospitalized patients with aspiration pneumonia, Staphylococcus aureus and gram-negative bacilli are common infecting pathogens.*

- *Fungal pneumonia* is seen in two basic populations: immunocompromised patients, and otherwise healthy patients exposed to an agent indigenous to a particular area.

- *Aspergillus* species are usually *opportunistic pathogens notorious for causing extensive lung necrosis and infarction,* in large measure related to their tendency toward invading blood vessel walls and initiating thrombosis of these infected vessels.

- *Blastomycosis, histoplasmosis, and coccidioidomycosis are fungal organisms that cause disease in otherwise healthy individuals (as well as in those who are immunocompromised).*

— *Regarding pneumonias in the immunocompromised patient population*

- "Routine" pneumonia is more severe than in immunocompetent patients with the same pathogen.

- One commonly sees *Mycobacterium tuberculosis* and *Mycobacterium avium-intracellulare* infections in immunocompromised patients.

- Immunocompromised patients have a marked vulnerability for viral (especially cytomegalovirus [CMV] and herpes simplex) and fungal pathogens (especially *Aspergillus* and *Candida* organisms).

— *Pneumocystis carinii pneumonia*

- *An unusual type of pneumonia until the advent of the AIDS epidemic*

- Nearly ⅔ of all AIDS patients have this infection at some point during the course of their disease

- Look for dyspnea, fever, and chest x-ray film findings of expanding, bilateral pulmonary infiltrates

- Histologically, an accumulation of foamy material within alveolar spaces and a minimal lymphoplasmacytic infiltrate within the pulmonary interstitium; cysts of this organism may be demonstrated within the intraalveolar foamy material (these cysts are 5 microns in diameter and are well demonstrated by Gomori's methenamine silver stain) (Fig. 13.2)

- Treatment—Bactrim

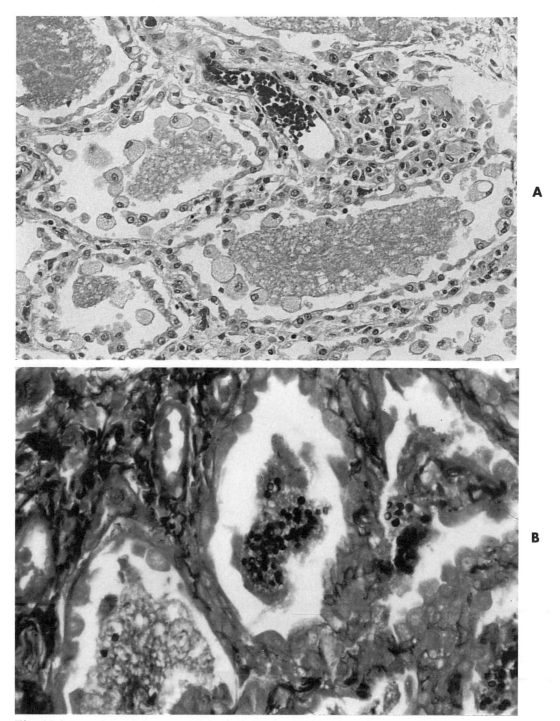

Fig. 13.2 *Pneumocystis carinii* pneumonia. **A,** Pulmonary alveoli contain a foamy material.
B, Within this foamy exudate are numerous *Pneumocystis carinii* cysts as demonstrated by this
Gomori-methenamine silver stain. (*A from Danjanov I, Linder J:* Anderson's pathology, *ed 10, St Louis, 1996, Mosby.*)

Box 13.2

> ### PATHOGENESIS OF BRONCHIECTASIS
>
> Bronchiectasis is predisposed by two main factors:
> **Interference with drainage of bronchial secretions**
> - Obstruction of proximal airway, e.g., tumor, foreign body
> - Abnormality in bronchial mucus viscosity, e.g., cystic fibrosis
> - Immotile cilia syndrome in which cilia are abnormal, leading to stagnation of secretions
>
> **Recurrent and persistent infection weakening bronchial walls**
> - Predisposed to by retention of secretions (as above)
> - Immunodeficiency states, particularly hypogammaglobulinemia
>
> In many cases in adults, no cause can be found (**idiopathic bronchiectasis**)

From Stevens A, Lowe J: *Pathology,* London, 1995, Times Mirror International.

- *Lung abscesses*—almost always caused by bacterial, fungal, or parasitic infection, complicating aspiration pneumonia, and bronchiectasis (see following); *one does not see abscess formation in uncomplicated viral infection*

  - Look for a cavity containing pus and surrounded by a rind of fibrous tissue
  - Abscess—may rupture into pleural space (to give empyema and pneumothorax [free air in pleural cavity]), erode into a blood vessel and produce a clinically significant bleed, and cause septicemia (and possibly lead to other, nonpulmonary sites of infection and abscess formation)

- *Bronchiectasis—abnormal dilation of a main bronchus*

  - Present with cough, hemoptysis, and abundant sputum expectoration
  - Most common site—base of lungs
  - Pathogenesis (Box 13.2)

■ **Chronic Obstructive Airways Disease (COAD), Also Called Chronic Obstructive Pulmonary Disease (COPD)**

- COAD consists of three *major entities* characterized by chronic reduction in the flow of air into and/or out of the lungs.
- This can happen from one of two basic mechanisms.

  - Airway narrowing with resultant increased resistance to airflow—*asthma and chronic bronchitis*
  - Reduction of outflow pressure caused by loss of lung's elastic recoil—*emphysema*

● Asthma

  - Most common cause of chronic reversible breathlessness, wheezing and coughing in the United States; 10% of children and 5% of adults have asthma and its incidence is on the *increase* in the United States
    - *Key lesions*—bronchospasm and mucus plugging of airways

- Known initiators of asthmatic attacks

  - Allergies
  - Infection (especially viral)
  - Irritating gases
  - Stress
  - Exercise
  - Certain drugs

● **Chronic bronchitis**

  - Associated with cigarette use
  - A clinically defined entity (sputum producing cough for at least 3 months/year over 2 consecutive years)
  - *Key lesion*—mucus plugging and airway luminal narrowing

● **Emphysema**

  - Associated with cigarette use
  - Defined as permanent dilation of the distal airspaces caused by the loss of tissue in the absence of scarring; affected structures are the respiratory bronchioles, alveolar ducts, and alveolar sacs; two major types: centriacinar—dilation of respiratory bronchioles; and panacinar—dilation of respiratory ducts, aveolar ducts, and alveoli

    - *Key lesions*—loss of elastic recoil and reduction in surface area available for gas exchange
    - Pathogenetic mechanisms—tissue destruction mediated by extracellular proteases, secreted by inflammatory cells, and absence/inactivation of protease inhibitors (such as seen in alpha$_1$-antitrypsin deficiency)

● **Summary points on COAD**

  - Components of asthma, chronic bronchitis, and emphysema are frequently seen together in the same patient.
  - Long-standing COAD can result in pulmonary hypertension and right sided heart failure (cor pulmonale).

■ **Restrictive Lung Disease**

- Characterized by reduction in lung compliance, that is, the ability of the lungs to expand and fill with air during each inspiratory (ventilatory) action
- *Key lesion*—abnormally rigid alveolar walls and interstitium, thereby necessitating a great deal of work to attempt inflation of the lungs; edema and fibrosis are the two main causes of restrictive lung disease, and both can result from alveolar wall damage
  - *Three stages of lung reaction in alveolar wall damage*

    - Alveoli fill with protein-rich exudate and RBCs; some of this protein is fibrin, which covers the inner surface of the alveolus to produce a *hyaline membrane.*
    - Interstitial edema and inflammation
    - Interstitial fibrosis

● **Adult respiratory distress syndrome (ARDS)**

  - An archetypal example of a disease involving alveolar wall damage
  - Has many potential intiating events (Box 13.3)

Box 13.3

CAUSES OF DIFFUSE ALVEOLAR DAMAGE

Infections
Viral
Extrathoracic sepsis

Trauma
Fat embolism
Lung contusion

Aspiration
Gastric acid
Near-drowning
Hydrocarbon fluids

Toxic Inhalants
Oxygen
Smoke
War gases
Oxides of nitrogen
Metal fumes
Other

Drugs and Toxins
Narcotics
Paraquat
Salicylates

Other
Radiation
Pancreatitis
Transfusion, cardiopulmonary bypass, etc.

From Damjanov I, Linder J: *Anderson's pathology,* ed 10, vol 1, St Louis, 1996, Mosby.

- *Clinical features of ARDS*
  - Precipitating event
  - Refractory hypoxemia (Pa_{O_2} less than 80 mm Hg on greater than 40% inspired oxygen)
  - Bilateral diffuse pulmonary infiltrates on chest x-ray film
  - Abnormally rigid lungs with reduced compliance (grossly, these lungs are heavy and beefy red)
- Summary of pathophysiology and clinical outcomes for ARDS (Fig. 13.3)
- **Chronic interstitial lung disorders**
  - These disorders have in common the fact that they involve inflammation centered in the alveolar walls.
  - A diverse group of entities may result in chronic interstitial lung disease.
  — *Usual interstitial pneumonitis (UIP)*
      - Idiopathic disorder seen mainly in patients over 50 years of age
      - May progress to "honeycomb" lung (see below)

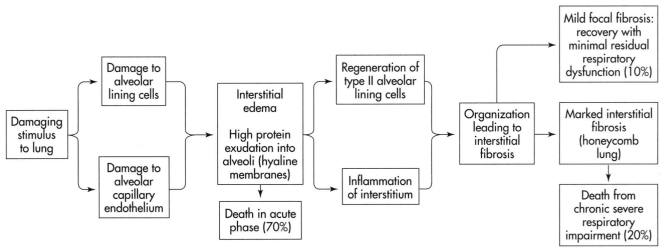

Fig. 13.3 Genesis and clinical scenarios in Adult Respiratory Distress Syndrome. *(From Stevens A, Lowe J:* Pathology, *London, 1995, Times Mirror International.)*

- Histologically, fibrosis of lung interstitial tissues

— *Dust-related fibrosis (pneumoconiosis)*

- Pneumoconiosis refers to lung disease caused by dust inhalation.
- Mostly, this involves inhalation of mineral dusts.
- Normally, dust particles are either physically removed from the respiratory tree (by being coughed out) or ingested by pulmonary macrophages.
- *However, certain inhaled material is toxic to macrophages, and this incites a cytokine-mediated inflammatory response that causes damage to lung tissue and, eventually, pulmonary fibrosis.*
- Main dusts associated with pulmonary fibrosis are silicates, iron oxide, and coal.

"Prototype" pneumoconiosis (silicosis)

- This is caused by inhalation of quartz (silicon dioxide) dust.
- It is seen in quarry, foundry, masonary, mining, and tunnel workers.
- Heavy, acute exposures can result in acute silicosis with pulmonary edema and alveolar damage.
- Prolonged exosure is associated with formation in lung of numerous fibrotic nodules; the nodules may enlarge and result in progressive massive fibrosis.
- *Note:* Patients with silicosis are at increased risk for acquiring tuberculosis.

Asbestos

- Asbestos exposure may result in several lung-related problems.

  - Benign pleural fibrous plaques
  - Chronic, progessive lung fibrosis
  - Malignant mesothelioma of pleura
  - Carcinoma of lung

- Asbestos exposure can cause interstitial fibrosis with subsequent pulmonary hypertension and cor pulmonale.

— *Autoimmune disorders*

- Rheumatoid arthritis, systemic lupus erythematosus (SLE), and scleroderma are sometimes accompanied by significant pulmonary interstitial fibrosis.

— *Goodpasture's syndrome*

- The genesis of this disease involves the production of autoantibodies that are reactive to lung alveolar and renal glomerular basement membranes.

- This results in alveolar damage with hemorrhage and hemoptysis; eventually, interstitial fibrosis may occur.

— *Granulomatous pulmonary disease*

- This may be associated with significant interstitial fibrosis in addition to the granulomatous process.

- Tuberculosis and sarcoidosis are examples of this category.

— *Pulmonary eosinophilic syndrome*

- Often associated with elevated blood eosinophil count and increased serum IgE level.

- *Main causes*

  - Allergic aspergillosis
  - Helminth infection (schistosomiasis, microfilariasis)
  - Idiopathic (Churg-Strauss syndrome).

— *Honey-combed Lung*

- *The end stage of chronic interstitial fibrosis*

  - In this scenario, one sees a lung consisting of large cystic spaces separated by dense, collagen-rich scarring.
  - Honey-combed lung represents the end stage of any type of process that causes chronic interstitial fibrosis.
  - Pulmonary hypertension and cor pulmonale are frequent complications.

■ Neoplastic Lung Lesions

- *The most clinically important of these is cancer, and the most common type of lung malignancy is carcinoma.*

- Prior to the widespread practice of cigarette smoking in the United States, primary lung cancer was a relatively uncommon event.

- Today, we are witnessing an increasing incidence of lung cancer related to cigarette use; *indeed, today lung cancer is the most common cause of **cancer death** in both males and females.*

- Risk of lung cancer development is directly related to length of smoking history and number of cigarettes smoked.

- In addition to cigarette smoking, there are other exposure-related factors for lung cancer.

  - Radon gas
  - Nickel

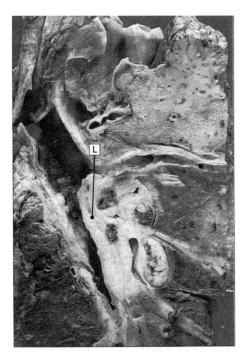

Fig. 13.4 Bronchogenic carcinoma. A large, centrally located lung carcinoma (*L*) protudes into the bronchial lumen and invades surrounding lung tissue. (*From Stevens A, Lowe J:* Pathology, *London, 1995, Times Mirror International.*)

- Iron oxides
- Chromium
- Asbestos
- Coal gas

• There are nearly 150,000 newly diagnosed lung cancer cases/year and 140,000 deaths/year caused by lung cancer in the United States.

● **Lung carcinoma**

• As stated earlier, the vast majority of primary lung cancer is carcinoma, and there are four main histologic types of carcinoma primary to the lung.

• *Note:* When extensively sampled, a substantial number of lung carcinomas show a mixture of two or more of the following histologic types (up to ½ in some series).

— *Squamous cell carcinoma*

• Usually arises centrally from one of the large bronchi (Fig. 13.4)

• Accounts for 35% of primary lung carcinoma

• Believed to be derived from metaplasia of respiratory epithelium into squamous epithelium, with subsequent development of squamous dysplasia and then carcinoma

• Relatively slow growing compared to other types of lung carcinoma

• Histologically, see malignant squamous cells, sometimes (but not always) associated with keratin production

— *Adenocarcinoma*

• Adenocarcinoma accounts for about 30% of primary lung carcinoma.

• These lesions tend to be located more in the periphery of the lung, *often arising in previous sites of scarring.*

• Prior to the widespread use of cigarettes by women, this histologic type was the one most commonly seen in women.

• Histologically, one sees malignant glandular structures.

• *Note:* One variant of adenocarcinoma, called bronchioloalveolar carcinoma, is well differentiated and, in its pure form, has a better prognosis than typical adenocarcinoma. This carcinoma tends to grow along preexisting alveolar septae and diffusely involve nearby lung tissue by aerogenous spread.

— *Small cell anaplastic (undifferentiated) carcinoma (oat cell carcinoma)*

• This type accounts for 20% of all lung carcinoma.

• *Its natural history is aggressive, with death caused by cancer within 6 to 12 months.*

• Lesions tend to be located centrally, arising from main bronchi.

• Well over 50% of patients have metastatic disease at the time that their lung carcinoma is diagnosed. Common sites are bone marrow, central nervous system, and liver.

• This type of primary lung carcinoma has neuroendocrine lineage (look for intracytoplasmic neurosecretory granules) and differentiation and is most often associated with ectopic hormone production (i.e., adrenocorticotropic hormone [ACTH], antidiuretic hormone [ADH], parathyroid hormone [PTH]) and other manifestations of the "paraneoplastic" syndrome.

• Histologically, one sees sheets of "small blue cells" with minimal cytoplasm, much associated necrosis, nulcear molding, and inconspicuous nucleoli.

• *Note:* For therapeutic and prognostic purposes, the separation of small cell anaplastic carcinoma (SCAC) from non–small cell anaplastic carcinoma is important. Surgery currently has a limited (though perhaps growing) role in SCAC; rather, this cancer is usually treated with systemic chemotherapy and/or radiotherapy, usually with excellent initial clinical responses. *However, 5-year survival in all SCAC, even with currently available therapeutic modalities, is only 5%.*

— *Large cell anaplastic carcinoma*

• A poorly differentiated carcinoma that does not satisfy the diagnostic criteria for any of the three types of carcinoma just discussed

• Constitutes 10% of lung carcinoma

• Prognosis poor, with wide cancer dissemination often present at time of diagnosis

• Histologically, nests and sheets of cells lacking specific differentiation features

General facts regarding lung carcinoma

• Spread of primary lung carcinoma can occur via local extension (i.e., into surrounding lung), lymphatic spread (usually first to peribronchial and hilar lymph nodes), hematogenous spread (bone, brain, liver, adrenals, eye, skin), and transcoelemic spread (wherein carcinoma cells seed the pleural cavity via malignant effusion).

• Symptoms and signs of lung carcinoma include cough, hemoptysis, dyspnea, chest pain, and wheezing.

• *Horner's Syndrome* includes ipsilateral ptosis (droopy eyelid), anhydrosis (loss of sweating), and small pupil; may be a problem when cancer invades cervical sympathetic chain tissue.

• Recurrent laryngeal nerve palsy may result from neoplastic extension and cause vocal cord paralysis with resultant speech deficit.

— *Other neoplasms involving lung tissue*

• *Relatively uncommon primary carcinomas* (e.g., clear cell pulmonary carcinoma)

• *Relatively uncommon primary lung sarcomas* (e.g., angiosarcoma)

• *Metastatic cancers*—Carcinomas, sarcomas, and lymphomas commonly secondarily involve the lung. Sarcomas of various types are particularly likely to metastasize to lung, as do renal cell carcinoma, hepatocellular carcinoma, and choriocarcinoma.

• *Carcinoid tumors*—a group of neuroendocrine neoplasms that covers a spectrum ranging from totally benign to low-grade cancer to an aggressive cancer that is histologically and clinically similar to small cell anaplastic carcinoma; may arise in or metastasize to lung

— *Pulmonary hamartomas*

• A benign lesion composed of tissues (mainly cartilage and respiratory epithelium) normally found within the lung; are not premalignant

◼ Pleural Based Disorders

• The lung surfaces, and the pleural cavity itself, are lined by a single layer of modified epithelial cells called mesothelial cells.

• These cells make a thin, watery fluid, participate in the resorption of this fluid, can proliferate in response to noxious stimuli, and have phagocytic capability.

● Pleural effusion

• Can be divided into one of two types based upon protein content and lactic dehydrogenase (LDH) enzyme levels

• Transudate—low protein content (less than 3 g/d), pleural fluid/serum protein ratio less than 0.5 and pleural fluid/serum LDH ratio less than 0.6

• Exudate—high protein content (greater than 3 g/d), pleural fluid/serum protein ratio greater than 0.5, and pleural fluid/serum LDH ratio greater than 0.6

— *Transudates tend to be seen in*

• Cardiac failure
• Hypoalbuminemia (from hepatic and/or renal disease)
• Vena caval obstruction

— *Exudates tend to be seen in*

• Infections (bacterial, [including tuberculosis] fungal, others)
• Cancer of lung/pleura

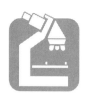

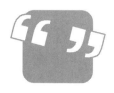

- Pulmonary infarction
- Autoimmune diseases (i.e., SLE, rheumatoid arthritis [RA])
- Intraabdominal diseases (i.e., pancreatitis, subphrenic abscess)

In addition to the above-mentioned pleural fluid analyses, further evaluation may include

- Cytologic examination of fluid, especially looking for malignant cells
- Microbiologic examination (smears, culture)
- Tissue biopsy, especially when one wants to exclude neoplastic and/or granulomatous disease

- **Pneumothoraces**

  - Pneumothorax refers to the situation of free air in the pleural space.
  - It may be spontaneous, traumatic, or iatrogenic (related to medical intervention).
  - Secondary spontaneous pneumothorax refers to a pneumothorax occurring in previously diseased lung (e.g., rupture of emphysematous bulla), whereas primary spontaneous pneumothorax occurs in previously healthy individuals.

- **Pleural Inflammation (pleurisy)**

  - Causes include

    - Infection (including bacterial, fungal, viral)
    - Renal failure
    - Autoimmune disorders

- **Neoplasms**

  - *The most common cancer to involve the pleura is metastatic carcinoma, usually from lung or breast.*
  - *Mesotheliomas* include a spectrum of mesothelial cell-based neoplasms ranging from benign to malignant.
  - Malignant mesotheliomas are related to asbestos exposure, and the latency period after exposure may last up to 50 years.

    - Malignant mesotheliomas may arise in pericardial and abdominal cavities but is *more common in the pleural cavity.*
    - Malignant mesotheliomas of the pleural cavity tend to encase the lung with a dense lesion that results in chest pain, dyspnea, and massive, recurring, bloody pleural effusion.
    - Currently available treatment for malignant mesotheliomas is not effective, and survival is very short for this cancer.

- **Congenital-Inherited Disorders**
- **Neonatal respiratory distress syndrome (NRDS)—hyaline membrane disease of newborn)**

  - *Key lesion*—deficiency of surfactant (normally produced by type II pneumocytes in the newborn's lungs)
  - *Most often associated with prematurity,* but also can be seen in infants of diabetic mothers (the excess insulin produced by such a fetus suppresses surfactant production)
  - 60% of pregnancies having a gestation of less than 28 weeks are affected by NRDS

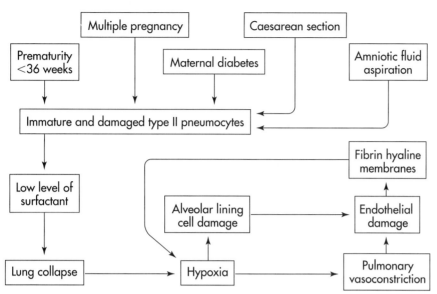

Fig. 13.5 Pathogenesis of Neonatal Respiratory Distress Syndrome (NRDS). Risk factors for NRDS are shown. The key lesion in NRDS is related to the fact that immature and/or damaged lung does not produce adequate amounts of surfactant, a lecithin rich lipid secreted by type II pneumocytes that reduces alveolar surface tension and keeps the alveoli open. In NRDS, the deficiency of surfactant results in alveolar collapse (atelectasis). The resultant hypoxic state causes damage to alveolar lining cells. Endothelial cells become damaged and leak plasma proteins (including fibrin) into the alveolar spaces; these proteins form the characterisic pink, "hyaline" membranes seen under the microscope. Subsequent events include organization of hyaline membranes and fibrosis. Overall, the process is essentially identical to that seen in diffuse alveolar damage. (*From Stevens A, Lowe J:* Pathology, *London, 1995, Times Mirror International.*)

- Mortality from NRDS—50% in infants weighing less than 1000 g
- Pathogenesis (Fig. 13.5)
- Treatment—synthetic surfactant and ventilatory support

— *Four main extrapulmonary complications of NRDS*

- Hypoxia-related intracerebral hemorrhage
- Failure of closure of patent ductus arteriosus
- Hypoxia-induced necrotizing enterocolitis
- Bronchopulmonary dysplasia

● **Immotile cilia syndrome**

- Associated with recurrent infection of the lower respiratory tract (and nasal sinuses) caused by abnormal respiratory epithelial cell cilia function; often this is related to a structural defect in the cilia, which do not act in their usual way to clear the respiratory tract of debris and organisms
- *Kartagener's Syndrome*—bronchiectasis, sinusitis, and situs inversus; airway problems caused by abnormal cilia structure and function

● **Cystic fibrosis (CF)**

- The most common lethal, hereditary disorder in Caucasians; 1:35 adult Caucasians carry this genetic defect
- Autosomal recessive inheritance
- Multisystem disease
- Lungs and pancreas particularly affected; also liver, male gonads, sweat glands

- *Key lesion*—production of a defective, thick mucous that is not easily cleared from the respiratory tract or pancreatic ducts; this results from a defective chloride channel in epithelial cells such that mucin produced by these cells is deficient in sodium and water; however, sweat sodium and chloride levels are elevated

- Pulmonary lesions—result from inspissation of mucous in airway structures

    - Increased lung infections, especially pneumonia from *Pseudomonas aeruginosa* and *Staphylococcus aureus*
    - *Bronchiectasis caused by repeated obstruction or infection of airways*
    - *Lung hyperinflation caused by air trapping behind mucous plugs; this predisposes to pneumothorax*
    - *Pulmonary hypertension and, eventually, cor pulmonale*
    - Prognosis not good, with typical survival until the late third to early fourth decade of life

● Alpha$_1$-antitrypsin (A1AT) defect

- A1AT defect includes a group of at least 60 genetic variants characterized by failure to produce normally active alpha$_1$-antitrypsin, which is a key protease inhibitor that is especially active against the destructive enzyme elastase.

- Alpha$_1$-antitrypsin is normally produced in the liver and has a molecular weight of 52 KD; normal phenotype is PiMM.

- The most abnormal phenotype has only 10% to 20% of normal A1AT activity and is associated *with cirrhosis and/or emphysema in a substantial number of patients* (see also Liver chapter).

MULTIPLE CHOICE REVIEW QUESTIONS

1. The most common cause of preventable death in hospitalized patients is which of the following?

    a. Myocardial infarction
    b. Renal infarction
    c. Hepatic infarction
    d. Splenic infarction
    e. Pulmonary thromboembolism

2. Bronchioloalveolar carcinoma is subtype of which of the following?

    a. Squamous cell carcinoma
    b. Adenocarcinoma
    c. Small cell anaplastic carcinoma
    d. Large cell anaplastic carcinoma
    e. Transitional cell carcinoma

3. A 65-year-old man with a long-standing cigarette smoking history presents with a cough and weight loss. You order a chest x-ray examination and this shows a large hilar mass. A pulmonologist performs bronchoscopy, and the pathologist's report describes a lesion composed of small round cells, with a very high nuclear/cytoplasmic ratio, inconspicuous nucleoli, nuclear molding, and no evidence for gland formation, prominent inter-cellular bridges or keratinization. Your patient has which of the following?

    a. Small cell anaplastic carcinoma
    b. Squamous cell carcinoma
    c. Adenocarcinoma
    d. Hamartoma
    e. Large cell anaplastic carcinoma

4. Which of the following organisms most commonly causes pulmonary infection in cystic fibrosis patients?

    a. *Histoplasma capsulatum*
    b. *Blastomyces dermatitidis*
    c. *Mycobacterium tuberculosis*
    d. *Pseudomonas aeruginosa*
    e. *Aspergillus flavus*

5. A 65-year-old man with a long-standing cigarette smoking history presents with severe shortness of breath. You suspect that he has ruptured an emphysematous bulla, and this is confirmed by further evaluation. This patient has which of the following?

    a. Primary empyema
    b. Secondary spontaneous pneumothorax
    c. Iatrogenic pneumothorax
    d. Iatrogenic empyema
    e. Pleurisy

Chapter 14

White Blood Cell Diseases

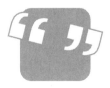

■ **Reactive Leukocyte Disorders**

• Cytopenia—deficiency of one of the formed elements of the blood (red cells, white cells, or platelets)

• Pancytopenia—decrease in all of the formed elements of the blood

• Normal reference ranges for leukocytes—varies with age, sex, race, and in response to a number of physiologic states (seasonal, diurnal, exercise, and others)

● Leukopenia

  • Decrease in white blood cells

  • Most commonly neutropenia (decreased neutrophils) and, less commonly, lymphopenia

  • The two general pathophysiologic categories (these can apply to all cytopenias)

    • Inadequate production

    • Accelerated loss or destruction

  • Inadequate production—marrow failure with hypocellularity or abnormal morphology of maturation sequence

    • Aplasia-hypoplasia—severe loss or absence of bone marrow cellularity; causes include drugs (direct toxic and idiopathic), marrow replacement (such as by tumor), idiopathic aplastic anemia (Fig. 14.1)

    • Ineffective hematopoiesis—cellular active bone marrow, but inability to mature and enter circulation; causes are megaloblastic anemia, rare inherited disorders, myelodysplasia

  • Increased destruction and consumption—usually compensatory hyperplasia of bone marrow

    • Immune—autoantibodies to neutrophils and their precursors

    • Nonimmune—infections, hypersplenism

● Leukocytosis

  • Increase in white blood cells

  • White cell differential—indicates which component is responsible

  — *Neutrophilia*

    • An increase in peripheral blood neutrophils

    • Common nonspecific response to

      • Infection—bacterial infections

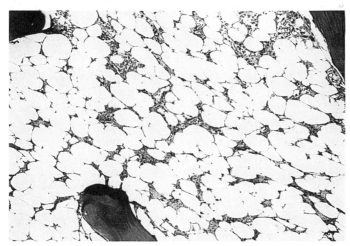

Fig. 14.1 Bone marrow hypoplasia. The marrow biopsy is markedly hypocellular with fat replacing the hematopoietic cells.
(*Damjanov I, Linder J:* Anderson's pathology, *ed 10, vol 1, St Louis, 1996, Mosby.*)

- Inflammation—any etiology, especially with tissue necrosis, trauma
- Some drugs—steroids, lithium, toxic reactions
- Other significant physiologic stresses—pregnancy, hemorrhage
- Metabolic derangements—ketoacidosis, thyrotoxicosis, eclampsia

- Must differentiate from neoplastic causes, especially chronic myeloid leukemia
- Morphology—neutrophil changes accompany increased numbers

  - Left shift—the presence of increased neutrophilic bands, myelocytes, and metamyelocytes in the peripheral blood commonly accompanies neutrophilia
  - Toxic granulation—increased prominence of azurophilic granules
  - Döhle's bodies—blue, inclusion-like areas in cytoplasm
  - Toxic vacuolization—clear cytoplasmic vacuoles correlate with sepsis

— *Lymphocytosis*

- Age-related, normal values higher in infants and children
- Causes

  - Epstein-Barr virus (EBV) infection or infectious mononucleosis
  - Other viral illnesses
  - Pertussis
  - Transient stress lymphocytosis preceding neutrophilia

- Must exclude neoplastic lymphoproliferative disorders, morphology most important

- Morphology

  - Reactive lymphocytes—also called atypical and variant lymphocytes, typical of EBV
  - Spectrum of changes, including increased cytoplasmic basophilia, enlarged nucleus, increased flowing cytoplasm with increased peripheral cytoplasmic basophilia, immunoblasts, and plasma cells
  - Confirmatory serologic tests and flow cytometry or genetic analysis—useful ancillary methods

— *Infectious mononucleosis*

- Ubiquitous self-limited infection by EBV usually occurring between 10 and 25 years of age in the United States
- Clinical—fever, pharyngitis, tender cervical adenopathy, splenomegaly, mild hepatitis
- Pathology—reactive (atypical) lymphocytosis, heterophile antibody, specific EBV antibodies

  - Antibody-negative causes—cytomegalovirus (CMV), human immunodeficiency virus (HIV), hepatitis, toxoplasmosis
  - Lymph nodes—diffuse hyperplasia, immunoblastic proliferation, Reed-Sternberg-like cells
  - Spleen—immunoblastic proliferation, infiltration of capsule
  - Heterophile antibody—agglutinating antibody against horse and sheep red cells that are absorbed by beef red cells but not guinea pig kidney cells, present in 95% of mononucleosis within 1 to 2 weeks

- Complications—splenic rupture, hemolytic anemia, thrombocytopenia, aplastic anemia, encephalitis
- Immunosuppressed patients—lymphoma, fatal persistent infection with lymphoproliferation

— *Eosinophilia*

- Most common causes—allergies, tissue-invasive parasites, drug reactions

— *Monocytosis*

- Often accompanies neutrophilia
- Other causes include—chronic infections, nonhematopoietic neoplasms, collagen vascular disorders, recovery from neutropenia

● **Functional defects of granulocytes**

- Inherited disorders—extremely rare, and only ones with morphologic findings are listed

- Chronic granulomatous disease—defective oxygen burst results in inability of neutrophils to kill catalase-producing organisms

  - Can have granulomas and pigmented histiocytes in tissues

- Pelger-Huët anomaly—benign, autosomal dominant (AD), bilobed or unsegmented neutrophil nuclei; acquired with myelodysplasia

- May-Hegglin anomaly—AD, blue cytoplasmic inclusions resembling Döhle bodies in all myeloid cells

- Chédiak-Higashi syndrome—autosomal recessive (AR), giant cytoplasmic granules
- Alder-Reilly anomaly—AR, marked azurophilic granules of all granulocytes, vacuolated and abnormally granulated lymphocytes, caused by several different types of mucopolysaccharide disorders

● **Reactive lymphadenopathy**

- Lymphadenopathy—local or generalized enlargement of lymph nodes
- Morphologic pattern on pathology useful to suggest etiology but, in most cases, pattern is nonspecific and without a specific etiology in 50% of cases
- HIV adenopathy includes several stages—initially, there is persistent generalized lymphadenopathy with marked follicular hyperplasia; this is followed by gradual reduction in lymphocytes and follicles to give a lymphocyte depleted appearance; late in the course, there may be enlargement of lymph nodes caused by lymphoma or Kaposi's sarcoma
- Metastases—common causes of local lymphadenopathy, the region a node is draining must be considered for this possibility and for sites of inflammation
- Several patterns of hyperplasia recognized (Fig. 14.2)

— *Follicular (Fig. 14.3)*

  - B cell immune response
  - Most common pattern
  - Pathology—enlargement and increased numbers of germinal centers

    - Architecture of node and organization of germinal centers is preserved vs. lymphoma.

  - Common causes—draining area of inflammation and chronic infection, rheumatoid arthritis, early HIV infection, Castleman's disease, toxoplasmosis, syphilis, nonspecific

— *Paracortical (interfollicular)*

  - A predominantly T cell immune response
  - Pathology—mottled expansion of areas between the germinal centers by immunoblasts and histiocytes that may expand to the entire node to give a diffuse pattern
  - Common causes—viral infection (EBV, CMV), drug reaction, draining skin disease (dermatopathic lymphadenopathy)

— *Mixed follicular and interfollicular*

  - Common causes—viral infection, toxoplasmosis, Kimura's disease

— *Sinusoidal*

  - Pathology—expanded medullary sinuses by histiocytes
  - Common causes—draining tumors, Langerhans' cell histiocytosis, Whipple's disease, postlymphangiogram

— *Necrotizing lymphadenitis and granuloma*

  - Common causes—cat-scratch disease, sarcoidosis, tuberculosis, fungal disease, leprosy

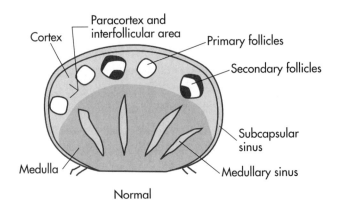

Normal

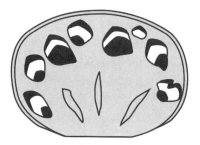

Follicular hyperplasia

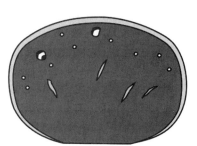

Paracortical (diffuse) hyperplasia

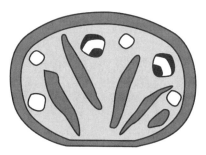

Sinusoidal hyperplasia

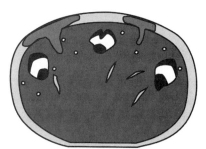

Mixed hyperplasia

Fig. 14.2 Patterns of reactive lymphoid hyperplasia.

— *Acute lymphadenitis*

- Cause—bacterial infection of the node or a node draining a bacterial infection
- Pathology—follicular hyperplasia with neutrophils, may form abscess

■ **Neoplastic White Cell Diseases**

- Most common malignancies of childhood and 7% of adult malignancies—derived from myeloid and lymphoid cells
- Divided broadly into lymphoid and myeloid (includes monocytic, megakaryocytic, and erythroid lineages)
- Leukemia—a malignancy of above lineage that primarily involves the bone marrow and blood, often causing a high white blood cell count (WBC)

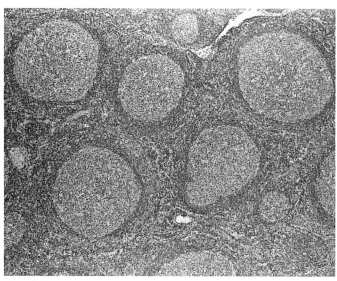

Fig. 14.3 Follicular hyperplasia. The number of follicles is increased, but they still retain their mixed and polarized composition, surrounded by mantle zones. (*Damjanov I, Linder J:* Anderson's pathology, *ed 10, vol 1, St Louis, 1996, Mosby.*)

- Lymphoma—a malignancy of lymphoid origin that predominantly involves the lymph nodes, spleen, thymus, tonsils, and other lymphoid regions

■ Myeloid Malignancies

- Comprise three related and overlapping groups—myeloid leukemia, myelodysplastic syndromes, and myeloproliferative disorders
- Nearly all arise in the bone marrow

● Acute myeloid leukemia (AML)

- A malignancy of the hematopoietic progenitor
- Most common acute leukemia of adults, with about 2/100,000 incidence
- Increased incidence with—Down syndrome, Fanconi's anemia, Bloom syndrome, neurofibromatosis, radiation exposure, benzene, alkylating agents, and epipidophylotoxin use

- Blast cell—a malignant cell that is undifferentiated or minimally differentiated having a high nuclear/cytoplasmic ratio, fine nuclear chromatin, and often prominent nucleoli
- Pathology—acute leukemia defined as over 30% blast cells in the bone marrow differential; 30% is an arbitrary but agreed upon number

    - Marrow packed with blast cells, replacing normal mix of fat and hematopoietic elements
    - Auer rods in the blast cells—pathogneumonic of AML
    - Auer rods—red refractile rodlike inclusions composed of crystallized granule components
    - Chloroma or granulocytic sarcoma—greenish tumors composed of blast cells occurring in patients with or who will soon have AML

Table 14.1 *Acute Myeloid Leukemia*

FAB DESIGNATION	BLAST MORPHOLOGY	SPECIAL FEATURES
M0 Undifferentiated	Primitive blasts	Surface markers necessary to recognize
M1 Minimal differentiation	Few granules, Auer rods	Myeloperoxidase positive
M2 Myeloid differentiation	Blast cells and some maturation to promyelocytes, Auer rods	Common type
M3 Promyelocytic	Hypergranular promyelocytes, clusters of Auer rods	DIC common
M4 Myelomonocytic	Myeloid and monocytic differentiation	Common type, cytochemistry helps identify
M5 Monoblastic	Promonocytes and blasts	Gum infiltrates
M6 Erythroleukemia	Marked dyserythropoiesis, erythroblasts, and myeloblasts	
M7 Megakaryocytic	Undifferentiated blasts, immunophenotype identifies lineage	Marrow fibrosis

FAB, French, American, and British; *DIC,* disseminated intravascular coagulation.

- Myeloblast cytochemistry—myeloperoxidase and Sudan black B positive, immunologic phenotype—CD13, CD33 positive
- Other cytochemistry and immunophenotypic markers useful in subclassification

- Classification based on the French-American-British (FAB) morphologic system (Table 14.1)
- With the addition of immunophenotyping and genetic evaluation classification is more reproducible and prognostically relevant
- Clinical—marrow failure caused by replacement by blast cells produces anemia, neutropenia, and thrombocytopenia (pancytopenia) with predictable symptoms

  - Leukemic cells—can infiltrate any organ to cause local symptoms
  - Chemotherapy—can induce remissions, some sustained
  - Long disease-free survival with marrow transplants (about 60%)

● Myelodysplastic syndromes (MDS)

- A group of myeloid malignancies more indolent than acute leukemia, characterized by ineffective hematopoiesis
- Increasing incidence with age, most common 60 to 70 years
- Clinical—symptoms of cytopenias

  - Survival dependant on—severity and complications of cytopenias, the rate of progression to acute leukemia (rate of increase in blast cells), and the presence of poor cytogenetic findings (loss or partial deletion of 5, 7, 20, and trisomy 8)
  - Progression to acute leukemia ranges from 8% to 60%

- Pathology—a hypercellular marrow, abnormal (dysplastic) maturation of myeloid, erythroid, and megakaryocytic lineages and failure of complete maturation leading to peripheral blood cytopenias (ineffective hematopoiesis)

  - Dysplastic features—hyposegmentation of granulocyte nuclei and

Table 14.2 *Myelodysplastic Syndromes*

FAB DESIGNATION	% BLAST IN MARROW	SPECIAL CRITERIA	LEUKEMIC TRANSFORMATION
RA Refractory anemia	<5	May have other cytopenias	Low
RAR Refractory anemia with ringed siteroblasts	<5	<15% ringed sideroblasts on iron staining 2° causes are alcohol, INH, congenital	Low
RAEB Refractory anemia with excess blasts	5-<20	Marked dysplasia common	Intermediate
RAEBIT Refractory anemia with excess blasts in transformation	20-<30	Survival similar to acute leukemia	High
CMML Chronic myelomonocytic leukemia	<20	High monocyte count in peripheral blood Similar to CML but lack Ph1 chromosome	Intermediate

FAB, French, American, and British; *INH,* isoniazid.

hypogranulation of granulocytes; megaloblastic-like changes, abnormal mitoses, binucleation and nuclear fragmentation of erythroblasts; giant sometimes hypogranular platelets

- Blast cells—may be increased but are less than 30% in the bone marrow

- Differential diagnosis—B_{12} and folate deficiency, antineoplastic drugs, alcohol, lead exposure, arsenic toxicity, rare congenital cases

  - Cytogenetic abnormalities present in MDS—useful in confirming the diagnosis

  - Classification by FAB morphologic types (Table 14.2)

● **Myeloproliferative disorders**

  - A group of hematopoietic stem malignancies more indolent than acute leukemia, characterized by marked bone marrow hypercellularity that can result in marrow fibrosis and markedly increased peripheral blood counts

    - Classified by the lineage most expanded in the peripheral blood
    - Maturation—normal or only mildly dysplastic
    - Progression to acute leukemia—may occur
    - Four basic types are recognized (Table 14.3)

  — *Chronic myeloid leukemia (CML)*

    - Predominantly granulocyte and monocyte expansion with the Philadelphia chromosome or molecular presence of the Bcr/Abl gene fusion product from the t9;22 translocation

    - Clinical—occurs at all ages with progressively rising incidence with aging

      - Progresses often to acute leukemia—inevitable with current median survivals of about 5 years

Table 14.3 *Myeloproliferative Disorders*

	CHRONIC MYELOID LEUKEMIA	POLYCYTHEMIA VERA	MYELOID METAPLASIA	ESSENTIAL THROMBOCYTHEMIA
Peripheral Blood				
Hb	↓	↑↑	↓	N-↓
WBC	↑↑ >30 × 10^9/L	↑ <20 × 10^9/L	<30 × 10^9/L	<20 × 10^9/L
Plts	↑, N, ↓	N or ↑	↑, N, ↓	↑↑↑ >600 × 10^9/L
Smear	Immature myeloid cells	Normal RBCs	Tear drop RBCs NRBC Myeloid percursors	Giant platelets
Bcr/abl	+	–	–	–

Hb, Hemoglobin; *WBC*, white blood count; *Plts*, platelets; *Bcr/abl*, Philadelphia chromosome; *RBC*, red blood cells; *N*, normal; *NRBC*, nucleated red blood cells.

- Pathology—packed marrow with increased myelopoiesis and initially low numbers of blast cells

  - Massive splenomegaly caused by extramedullary myelopoiesis common with splenic pain and infarcts
  - Acute leukemia—may be of myeloid type (70%) or lymphoid (30%) demonstrating this is truly a malignancy of the pluripotential stem cell

— *Polycythemia vera (PV)*

  - Marked increase in the red cell mass with low erythropoietin (EPO) levels
  - Must exclude secondary causes of high hemoglobin—hypoxia, cyanotic cardiac disease, dehydration or extremes of plasma volume relative to hemoglobin levels, and rare tumors that secrete EPO
  - Clinical—high red blood cell count (RBC) causes hyperviscosity of the blood, producing headache, dizziness, heart failure
  - Complication—hyperuricemia and gout, pruritus, thrombosis
  - Pathology—widespread organ congestion, especially liver and spleen

    - Bone marrow hypercellularity
    - Progressive to spent phase at about 10 years resembling myelofibrosis
    - About 2% transformation to AML

— *Myeloid metaplasia with myelofibrosis*

  - Marked bone marrow fibrosis and scarring secondary to a primary myeloproliferative malignancy
  - Pathology—marrow fibrosis (Fig. 14.4)

    - Marked hepatosplenomegaly caused by extramedullary hematopoiesis
    - Maturation of blood cells fairly normal
    - Peripheral blood—tear drop shaped RBC, nucleated RBC, early myeloid cells, and giant platelets (commonly referred

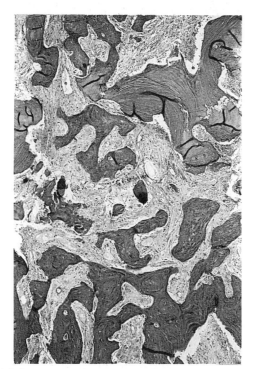

Fig. 14.4 Bone marrow fibrosis. The marrow hematopoietic space is replaced by fibrosis and osteosclerosis. (*Damjanov I, Linder J:* Anderson's pathology, *ed 10, vol 1, St Louis, 1996, Mosby.*)

to as myelophthisic or leukoerythroblastic and associated with marrow fibrosis or replacement caused by any process)

- Clinical—intermediate course, transformation to AML in 5% to 10% of cases
- Complications—thrombosis, hemorrhage, infections, transfusion dependence, portal hypertension

— *Essential thrombocythemia*

- Indolent myeloproliferative disorder in which high platelets predominate
- Diagnosis of exclusion from other myeloproliferative disorders and secondary reactive causes of thrombocytosis
- Secondary causes—hemorrhage, chronic inflammatory disorders, other malignancies, iron deficiency, and postsplenectomy
- Clinical—more common in elderly but can occur in anyone after 20s

    - Produces both thrombosis and, paradoxically, hemorrhage
    - Less commonly progresses to leukemia or fibrosis

■ **Lymphoid Malignancies**

- Include lymphoid leukemia, lymphoma, and plasma cell diseases
- Primarily involve lymph nodes and other lymphoid regions, can arise in

any body site or organ and also frequently invade the bone marrow and peripheral blood to produce leukemia

● **Lymphoid leukemia**

— *Acute lymphoblastic leukemia*

• Malignancy of primitive blast cells that show lymphoid differentiation

• Most common leukemia of childhood, peak 2 to 10 years old

• Clinical—symptoms of cytopenias, joint pain, infiltration of the testes and central nervous system (CNS) provides sites of extramedullary relapses

• Most frequently arises in the bone marrow; however, if nodes or thymus is the primary site and marrow involvement is absent or limited, it is often classified as non-Hodgkin's lymphoblastic lymphoma

Pathology

MORPHOLOGIC CLASSIFICATION IS BY THE FAB

• FAB L1—uniform small blasts (2× size of lymphocytes), scanty cytoplasm, mostly round regular nucleus equal microblasts, common in children

• FAB L2—larger, more variable blasts, prominent nucleolus, identical to myeloid blasts but no Auer rods, common in adults

• FAB L3—larger blasts, abundant basophilic cytoplasm often with vacuoles, several prominent nucleoli, leukemic phase of Burkitt's lymphoma or small noncleaved non-Hodgkin's lymphoma (NHL)

IMMUNOLOGIC CLASSIFICATION—ABOUT 85% B PHENOTYPE, 15% T PHENOTYPE

• T cell (15%)—TdT (terminal deoxyribonucleotydyl transferase), cytoplasmic CD3, CD2, CD7, CD5, L1, and L2 morphology

• Early B precursor (65%)—TdT, CD10, CD19, CD22, lack cytoplasmic (cIg) and surface (sIg) immunoglobulin, L1 and L2 morphology

• Pre-B cell (20%)—TdT, CD10, CD19, CD20, CD22, cIg, L1, and L2 morphology

• B cell (1%)—CD10, CD19, CD20, CD22, sIg, lack TdT, L3 morphology

PROGNOSTIC VARIABLES

• Poor prognosis—high WBC, males, outside ages 3 to 8 years, solid tumor masses (lymphoma presentation)

• Cytogenetics—most important prognostic variable

  • Good prognosis—hyperdiploidy N greater than 50
  • Intermediate—N 46 to 50
  • Poor—N less than 46 or a specific translocation

• Important specific translocations

  • 8;14, 8;22, 8;2—involve the c-myc oncogene and the immunoglobulin heavy, lambda and kappa genes, respectively, strong association with L3 morphology and Burkitt's lymphoma

- 9;22—5% of childhood acute lymphoblastic leukemia (ALL) and 25% of adult ALL, slightly different molecular structure than CML and usually not preceded by CML
- 1;19—pre-B phenotype
- 11q23;variable partners—less than age 1 year, may have both myeloid and lymphoid differentiation

CLINICAL

- Poor risk—transplantation or aggressive multi-agent chemotherapy
- Good risk—80% survival with standard chemotherapy

— *Chronic lymphocytic leukemia*

- An indolent malignancy of mature-appearing, usually B lymphocytes
- Caucasian (very rare in Asian populations), greater than 50 years old, most common leukemia in North America (NA) and Europe
- Complications—autoimmune hemolytic anemia, hypogammaglobulinemia (infections common cause of death), marrow replacement causing cytopenias
- Pathology

  - Mature-appearing small lymphocytes with condensed chromatin and scanty cytoplasm in the peripheral blood and marrow
  - Peripheral blood (PB) smear may have many broken cells called smudge cells
  - Infiltrate lymph nodes and spleen in a diffuse pattern identical to small lymphocytic lymphoma
  - Immunology—95% B cell type, monoclonal sIg, pan B markers, CD23, CD5 (usually a T cell marker but abnormal expression in chronic lymphocytic leukemia [CLL]),
  - May progress to large cell lymphoma (Richter's syndrome) or a more accelerated disease with increased numbers of lymphocytes with more cytoplasm and prominent nucleoli (prolymphocytes)

- Cytogenetics—trisomy 12 (poor prognosis), abnormal 13q
- Rai Staging System:

  - 0—peripheral blood and bone marrow involvement
  - I—with enlarged nodes
  - II—with enlarged liver or spleen
  - III and IV—with anemia or thrombocytopenia
  - Survival—greater than 10 years for stage I, 6 years stage II and III, and 2 years for III and IV

- Not curable, and treatment is for bulky symptomatic disease and complications

— *Hairy cell leukemia*

- Rare, indolent B cell leukemia of middle-aged males

- Clinical—pancytopenia, splenomegaly, and hairy cells in PB and marrow
- Pathology

    - Hairy cells—medium-sized lymphocytes with moderate cytoplasm and cytoplasmic projections (hairs) that may be rare in PB
    - Bone marrow—hairy cells are uniformly spaced with nuclei lying centrally in clear cytoplasm resembling fried eggs or chicken wire, marrow fibrosis accompanies the infiltrates
    - TRAP (tartrate resistant alkaline phosphatase) positive

    - Immunophenotype—pan B, sIg and CD25, CD11c and CD103
    - Clinical—effective treatment with new purine analogues

■ **Lymphoma**

- Incidence risen at 3% to 4% per year since 1970
- Lymphoma are further divided into Hodgkin's disease (HD) and NHL
- NHL and leukemia overlap, and their division often artificial
- All NHL—may have malignant cells infiltrating the bone marrow and circulating in the peripheral blood
- All B cell lymphoma—may secrete a monoclonal immunoglobulin detectable in the serum
- Epidemiologic associations—EBV, human T-cell leukemia/lymphoma virus (HTLV)-1, immunodeficiencies, radiation, pesticides, herbicides, hair dyes, organic solvents, and familial

    - Treatment—depends on the histologic type and extent of disease

● **Stage—systematic means of assessing the extent and spread of a tumor**

    — *Ann Arbor staging system*
        1. Stage I—single site or nodal region
        2. Stage II—two node regions on the same side of the diaphragm
        3. Stage III—lymph node regions above and below the diaphragm
        4. Stage V—extranodal sites of involvement, especially common in the marrow and liver.

    - Two more levels are added to the number for final stage designation

        - A—no symptoms
        - B—fever, drenching night sweats or weight loss

    - In general, higher stages treated with chemotherapy and more aggressive approaches, lower stages with radiotherapy

● **Non-Hodgkin's Lymphoma**

    - All ages—affected with increasing incidence with age, males more frequently
    - The separation of some NHL from their leukemic counterpart—largely by arbitrarily established cutoff points for PB and marrow involvement
    - NHL—a large number of diverse diseases with behavior ranging from slowly progressing or indolent to rapidly growing aggressive types

Box 14.1

CLASSIFICATION OF NON-HODGKIN'S LYMPHOMA

Indolent
Small B-cell lymphocytic lymphoma (SLL/CLL)
Mantle cell lymphoma (MCL)
Follicle center lymphoma (FCL)
Mucosal associated lymphoma (MALT) or Monocytoid
  (marginal zone) B cell lymphoma (MZL)
Mycosis fungoides/Sézary syndrome (MF/SS)

Aggressive
Diffuse large B cell lymphoma
Peripheral T cell lymphoma
Burkitt's lymphoma
Precursor B and T lymphoblastic lymphoma-leukemia

- Indolent types—have a longer natural history but not curable by current standard treatment
- Many aggressive lymphoma may be cured by standard treatments
- Clinical

   - ⅔ arise in lymph nodes, about ⅓ at extranodal (EN) sites in any organ
   - GI tract—the most common EN site
   - About ⅓ may have PB involvement

- Classification (Box 14.1)—evolving with refinements resulting from application of immunophenotyping, genetics, and morphology
- Currently at least 30 entities recognized by the recent international lymphoma study group proposal that unites all lymphoid malignancy regardless of whether they present a lymphoma or leukemia
   - 80% of cases represented in the simplified scheme (see Box 14.1)
   - General morphologic rules for prognosis

      - Nodular or follicular low magnification pattern behaves indolently
      - Small cytologic nuclear size with mature chromatic pattern behaves indolently
      - Large nuclear size or cells with fine chromatin (lymphoblast-like) behave aggressively

- Indolent lymphoma—may evolve or transform to a more aggressive type with a corresponding change in their morphology
- Genetic and immunologic studies—may be required for diagnosis and precise classification
   - 80% of NHL are B cell in origin

— *B small lymphocytic lymphoma*

   - The lymphomatous counterpart of CLL

— *Follicle center cell lymphoma*

   - B cell lymphoma that mimics the normal follicle in both pattern and the cytologic spectrum

- Common in Europe and North America but rare in Asia, adults greater than age 40 years, usually with high stage and marrow involvement at presentation
  - Pathology
    - Morphology—resembles normal lymph node with nodules of malignant cells with a spectrum of small cleaved to large transformed (large noncleaved, large cleaved, and immunoblast) cells
    - Characteristic t14;18 involving the IgH gene and chromosome 18 Bcl-2 gene
    - Immunology—monoclonal sIg, pan B antigens
    - Over express Bcl-2 protein that is thought to inhibit apoptotic cell death

  - Clinical
    - Indolent behavior with 7 to 10 year median survival, not curable by standard treatment
    - Can progress to diffuse large B cell lymphoma

— *Mantle cell lymphoma*
  - A moderately common B cell NHL
  - Has the poorest survival of all indolent lymphoma
  - Common after age 60 years with a disseminated disease
  - May involve the GI tract (malignant lymphomatous polyps) and Waldeyer's ring
  - Median survival 3 to 5 years with a relentlessly progressive course
  - Can evolve to an aggressive type that is morphologically similar to lymphoblastic lymphoma

  - Pathology
    - Small-sized cells, little cytoplasm, irregular nuclear membranes between small lymphocytic and small cleaved
    - May form broad rings around benign germinal centers giving malignant mantle zones, or be more diffuse
    - Cytogenetics—t11;14 very characteristic involving IgH gene and cyclin D1 on chromosome 11
    - Immunophenotype—pan B cell also with CD5 expression as CLL but lacks CD23
  - No effective treatment

— *Mucosal associated lymphoma (MALT) or Monocytoid (marginal zone) B cell lymphoma*
  - These are common in the GI tract, especially the stomach and have been discussed in this location (see Head and Neck chapter)
  - Pathology—in lymph nodes the proliferation produces an expansion of the node by a mixture of small B cells with abundent cytoplasm (monocytoid B cells), plasmacytoid cells, and large transformed cells, this may surround and invade the benign remaining germinal centers

- These are also known as marginal zone lymphomas by their pattern in the spleen
- The marginal zone is the zone that surrounds the mantle zone
- Immunology—pan B cell, monoclonal sIg and cIg in the plasmacytoid cells

- Clinical—nodal based monocytoid B cell lymphoma have a high incidence in women with underlying Sjögrens disease and a cervical node site

- Indolent behavior

— *Mycosis fungoides/Sézary syndrome (MF/SS)*

- Skin-based T helper cell lymphoma
- Clinical—erythrodermia, skin plaques, and nodules
- Pathology—clusters of malignant cells with cerebriform nuclei in the epidermis forming Pautrier's abscesses

- Sézary syndrome—generalized erythrodermia with leukemic phase of circulating cerebriform cells

- Clinical—very indolent, not curable
- May progress to larger cell type with involvement of other organs
- Local skin treatment

— *Diffuse large B cell lymphoma*

- A group of B cell lymphomas with large nuclear size and diffuse growth pattern
- Common in adults and children
- Clinical—rapidly enlarging lymph node (LN) or EN mass (especially stomach) (Fig. 14.5)
- Pathology—large morphologically undifferentiated cells resembling large cell types seen in germinal centers

- Varying numbers of small lymphocytic cells—may be present that are reactive T cells or part of the neoplastic clone
- Differential diagnosis—includes other poorly differentiated neoplasms
- Immunology—B cells with monoclonal sIg
- 20% have t14;18, 30% t3q27; various partners (Bcl-6 on 3q27)

- Clinical—International Prognostic Index (IPI) now used for staging

- Poor risk IPI factors—age greater than 60 years; LDH greater than normal; stage greater than II; performance status greater than 1 (patient bedridden greater than ½ day or more) more than 1 extranodal site
- About 50% long-term survival with current chemotherapy

— *Peripheral T cell lymphoma*

- Heterogeneous group of T cell lymphoma

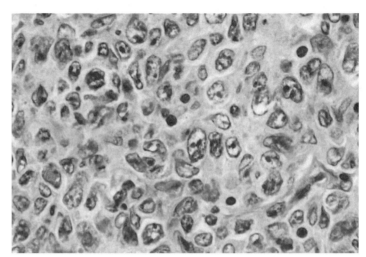

Fig. 14.5 Diffuse large cell lymphoma. The lymph node is replaced by large malignant lymphoid cells. (*Damjanov I, Linder J: Anderson's pathology, ed 10, vol 1, St Louis, 1996, Mosby.*)

- Pathology—most common types resemble diffuse large B cell lymphoma (DLBCL)

  - T cell phenotype usually with CD4

- Clinical—grouped with DLBCL for treatment

— *Burkitt's lymphoma*

- Aggressive B cell NHL common in children
- The lymphomatous counterpart to ALL L3
- Endemic type—tropical Africa with involvement of mandible
- Sporadic type—often abdominal mass in ovary or ileocecal bowel

  - Most common lymphoma in HIV

- High association with EBV
- Pathology—identical to ALL L3, in tissue are medium-sized cells with 2 to 5 prominent small nucleoli, squared off cytoplasm, and a high mitotic rate with many phagocytic histiocytes (gives a starry sky pattern)

— *Precursor T and B lymphoblastic lymphoma/leukemia*

- Lymphomatous counterpart of ALL
- Precursor T phenotype more commonly presents with lymphoma (85%)

  - Older male children with mediastinal masses arising in the thymus

● Hodgkin's disease (HD)

- A malignant disorder arising primarily in lymph nodes, characterized by Reed-Sternberg (RS) cells that are currently thought to arise from hematolymphoid cells, most likely T and B cells

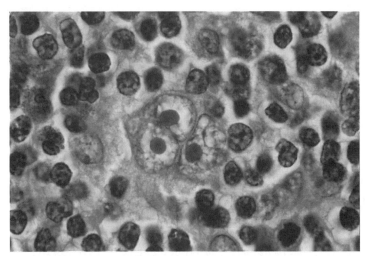

Fig. 14.6 Classic Reed-Sternberg cell. There is a multinucleated cell that has huge inclusion-like nucleoli. (*Damjanov I, Linder J:* Anderson's pathology, *ed 10, vol 1, St Louis, 1996, Mosby.*)

- Reed-Sternberg cells—huge pleomorphic malignant cells with polylobated nuclei or that are binuclear and contain large prominent eosinophilic nucleoli classically resembling two owls' eyes (Fig. 14.6)

    - In the correct cellular background, RS cells diagnostic of Hodgkin's disease

- Classification—by the Rye system include the various types of RS cells and the background stromal reaction and cellular composition

- Lymphocyte predominant—has few classic RS cells, but has the L and H variant associated with background small lymphocytes

    - Rare form that is indolent, clearly arises from B cells

- Nodular sclerosis—80% of HD in NA

    - Has the lacunar variant of the RS cell usually in a background of mature lymphocytes, eosinophils, and plasma cells
    - Dense fibrous (sclerotic) bands are formed that divide the node into nodules
    - Lacunar cells—RS cells sit in halos of clear or retracted cytoplasm
    - Commonly in females, above the diaphragm especially the mediastinum, and in younger individuals

- Mixed cellularity—more common outside North America and Europe

    - Diffuse pattern of RS cells in mixed cellular background
    - Unclassifiable cases go in this type

- Lymphocyte depletion—rarest type in which background lymphocytes are reduced because of large numbers of RS cell or diffuse fibrosis

    - Hard to differentiate from some diffuse large cell NHL

- Clinical—staging by Cotswald modification of Ann Arbor System

- Painless enlargement of lymph nodes common in stages I and II
- B symptoms common in stage III and IV
- Bimodal age distribution with peak in children and young adults and again in middle age
- Survival—nearly 100% for stages I and II
- Radiotherapy—effective for lower stages

- Hodgkin's disease spreads along lymph node chains in a sequential manner and less commonly involves the marrow
- EBV—strongly implicated in the pathogenesis and may be demonstrated in many RS cells

■ **Plasma Cell Diseases**

● **Multiple myeloma**

- A clonal proliferation of B lymphoid cells maturing to abnormal but recognizable plasma cells
- Pathology—eccentric nucleus, clock face type of chromatin and basophilic cytoplasm

  - Bone marrow-based proliferation with multifocal sheets and clusters of atypical plasma cells, demonstrable as monoclonal by restriction of light chain expression to either lambda or kappa
  - May cause pathologic fracture or be visible as multiple discrete lytic lesion of the bone on x-ray film

- Plasmacytoma—an isolated mass composed of malignant plasma cells

  - Osseous plasmacytoma—almost always progress to systemic multiple myeloma but only 30% of soft tissue extramedullary plasmacytoma do

- Plasma cells of multiple myeloma (MM) secrete a monoclonal immunoglobulin into the plasma in 99% of cases

  - Detected as a discrete band on serum protein electrophoresis
  - IgG 50%, IgA 25%, IgM 10% and light chains only in 15%
  - Light chains not detected in the serum but excreted in the urine where they are also known as Bence Jones proteins
  - Amyloid light chain (AL) is found in about 10% of MM

- Occurs with rising incidence after age 50 years
- Clinical—bone pain, anemia, and fatigue are common, also infection, hypercalcemia, renal disease, and fractures
- Not considered curable with current standard treatment, with survival 2 to 5 years
- Minimal criteria for diagnosis are—biopsy of a plasmacytoma or over 10% atypical plasma cells in the bone marrow with no reactive cause for the plasmacytosis and one of monoclonal serum immunoglobulin, monoclonal urine immunoglobulin, or lytic bone lesions

● **Waldenström's macroglobulinemia**

- A lymphoma with marked plasmacytoid differentiation arising most frequently in the bone marrow that produces a monoclonal IgM protein that can cause hyperviscosity syndrome

- **Monoclonal gammopathy of undetermined significance (MGUS)**
  - 1% to 3% of monoclonal proteins detected in the serum found in healthy asymptomatic individuals over the age of 50 years
  - About 20%—will develop multiple myeloma during the next 10 to 15 years
  - May have mild marrow plasmacytosis, but do not fulfill the criteria of MM

■ Langerhans' Cell Histiocytosis

- A clonal proliferation of the marrow-derived antigen presenting Langerhans' cell
- Pathology—clusters of Langerhans' cells having distinctive, irregular folded nuclei and moderate amounts of cytoplasm

  - Special features include—CD1a positive and the finding of Birbeck granules by electron microscopy (rough endoplasmic reticulum having a tennis racquetlike structure)

- Three overlapping clinical disorders

  - Unifocal (eosinophilic granuloma)—indolent with single focus of Langerhans' cells usually in the bone (skull) or lung in adults, most common form
  - Multifocal unisystem (Hand-Schüller-Christian disease)—younger children usually with multisite bone involvement
  - Multifocal multisystem (Letterer-Siwe disease)—infants and young, usually male, children involving skin, bone, liver, and other sites, producing organ dysfunction; may be progressive with poor outcome

MULTIPLE CHOICE
REVIEW QUESTIONS

1. A 14-year-old male has a rapidly growing mediastinal mass. Biopsy of the mass showed that it was composed of neoplastic cells with a high mitotic rate; slightly larger than normal lymphocytes, fine chromatin, and slightly lobulated nuclei. These were positive for terminal transferase (TdT). Small numbers of malignant cells were also present in the bone marrow. The diagnosis is which of the following?

   a. Burkitt's lymphoma
   b. Lymphoblastic lymphoma
   c. Diffuse large B cell lymphoma
   d. Hodgkin's disease, nodular sclerosis type
   e. Small lymphocytic lymphoma/chronic lymphocytic leukemia

2. The most indolent behavior would be expected of which of the following non-Hodgkin's lymphoma?

   a. Burkitt's lymphoma
   b. Mantle cell lymphoma
   c. Lymphoblastic lymphoma
   d. Small lymphocytic lymphoma
   e. Diffuse, large B cell lymphoma

3. A 19-year-old college student has recent onset of fever and sore throat. Generalized lymph node enlargement and mild splenomegaly are detected. The peripheral blood shows lymphocytosis with atypical lymphocytes. This patient most likely has which of the following?

   a. Chronic lymphocytic leukemia
   b. Infection with *Streptococcus pyogenes*
   c. Infection with Epstein-Barr virus
   d. Hodgkin's disease
   e. Human immunodeficiency virus infection

4. The finding of Auer rods in a leukemic blast indicates a diagnosis of which of the following?

   a. Acute lymphocytic leukemia
   b. Chronic lymphocytic leukemia
   c. Hairy cell leukemia
   d. Chronic myelogenous leukemia
   e. Acute myelogenous leukemia

5. Myeloid metaplasia with myelofibrosis is a likely complication of which of the following?

   a. Chronic lymphocytic leukemia
   b. Myelodysplasia, refractory anemia
   c. Hairy cell leukemia
   d. Polycythemia vera
   e. Hodgkin's disease, nodular sclerosis

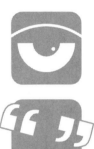

Chapter 15

Red Blood Cell Diseases

■ General Concepts

- Red cells produced in the bone marrow from progenitor cells under the influence of cytokines, especially erythropoietin in the later stages of development
- Mature red blood cells (RBCs) function—to hold and protect hemoglobin as it transports oxygen to tissue
- Anemia—decrease in the peripheral blood (PB) hemoglobin concentration below the normal for age, sex, and physiologic state (altitude of residence, pregnancy state, and others)
- Complete blood count (CBC)—automated cell counting instrument generated values for the hemoglobin (Hb), red blood cell count (RBC), red cell size (mean cell volume [MCV]) and size variability (red cell size distribution width, RDW), average amount of hemoglobin in red cells (mean cell hemoglobin [MCH], and mean cell hemoglobin concentration [MCHC]), in addition to a white blood cell count (WBC), often a WBC differential (classification of the relative frequencies of each type of leukocyte), and a platelet count
- RBCs—develop over 5 to 7 days in the marrow, first giving rise to reticulocytes which persist in the circulation for about 24 hours
- Reticulocytes—bluish colored RBCs on Romanovsky's type stains (routine PB stain) that still contain some rough endoplasmic reticulum (RER) remaining from the production of hemoglobin

  - Polychromasia—increased numbers of bluish RBCs seen on PB microscopic evaluation

- Reticulocyte count—enumeration of reticulocytes performed by staining RBCs with a dye that detects the RER and counting either by microscope or on one of a number of special flow instruments
  - In a patient with anemia

    - A reticulocyte count will be elevated in the face of an active marrow trying to compensate for excess RBC loss or destruction.
    - A reticulocyte count will be inappropriately low or zero when the marrow is not producing RBCs properly.

- Using the CBC, reticulocyte count, and morphology of the peripheral blood—most common causes of anemia can be deduced, and definitive diagnostic tests, such as bone marrow examination and other specialized tests, performed if needed
- Two approaches to anemia are by mechanism (pathophysiologic) (Box 15.1) and by RBC morphology (Box 15.2) with both often combined in practice

Box 15.1

COMMON MECHANISMS OF ANEMIA

Decreased Production

Failure of red cell production
   Part of general marrow failure
      Congenital
      Aplastic anemia
      Nutritional
         B_{12}, folate
      Marrow replacement
   Limited to red cell production
      Congenital
      Autoimmune
      Human Parvovirus infection
Failure of hemoglobin production
   Thalassemia
   Nutritional
      Iron deficiency
      Chronic disease

Shortened Red Cell Survival

Increased Destruction
   Hemolytic anemias
Blood loss

Box 15.2

COMMON RED CELL MORPHOLOGIES AND CAUSES

Hypochromia-Microcytosis
   Iron deficiency
   Thalassemia
Spherocytes
   Immune
      Autoimmune hemolytic anemia
      Hemolytic disease of the newborn
   Nonimmune
      Hereditary spherocytosis
Macroovalocytes
   Megaloblastic anemia
Acanthocytes
   Severe liver disease
Target cells
   Liver disease
   Hemoglobinopathies
Irreversible sickle cells
   Sickle cell anemia
Inclusions
   Malarial parasites
   Howell-Jolly bodies—hyposplenism
   Crystals of hemoglobin C
Schistocytes
   Disseminated intravascular coagulation, thrombic
      thrombocytopenia purpura, mechanical heart valve

■ Disorders of Red Cell Production

● Aplastic anemia

- Failure of bone marrow hematopoiesis
- Rare disorder, occurs at any age with symptoms of pancytopenia
- Congenital causes—Fanconi's anemia, Schwachmann-Diamond
- Acquired causes—most idiopathic, some with infections (hepatitis C), drug reactions (chloramphenicol), toxins (benzene), radiation, and others
- Pathology—bone marrow is empty, with the marrow space occupied by fat lacking hematopoietic activity (normal is about 50% cellularity) (see Fig. 14.1)
- Pure red cell aplasia can be seen with congenital Blackfan-Diamond, thymoma, parvovirus infection, and other disorders

    - All—show striking absence of erythroblasts in the marrow
    - Parvovirus—may see rare nuclear inclusions the few remaining early erythroblasts

- Red cell production—may be impaired with abnormalities of red cell development in congenital dyserythropoietic anemia and acquired myelo-dysplastic syndromes
- Red cell production—decreased by diseases that replace the bone marrow space

    - Common causes—malignancy (both hematologic and metastatic), granuloma, fibrosis, storage diseases (Gaucher's), and others
    - Pathology—PB often shows some or all of normochromic normocytic anemia, nucleated RBCs, early myeloid cells, and, occasionally, tear drop RBC; this is referred to as leukoerythroblastic or myelophthisic anemia

- Fanconi's anemia

    - Rare autosomal recessive (AR) congenital anemia, presenting between 5 to 10 years old
    - Accompanied by skeletal abnormalities, including hypoplastic thumbs, renal and skin abnormalities
    - Chromosomes—exhibit abnormal fragility during cell culture

● Megaloblastic anemia

- Anemia or pancytopenia caused by altered DNA synthesis resulting from deficiency of B_{12}, folate or rarely inherited metabolic defects in the purine and pyrimidine pathways
- Pathology—morphologic changes in the marrow and PB are the same for all causes

    - PB—large oval-shaped RBCs called *macroovalocyte,* decreased reticulocytes, hypersegmentation of granulocyte nuclei (5 and 6 lobes) with varying anemia, neutropenia, thrombocytopenia, or pancytopenia
    - Marrow—hypercellular marrow, but ineffective hematopoiesis and cellular destruction in the marrow; erythroblasts are enlarged with arrested immature nuclei called *megaloblasts;* the cytoplasm, however, matures normally, giving nuclear-cytoplasmic dysynchony;

granulocyte precursors are also enlarged with abnormal nuclei (giant metamyelocytes and bands)

- B_{12} deficiency

    - Absorption—(1) binding of dietary B_{12} to intrinsic factor (IF) produced by gastric parietal cells, (2) occurs in the small bowel and is dependent on the release of B_{12} from R binder proteins by normal digestion and pancreatic function, (3) B_{12}-IF absorbed in the terminal ileum by binding of the IF to specific receptors

    - B_{12} present in all animal products, and all diets, except strict vegan, is sufficient for intake

    - Malabsorption—the most common cause of deficiency most frequently caused by pernicious anemia

    - Pernicious anemia—B_{12} malabsorption caused by autoimmune gastritis that destroys the ability to produce IF and produces antibodies to IF, elderly of Northern European extraction, insidious onset, association with other autoimmune disease, including autoimmune thyroiditis and Addison's disease

    - Defects at other absorption steps also seen caused by gastrectomy, ileal defects (resection, inflammation, neoplasm), rare parasites (*Diphyllobothrium latum* consumes the B_{12}), blind loop syndrome, and some proximal causes of malabsorption, such as pancreatic insufficiency or duodenal disease

    - Clinical—may develop irreversible posterior and lateral spinal column degeneration, producing ataxia and sensory changes

    - Can measure B_{12} levels, but a response to therapy also useful in diagnosis

- Folate deficiency

    - Absorption—dependent on intact jejunal deconjugase function
    - Dietary sources—largely fresh leafy vegetables
    - Lack of dietary intake—the most important causes of deficiency
    - Alcoholics, drug addicts, and those of low socioeconomic status at high risk of poor dietary intake
    - Pregnancy-lactation, hemolytic anemia, and infants have higher requirements
    - Overcooking destroys folate, and some drugs (dilantin, alcohol) impair absorption
    - Clinical—no neurologic changes, can measure serum levels (reflect short-term diet), red cell levels (reflect levels at the time of erythropoiesis), or monitor response to treatment

■ **Defective Hemoglobin Production**

- The most common causes of anemia worldwide
- Causes—predominantly thalassemia and iron deficiency
- ● Iron deficiency anemia
    - *Simple iron kinetics*
        - A daily western dietary contains about 10 to 20 mg of iron.
        - About 1 to 2 mg is absorbed in the duodenum, and this is the regulated step.

- More iron is absorbed with anemia regardless of the cause of anemia.
- Iron circulates bound to transferrin, and the amount of iron and transferrin varies with iron status.
  - Typical iron deficiency has low serum iron/high transferrin.
- Most iron circulates as hemoglobin but is also present in other body enzymes and stored in histiocytes, especially in the marrow.
  - Stores vary from about 1 to 5 g in adults (males much higher).
  - Serum ferritin measurement is an indirect assessment of iron stores but may be spuriously elevated with inflammation and liver disease.
  - Iron staining of a bone marrow aspirate to demonstrate iron in the histiocytes is the gold standard for storage assessment.
  - A large amount of iron from the degradation of senescent. RBCs is recycled to developing RBCs in the marrow daily.

— *Causes of iron deficiency*
  - The most common cause worldwide is dietary deficiency.
    - Common during infancy and pregnancy in North America and Europe
  - The most important cause in North America and Europe is chronic blood loss.
    - Occult gastrointestinal tract loss caused by malignancy or ulcer
    - In females genital tract loss from menorrhagia or malignancies
      - 1 ml of RBCs—contains about 1 mg of iron, almost the entire amount absorbed per day
  - Malabsorption is less common usually because of diseases affecting duodenal absorption, such as sprue, gastrectomy, or pancreatic insufficiency.

— *Pathology*
  - Microcytic-hypochromic anemia with a low reticulocyte count
  - Lack of iron stores in the bone marrow on Prussian blue staining
  - May be associated with atrophic glossitis, finger nail spooning, and esophageal webs

— *Clinical*
  - Fatigue and dyspnea common
  - With iron administration—reticulocyte response in 3 to 7 days with correction of anemia over next 6 weeks
  - Must identify cause of deficiency

- **Anemia of chronic disease**
  - A common group of anemias that appear multifactorial in pathogenesis occuring with a number of persisting illnesses
  - In North America probably the second most common cause of anemia

after iron deficiency and the most frequent cause in a hospital population

- Occurs 1 to 2 months during illness
- Likely caused by cytokines, especially tumor necrosis factor (TNF), interleukin (IL)-1, and IL-6 producing decreased erythropoiesis, shunting of iron to macrophages, low transferrin levels, and low serum iron
  - Pathology

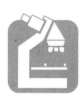

  - Anemia with normal appearing red cells (normochromic-normocytic)
  - Low reticulocyte count, low serum iron-low transferrin with increased iron stores in the bone marrow by Prussian blue staining

- Common causes—collagen-vascular diseases, chronic infections, malignancies

- Thalassemia
  - Inherited hemoglobinopathies, characterized by decreased synthesis of one of the globin chains
  - Most common hemoglobinopathies, and most common inherited cause of anemia
  - Most frequent in African, Asian, and Mediterranean populations
  - The mild clinical form—known as thalassemia trait
    - Mild microcytic-hypochromic anemia often with increased RBC, target cell, and normal or increased iron stores
    - Usually represents a heterozygous or carrier state

— *Alpha thalassemia*
  - Four phenotypes—can be recognized that result from a huge number of genetic defects causing decreased alpha globin chain production
    - Clinical findings—correlate to the number of the four alpha globin genes that remain functional
  - Alpha genes—are on chromosome 16, and exist as two closely tandem-linked copies on each allele
  - One gene defective—silent carrier, no clinical effect
    - Can be detected by genetic DNA analysis
  - Two gene defect—can be *cis* (common Asian form) or *trans,* produces thalassemia trait
  - Three-gene defect—Hemoglobin H disease
    - Hb H—composed of beta chain tetrameres that form from the excessively produced beta chains relative to the alpha chains
    - Hb H demonstrated by incubated reticulocyte stain showing H inclusion bodies that are multiple, dark, red cell inclusion resembling a golf ball
    - Severe anemia with hypochromia and nucleated RBC (NRBC) in the PB

- Excess beta chains—also produce a chronic hemolytic anemia with expansion of marrow causing bone deformities and large spleen
- Seen predominantly in Asians

- Four-gene defect—Bart's Hb Hydrops Fetalis
  - No alpha chains produced, and the predominant hemoglobin, Bart's Hb consists of four gamma chains
  - Seen predominantly in Asians
  - Bart's Hb—fails to transport oxygen, resulting in heart failure, anasarca (hydrops), and intrauterine death

— *Beta thalassemia*
  - Multiple genetic defects result in underproduction of beta globin chains.
    - A single beta globin gene present on chromosome 11 in a gene complex that also has the gamma and the delta globin chains
    - B^0—the affected allele produces no beta chains
    - B^+—the affected allele produces reduced amounts of beta chains
  - Heterozygotes with B^+ or B^0 beta thalassemia have thalassemia trait phenotype (see preceding).
    - Elevated Hb A_2 (alpha2, delta2) levels—diagnostic
  - Homozygotes for B^0 have no beta gene production and have the phenotype of beta thalassemia major.
    - Only Hb F and A_2 are produced
    - As fetal Hb production decreases after birth, is progressively severe anemia
    - PB—severe hypochromia and microcytosis with NRBC
    - Massive expansion of erythropoiesis—causes bone deformities and splenomegaly
    - Survival—requires chronic transfusion; secondary hemochromatosis causes cirrhosis, cardiomyopathy, and death by 20s
  - Inheritance of combinations of B^+ and B^0 genes produces a phenotype between the mild thalassemia trait and the severe thalassemia major.

■ **Hemolytic Anemia**
- Decreased survival of the RBC in circulation less than the normal 120 days that may produce anemia if the rate of destruction is greater than the ability of the bone marrow to compensate (Box 15.3)

● Sickle cell anemia
- A homozygote for beta 6 substitution of valine for glutamic acid that produces episodic hemolysis, microvascular obstruction, and infarction as the result of irreversible polymerization of the abnormal Hb under low oxygen conditions

Box 15.3

CAUSES OF HEMOLYTIC ANEMIA

Inherited
  Membrane
    Spherocytosis
    Elliptocytosis
  Enzyme
    G6PD
  Hemoglobinopathy
    Hb S
    Hb C
Acquired
  Immune
    Autoimmune hemolytic anemia
    Delayed transfusion reaction
    Hemolytic disease of the newborn
  Nonimmune
    Drugs
      Oxidant stress—dapsone
    Infection
      Malaria
    Physical agents
      Burns
      Clostridial toxin
      Disseminated intravascular coagulation, thrombic thrombocytopenia purpura, hemolytic uremic syndrome
      Mechanical heart valve
    Paroxysmal nocturnal hemoglobinuria (PNH)

- Hb S allele present in 8% of African Americans, and the homozygous state in 0.2%
  - Pathology—begin to occur as the amount of Hb F falls after birth
    - PB—anemia and irreversibly sickled cells, elevated reticulocyte count (Fig 15.1)
    - Hb S detected by antibody test, solubility test, and on Hb electrophoresis
    - Infarctive crisis—caused by vascular obstruction producing infarction; common sites are bones (avascular necrosis), spleen (atrophy and autosplenectomy), renal (concentration defect and papillary necrosis), cutaneous ulcers, central nervous system strokes, retinopathy, and acute chest syndrome
    - Iron overload and gallstones result from the chronic hemolysis
  - Other complications
    - Aplastic crisis—usually caused by infection by human parvovirus
    - Osteomyelitis—commonly caused by *Salmonella* organisms

- **Hemoglobin C disease**
  - A mild chronic hemolytic anemia caused by beta 6 substitution of lysine for glutamic acid
  - Second most common abnormal hemoglobin in North America, with about 2% of African-Americans carriers

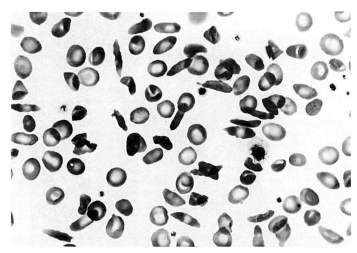

Fig. 15.1 Sickle cell anemia. Numerous hyperchromatic, pointed, irreversibly sickled cells are present. *(Damjanov I, Linder J: Anderson's pathology, ed 10, vol 1, St Louis, 1996, Mosby.)*

- Pathology
  - PB—mild anemia, elevated reticulocyte count, target cells, and occasional Hb C crystals visible after splenectomy
  - Splenomegaly
  - Hb C identified by antibody test or hemoglobin electrophoresis
- Interacts with Hb S in double heterozygote state
- **Hereditary spherocytosis**
  - Predominantly autosomal dominant (AD) disorder of the RBC membrane resulting in formation of spherocytes and a chronic hemolytic anemia caused by defects in spectrin, ankyrin, and protein 4.2
    - All—involve the stabilization of spectrin
    - Recurrent passage of the RBC through the spleen results in loss of membrane
    - Pathology—Fig. 15.2
      - Spherocytic RBCs that lack central pallor, increased reticulocyte count, and a negative direct antiglobulin (Coombs') test
      - Osmotic fragility test—identifies the spherocytes as a population of RBCs sensitive to lysis in low ionic strength
      - Splenomegaly caused by congestion of splenic cords
    - Complications—aplastic crisis, gallstones
    - Clinical—splenectomy decreases the hemolysis effectively
- **Enzyme defects**
  - Glucose-6-phosphate dehydrogenase deficiency—common on a worldwide basis
  - Occurs in 10% of African Americans in an X-linked fashion; also common in Mediterranean and Asian groups
    - Degree and severity of the deficiency—varies widely
    - With exposure to various oxidant stresses, usually drugs such as

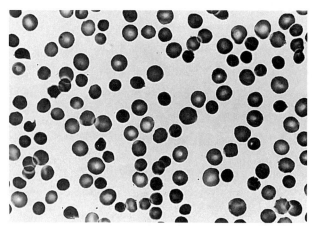

Fig. 15.2 Hereditary spherocytosis. Numerous small, hyperchromatic spherocytes are present. (*Damjanov I, Linder J:* Anderson's pathology, *ed 10, vol 1, St Louis, 1996, Mosby.*)

sulfonamides, primaquine, or nitrofurantoin—the hexose monophosphate shunt cannot maintain hemoglobin in a reduced state

• Clinical—episodic hemolysis, jaundice, and black-colored urine, occasionally neonatal jaundice, favism (severe sudden hemolysis on exposure to fava beans), and chronic hemolysis

• Hemoglobin precipitates—form on the RBC membrane and are pitted by the spleen-producing hemolysis

• Pathology

• Can identify the hemoglobin precipitates as Heinz bodies with reticulocyte stains, but no typical morphology on routine PB stains

• Reticulocyte response—follows hemolysis

• Can assay for enzyme, but beware of elevated levels in reticulocytes causing false-negative results

● **Other causes of hemolysis**

— *Angiopathic hemolytic anemia*

• Hemolysis caused by RBC trauma frequently presumed because of microthrombi fibrin strands fragmenting the RBC

• Causes—artificial aortic valves, march hemolysis, malignant hypertension, eclampsia, disseminated intravascular coagulation (DIC), thrombotic thrombocytopenic purpura (TTP), and hemolytic uremic syndrome (HUS)

• Pathology—PB—numerous RBC angular fragments (schistocytes) irregular shapes, helmet cells, thrombocytopenia common (Fig. 15.3)

— *Malaria*

• Most common acquired hemolytic anemia worldwide caused by plasmodium parasitization of RBC

• Tropical distribution with variety of species

• Cyclical hemolysis producing fever and chills

• Diagnosis by identification of various developmental forms in the RBC on routine blood smears

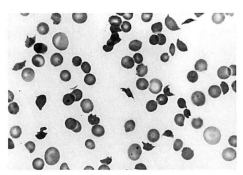

Fig. 15.3 Angiopathic hemolytic anemia. Pointed and angular red cell fragments or schistocytes are present. *(Damjanov I, Linder J:* Anderson's pathology, *ed 10, vol 1, St Louis, 1996, Mosby.)*

— *Autoimmune hemolytic anemia*

- Acquired RBC destruction caused by antibody recognition of surface antigens resulting in complement lysis or opsonization and phagocytosis in the spleen
- Autoimmune hemolytic anemia (AIHA) can occur at any age but more common with aging
- Causes—idiopathic, malignancies (especially lymphoid), drugs (dopa), autoimmune diseases, and certain infections (EBV and mycoplasma)
- Warm autoimmune hemolytic anemia—caused by antibodies reactive at 37° C, most common type

  - Clinical—abrupt onset of jaundice, splenomegaly, and anemia, usually idiopathic etiology
  - Pathology—spherocytes, anemia, reticulocytosis, and positive direct antiglobulin test (DAT)
  - Usually caused by IgG antibodies with no complement on RBCs

- Cold autoimmune hemolytic anemia—caused by antibodies reactive at 4° C

  - Postinfectious—children and young adults, acute onset but usually self-limited, after EBV, cytomegalovirus (CMV), and mycoplasma
  - Cold agglutinin disease—older patients often with underlying non-Hodgkin's lymphoma (NHL), may have Raynaud's disease, livido reticularis, and exacerbation of hemolysis with cold exposure
  - Pathology—usually caused by an IgM antibody, and the DAT is positive for complement on the RBC surface, PB—agglutination of the RBC in the smear, reticulocytosis

- Paroxysmal cold hemoglobinuria—rare acute hemolysis after exposure to cold caused by a cold reacting IgG that fixes complement at reduced temperature followed by hemolysis with warming; antibody referred to as the Donath-Landsteiner antibody; historically seen in tertiary syphilis, but now common in children postviral illnesses

MULTIPLE CHOICE REVIEW QUESTIONS

1. A normochromic normocytic anemia, low serum iron and iron binding capacity, and abundant iron in the bone marrow macrophages are most characteristic of which of the following?

   a. Iron deficiency anemia
   b. Anemia of chronic disease
   c. Malaria
   d. Glucose 6-phosphate dehydrogenase deficiency (G6PD)
   e. Beta thalassemia

2. The combination of normochromic/normocytic anemia and nucleated red blood cells in the peripheral smear is most typical of which of the following?

   a. Myelophthisic anemia
   b. Iron deficiency anemia
   c. Hereditary spherocytosis
   d. Hemoglobin C disease
   e. Alpha thalassemia

3. A 70-year-old woman noted fatigue, shortness of breath and burning feet. An unsteady gait was observed. The MCV (mean red cell volume) was 110 femtoliters (normal 82-96) and hypersegmented neutrophils were seen on smear. Antiparietal cell antibodies were detected in the serum. It is most likely that this patient has deficiency of which of the following?

   a. Folic acid
   b. Niacin
   c. Thiamine
   d. Vitamin C
   e. Vitamin B_{12}

4. Most hereditary spherocytoses are characterized by a decreased amount of which of the following?

   a. Alpha globin
   b. Beta globin
   c. Glucose 6-phosphate dehydrogenase
   d. Spectrin
   e. Complement resistance

5. Decreased synthesis of beta globin chains with normal synthesis of alpha chains is found in which of the following?

   a. Sickle cell anemia
   b. Alpha thalassemia
   c. Beta thalassemia
   d. Hemoglobin C disease
   e. Hemoglobin H disease

Chapter 16

Bleeding Disorders

■ Thrombosis

- Maintaining the blood in a fluid state is achieved by the interaction of the vascular endothelium, blood anticoagulant proteins, and platelets.

- Important platelet inhibitors produced by the endothelium are prostacycline (PGI_2), and nitric oxide.

- There are three main anticoagulant pathways: antithrombin III (AT III), protein C pathway, and plasminogen.

  - AT III

    - Binds irreversibly to several coagulant factors, most importantly thrombin and activated factor X (Xa)
    - Binding—enhanced by heparin-like substances on the endothelial surface or administered theraputic heparin
    - Pathway—continuously active

  - Protein C pathway

    - Involves protein C, protein S, factor V, thrombomodulin, and thrombin
    - Some thrombin produced from the coagulation cascade—binds to endothelial thrombomodulin
    - Complex of thrombin-thrombomodulin—activates protein C (APC)
    - APC—inactivates VIIIa and Va in complex with the endothelial surface and the cofactor protein S
    - Activation—occurs with production of thrombin (coagulation)

  - Fibrinolysis

    - Also occurs in concert with coagulation
    - Plasminogen—activated by plasminogen activators (especially tissue plasminogen activator [tPA] produced by the endothelium) in the fibrin meshwork to plasmin where it cleaves fibrin
    - In the plasma alpha-2 antiplasmin—rapidly inactivates any free plasmin away from a clot unbound to fibrin
    - Plasminogen activator inhibitor-1 (PAI-1)—inactivates plasminogen activators in the plasma, further limiting the formation and action of plasmin to the area of a fibrin clot

- Predisposition to thrombosis can be divided into factors producing vessel (endothelial) injury, stasis, and changes in the blood promoting clotting, collectively known as Vichow's triad.

  - Endothelial injury may be from surgery, trauma, hemodynamic stress cho-

Table 16.1 *Useful Bleeding Features*		
BLEEDING PATTERN	**COAGULATION ABNORMALITY**	**PLATELET-VESSEL ABNORMALITY**
Petechia	No	Yes
Hemarthrosis	Yes	No
Time after injury	Delayed	Immediate
Sites of bleeding	Intramuscular	Skin and mucosa
	Visceral	
	Deep hematoma	

lesterol, viruses, immune complexes, hyperhomocytinemia, diabetes, hypertension, antiphospholipid antibodies, smoking, hyperlipidemia, or other factors.

- Endothelial injury—most important in arterial thrombosis
- Polycythemia, paroxysmal nocturnal hemoglobinuria (PNH); other myeloproliferative disorders also predisposed to arterial thrombosis

- Venous thrombosis is more common in the setting of stasis, especially immobilization of the lower limbs, pregnancy, and abnormalities of the proteins involved in the anticoagulation pathways.

- Anticoagulant proteins—usually display autosomal dominant (AD) inheritance with variable penetrance
- Acquired forms seen in liver disease and with administration of some drugs
- Important deficiencies are—factor V Leiden (a mutation in factor V that interferes with its inactivation by APC, may account for 40% to 50% of thrombosis predisposition), proteins C, S, and AT III deficiency (collectively possibly 15% of unexpected thrombosis)
- Dysfibrinogenemia, plasminogen deficiency, and abnormalities of tPA and PAI-1—less common, the latter two are of unknown frequency

- Pathology of thrombosis—discussed in hemodynamic disturbances

■ Bleeding Disorders

- Hemostasis is dependent on vessels, platelets, and the coagulation system.
- Bleeding disorders result from abnormalities in each of these and the fibrinolytic system.
- The pattern of bleeding is useful in determining the etiology of bleeding (Table 16.1).
- Coagulation system is diagrammed in Fig. 16.1.
- General coagulation tests

  - Thrombin time (TT) assesses the amount and quality of fibrinogen.
  - Prothrombin time (PT) assesses the extrinsic pathway and the common pathway.
  - Activated partial thromboplastin time (aPTT) assesses the intrinsic pathway and the common pathway.

- Coagulation disorders can be divided broadly into factor deficiencies and inhibitors.

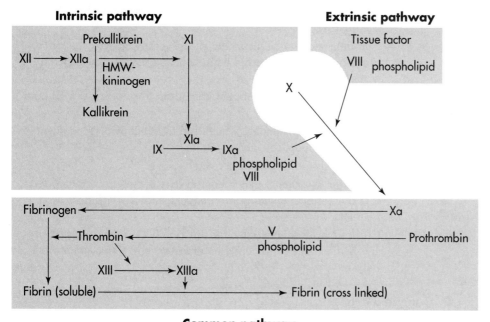

Fig. 16.1 Coagulation cascade. *(Modified from Damjanov I, Linder J: Anderson's pathology, ed 10, vol 1, St Louis, 1996, Mosby.)*

- Factor deficiencies may be inherited or acquired.
- **Acquired deficiencies**
  - Liver disease
    - The liver is the source of all factors except VIII and von Willebrand factor (VWF).
    - With severe liver disease, the Vitamin K factors are depleted first as carboxylation is affected, V is preserved until late stages.
    - VIII and VWF may be increased.
    - Fibrinogen produced in liver disease can be abnormal and dysfunctional.
    - Laboratory test values include elevated PT, aPTT, and TT, platelets can be low from hypersplenism.
  - Vitamin K deficiency
    - Vitamin K—the cofactor in liver carboxylation of II, VII, IX, and XII that forms the calcium binding site
    - Causes—fat malabsorption, diet low in leafy vegetables, neonates, and Coumadin administration
    - Hemorrhagic disease of the newborn—bleeding at day 2 to 7 caused by Vitamin K deficiency in neonates, prevented by prophylactic administration at birth
    - Laboratory—PT is the most sensitive to Vitamin K deficiencies because of its dependence on VII, which has the shortest half life of about 4 hours
  - Disseminated Intravascular Coagulation (DIC)

- Syndrome resulting from uncontrolled activation of thrombin in the microvasculature
- Common causes—tissue factor release (promyelocytic leukemia, obstetrical accidents, other malignancies), vascular endothelial damage (sepsis, shock)
- Coagulation factors consumed, including fibrinogen, V, VIII, and platelets
- Microthrombi generated, which lead to ischemic organ damage and microangiopathic hemolysis
- Fibrinolysis—may also be activated
- Laboratory—changes depend on severity of the process, elevated PT, aPTT, fibrin degradation products, and TT with decreased platelets
- Clinically—produces organ dysfunction because of microthrombi and hemorrhage from depletion of factors and activation of fibrinolysis

● **Inherited deficiencies**

- Deficiencies of VIII and IX only common significant disorders
- Both are X-linked
- Clinical—males with classic factor deficiency bleeding (see Table 16.1), the severity dependent on the levels of coagulation factors
- Laboratory—mild deficiencies of VIII and IX may have normal aPTT, but it is prolonged in most patients; specific factor assays assign the correct diagnosis
- Most other factor deficiencies—produce prolongation of the PT, aPTT, or both, depending on their site in the coagulation cascade (see Fig. 16.1) permitting tentative identification and selection of specific factor assays
- Notable exceptions to the above—mild deficiencies above the sensitivity of the common screening coagulation tests; factor XIII, which is not included in any of the screening tests; and VWF deficiency

● **Coagulation inhibitors**

- Specific antibodies
  - Occur in hemophiliacs in response to antigens given with factor replacement treatment or as autoimmune disorders in elderly
  - Cause severe, difficult-to-control hemorrhage
  - Laboratory—extremely long coagulation tests; specific factor assay identifies the antibody targeted factor

- Lupus anticoagulant
  - Antiphospholipid antibodies—interfere with the phospholipid used in coagulation tests, mostly affecting the aPTT, causing prolongation
  - Occur with systemic lupus erythematosus (SLE), drugs (procainamide, antipsychotics), HIV, postviral illness, or idiopathic
  - Generally do not bleed, but have an increased incidence of thrombosis

■ **Platelets Disorders**

- The screening tests for platelet disorders—a platelet count and a careful history and physical examination
- Other common follow-up tests are a bleeding time, platelet function or aggregation studies, a bone marrow, and peripheral blood film examination

● Quantitative platelet disorders

- Spurious thrombocytopenia—may be seen with a partially clotted blood sample, platelet clumping (an antibody-mediated phenomena usually dependent on the ethylenediaminetetraacetic acid [EDTA] anticoagulant) or platelet satelitism (rings around neutrophils)
  - Production failure
    - All general causes of marrow failure (see White Blood Cell Diseases chapter and Red Blood Cell Diseases chapter)
    - Rare inherited specific megakaryocyte aplasia
    - Heavy alcohol abuse—a fairly common cause of suppression that recovers spontaneously 5 to 7 days after abstinence
  - Increased destruction
    - May be immune or nonimmune
  - Immune
    - Immune thrombocytopenic purpura (ITP)—an antibody-mediated destruction of platelets analogous to autoimmune hemolytic anemia
    - Causes—idiopathic, drug induced, collagen vascular diseases, post-infectious, or with lymphomas
    - In the hospital heparin-associated thrombocytopenia—an important cause that can result in massive thrombosis
  - Nonimmune
    - Thrombotic thrombocytopenic purpura and hemolytic uremic syndrome (TTP, HUS)—uncommon disorders of fever, uremia, micro-angiopathic anemia, thrombocytopenia, and, with TTP neurologic symptoms; caused by platelet microvascular thrombi, may be seen with verrotoxin producing *Escherichia coli* infection, and idiopathically
    - DIC (see preceding)

● Qualitative platelet disorders

- Present with classic finding of platelet-vessel bleeding (see Table 16.1)
- von Willebrand disease
  - Fairly common (possibly the most common inherited bleeding disorder) deficiency of VWF produced by the endothelium
  - Results in both platelet bleeding caused by the lack of this adhesion protein and coagulation pattern bleeding in some patients as VWF is the transport protein for VIII in the plasma
  - Deficiency—may be the entire absence of VWF or lack of the most functional high molecular weight multimers
  - Laboratory—levels of VWF vary over time, may see prolonged

aPTT, low factor VIII levels, low VWF levels, absence of high molecular weight (HMW) VWF, prolonged bleeding time, and abnormal platelet aggregation with ristocetin

- Aspirin and drug effects
  - Most common causes of mild platelet dysfunction
- Glanzmann's thrombasthenia
  - Rare inherited abnormality of platelets caused by deficiency of fibrinogen receptor IIb-IIIa
  - Normal platelet count and morphology but prolonged bleeding time and, in some patients, severe bleeding history
- Bernard-Soulier disease
  - Rare inherited abnormality of platelet glycoprotein Ib
  - Mild thrombocytopenia and giant platelets, prolonged bleeding time

- Other inherited platelet abnormalities include—storage pool defects (abnormal platelet granule contents, especially adenine diphosphate [ADP]) and abnormalities in the release of granule contents (complex diverse group often referred to as aspirin-like defects)

  - Prolonged bleeding times, normal platelet counts

■ Vessel Abnormalities

- Uncommon; only the bleeding time may be prolonged with normal platelet function studies

- Disorders include—vasculitis, septicemia, other infections (Rocky Mountain Spotted Fever), scurvy, Ehlers-Danlos syndrome, Cushing's syndrome, hereditary hemorrhagic telangiectasia, amyloidosis

Multiple Choice Review Questions

1. Hemorrhagic disease of the newborn (Vitamin K deficiency) causes bleeding primarily because of which of the following?

    a. Decreased synthesis of clotting factors
    b. Decreased platelet function
    c. Decreased platelet production
    d. Increased platelet destruction
    e. Synthesis of abnormal vascular collagen

2. The predominant aspirin effect resulting in a predisposition to bleeding is that it does which of the following?

    a. Decreases synthesis of clotting factors
    b. Decreases thrombin activity
    c. Decreases platelet production
    d. Decreases platelet function
    e. Damages vascular endothelium

3. A young woman presents with heavy menorrhagia and easy bruising. A platelet count is normal. The most appropriate test of platelet function is which of the following?

    a. Bleeding time
    b. Prothrombin time
    c. Thrombin time
    d. Activated partial thromboplastin time
    e. Fibrinogen level

4. Which of the following is an important inhibitor of platelet in vivo?

    a. Prostacyclin (PGI_2)
    b. Epinephrine
    c. Adenosine diphosphate
    d. 5-Hydroxytryptamine
    e. Thrombin

5. The conversion of fibrinogen to fibrin is the result of activation of which of the following?

    a. Prothrombin
    b. Factor X
    c. Plasminogen
    d. Factor XIII
    e. Thrombomodulin

Chapter 17

Transfusion Medicine

- Blood groups—inherited polymorphism in proteins, glycoproteins, and glycolipids on the red cell membrane carried by genes inherited in an allelic manner or as groups of tightly linked genes, to which individuals may raise alloantibodies in response to exposure

- Sensitization—exposure of blood groups antigens to an individual that allows that formation of alloantibodies

  - Mechanisms of exposure—for ABO (blood group) cross-reactive antigens in the environment; for most others, transfusion, pregnancy (fetal to maternal), and transplantation of organs

- Importance of blood groups—safe blood transfusion, organ transplantation, hemolytic disease of the newborn

◼ Important Blood Groups

- ABO and Rh blood group systems are the most important of the over 200 antigens
- Most are expressed as autosomal codominant traits

◼ ABO System

- Dominant antigens involved in blood transfusion
- Antigens—complex carbohydrates carried on red cell glycoproteins, glycolipids, and other tissues and fluids
- Antibodies to the ABO antigens—"natural" occurring in all normal individuals after the first year of life because of sensitization by similar antigens present in the environment, likely GI tract bacteria
- Natural antibodies are IgM class and can

  - Agglutinate red cells in a test tube (the basis of cross matching)
  - Fix complement in vivo, causing acute hemolytic transfusion reactions

- ABO types and their naturally occurring antibodies given in Table 17.1
- Genetics of the ABO system well characterized and depends on two genes
- H transferase—a fucosyltransferase that makes the precursor H substance and A, B, and O glycosyltransferases—alleles at chromosome 9 locus

  - A transferase—adds a terminal N-acetylgalactosamine sugar
  - B transferase—adds a terminal galactosamine sugar
  - O transferase—a truncation mutation without transferase activity that adds no terminal sugar
  - Other transferases—generally of altered substrate affinity and cause less or altered sugar addition, leading to weaker subgroups of A or B

Table 17.1 *ABO Antigens and Antibodies*

ABO GROUP	RBC ANTIGEN	NATURAL SERUM ANTIBODY
O (45%)*	None (H)	Anti-A, anti-B, anti-A,B
A (40%)	A	Anti-B
B (10%)	B	Anti-A
AB (5%)	A and B	None

*Approximate frequencies in North American Caucasians.

Table 17.2 *ABO Inheritance*

ABO GROUP (PHENOTYPES)	ACTIVE GENES	POSSIBLE GENOTYPES
O	H transferase	O/O
A	H and A transferases	O/A, A/A
B	H and B transferases	O/B, B/B
AB	H, A, and B transferases	A/B

- Simple mendelian inheritance—will determine the ABO group (Table 17.2)
- A_2—the only common subgroup found in 20% of A and AB subjects
  - About 2% of A_2 and 25% of A_2B—make anti-A_1
  - Anti-A_1—seldom reacts at 37 degrees, and rarely results in clinical problems other than to delay finding compatible blood
- People rarely lack the H transferase—Bombay phenotype
  - Phenotype as group O but also lack H antigens
  - Make anti-H, anti-A,B, anti-A, and anti-B and can have severe hemolytic transfusion reactions
- Clinical importance
  - All people have natural IgM antibodies to ABO groups and may have IgG antibodies from pregnancy or other exposure.
  - These can fix complement at 37° C.
  - Transfusion of non-ABO compatible blood can cause immediate intravascular red cell hemolysis.
  - This produces shock, renal failure, DIC, and sometimes death.
  - ABO antigens are present on other tissue including platelets, vascular endothelium, various epithelium, plasma, and secretions.
  - In solid organ transplantation, ABO matching is important and preformed antibodies may cause hyperacute rejection.

■ **Rh System**

- Next to the ABO antigens, Rh antigens are the most immunogenic and will cause the formation of antibodies upon exposure in 80% of patients.

- Exposure is usually from transfusions and pregnancy.
- The commonly recognized antigens include D, C, E, c, and e, with the absence of D, usually referred to as d.
- There are many rare members of this antigen system.
- The antigens are encoded by two tandem, tightly linked genes on chromosome 1 that probably represent a gene duplication event.
- One gene encodes for the C/c and E/e polymorphism, and one for the presence of D (note: there is no d allele, and d really means the absence of D antigen).
- The two membrane lipoproteins assemble to form a membrane complex that may function in ion regulation.
- Practically, the two genes can be considered as a single allele, such as CDe (the most common allele in Caucasians, 41%) and cde (the next, 39%).
- In the simplest form, individuals are Rh positive (D antigen) or negative, and, for transfusion blood-typing purposes, this is all that is routinely considered.
- For Caucasians approximately 85% are Rh(D) positive, with higher frequencies in other geographic groups.
- Clinical importance

  - Antibodies can cause hemolytic disease of the newborn and delayed transfusion reactions.
  - Antibodies are not naturally occurring and require sensitization with transfusion, pregnancy, or other exposure to blood, such as needle sharing.
  - Anti-D is the most common antibody to develop in individuals who lack this antigen, but anti-C, -c, -E, and -e and combinations are seen. (Note: there is no anti-d, as this is the lack of D antigen seen with a nonfunctional D gene.)
  - Rare individuals have no functional Rh genes. They express no Rh membrane proteins and have a congenital hemolytic anemia with spherocytes and stomatocytes.

Other Important Antigens

- Other antigens are clinically important if they cause hemolytic disease of the newborn, hemolytic transfusion reactions, or if they delay the timely provision of blood products from the blood bank because of difficulties in the cross-matching process.
- The more problematic antigen systems (abbreviations in parenthesis) include Kell (K), Duffy (Fy), Kidd (Jk), Lewis (Le), MNSs blood group, P (P$_1$), and Lutheran (Lu).

Mechanisms of Immune Red Cell Destruction

- Intravascular—caused by complement lysis by IgM antibodies or less commonly IgG antibodies that can fix complement

  - Most important mechanism for ABO antibodies and immediate hemolytic transfusion reactions

- Extravascular—caused by the mononuclear phagocyte engulfing and destroying the red cells opsonized by IgG through the Fc gamma receptors

  - Occurs predominantly in the spleen

- Direct antibody-dependent cell-mediated cytotoxicity possibly also involved
- Is the mechanism for delayed hemolytic transfusion reactions and hemolytic disease of the newborn (HDN)

■ Hemolytic Disease of the Newborn

- IgG produced by mother is normally transported across the placenta, providing immunologic protection to the neonate.
- Fetal red cells can enter the mother's circulation and may cause antibody production to red cell antigens inherited from father that mother lacks.
- Antibodies to fetal red cells can cross the placenta and cause hemolysis of fetal red cells.

  - Fetal red cell entry occurs at any time during pregnancy but is more common in later trimesters, with trauma or obstetric emergencies, such as abruption, and always occurs at parturition.
  - Mothers may be sensitized in a first pregnancy.
  - High levels of antibody can develop in a second pregnancy affecting the fetus if it also carries the same paternal antigen.
  - Antibodies to Rh and ABO antigens are the most common.

- Severe hemolysis can produce marked anemia, hepatosplenomegaly, edema, congestive heart failure, and intrauterine death.

  - Hydrops fetalis—intrauterine death with severe fetal edema
  - Erythroblastosis fetalis—historic synonym for hemolytic disease of the newborn, referring to the large numbers of erythroblasts in the neonatal peripheral blood in response to hemolysis

- Less severe hemolysis may allow survival till birth, but ongoing hemolysis after birth can overwhelm the neonatal liver's capacity to metabolize the bilirubin produced from hemoglobin degradation.
  - The resulting unconjugated hyperbilirubinemia can cause kernicterus.

    - In utero the maternal liver metabolizes most of the bilirubin.
    - Kernicterus is the toxic effect of high levels of bilirubin on immature brain tissue that untreated may produce choreoathetosis, mental retardation, and death.
    - This can be treated by phototherapy and exchange transfusion before the bilirubin levels reach critical levels.

- HDN caused by D Rh antigen is preventable with administration of anti-D antibody to nonsensitized Rh negative mothers during pregnancy and at delivery.

  - Prior to this program Rh-caused HDN was quite common.
  - This passive immunity seems to prevent primary immunization caused by exposure to D cells, perhaps the result of their rapid destruction bypassing the usual antigen-presenting cells.

- HDN caused by ABO antibodies is milder than Rh disease, seldom causing significant problems, aside from mild anemia and jaundice.
  - Other clinically significant antigens listed above can also cause HDN.

■ **Blood Banking Basics**

- Use of all blood products should be considered potentially hazardous, and these risks should be weighed against the potential benefits.

● **Compatibility Testing**

- All blood products are tested and assigned an ABO group and Rh status (positive for D or negative) when this is important for a product's safe transfusion.
  - All recipients' red cells and serum are tested to
    - Assign their ABO and Rh types
    - See if they have unexpected antibodies to any of the clinically significant blood antigens, in addition to the expected naturally occurring ABO antibodies (serum screening test)
- Using the patient blood type—ABO and Rh type-specific blood can then be selected for transfusion.
  - Compatibility is verified by
    - Confirming the ABO group compatibility with either an immediate agglutination test or full crossmatching of patient serum against the red cells in the unit (using an *indirect* antiglobulin or Coombs' test) for recipients who have unexpected antibodies in the serum screening test
    - Maintaining and enforcing stringent regulations regarding identification of the patient, the patient sample that was tested, and the unit of red cells at the time of transfusion
- Most acute hemolytic transfusion reactions are caused by errors in patient identification or clerical errors (misread label or similar type of error) that result in a transfusion of the incorrect ABO type.

● **Antiglobulin Test (Coombs' Test)**

- The basic test in the blood bank, in addition to observing for RBC agglutination
- Direct antiglobulin test—detects antibody bound to the red blood cells being tested (indicates in vivo bound antibody) and performed by
  - Washing patients' red cells
  - Adding the antihuman globulin reagent (AHG or Coombs' serum)
  - Observing for agglutination
  - If antibodies or components of complement were on the red cells being tested—the anti-immunoglobulin or anticomplement antibodies in the AHG would bind to these and cause agglutination
  - Antibody bound to red cells in vivo—may be cause of hemolytic disease of the newborn, hemolytic transfusion reactions, autoimmune hemolytic anemias, and some drug-induced hemolytic anemias
- Indirect antiglobulin test—detects antibody in the serum being tested and is performed by
  - Incubating test serum with indicator red cells (whose antigen phenotype is known) or with the RBCs of the unit to be transfused to allow binding of any antibody present in the serum being tested

- Washing and adding AHG
- Observing for agglutination
- Agglutination of the indicator cell—indicates the serum contained antibodies that bound to antigens on the indicator cell
- Antibody in the test serum—indicates prior sensitization to an RBC antigen and the need to transfuse red cells that lack this antigen to allow them to survive in the recipient
- Antibodies to the RBCs in the unit to be transfused—indicate incompatibility of that unit, and it can not be safely transfused into that patient

- Human leukocyte antigen (HLA) testing—uses some similar methods, except lymphocytes are substituted for red cells

MULTIPLE CHOICE
REVIEW QUESTIONS

1. The best alternative choice for the transfusion of a Group B patient when no Group B products are available is which of the following?

   a. Group A packed cells
   b. Group AB packed cells
   c. Group AB whole blood
   d. Group O packed cells
   e. Group O whole blood

2. The requirement of a red cell antibody screen in pre-transfusion testing is to do which of the following?

   a. Assure probable transfusion compatibility of ABO group specific blood
   b. Determine a patient's ABO type
   c. Determine a patient's Rh phenotype
   d. Detect naturally occurring anti-A or anti-B
   e. Detect a positive direct antiglobulin test

3. A normal individual with no antibodies against both A and B red blood cell antigens is most likely which of the following?

   a. Group O
   b. Group B
   c. Group AB
   d. Group A
   e. Bombay phenotype

4. A child has group O, Rh negative blood type and the mother is Group B, Rh negative. Assuming no subgroups or null alleles, which of the following is the blood type that would best exclude a man of being the father?

   a. Group A, Rh positive
   b. Group AB, Rh negative
   c. Group O, Rh positive
   d. Group O, Rh negative
   e. Group B, Rh positive

5. Which of the following are antibodies that react with the Jk^a antigens?

   a. Present in Jk^a-positive individuals
   b. Directed against the patient's glycolipid structures
   c. Produced by transferases such as galactosyl-transferase
   d. Usually IgM
   e. The result of transfusion or pregnancy

$\mathbb{C}$hapter 18

Head and Neck

■ **Oral Cavity and Oropharnyx (Excluding Dental Conditions)**

● Congenital

- Cleft lip and palate—most common congenital malformations

- Branchial cleft cyst and fistula—developmental persistence of branchial arches from the parotid region to the lateral neck, usually lined by squamous epithelium, filled by clear fluid, and many associated with lymphoid tissue

- Developmental thyroid abnormalities—lingual thyroid and cysts from the thyroglossal duct anywhere midline from the base of tongue to thyroid gland

● Inflammatory conditions

- Infections—extremely frequent in the oropharnyx

- Infections by site—lips-cheilitis, gums-gingivitis, tongue-glossitis, anterior oral mucosa-stomatitis, posterior mucosa-pharyngitis and tonsillitis

- Specific entities of note

- Bacterial pharnygitis—especially betahemolytic streptococci with the nonsuppurative sequelae of scarlet fever, glomerulonephritis, and rheumatic fever

- Necrotizing ulcerative gingivitis (Vincent's disease)—ulcerating infection caused by normal gingival floral including *Bacteroides intermedius, Fusobacterium necrophorum,* and *Borrelia vincentii*

- Inflammatory conditions of note

- Recurrent aphthous ulcers—likely the most common oral mucosal disorder, unknown etiology, small shallow ulcers with fibrinopurulent exudate and underlying acute inflammation

- Many skin disorders and systemic diseases—may affect the oropharnyx including lichen planus, erythema multiforme, systemic lupus erythematosus (SLE), pemphigus vulgaris, pemphigoid, human immunodeficiency virus (HIV)-acquired immunodeficiency syndrome (AIDS) complications and Crohn's disease

● Tumors and tumorlike lesions

— *Fibrous hyperplasia*

- A reactive condition—thought caused by chronic trauma, such as dentures

- Can be focal, generalized, or papillary

- Papillary usually on the hard palate of denture wearers, and generalized seen with dilantin use
- Pathology—nondysplastic squamous epithelium that may be thickened with parakeratosis or orthokeratosis overlying collagenized lamina propria that may be inflamed
  - Not considered to be premalignant

— *Oral papillomas*
- Variety of lesions united by their gross exophytic papillary appearance
- Squamous papilloma—most common oral neoplasm
  - Usually tongue, palate, gingiva, and lips
  - Pathology—papilla of stratified squamous epithelium on fine fibrovascular cores
  - Varying numbers contain human papilloma virus (HPV)
- Other lesions include—verruca vulgaris, condyloma acuminatum, and upper aerodigestive (juvenile) papillomatosis

— *Mucoceles*
- General term for cyst or cystlike lesion resulting from accumulation of mucous
- Mucous extravastation—most common intraoral mucoceles resulting from rupture of a minor salivary gland, most common in the lower lip from trauma, not lined by epithelium
- Mucous retention cyst—a true cyst lined by salivary gland epithelium caused by mucous collection from duct obstruction
- Ranula—any type of mucocele in the floor of the mouth

— *Fibroma*
- Common lesion caused by chronic irritation
- 20- to 40-year old on lateral tongue, buccal and labial mucosa, or gingival margin
- Pathology
  - Gross—small less than 1 cm nodule
  - Microscopic—thinned or ulcerated epithelium over hypocellular dense collagen bundles and fibroblasts

— *Pyogenic granuloma*
- Most likely hyperplastic granulation tissue rather than true neoplasm, although some consider it a hemangioma
- Contains no granulomatous inflammation or suppuration
- Possibly a response to trauma or injury, also common in pregnancy
- Pathology
  - Gross—rapidly enlarging polypoid mass
  - Microscopic—ulcerated or atropic epithilium over edematous, myxoid stroma rich in capillaries
- Not infrequently recurs after excision

— *Granular cell tumor*

- Tumor of Schwann cells arising in skin and mucous membranes, with the most frequent site the tongue
- Pathology

  - Gross—firm, painless submucosal nodule
  - Microscopic—large cells with central, small, round nuclei and abundant pink cytoplasm

- Most—benign but can recurr with incomplete excision or be multiple

— *Premalignant lesions*

Leukoplakia

- Clinical term meaning white patch on a mucous membrane that does not rub off and that is not found to be another specific histologic disorder on biopsy (many disorders present as white patches including—candidiasis, lupus erythematosus, lichen planus, and squamous cell carcinoma)
- Commonly biopsied lesion of 50- to 70-year-old males
- About 5%—have simultaneous malignancy in the biopsy; about 5% will have malignancy on subsequent biopsy
- Lesions with reddened areas and on the floor of mouth, lateral underside of tongue, and the lips highest risk for carcinoma
- Pathology—"leukoplakia" does not indicate a specific histologic diagnosis

  - Nondysplastic keratosis—most cases will be of this histologic type composed of combinations of hyperorthokeratosis, hyperkeratosis, and acanthosis without atypia
  - Dysplastic keratosis—mild to severe epithelial dysplasia
  - Carcinoma in situ—complete loss of maturation sequence from bottom to top of epithelium, but no invasion through basement membrane

Erythroplakia (erythroplasia of Queyrat)

- Velvety red patches on mucous membrane not found to be caused by another specific condition clinically or with biopsy (many disorders present as red lesions—hemangioma, gingivitis, pyogenic granuloma, candidiasis, squamous carcinoma, lymphoma and leukemia, Kaposi's sarcoma, and other tumors)
- Like leukoplakia, erythroplakia—does not indicate a specific histologic diagnosis, but most are found to be squamous cell carcinoma or dysplasia
- Demographics and sites of involvement similar to squamous carcinoma
- Pathology

  - Microscopic—90% invasive squamous cell carcinoma, carcinoma in situ, and severe dysplasia; 10% mild or moderate dysplasia (Fig. 18.1)

- Areas of erythroplakia—should be completely excised and subject to entire histologic examination

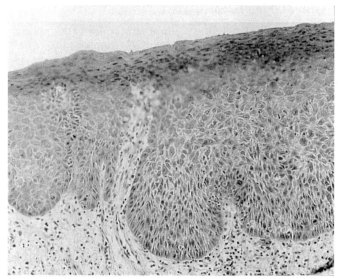

Fig. 18.1 Erythroplakia. This oral biopsy from a velvety red patch has loss of sequential maturation of the squamous cells (from top to bottom) but does not invade the underlying connective tissue, consistent with a squamous cell carcinoma, in situ. (*Damjanov I, Linder J:* Anderson's pathology, *ed 10, vol 2, St Louis, 1996, Mosby.*)

— *Malignant lesions*

- Squamous carcinoma—is the most frequent oral malignancy followed by salivary gland carcinomas and, distantly, lymphoma

Squamous cell carcinoma

- Strongly associated with tobacco and alcohol use
- 2% to 3% of all carcinomas, 2:1 male predominance, occurring after age 50 years
- 5-year survival rate—about 50% overall
- Sites—30% tongue, 15% lip, and 15% floor of mouth
- Pathology—squamous carcinoma of varying degrees of differentiation

  - Verrucous carcinoma—less common, well-differentiated squamous cell carcinoma, may be underdiagnosed as benign, common with chewing tobacco and snuff use

■ **Salivary Glands**

● Salivary gland tumors

- Benign tumors—relatively more common in larger salivary glands with benign to malignant ratio falling as glands get smaller

— *Pleomorphic adenoma (benign mixed tumor)*

- The most common tumor (greater than 50%), most frequent in parotid
- All ages but peaks at 40 years, female:male is 3 to 4:1
- Smooth, painless, hard, slow-growing mass
- Pathology

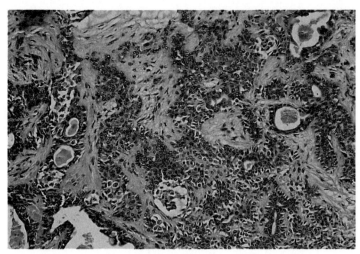

Fig. 18.2 Pleomorphic adenoma. Benign ductlike structures lie in a fibromyxoid stroma. (*Damjanov I, Linder J:* Anderson's Pathology, *ed 10, vol 2, St Louis, 1996, Mosby.*)

- Gross—encapsulated but with small protruding nodules
- Microscopic—variable mix of epithelial (ductal and myoepithelial cells) and mesenchymal components (fibrous, myxoid, or cartilage-like stroma) (Fig. 18.2)

- Benign but excision must include a cuff of normal tissue to prevent

— *Warthin's tumor (papillary cystadenoma lymphomatosum) local recurrence*

- Benign tumor of the parotid
- Male predominance, age greater than 40 years
- Pathology

  - Microscopic—two-cell layer of eosinophilic (oncocytic) columnar cells lining cysts and papillary projections with a stroma of lymphoid tissue and germinal centers

— *Mucoepidermoid carcinoma*

- Most common malignant tumor of salivary glands in the United States
- Occurs at all ages, but incidence increases with age
- May arise post-irradiation
- Pathology

  - Microscopic—mixture of squamous epithelium, mucinous glandular elements, and intermediate cells with features of both
  - Behavior depends on the amount and degree of differentiation in the squamous component
  - Indolent—well-differentiated, more prominant mucinous and cystic areas
  - Aggressive—resemble squamous carcinoma arising at any site, scanty intracellular mucin

— *Adenoid cystic carcinoma*

- Most frequent salivary gland malignancy in Europe
- More common in minor salivary glands
- Pathology—extensive local invasion, tracking along nerve bundles
  - Microscopic—small cells with compact, dark nuclei and scanty cytoplasm
  - Characteristic cribriform pattern: Swiss cheese or sievelike with hyaline or mucoid material forming the holes
- Difficult to excise, poor outcome at 20 years

— *Acinic cell carcinoma*

- An uncommon, low-grade malignancy, most frequently of parotid glands that mimics appearance of an acinus

● Sialadenitis

- Inflammation of the salivary gland—may be result of obstruction, radiation, autoimmunity, or microbial pathogens

— *Infectious sialadenitis*

- Acute suppurative sialadenitis—usually caused by ascending *Staphylococcus aureus* or streptococci, causing typical acute inflammation
  - Granulomatous inflammation—*Mycobacterium tuberculosis*
  - Mumps sialadenitis—common but rarely biopsied, lymphocytic infiltration

— *Sjögren's syndrome*

- An autoimmune sialadenitis that results in xerostomia (dry mouth)
- Pathology—myoepithelial sialadenitis with the benign lymphoepithelial lesions
  - Dense lymphocytic infiltrates replace the glands
  - Duct epithelial and myoepithelial cells proliferate, producing the pathognomonic epimyoepithelial islands

— *Sialolithiasis*

- Calcified stones in the ducts of salivary glands
- Etiology—unknown and not associated with metabolic disorders of calcium or phosphorus
- Most frequent in the submandibular gland
- Episodic swelling and pain that predisposes to recurrent infection
- End-stage atrophy with scarring

■ **Nose and Nasopharynx**
● Inflammatory disorders

- Most common disorders of the nose and paranasal sinuses.
- Most common nasal symptom is rhinitis.

— *Sinusitis*

> • Most frequent etiologies are viral illness, such as the common cold or seasonal allergies.
>
> • Bacterial sinusitis may develop with allegies, cilliary dysfunction, abnormal immune status, obstruction of the sinus drainage, and rarely with viral infections.
>
> • *Haemophilus influenzae* and *Streptococcus pneumoniae* are common pathogens in acute sinusitis.
>
> • Cultures of chronic sinusitis often yield no specific organism.

— *Mucocele*

> • An expansile collection of mucous, serous fluid, and debris in the sinus that may erode bone
>
> • Result of chronic sinusitis and obstruction

— *Wegener's granulomatosis*

> • A necrotizing vasculitis predominantly involving the upper and lower respiratory tracts and kidneys
>
> • Pathology—microscopic—necrotizing, granulomatous vasculitis
>
> > • Infective causes—must be excluded before diagnosis can be made
> >
> > • Associated with an antineutrophil cytoplasmic antibody directed against a neutrophil serine protease, proteinase 3

● **Benign tumors**

— *Nasal polyps*

> • Reactive lesions caused by chronic inflammation or allergies (many eosinophils)
>
> • Rare causes—cystic fibrosis and Kartagener's syndrome (situs inversus, chronic sinusitis, bronchiectasis, and male infertility caused by abscence of ciliary dynein arms)
>
> • Microscopic—edmatous, chronically inflammed (plasma cells and eosinophils) submucosa covered by respiratory epithelium

— *Juvenile nasopharyngeal angiofibroma*

> • Benign tumor of the nasopharynx limited to teenage and young adult males
>
> • Microscopic—irregular, angular vascular channels in a variably cellular fibrous stroma
>
> • Clinical—locally invasive, they may bleed profusely with surgery

— *Papilloma*

> • Benign tumor occurring in middle-aged males associated with human papilloma virus (HPV) types 6 and 11
>
> • Microscopic—composed of nonkeratinizing squamous epithelium growing in an endophytic (inward) or exophytic (polyploid) manner (Fig. 18.3)
>
> • Clinical—rapid expansile growth can be seen with frequent recurrence and some cases of progression to squamous cell carcinoma

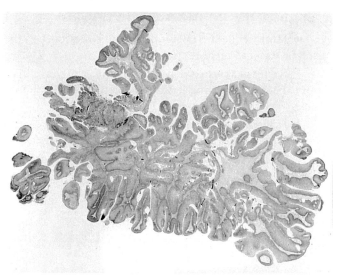

Fig. 18.3 Papilloma. An irregular, spiky growth of fibrovascular cores covered by cells resembling the normal basal layer cells is present. (*Damjanov I, Linder J:* Anderson's pathology, *ed 10, vol 1, St Louis, 1996, Mosby.*)

● **Malignant Tumors**

— *Squamous cell carcinoma*

• Most common malignant tumor of the nasopharynx *Nasopharyngeal carcinoma (NPC)*

• Undifferentiated squamous carcinoma with lymphoid-rich stroma (lymphoepithelioma)—the most common malignancy of the nasopharynx

• Most frequent in males, greater than 50 years old, high incidence in southeast China

• Associated with human leukocyte antigens (HLA) A2, B17, and Bw46 and a strong link to Epstein-Barr virus (EBV)

• May initially present as a cervical lymph node metastasis

• Microscopic—syncitial sheets of undifferentiated cells with vesicular nuclei and prominant nucleoli amongst a stroma typically rich in small, mature lymphocytes (the lymphocytes are reactive not neoplastic)

• Clinical—radiosensitive, presents at high stages, about 50% 5-year survival

— *Olfactory neuroblastoma*

• Malignant tumor arising from neuroepithelial element associated with the cribriform plate

• Occurs at any age, with a mean of 40 years

• Microscopic—may be similar to neuroblastoma of the adrenal with small monotonous cells and little cytoplasm showing neural differentiation (fibrillar background, true or pseudorosettes) or sheets of undifferentiated malignant cells resembling small cell carcinoma

- Electron microscopy—axonal processes containing neurosecretory granules
- Immunolohistologic—neurofilament and S 100 protein
- Clinical—can be aggressive, with survival in the 50% range at 5 years after combined surgical and radiotherapy treatment

Ear

Chondrodermatitis nodularis helicis

- Persistent, small, tender ulcerated nodules on the helix portion of the outer ear
- Microscopic—cartilaginous degeneration with overlying chronic inflamation and marked acanthosis of the adjacent skin margins

Otitis media

- Acute serous—usually caused by obstruction of the eustachian tube; common in early childhood with viral upper respiratory tract infection; may become secondarily bacterially infected
- Acute suppurative—common infection of childhood, usually *Haemophilus influenzae* or *Streptococcus pneumoniae;* spread to contiguous structures may cause complications, including osteomyelitism, labyrinthitis, meningitis, and destruction of the facial nerve
- Chronic serous—may be caused by chronic obstruction of the eustachian tube (note carcinoma of the nasopharnyx in adults causing unilateral disease) or recurrent-inadequately treated suppurative disease; characterized by increased mucinous cells and glands in the middle-ear mucosa
- Chronic suppurative—secondary to acute with destruction on middle-ear structures and perforation on the tympanic membrane or de novo caused by *Proteus* organisms or *Pseudomonas aeruginosa;* granulation tissue may form polypoid structures (aural polyp) that protrude through eardrum perforations; may develop cholesteatoma

Cholesteatoma

- An epidermoid cyst in the epitympanic recess and mastoid antrum associated with tympanic perforation and migration of the squamous epithilium in the middle ear
- Microscopic—a squamous epithilial-lined, keratin-filled cyst with an expansile destructive behavior

Otosclerosis

- An important primary cause of deafness
- May be bilateral and hereditary, with a female tendency
- Microscopic—replacement of petrous bone around the oval window by irregular woven bone that resembles Paget's disease, fusion (ankylosis) of the stapes to the petrous bone in some cases results in conductive deafness
- Clinical—surgical insertion of stapes prosthesis

Ménière's disease

- Characterized by tinnitus, paroxysmal vertigo, and unilateral deafness
- Pathogenisis—marked distension of the endolymphatic system by excess fluid (hydrops)
- Etiology unknown

- **Acoustic neuroma**
  - A schwannoma of the eighth cranial nerve that, when bilateral, is a feature of neurofibromatosis 2
  - Neurofibromatosis 2—not associated with cutaneous lesions, autosomal dominant, and carried by a gene on chromosome 22q11
- **Paraganglioma (chemodactoma)**
  - Locally aggressive tumor of the middle ear derived from the jugulotympanic paraganglia
  - More common in females
  - Microscopic—resembles the carotid body
- **Rhabdomyosarcoma**
  - May be seen in the middle ear as a common childhood site

MULTIPLE CHOICE
REVIEW QUESTIONS

1. Local infection of the oral cavity is more frequent with all *except* which of the following?

   a. Diabetes
   b. Systemic antibiotic therapy
   c. IgA deficiency
   d. Sjögren disease
   e. Colonization by *Corynebacterium diphtheriae*

2. Pyogenic granuloma is which of the following?

   a. A gingival lesion due to *Streptococcus pyogenes*
   b. Characterized by giant cells and caseous necrotizing granuloma
   c. Caused by a fungal infection, usually *Corpus albicans*
   d. Common in the first trimester of pregnancy
   e. Common in hyperparathyroidism

3. Which of the following is *true* of squamous cell carcinoma in the oral cavity?

   a. It rarely occurs in this location.
   b. It is frequent in tobacco users.
   c. It is frequently proceeded by aphthous stomatitis.
   d. It is common in females.
   e. It rarely arises in more than one site.

4. Nasopharyngeal angiofibroma occurs in which of the following?

   a. Infancy and childhood
   b. Elderly males
   c. Elderly females
   d. Teenage males
   e. Teenage females

5. Oral leukoplakia may be the clinical appearance of all *except* which of the following?

   a. Squamous cell carcinoma
   b. Thrush
   c. Aphthous stomatitis
   d. Lichen planus
   e. Benign hyperkeratosis

Chapter 19

Gastrointestinal Tract

■ **Esophagus**

● Diseases of the lumen and motor functions

— *Tracheoesophageal fistula, atresia and stenosis*

• Atresia alone—rare, and 90% occur with a fistula

• 50% associated with vertebral defects, anal atresia, renal dysplasia, and congenital heart disease

• Most common type—upper esophageal blind pouch separated from the lower portion by an area of atresia with lower portion attached to the trachea

• Aspiration—occurs after the upper pouch fills with feeding or secretions

• Congenital stenosis—rare; acquired type more frequent

— *Webs and rings*

• Narrowing of the lumen produced by hyperplasia of the squamous epithelium showing glycogen acanthosis

• Plummer-Vinson (Paterson Kelly) syndrome—triad of cervical esophageal web, iron deficiency anemia, and glossitis

• Rare, occurs in women, and has an increased incidence of carcinoma

• Schatzki's ring—gastroesophageal (GE) junction ring, found on radiologic studies, may have some chronic inflammation and fibrosis of the submucosa

— *Diverticula*

• Diverticulum—any out-pouching of the gastrointestinal tract wall

• True diverticula—have all four layers (mucosae, submucosa, muscularis, and serosa), but false diverticula lack the muscularis propria in the wall

• Zenker's diverticula—at the cricopharyngeus muscle

• Midesophageal—at the bifurcation of the trachea, sometimes caused by scarring of mediastinal lymph nodes, historically caused by tuberculosis, but now mostly caused by motor dysfunction

• Lower esophageal—younger age group, associated with achalasia or spasm

• Intramural—dilated openings of submucosal glands, no functional significance

272

- Clinical—large diverticula may fill with food, cause obstruction or reflux; surgical correction if symptomatic

— *Hiatus hernia*

- Protrusion of the stomach above the diaphragm through an enlarged esophageal hiatus
- Sliding—90%, rarely symptomatic or necessitating surgery
- Paraesophageal—rolling up of the gastric fundus beside the esophagus

  - Requires surgery even when asymptomatic, because of the risk of strangulation

— *Esophageal motor disorders*

Systemic diseases

- Upper esophagus—has skeletal muscle and may be affected by myasthenia gravis, amyloidosis, dermatomyositis, and myxedema
- Lower esophagus—has smooth muscle and may be affected by scleroderma, alcoholism, and diabetes

Neurologic disease

- Esophageal dysfunction occurs with strokes and amyotrophic lateral sclerosis

Achalasia

- Failure of the lower esophageal sphincter to relax and the absence of peristalsis on swallowing
- Represents a loss of myenteric ganglion cell function
- Ganglion cells may be absent histologically, reduced in number, involved by chronic inflammation, or normal
- Food— retained and esophagus dilates
- Predisposition to carcinoma
- Chagas' disease—may cause achalasia because of the destruction of the ganglion cells by *Trypanosoma cruzi*

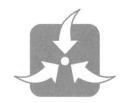

● **Esophageal rupture and tears**

- Mallory-Weiss syndrome—tear in the wall at the GE junction, usually from forceful vomiting
- Boerhaave's syndrome—perforation of the esophagus

● **Inflammation**

— *Reflux esophagitis*

- Caused by exposure of the esophageal mucosa to gastric juice
- Occurs transiently after meals, but recurrent chronic exposure produces inflammation through the action of pepsin, gastric acid, and possibly bile
- Associated with sliding hernia, alcohol, pregnancy, smoking, diabetes, and systemic sclerosis
  - Clinical—heartburn
  - Pathology

    - Basal cell hyperplasia, elongation of the papillae with capillary proliferation

- Eosinophils—may be seen, and neutrophils accompany ulceration
- Fibrosis and stricture—may result from chronic inflammation
- Metaplasia of the squamous mucosa to a gastric or intestinal type (Barret's esophagus) can occur

- Barret's esophagus—associated with a greatly increased incidence of adenocarcinoma

— *Infectious esophagitis*

- Usually immunocompromised patients
- Herpetic esophagitis with leukemia and lymphoma, cytomegalovirus with human immunodeficiency virus (HIV) infection and *Candida* organisms with chemotherapy, HIV and immunosuppression posttransplantation

— *Chemical and physical agent esophagitis*

- Extremely hot liquids, alcohol, and radiation—may cause inflammation, as can ingestion of any caustic acid or alkaline substance, with suicide or accidental poisoning episodes

● **Esophageal varices**

- Venous shunts from the portal circulation via the gastric veins through the lower esophageal anastomosis to the systemic drainage
- Caused by portal hypertension
- Because of the superficial submucosal location of the dilated veins—rupture can occur with massive hemorrhage

● **Benign tumors of the esophagus**

- Leiomyomas most frequent, composed of smooth muscle from the muscularis propria
- Squamous papilloma—mucosal tumor associated with human papilloma virus (HPV) types 11 and 6

● **Malignant tumors of the esophagus**

— *Squamous carcinoma*

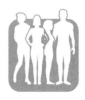

- Most common esophageal malignancy (60%)
- United States 6/100,000, male preference, 50 to 60 years of age and African Americans
- Extreme regional variation worldwide, with parts of China, Iran, India South Africa, Sri Lanka, and Singapore having high incidence
- Diet and environment factors—suggested by the geographic distribution, but no specific association for any agent has been identified
- Strongest link—cigarette smoking, with weaker links to alcohol, achalasia, celiac sprue, esophageal webs, esophagitis, and strictures
- Clinical—symptoms occur late, only 25% of patients are surgical candidates, 5-year survival is only 10%
- Pathology

- Occurs in the middle and lower thirds
- Gross—may be polypoid (most common at 60%), ulcerated, or infiltrating with mixed patterns common
- Microscopic—usually moderately differentiated with squamous origin indicated by the presence of intercellular bridges or squamous pearls in the well-differentiated areas
- Spread—by transmural invasion, then metastasis to regional nodes—cervical for upper ⅓, mediastinal for the mid-⅓, and gastric and celiac for the lower ⅓

— *Adenocarcinoma*

- Associated with Barrett's esophagus
- Increasing in frequency (now 40% of esophageal malignancies)
- Pathology

  - Gross—ulcerated masses at the GE junction
  - Microscopic—tumor glands similar to gastric and intestinal carcinoma
  - Some represent proximal extension of gastric carcinoma

■ **Stomach and Duodenum**

● Developmental abnormalities

— *Diaphragmatic hernias*

- Weakness or absence of part of the diaphragm—can result in herniation of the abdominal contents into the thorax

— *Congenital pyloric stenosis*

- Males, 0.3% to 0.4% of births, some familial tendency
- Clinical—projectile vomiting at 2 to 4 weeks
- Pathology—muscular hypertrophy of the pylorus

● Gastritis

- Diffuse or localized inflammation of the stomach

— *Acute gastritis*

- Also known as erosive gastritis
- Most common cause—chemical gastritis caused by excessive alcohol, bile reflux, and nonsteroidal anti-inflammatory drugs
- Other causes—ischemia (shock and hypotension), congestion from portal hypertension and cirrhosis, infectious agents in HIV patient, and systemic sepsis
- Common end pathway—loss of the mucosal barrier to gastric acid and pepsin
- Pathology

  - Hyperemia and acute inflammation
  - Superficial ulceration, loss of the mucosa, and focal hemorrhage
  - Stress ulcers—acute gastritis occurring with head trauma (Cushing's ulcers) and burns (Curling's ulcers)

— *Chronic gastritis*

Autoimmune gastritis

- Autosomal dominant (AD) with incomplete penetrance with high prevalence in people of northern European extraction
- Autoantibodies to parietal cells and their components, including intrinsic factor
- Pathology

  - Progressive mucosal atrophy in the body and fundus with chronic inflammation and metaplasia

- Clinical—complications are pernicious anemia and gastric carcinoids

Chronic active (Helicobacter pylori) gastritis

- Most common cause of gastritis
- Common asymptomatic infection, with highest prevalence in lower socioeconomic groups
- Pathology

  - Gross—antrum and body
  - Microscopic—chronic inflammatory cell infiltrate in the laminal propria, neutrophils and eosinophils in the epithelium, and numerous S-shaped *Helicobacter* organisms in the superficial mucous (Fig. 19.1)

- Complications—atrophic gastritis, duodenal ulcer, gastric ulcer, gastric carcinoma, and gastric lymphoma

  - Atrophic gastritis—thinning of the mucosa, loss of gastric glands, and the development of intestinal metaplasia of the epithelium
  - Intestinal metaplasia—a marker for increased risk of carcinoma

● Ulceration

- Loss of mucosa that extends below the muscularis mucosae

— *Peptic ulcer*

- Chronic ulceration in areas of exposure to acid-pepsin digestive juices
- 98%—single ulcers in the duodenum or stomach (4:1 ratio)
- Duodenal sites more common in males
- Epidemiology—low socioeconomic status, closely parallels *H. pylori* and chronic gastritis
- Possibly caused by chronic decrease in mucosal barrier to acid-pepsin
- Pathology

  - Gross—clean, round, sharply punched-out ulcers in first part of the duodenum or the lesser curvature of the stomach
  - Microscopic—superficial fibrin and necrotic debris overlying acute inflammation and granulation tissue with a deep zone of fibrosis and scarring

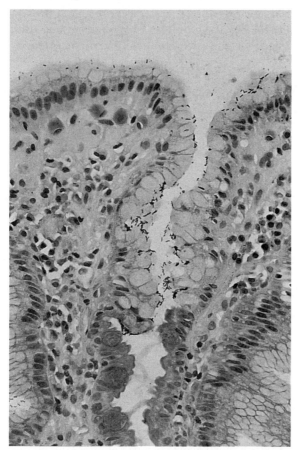

Fig. 19.1 Gastritis. This special stain demonstrates large numbers of *Helicobacter* organisms adherent to the surface mucous cells. (*Damjanov I, Linder J:* Anderson's pathology, *ed 10, vol 2, St Louis, 1996, Mosby.*)

- Complications—hemorrhage, penetration or perforation, obstruction
- Zollinger-Ellison syndrome—hyperacidity and ulcers caused by tumors producing gastrin
  - Suspect with multiple ulcers
  - 75% pancreatic, 20% duodenal tumors
  - 50% occur in multiple endocrine neoplasia (MEN) type 1

● **Polyps**
- A polyp is a mass lesion projecting above the level of the nearby mucosa.
- 90% of gastric polyps are non-neoplastic, either inflammatory or reactive.
- Inflammatory polyps are composed of granulation tissue.
- Hyperplastic polyps are the most common gastric polyp.
  - Etiology unknown, but may be caused by regenerative hyperplasia (also called *regenerative polyps*)
  - Frequent in chronic gastritis setting

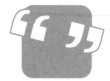

- Pathology—dilated and branching glands lined by nondysplastic foveolar epithelium in an edematous stroma with chronic inflammation, some smooth muscle, and cystic glands
- No malignant potential

- Adenomas

  - Incidence increases with age and male sex and parallels gastric carcinoma
  - Usually located in the antrum
  - True neoplasms with a malignant potential
  - Pathology—may be flat or pedunculated, composed of proliferating glands that show varying degrees of dysplasia, foci of invasive carcinoma may be present

- **Gastric adenocarcinoma**

  - 90% to 95% of gastric malignancies (lymphomas represent about 4%, carcinoid about 3%)
  - Second most common cancer worldwide, but incidence is declining

  — *Early gastric cancer*

    - Adenocarcinoma locally confined to the mucosa or submucosa regardless of whether there is lymph node metastasis or not
    - Important, as they have a 90% to 95% survival at 5 years with treatment

  — *Advanced gastric cancer*

    - Invasion into the muscularis propria
    - Has a much poorer survival of only 10% at 5 years if there is any nodal spread

  — *Invasive carcinoma*

    - 50% in antrum, 25% in the cardia
    - Pathology—polypoid-fungating, ulcerated, or diffusely infiltrating
    - Intestinal type

      - Forming glands resembling colonic carcinoma
      - Declining incidence in North America and the world
      - Common in Asia, Japan, Latin America, and parts of northern Europe
      - Associated with *H. pylori* and possibly other environmental or dietary factors
      - Associated with chronic atrophic gastritis, gastric adenomas, and partial gastrectomy, especially when intestinal metaplasia and cellular atypia are present
      - No increased risk with chronic gastric ulcer

    - Diffuse type

      - An infiltrating pattern of single or loosely cohesive cells that may show a signet ring cell morphology
      - Poor prognosis
      - No association with *H. pylori* or chronic gastritis

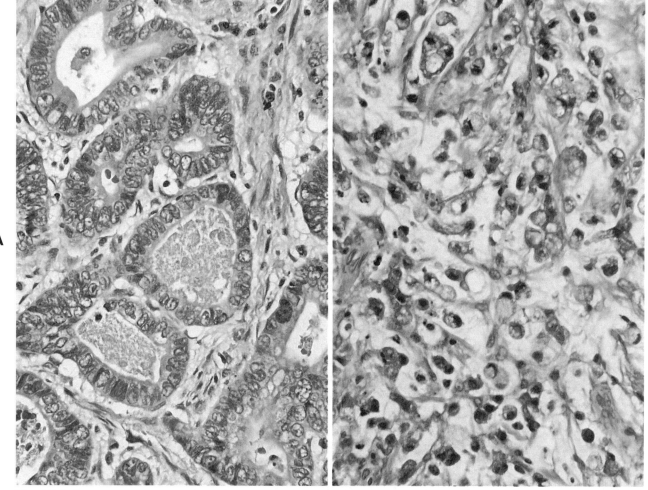

Fig. 19.2 Gastric carcinoma. The intestinal type forms circular gland structures **A,** while the diffuse type consists of single cells, some with a signet ring morphology **B.** (*Damjanov I, Linder J:* Anderson's pathology, *ed 10, vol 2, St Louis, 1996, Mosby.*)

- Stable incidence
- Occurs at an earlier age, and there is no male tendency (Fig. 19.2)

● Other tumors

- Stomach—the most frequent site of lymphoma and stromal tumors of the GI tract (discussed later with intestinal tumors)

■ **Small and Large Intestines**

● Congenital abnormalities

— *Small intestine*

- Omphalocele—persistent small bowel outside the abdominal cavity through an incomplete abdominal wall
- Umbilical hernia—a lesser defect in the wall, with protrusion of the intestine

Meckel's diverticulum

- Remnant of the vitelline duct
- Most common congenital anomaly of the bowel

- Rule of 2s—2% incidence, 2 feet from the caecum in ileum, 2 inches long, and 2% symptomatic
- Clinical—pain or hemorrhage from peptic ulceration (50% have ectopic gastric epithelium), intussusception, or perforation

— *Large intestine*

Malrotation

- Both large and small bowel includes situs inversus and Kartagener's syndrome
- Complications—diagnostic confusion by alteration of the pain patterns of acute conditions, such as appendicitis and predisposition to volvulus

Congenital megacolon (Hirschsprung's disease)

- Lack of submucosal (Meissner's) and myenteric (Auerbach's) ganglion cells resulting in obstruction caused by lack of coordinated muscular action
- Familial tendency, and more frequent with Down syndrome
- Pathology

    - Gross—aganglionic segment is contracted and the proximal colon dilated
    - Aganglionic portion—begins at rectum and progresses proximally a variable distance, but usual extent is to the sigmoid (90%)

- Clinical—obstruction, megacolon, and perforation

- **Colonic diverticular disease**

    - Common out-pouching of colonic mucosa; when multiple, referred to as diverticulosis
    - Common in North America and Europe, and increase after age 40 years to a prevalence of 50% in the elderly
    - May be associated with low-fiber diet, resulting in increased intraluminal pressure
    - Pathology—forms as two rows alongside the antimesenteric tinea coli at weak points in the muscularis where it is perforated by arteries

        - Accompanied by muscularis hypertrophy
        - Flask-shaped protrusions about 1 cm in size, often containing a fecalith
        - Lined by mucosa and attenuated submucosa

    - Clinical—asymptomatic with complications in about 10%

        - Inflammation (diverticulitis that can form a mass mimicking carcinoma), perforation, and bleeding

    - Diverticula of the small bowel are rare

- **Circulatory disorders**

    - Rich collateral circulation between branches of the celiac trunk, superior mesenteric and inferior mesenteric

    — *Ischemic disorders*

        - Arterial causes—atherosclerosis, emboli, thrombosis, hypotension, mechanical (volvulus, hernia, intussusception)

- Venous causes—mechanical, hypercoagulable states (inherited, such as deficiencies of protein C, S, and antithrombin III, and acquired, such as carcinoma, paroxysmal nocturnal hemoglobinuria [PNH], hyperviscosity, and others)
- Clinical—abdominal pain, bloody diarrhea, shock
- Features vary with cause, duration, and severity
- Acute reversible ischemia

  - Caused by transient, less severe ischemia (hypotension, disseminated intravascular coagulation [DIC], recurrent mild mechanical obstruction)
  - At the splenic flexure in colon or at sites of circulatory compromise caused by atherosclerosis
  - Epithelial necrosis (most sensitive to ischemia), mucosal edema, hemorrhage and congestion of submucosal vessels, surface inflammatory pseudomembrane, and superficial ulceration
  - Can repair without any evidence

- Acute transmural ischemia

  - Prolonged and complete occlusion of a major vessel
  - More common in small bowel with venous occlusion, prolonged mechanical obstruction, thrombosis, or embolus
  - Gross—dusky segmental hemorrhagic necrosis
  - Microscopic—hemorrhagic coagulative necrosis extending through the muscularis propria with early bacterial flora invasion, gangrene, and perforation (high mortality)

- Chronic ischemia

  - Ulceration, fibrosis, strictures, and stenosis

— *Angiodysplasia*

- Vascular telangiectasia (dilations) causing acute or recurrent colonic hemorrhage, more commonly in the elderly
- Cecal and ascending colon
- Pathology—cluster of dilated capillaries and venules arising from a feeding arteriole in the lamina propria and submucosa
- Angiography—the best way to identify

— *Hereditary hemorrhagic telangiectasia (Osler-Weber-Rendu disease)*

- Young patients with telangiectasia of lips and mouth, nosebleeds, and family history

— *Hemorrhoids*

- Common dilation of the veins (varices) in the internal and external hemorrhoidal venous plexuses
- May be the result of pregnancy, portal hypertension, genetic predisposition, or possibly recurrent straining with defecation
- Internal (above the dentate line) and external (below the dentate line)
- Complications—thrombosis, bleeding, prolapse, strangulation

- **Intestinal obstruction**
  - *Hernias*
    - Protrusion of the bowel through a defect in the peritoneal wall into a mesothelial-lined sac
    - Sites—inguinal, femoral, umbilical, incisional (surgical)
    - Incarceration—entrapment of the bowel within the hernia sac
    - Strangulation—ischemia and ischemic necrosis of an incarcerated hernia
    - Hernias—the most common cause of small bowel obstruction
  - *Intussusception*
    - Telescoping of a proximal segment of bowel into the adjacent segment
    - In children—usually no apparent underlying cause
    - In adults—occurs with an intraluminal mass (polyp or carcinoma)
    - The intussusceptum—the invaginating bowel; the intussesceptiens—the ensheathing part
    - Complication—obstruction, hemorrhage, infarction if not reduced
  - *Volvulus*
    - Twisting of the bowel (or organ) on its vascular pedicle
    - Obstruction and infarction of the involved segment
    - More common in the small bowel and sigmoid colon
  - *Adhesions*
    - Common cause of obstruction in adults
    - Result of previous intraabdominal operations
  - *Other causes of obstruction*
    - Neoplasms—most common cause of large bowel obstruction in adults
    - Strictures, intraluminal masses (gallstones, fecaliths, foreign bodies), imperforate anus, meconium ileus (cystic fibrosis) infarction, neurogenic (amyloid, Hirschsprung's disease, diabetes)

- **Infectious conditions**
  - Major worldwide health problem and cause of infant mortality
  - Bacterial, viral, and parasitic pathogens—may all produce diarrhea
  - Cultures and stool examination for parasites—the gold standard for diagnosis, in conjunction with endoscopy and biopsy in a number of instances
  - *Bacterial enterocolitis*
    - Routes of spread: fecal-oral, contaminated food or water, and direct contact
    - Pathogenesis of diarrhea exemplified by *Escherichia coli*
    - Enteropathogenic—unclear mechanism of diarrhea
      - Diagnosis by *E. coli* serotypes
      - Microscopic—no changes except bacteria on epithelial cells
    - Enterohemorrhagic—0157:H7 strain of *E. coli*

- From undercooked beef
- Children and elderly with dysentery-like illness
- Produces a Shiga-like toxin (verotoxin)
- Complications—hemolytic uremic syndrome
- Microscopic—range of changes from mild infective colitis, resembling ischemic colitis and resembling pseudomembranous colitis

- Enterotoxigenic—toxins stimulate fluid secretion by epithelial cells similar to cholera toxin

  - Microscopic—no changes

- Enteroaggregative—aggregates of adherent *E. coli* produce a toxin

  - Microscopic—no changes

- Enteroinvasive—dysenteric illness similar to shigellosis

  - Microscopic—colitis

— *Acute self-limited colitis*

  - Histologic changes produced by nontyphoid *Salmonella* and *Shigella* organisms, *Campylobacter jejuni, E. coli, Clostridium difficile,* and rarely *Yersinia enterocolitica*

  - Microscopic—normal crypt architecture, neutrophil infiltration, mucin depletion; more prominent closer to luminal surface, crypt abscesses rare

— *Pseudomembranous colitis*

  - Most common cause—*C. difficile,* but may be caused by ischemia, verotoxin *E. coli,* and *Shigella* organisms.
  - Pathogenesis—clostridial toxins A and B
  - Clinical—postantibiotic diarrhea
  - Pathology—cream to greenish flat-topped plaques

    - Microscopic: fibrin, neutrophils and mucin appear to erupt from intercrypt surface epithelium

— *Amebiasis*

  - *Entamoeba histolytica,* the most common human pathogenic protozoa

  - Large intestinal trophozoites undergo division or produce cysts; cysts shed in the feces are ingested, pass through to the large bowel where they excyst to form new trophozoites

  - Pathology—flask-shaped ulcers with amoeba (trophozoites) that ingest red cells

  - Complications—dissemination especially to liver and brain, perforation, megacolon, strictures, colitis

- **Idiopathic inflammatory bowel disease**

  — *Ulcerative colitis*

    - A chronic, idiopathic, inflammatory disorder of the large bowel that extends proximally from the anus to involve all or part of the rectum and colon in a continuous, uninterrupted fashion

Box 19.1

CROHN'S DISEASE VERSUS ULCERATIVE COLITIS

Features Suggestive of Crohn's Disease
Focal mucosal inflammation
Terminal ileal inflammation
Linear ulceration or cobblestone mucosal appearance
  (gross)

Features Highly Suggestive of Crohn's Disease
Aphthoid ulcers
Proximal areas of inflammation separated by normal
  mucosa (skip zones)

Pathognomonic Features of Crohn's Disease
Noncaseating granuloma
Subserosal lymphocytic inflammation (transmural in-
  flammation)
Fistulas other than anal

Modified from Damjanov I, Linder J: *Anderson's pathology,* ed 10, vol 2,
St Louis, 1996, Mosby.

- Common in North America and Europe, with an incidence of
2 to 15/100,000

- Peak onset 15 to 25 years old, with second peak in elderly years

- More common in Caucasians, especially Jews

- Familial predisposition and association with human leucocyte
antigen (HLA) DR2

- Pathogenesis—unknown, but thought to be chronic autoimmune injury following some unidentified initiating injury

- Extent—always involves anus and rectum—alone (ulcerative
proctitis), 10%; with left colon, 40%; to right colon, 30%; and pan-
colitis, 20%

Pathology (Box 19.1)

- May be active (i.e., with neutrophils), inactive (quiescent), or
fulminant

- Gross—uninterrupted involvement from anus proximal, variable ulceration and hemorrhage, toxic dilation of colon with fulminant, flattened appearance with inactive phase; all may have pseudo-
polyps (thin projections of mucosa produced by regenerative growth
of mucosa undermined by inflammation)

- Microscopic

  - Active and fulminant—inflammation predominantly in the
    mucosa, neutrophils infiltrate and distend crypts (crypt ab-
    scess), abnormal regenerative crypt architecture with branch-
    ing, shortening, irregularity, and dilation

  - Chronic—loss of neutrophils, increase in lamina propria lym-
    phocytes, eosinophils and plasma cells, abnormal crypt archi-
    tecture with short, branched crypts, follicular hyperplasia
    common in the rectum (follicular proctitis)

- Differential diagnosis—Crohn's disease, infectious colitis

- Clinical—recurrent diarrhea, hematochezia, crampy pain, fever, and anemia
- Complications—toxic megacolon, ischiorectal abscess, dysplasia-carcinoma (see following), arthritis, uveitis, iritis, pyoderma gangrenosum, erythema nodosum, and primary sclerosing cholangitis (80% of cases have ulcerative colitis)
  - Dysplasia-carcinoma—tenfold risk
    - Key variables—extent of disease (no increase with rectal only, highest risk with pancolitis) and duration (begins after 10 years and may reach 30% at 25 years)
    - Finding severe epithelial dysplasia on biopsy—a marker for high risk to develop carcinoma
    - Surveyance colonoscopy—may be useful

— *Crohn's disease*

- A chronic idiopathic inflammatory disease of the gastrointestinal tract characterized by ulceration, frequent involvement of the terminal ileum, and a relapsing course
- Less common than ulcerative colitis, with peak incidence in the second and third decades and a familial tendency
  - Etiology—unknown
- Extent—may involve any area of the GI tract, but small bowel (especially terminal ileum) is involved in over 70% of cases, with the colon alone in about 20%

Pathology (see Box 19.1)

- Gross—segmental involvement with discontinuous lesions (skip lesions), thickening of the bowel wall and narrowing of the lumen, creeping of the mesenteric fat over the bowel wall; deep linear ulcers and fissures impart cobblestone appearance; anal fissure common; strictures, fistulae, peritoneal fibrosis, and adhesions are common

- Microscopic—transmural inflammation with lymphoid follicles and noncaseating granuloma, begins with small aphthous ulcers over lymphoid follicles, ulcers and fissures have acute inflammation (Fig. 19.3)
  - Clinical—diarrhea and abdominal pain
  - Complications—fistulae, obstruction, some increased risk of carcinoma, ankylosing spondylosis, anterior uveitis
  - Differential diagnosis—ulcerative colitis, ischemic colitis, diverticulitis, with fistulae, irradiation injury

— *Malabsorption*

- Clinical—bulky stools and steatorrhea, malnutrition, vitamin deficiency
- Mechanism
  - Decreased intraluminal digestion—postgastrectomy syndrome, pancreas and liver (destructive disease and loss of secretory function), bacterial overgrowth, parasites, drugs (cholestyramine)
  - Impaired transport—lymphatic obstruction, congestive heart failure

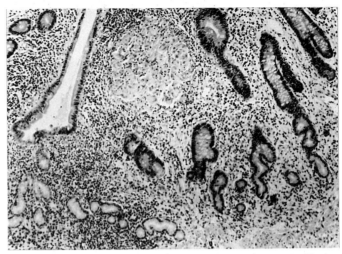

Fig. 19.3 Crohn's disease. The colonic lamina propria is filled by a chronic inflammatory infiltrate that includes a non-caseating granuloma. (*Damjanov I, Linder J:* Anderson's pathology, *ed 10, vol 2, St Louis, 1996, Mosby.*)

- Loss of intestinal mucosal function—injury and mucosal loss

— *Intestinal disease causing malabsorption*

- Biopsy—has varying utility in diagnosis
- Biopsy diagnosis possible in Whipple's disease, abetalipoproteinemia, celiac disease, agammaglobulinemia, lymphoma, eosinophilic gastroenteritis, systemic mastocytosis, amyloidosis, lymphangiectasia, Crohn's disease, infections, collagen vascular disease, postsurgical changes, enterocyte enzyme deficiencies, and other disorders
- Celiac disease (gluten enteropathy, celiac sprue)

  - Pathogenesis—involves dependence on exposure to gluten or gliadin components of wheat, resolution with removal from the diet, and familial tendency with increased incidence of HLA DR3 and DQ2
  - Diagnosis—based on clinical, immunological, and biopsy findings
  - Pathology—severe atrophy of intestinal villi with lengthening and hyperplasia of the crypts, increased interstitial chronic inflammatory cells
  - Increased risk of intestinal lymphoma of T cell type in patients over 50 years
  - Histology—similar to tropical sprue or postinfectious sprue
  - Changes revert to normal with dietary restriction of wheat products

— *Acute vermiform appendicitis*

- About an 8% lifetime risk of developing appendicitis, with peak incidence in the 15- to 25-year-old age group
- Pathogenesis likely multifactorial

- 40% have obstruction usually by a fecalith, but also foreign bodies, tumors, nematodes, and calculi
- Unobstructed cases sometimes associated with lymphoid hyperplasia, viral infections, but most have no obvious cause

- Clinical—periumbilical pain that later localizes to the right lower quadrant, loss of appetite, fever, leukocytosis, and abdominal tenderness in the region of the appendix

  - Frequent atypical presentations, 15% to 25% misdiagnosis is not uncommon
  - Differential diagnosis—mesenteric lymphadenitis, gastroenteritis, ectopic pregnancy, endometriosis, salpingitis, ovulatory pain, Meckel's diverticulitis, and intussusception

  - Pathology—serosal congestion, edema, and exudate

    - Microscopic—neutrophilic infiltration and mucosal ulceration
    - Complications—suppuration, gangrene, perforation, abscess formation, sepsis

— *Tumors of the small and large intestines*

  - Most—epithelial; colorectal carcinoma—second most common site of cancer after lung

- **Nonneoplastic polyps (Fig. 19.4)**

  — *Hyperplastic*

    - Common in Europe and North America, occurs at all ages
    - Pathology—arise in large bowel, may be multiple, small size, typically up to 5 mm

      - Composed of serrated, saw-toothed epithelium that may show hyperplasia of the crypts and metaplasia but no dysplasia

    - Not considered any increased risk of carcinoma

  — *Juvenile polyps*

    - Hamartomas
    - Common in first 5 years of life
    - Pathology—usually solitary, most frequently rectal, up to 2 cm in diameter, composed of cystic, dilated glands in excess laminal propria that can have chronic inflammation

      - Clinical—may ulcerate and bleed or autoamputate and pass with stool
      - Juvenile polyposis—greater than 10 polyps, may be familial (AD) or sporadic (75%), may develop malignancy (10%)

  — *Peutz-Jeghers polyp*

    - Rare AD syndrome of hamartomatous polyps
    - Polyps most common in the stomach and small bowel
    - Melanotic mucosal and cutaneous pigmentation around the oral cavity, genitalia, and palms
      - Polyps—not premalignant

Common intestinal polyps

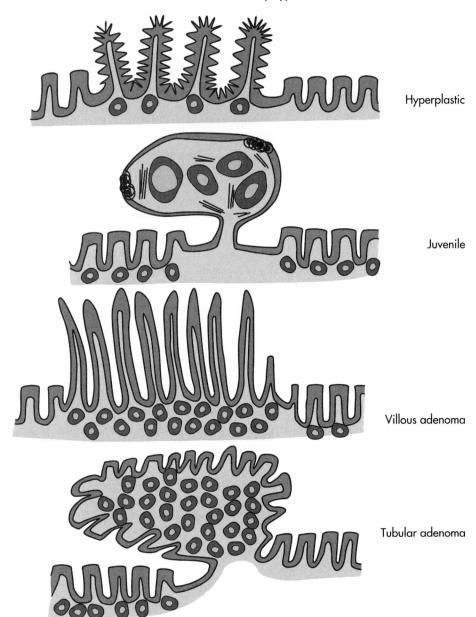

Hyperplastic

Juvenile

Villous adenoma

Tubular adenoma

Fig. 19.4 Common intestinal polyps.

- Increased risk of carcinoma of the pancreas, breast, lung, ovary, and uterus
- Pathology—large pedunculated polyps composed of arborizing stroma and smooth muscle surrounding normal glands with prominent mucus glands

— *Other hamartomatous polyps*

- Cowden's syndrome—AD, polyps, and cutaneous lesions (trichilemmomas), with increased risk of breast carcinoma in females (50%)

- Adenomatous polyps (see Fig. 19.4)

  - Neoplastic premalignant proliferations of dysplastic epithelium
  - Incidence about 25% to 50% at age 60 years, with equal sex distribution
  - Pathology—brown raspberry-like lesions of varying size

    - Microscopic—composed of glandular epithelium with crowded cells and varying degrees of dysplasia
    - Tubular—glands that appear tubular and round on section
    - Villous—mainly elongated villi
    - Tubulovillous—mixture of tubules and villi
    - Colon most common site, with ⅓ in the rectosigmoid

  - Clinical—may be asymptomatic, bleed causing anemia, or rarely cause hypokalemia or hypoproteinemia from hypersecretion (usually massive villous adenomas)

- Adenomatous polyp syndromes

  — *Familial adenomatous polyps (FAP)*

    - Autosomal-dominant adenomatous polyposis coli (APC) gene mutations at 5q21
    - Minimum of 100 usually tubular colonic polyps with polyps at other GI sites as well
    - 100% of cases will progress to adenocarcinoma by about age 40 years
    - Develop polyps after puberty
    - Prophylactic colectomy and screening of first-degree relatives management of choice
    - Gardner's syndrome

      - Variant of FAP with intestinal polyps, multiple osteomas, epidermal cysts, and fibromatosis

    - Turcot's syndrome

      - Possibly a rare variant of FAP with polyps and brain tumors

  — *Adenoma-carcinoma sequence*

    - Demographics and distribution of polyps and carcinoma—similar
    - Peak incidence of polyps antedates carcinoma
    - Foci of early carcinoma—common in polyps, but uncommon de novo elsewhere in the epithelium
    - Risk of carcinoma—proportional to the number of polyps
    - Genetic studies indicate consistent progressive accumulation of mutations in several suppressor genes (APC, mutated in colorectal carcinoma [MCC] gene and deleted in colorectal carcinoma [EDCC] gene) and k-ras and p53 with progression from adenoma to carcinoma

- Other inherited colorectal cancer predisposition

  - May have adenomatous polyps but fewer than 100
  - Lynch syndrome—hereditary nonpolyposis colorectal cancer

    - May account for 10% of all colorectal carcinoma

- Lynch 1—right-sided carcinoma by about mid-fifth decade
- Lynch 2—endometrial cancer, adenocarcinoma of the stomach, small bowel, ovary, pancreas and biliary tract, transitional carcinoma of ureter, and renal pelvis
- Caused by mutations in the DNA mismatch repair genes (hMSH2, hMLH1)

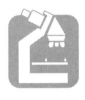

- **Colorectal carcinoma**
  - High rates in North America
  - Peak incidence 60 to 70 years old, with similar sex incidence except for 2:1 male rectal carcinoma rate
  - Dietary factors, such as low vegetable fiber content, high content of refined carbohydrates and fat, and possible decreased intake of certain micronutrients postulated as pathogenic links
  - Pathology
    - Grossly—polypoid in the right colon and constricting annular napkin rings in the distal colon
    - Microscopic—almost all are adenocarcinomas (98%) ranging from well to poorly differentiated
  - Prognosis
    - Stage dependent
    - Limited to mucosa—100% 5-year survival
    - Penetrating through the muscularis propria—80% 5-year survival
    - Penetrating through the muscularis propria with lymph node spread—20% to 40% 5-year survival (Fig. 19.5)

- **Small intestinal neoplasms**
  - Uncommon site, accounting for only 5% of gastrointestinal malignancies
  - Benign tumors, usually leiomyomas, adenomas, and lipomas, slightly more common than malignant
  - Malignant tumors—about an equal mix of adenocarcinoma and carcinoid

- **Carcinoid tumors**
  - Arise from the GI tract neuroendocrine cells
  - All are malignant with the risk of spread dependent on site (rectal and appendicele less likely to spread) and penetration of the muscularis propria
    - Pathology

      - Appendix most common site, followed by small bowel, rectum, stomach and colon; gastric and ileal may be multicentric
      - Gross—submucosal or intramural yellow-tan masses up to several centimeters in diameter
      - Microscopic—nests, trabeculae, glands, or sheets of regular cells with round to oval nuclei, stippled chromatin, and scanty cytoplasm
      - Immunohistochemically—can demonstrate chromogranin-, synaptophysin-, and neuron-specific enolase granule components and specific GI hormones

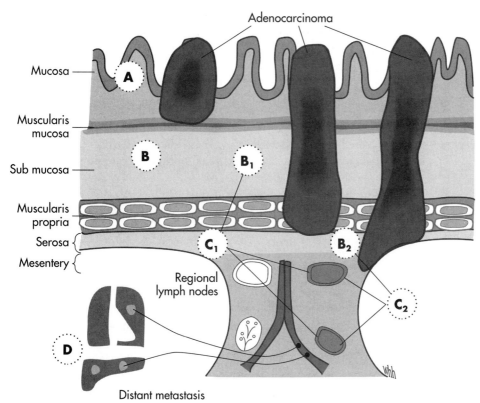

Mucosa

Muscularis
mucosa

Sub mucosa

Muscularis
propria

Serosa

Mesentery

Adenocarcinoma

Regional
lymph nodes

Distant metastasis

Fig. 19.5 Astler-Coller staging for colorectal carcinoma. A B_1 tumor with regional lymph node metastasis is staged C_1, and a B_2 tumor with nodal metastasis is staged C_2. Alphas indicate stage.

- Clinical—often asymptomatic

  - May produce specific hormone, causing Cushing's syndrome (adrenocorticotropic hormone [ACTH]), hyperinsulinism, or Zollinger-Ellison (gastrin) syndrome
  - 5-year survival is 90%

- Carcinoid syndrome

  - 1% of all carcinoid, and about 20% with widespread metastasis
  - Vasomotor instability, intestinal hypermobility, bronchoconstriction all in episodic attacks
  - Hepatomegaly and systemic fibrosis, especially right-sided cardiopulmonary
  - Caused by hyperproduction of serotonin and its metabolites

- **Mesenchymal tumors**

  - Submucosal lipoma most common, occurring in the bowel most often

— *Spindle cell stromal tumors*

  - Arise from the muscularis propria
  - Most leiomyoma or leiomyosarcoma
  - Some with neural differentiation or lacking differentiation referred to as GI stromal tumors
  - Pathology

    - Gross—variably sized nodules or polypoid masses

- Microscopic—spindle cells in fascicles, epithelioid cell type in the stomach

- Clinical—larger size and higher mitotic rate predict poorer behavior

● **Gastrointestinal lymphoma**

- GI tract—the most common site of extranodal lymphoma, but only accounts for 1% to 3% of gastrointestinal tract malignancies

- Increased frequency, with *H. pylori* associated gastritis, celiac sprue, immunodeficiency, Mediterranean regions, and post-organ transplant immunosuppression

- Stomach—the most common GI tract site

- Indolent lymphoma of mucosal-associated lymphoid tissue (MALT lymphoma)

  - Associated with *H. pylori* infection in the stomach
  - Arise from B cells
  - Clinical—tends to remain localized and have long survival; early may treat with antibiotics against *H. pylori*
  - Lack the genetic findings of the more common nodal-based indolent lymphoma
  - Pathology—key features are lymphoepithelial lesions (invasion of the lymphoma cells into the gastric crypts), mixture of small lymphoid cells that includes small lymphocytes, lymphocytes with abundant cytoplasm, and round to irregular nuclei (monocytoid B cells), plasmacytoid cells, and large transformed cells

- Large cell lymphoma of the GI tract

  - May arise anywhere, but stomach is the most common site
  - Sometimes represent transformation of a MALT lymphoma
  - Pathology—rapidly growing masses, composed of large undifferentiated cells with a high nuclear/cytoplasmic ratio, must differentiate from carcinoma, carcinoid, and other undifferentiated tumors

- Sprue-associated lymphoma

  - Younger individuals with a history of malabsorption
  - Proximal small bowel
  - Arise from T cells
  - Clinical—poor prognosis

- Immunoproliferative small intestinal disease (Mediterranean lymphoma)

  - Children and young adults in the Mediterranean, Middle East
  - B cell lymphoma
  - Special type of MALT lymphoma, with more plasma cell and plasmacytoid differentiation that produces abnormal alpha heavy chains
  - Clinical—early on may respond to broad spectrum antibiotics, but may progress to a more aggressive large cell lymphoma with poor outcome

- **Appendix**
  - Dilation of the appendix by mucinous secretions—known as a mucocele
    - Mucosal hyperplasia (resembling hyperplastic polyps)—likely an uncommon cause
    - Mucinous cystadenoma—common, may rupture in one fifth of cases; appendectomy is curative
    - Mucinous cystadenocarcinoma—penetrating invasion of the wall of the appendix, may implant on the peritoneum with rupture (ovary common sites)
  - Pseudomyxoma peritonei—ascites composed of gelatinous mucous
    - May result in rupture of mucinous cystadenoma, cystadenocarcinoma of appendix, or from other sites
    - Worse prognosis—if it arises from an adenocarcinoma, contains epithelium in the mucous, or is widespread as opposed to localized

MULTIPLE CHOICE REVIEW QUESTIONS

1. Intestinal intussusception in a middle-aged person is most likely associated with which of following?

   a. An adenomatous polyp
   b. No other intestinal diseases
   c. Acute dysentery
   d. Crohn's disease
   e. A carcinoid tumor

2. The most common site of peptic ulceration is which of the following?

   a. Esophagus
   b. Stomach
   c. Duodenum
   d. Jejunum
   e. Ileum

3. The most common malignant neoplasm of the esophagus is which of the following?

   a. Leiomyosarcoma
   b. Small cell carcinoma
   c. Squamous cell carcinoma
   d. Adenocarcinoma
   e. Metastatic carcinoma from another organ

4. Hamartomatous intestinal polyps are typical of which of the following?

   a. Turcot syndrome
   b. Familial polyposis coli
   c. Gardner's syndrome
   d. Peutz-Jeghers syndrome
   e. Lynch's syndrome

5. A higher risk of developing colorectal carcinoma is present with all *except* which of the following?

   a. Ulcerative colitis
   b. Familial adenomatous polyposis
   c. Gardner's syndrome
   d. Peutz-Jeghers syndrome
   e. Turcot syndrome

Chapter 20

Liver, Gallbladder, Extrahepatic Biliary Tract, and Pancreas

LIVER

- This is a genuine "master organ" with numerous critical roles necessary for maintaining life.

  - Major storage site for glycogen (along with skeletal muscle)
  - Major site for gluconeogenesis
  - Site of cholesterol synthesis
  - Production site for numerous plasma proteins including albumin (albumin necessary to maintain normal plasma oncotic pressure)
  - Production site for coagulant and anticoagulant proteins
  - Inactivation site for endogenous enzymes/proteins (e.g., activated coagulant proteins)
  - Bile production site
  - Major extramedullary hematopoiesis site in utero and early postnatal life and in adults during pathologic states (e.g., myeloproliferative disorders)
  - Detoxification site for drugs, toxins, medications, hormones (e.g., estrogen)
  - Vitamin storage and metabolism (e.g., vitamin A)
  - Site of urea cycle (important in protein catabolism)

- Normal adult liver resides in right upper quadrant and weighs approximately 1500 g with greatest overall dimensions of $20 \times 15 \times 10$ cm; it has two major lobes (right and left) and two smaller lobes (caudate and quadrate).

HISTOLOGIC "GAME PLAN" OF THE LIVER

Classical microscopic units are hexagon-shaped lobules with a central (efferent) vein. Radiating outward from this are the "one-cell"-in-thickness hepatic plates composed of hepatocytes (the main "business" or parenchymal cell of the liver). At the periphery of each lobule are up to six portal areas, each of which contains collagen-rich fibrous tissue, bile ducts (each lined by a single layer of cuboidal cells), arteries, branches of the portal vein, autonomic nerve fibers, lymphatic channels, and inflammatory cells (lymphocytes, macrophages, and mast cells). *Note:* The hepatic plates are separated by blood vessel channels known as sinusoids; these are lined by endothelial cells and Kupffer cells (a type of macrophage). Cells of Ito lie between sinusoidal endothelial cells and hepatocytes in locations known as Disse's spaces; cells of Ito store lipids and vitamin A and produce collagen.

A more recent development in describing hepatic microanatomy involves the concept of the functional hepatic acinus. This concept takes into account the liver's microcirculation.

- Liver divided into zones (using portal areas as a central "starting" point)

  - *Zone 1* consists of liver tissue nearest to the portal area. It is least sensitive to ischemia or nutritional deficit but most sensitive to effects of toxins.
  - *Zone 2* is intermediate between zones 1 and 3 in location and in vulnerability to ischemia and toxins.
  - *Zone 3* is the liver tissue surrounding the central vein. It is *most susceptible* to ischemic damage and nutritional deficit but most resistant to toxic insult.

- *Note:* Hepatic blood flow occurs from the portal areas, through the sinusoids to the central veins; approximately ⅓ of the liver's blood supply is from the hepatic artery, while the remainder comes from the portal vein.

■ **Bile Metabolism**

- Bile is composed of

  - Water-insoluble hydrophobic lipids (*phospholipids* and *cholesterol*)
  - Detergents that solubilize lipids (bile salts, including sodium glycocholate and taurocholate)
  - Proteins (serum proteins, hepatocyte enzymes, bile-specific proteins)
  - Bilirubin IX (80% appears in bile as diglucuronide conjugate, while 18% is in the monoglucuronide form and 2% is unconjugated)

- *Note: Bile* has a key role in the solubilization of lipids and absorption of lipid materials by the small intestine—especially the fat soluble vitamins (D, A, K, E).

■ **Bilirubin Metabolism**

- Most bilirubin is produced as a result of the breakdown of "worn out" red blood cells (RBCs), *mainly in the spleen.*
- Heme → Biliverdin → Bilirubin.
- Bilirubin produced in the mononuclear-phagocyte system (MPS), especially in the spleen, is transported to the liver via the bloodstream. (It binds tightly to albumin).
- Hepatocytes take up the bilirubin brought to them by the sinusoidal blood.
- The vast bulk (98%) of this bilirubin is conjugated to glucuronic acid (mostly diglucuronic acid conjugation, but some monoglucuronic acid conjugation) by the enzyme uridine diphosphate glucuronyl transferase (UDPGT).
- Bilirubin (mostly conjugated) is secreted into the bile canaliculi by hepatocytes.
- In the small bowel, conjugated bilirubin is broken down into glucuronides and free bilirubin; gastrointestinal tract bacteria convert the bilirubin to urobilinogens.
- Oxidation to urobilin (stercobilin) is the next step.
- *Note:* The vast majority of bilirubin presented to the small bowel is converted to urobilinogen and urobilin (stercobilin). But a smaller amount (20% of

bilirubin) is reabsorbed by the small bowel and colon, and, from there, it is transported back to the liver's hepatocytes.

- Some conjugated bilirubin also reaches the kidneys and appears in the urine.

■ **Basic Bilirubin Facts** Elevation of blood bilirubin levels results in *jaundice (icterus)* when bilirubin levels are above 2.5 mg/dl. Elevated blood bilirubin levels can be divided into unconjugated and conjugated types.

- *Unconjugated bilirubin*

  - Not attached to glucuronide molecule(s) and is lipid soluble
  - Tightly bound to plasma albumin
  - Not excreted into urine

- *Note:* Infants have an immature blood-brain barrier that allows the lipid-soluble unconjugated bilirubin to cross into brain tissue; unconjugated bilirubin is toxic to the brain and, in the face of high-serum unconjugated bilirubin levels, can become deposited in the basal ganglia, where it results in neurologic problems known as *kernicterus.*

- *Conjugated bilirubin*

  - Water soluble
  - Nontoxic to tissues
  - Loosely albumin bound
  - Easily excreted into urine

● Unconjugated hyperbilirubinemia

- Excess bilirubin production (most commonly seen in RBC hemolytic states but also after absorption of large hemorrhages and in ineffective hematopoiesis)
- Abnormal hepatocyte uptake of bilirubin presented to it by the sinusoidal blood flow (e.g., medication effect)
- Abnormal conjugation with glucuronide (Gilbert syndrome, Crigler-Najjar syndrome, physiologic jaundice of the newborn)

● Conjugated hyperbilirubinemia

- *Reduced hepatocyte secretion of conjugated bilirubin* (Dubin-Johnson syndrome, Rotor's syndrome, drug induced, intrinsic hepatocyte disease [such as viral hepatitis], primary biliary cirrhosis, sclerosing cholangitis)
  - *Extrahepatic biliary tract obstruction*

    - Calculi
    - Neoplasms
    - Extrahepatic biliary atresia

- *Note:* Cholestasis refers to the situation in which hepatocyte secretion of conjugated bilirubin is blocked at any of several levels, including the hepatocyte cell membrane, bile canaliculus, intrahepatic bile ducts, and the extrahepatic biliary tree.

■ **Evaluation of the Patient with Liver Disease**

● History and physical examination (critical starting point)

- Inquire for symptoms of fatigue, malaise, weight loss-gain, anorexia, pruritus ("itching" is a prominent symptom in patients with cholestasis [or obstruction to bile outflow]), jaundice, right upper-quadrant pain, light-colored stools, dark-colored urine, transfusion history, injection drug use, occupational history, travel history, medication use, history of familial liver disorders, animal exposure.

- Examine for scleral icterus and jaundice (yellow discoloration of the skin).
- Look carefully for skin excoriation (may indicate pruritis, possibly from underlying cholestasis).
- In men, look for gynecomastia and testicular atrophy as signs of hepatic cirrhosis.
- Palpate liver, assessing its size, consistency, and any associated pain to palpation.

● **Blood tests**

- Serum bilirubin levels (both conjugated to glucuronic acid [conjugated or direct] and unconjugated to glucuronic acid [unconjugated or indirect])
- Serum enzymes (especially alanine aminotransferase [ALT], aspartate aminotransferase [AST], alkaline phosphatase [AP] and γ-glutamyl transpeptidase [GGT])
- *Note:* ALT and AST are mainly elevated in diseases that affect primarily the hepatocytes, while AP and GGT are most significantly elevated in disorders of the bile ducts and other elements of the biliary tree; they are also often elevated when the liver is involved by an infiltrative process or mass lesion(s).
- *Serum albumin level—liver is the sole source of this protein, which is absolutely crucial to maintain normal blood plasma oncotic pressure and avoid generalized body edema*
- Elevated serum ammonia levels seen in liver failure
- Prothrombin time—a test of coagulation function; depends upon proteins (enzymes) synthesized in the liver that participate in the extrinsic coagulant cascade
- Serum antibody levels, such as antimitochondrial antibody ([AMA] seen in 90% of primary biliary cirrhosis patients), serum antismooth muscle antibody (seen in 70% of patients with "chronic active hepatitis" caused by hepatitis B infection), and antibodies directed against specific agents (e.g., hepatitis B core antigen antibody, hepatitis B surface antigen antibody, hepatitis C antibody, hepatitis A antibody)
- Detection of viral-associated protein (e.g., hepatitis B surface antigen) and nucleic acid (RNA and DNA) may also be performed on blood specimens

● **Radiographic studies**

- Magnetic resonance imaging (MRI) or computed tomography (CT) for evaluation of focal hepatic lesions

● **Liver biopsy**

- Usually obtained percutaneously and consists of a small core of hepatic tissue; larger (wedge) biopsies may be obtained at laparoscopy and laparotomy

● **General histologic patterns of significant liver damage**

— *Types of necrosis (Table 20.1)*

- Coagulative—similar to coagulative necrosis elsewhere; one

Table 20.1 *Acute Necroinflammatory Disease*

Pattern of Injury	Morphology of Lesions	Etiologic Examples
Spotty necrosis	Apoptosis with or without ballooning	Viral hepatitis B, C, A, rubella, rubeola, drug induced
	Apoptosis with or without ballooning with or without cholestasis and granulomas	Drug induced (such as phenylbutazone, phenytoin)
Spotty necrosis and sinusoidal lymphocytosis	Apoptosis with or without ballooning	Infectious mononucleosis, CMV mononucleosis, drug induced (such as phenytoin, dapsone)
Spotty-patchy necrosis	Coagulative necrosis	Hepatitis due to Rift Valley, Lassa, Ebola, Coxsackie, dengue viruses
Patchy and confluent necrosis	Coagulative necrosis	Herpes virus hepatitis, varicella-zoster hepatitis, adenovirus hepatitis
Submassive (zonal) necrosis		
Zone 3	Ballooning	Viral hepatitis B, drug induced (such as halothane, methyldopa, isoniazid), toxic (such as CCl_4 and steatosis)
	Ballooning and Mallory bodies with or without steatosis	Alcoholic hepatitis; pseudoalcoholic hepatitis
	Coagulative necrosis	Ischemic necrosis, drug induced (such as acetaminophen) toxic (such as mushroom toxicity)
Zone 2	Coagulative necrosis	Yellow fever hepatitis
Zone 1	Ballooning	Viral hepatitis A, infectious mononucleosis, drug induced (such as halothane), toxic (such as phosphorus poisoning)
	Ballooning and Mallory bodies	Amiodarone injury
	Coagulative necrosis	Toxic injury (such as $FeSO_4$ toxicity in children), adenovirus hepatitis
Massive necrosis	Ballooning	Viral hepatitis (B with or without D coinfection, hepatitis A, hepatitis C), drug induced (such as halothane, phenytoin)
	Coagulative necrosis	Ischemic necrosis, viral infections (such as echovirus hepatitis), drug induced (acetaminophen), toxic injury (such as mushroom toxicity)
Microvesicular steatosis, panacinar	Spotty necrosis	Alcohol, drug induced (such as tetracycline, valproate), toxic (such as Jamaican vomiting sickness), fatty liver of pregnancy

From Damjanov I, Linder J: *Anderson's pathology,* ed 10, vol 2, St Louis, 1996, Mosby.
CMV, Cytomegalovirus.

sees "ghostlike" outline of cells with essentially no residual nuclear staining

• Apoptosis—individual cell necrosis

• Piecemeal necrosis—death of hepatocytes about the periphery of portal tracts (may be seen in chronic hepatitis B with activity [formerly called "chronic active hepatitis"])

— *Types of hepatocyte degeneration (see Table 20.1)*

• Ballooning degeneration—hepatocyte swelling (sometimes to several times normal size); cell membranes become indistinct and sometimes disintegrate; nuclei disappear (karyolysis)

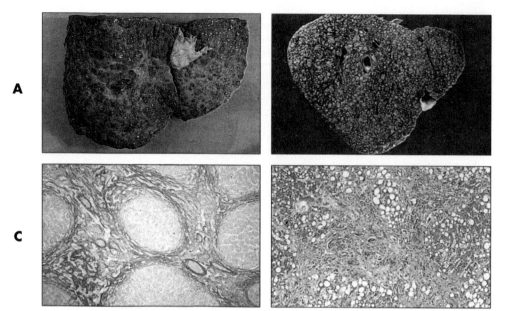

Fig. 20.1 Cirrhosis of the liver. **A,** Surface of liver, showing "pebbly" appearance. **B,** Cut section demonstrates nodules separated by bands of fibrous tissue. **C,** Photomicrograph showing nodules of regenerating hepatocytes separated by bands of fibrous tissue. **D,** Fatty change within hepatocytes (clear spaces) of a liver with cirrhosis caused by alcoholism. (*From Stevens A, Lowe J:* Pathology, *London, 1995, Times Mirror International.*)

- Steatosis—intrahepatocyte accumulations of lipid material
- Mallory bodies—intrahepatocyte cytoplasmic inclusions of cytoskeleton filament material

— *Cirrhosis*

- An irreversible form of chronic liver disease, *cirrhosis represents the end stage of many different processes afflicting the liver.*
- Cirrhosis may be defined as having three essential components: long-standing damage to liver cells, chronic inflammation/initiated diffuse fibrosis (scarring), and the formation of nodules composed of regenerative hepatocytes (Fig. 20.1).

— *Classification of cirrhosis*

Morphologic—based upon size of the nodules formed—a system without a great deal of modern day clinical relevance

- *Micronodular*—often seen as sequela to alcohol-induced liver damage; nodules less than 3 mm in diameter
- *Macronodular*—often seen after hepatic necrosis; nodules greater than 3 mm in diameter
- *Mixed*—combination of above

Etiologic

- Alcohol associated (65% of cases in United States)
- Viral hepatitis sequela (10%)
- Cryptogenic (idiopathic) (10%)
- Biliary (5%)

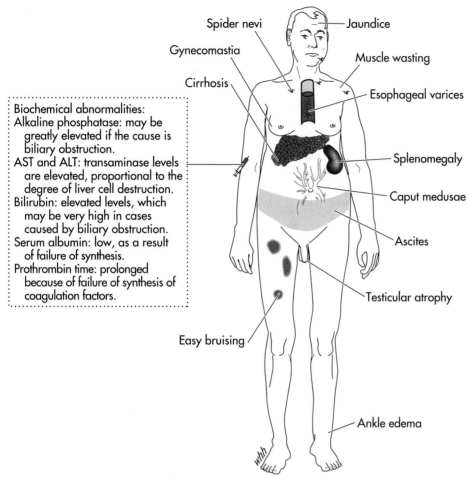

Biochemical abnormalities:
Alkaline phosphatase: may be
  greatly elevated if the cause is
  biliary obstruction.
AST and ALT: transaminase levels
  are elevated, proportional to the
  degree of liver cell destruction.
Bilirubin: elevated levels, which
  may be very high in cases
  caused by biliary obstruction.
Serum albumin: low, as a result
  of failure of synthesis.
Prothrombin time: prolonged
  because of failure of synthesis of
  coagulation factors.

Spider nevi — Jaundice
Gynecomastia
Cirrhosis — Muscle wasting
Esophageal varices
Splenomegaly
Caput medusae
Ascites
Testicular atrophy
Easy bruising
Ankle edema

Fig. 20.2 Clinical ramifications of cirrhosis. Observed clinical abnormalities are caused by the effects of hepatocyte dysfunction as well as portal hypertension. For example, impaired metabolism of endogenous estrogen in men results in testicular atrophy, gynecomastia, and the formation of vascular lesions on the skin (spider nevi). Ascites and edema are caused by low serum albumin while esophageal varices, caput medusae, and splenomegaly are caused by portal hypertension. Bruising/bleeding problems are caused by reduced clotting factor production.

- Primary hemochromatosis (5%)
- Others (5%)
  - Wilson's disease
  - Alpha$_1$-antitrypsin deficiency
  - Storage diseases of childhood
  - Cystic fibrosis
  - *Note:* In hepatic cirrhosis, collagen types I and III extend outward from their normal portal tract locale and become deposited in fibrous bands throughout the liver; this results in disruption of normal blood flow patterns and the appearance of portal hypertension.

● **Clinical features of cirrhosis (Fig. 20.2)**
  - None (asymptomatic or clinically silent)
  - Nonspecific symptoms

- Specific signs of portal hypertension and/or hepatic failure (see following sections)

— *Features of portal hypertension*

- Ascites (accumulation of fluid in peritoneal cavity)—a transudate
- Collateral vascular channels develop, resulting in esophageal, periumbilical (caput medusae), and hemorrhoidal varices
- Splenomegaly (normally, the spleen has a mass of 100 to 200 g but may enlarge to 1000 g in portal hypertension)

— *Causes of portal hypertension*

- *Prehepatic*

  - Obstruction or narrowing of portal vein before it enters the liver
  - Massive splenomegaly and shunting of excess blood into splenic vein

- *Hepatic*

  - Cirrhosis
  - Nodular hyperplasia
  - Schistosomiasis infection
  - Granulomatous disease, such as tuberculosis and sarcoidosis

- *Posthepatic*

  - Budd-Chiari syndrome—thrombosis of major hepatic veins and inferior vena cava
  - Right sided heart failure
  - Constrictive pericarditis
  - Venoocclusive disease

— *Manifestations of hepatic failure*

- Jaundice (inability to process bilirubin by liver)
- Hepatic encephalopathy, often with asterixis ("liver flap")
- Renal failure (caused by shunting of blood away from kidney)
- Bleeding caused by coagulation protein deficiencies (almost all of these factors are produced in, and inactivated by, the liver) and disseminated intravascular coagulation (DIC)
- Hypoalbuminemia and reduced plasma oncotic pressure resulting in generalized edema
- Reduced immune surveillance and increased susceptibility to infection
- Portal hypertension
- Increased risk of portal vein thrombosis
- Reduced ability to detoxify and metabolize drugs and hormones
- In males, gynecomastia and testicular atrophy may be seen

— *Hepatic "storage diseases"*

Bilirubin related

DUBIN-JOHNSON SYNDROME

- Autosomal recessive inheritance
- Caused by impaired adenosine triphosphate (ATP)-dependent

transport system that is involved with the transfer of organic anions, including bilirubin diglucuronide, out of hepatocytes and into bile; *bilirubin in Dubin-Johnson Syndrome (D-JS) is conjugated normally but is not effectively secreted into the bile*

- Livers in D-JS are black, caused by accumulation of lysosomal pigments comprised of protein breakdown products that, like bilirubin diglucuronide, are not effectively secreted into bile

ROTOR'S SYNDROME—VARIANT OF D-JS

GILBERT'S SYNDROME

- Autosomal recessive disorder characterized by chronic, mild, unconjugated hyperbilirubinemia; patients are usually asymptomatic

- Defect—*mild anomaly* of the glucuronyl transferase system; exact mechanism incompletely understated; probably also involves defect in hepatocyte uptake of unconjugated bilirubin

- 7% of population have this defect, and many are not aware of it

CRIGLER-NAJJAR SYNDROME

- Autosomal recessive disorder

- Like Gilbert's—characterized by unconjugated hyperbilirubinemia

- Defect—complete or partial absence of enzyme glucuronyl transferase

- Type I—severe and usually results in childhood death

- Type II—associated with less severe disease that is usually nonfatal

- Condition is associated with the deposition of lipidsoluble unconjugated bilirubin in the brains of infants, causing kernicterus

Iron storage disorders

HEREDITARY (PRIMARY OR IDIOPATHIC) HEMOCHROMATOSIS

- Autosomal recessive inheritance, *defect is located on chromosome 6.*

- In this disorder, a complex, iron-laden storage protein called *hemosiderin* accumulates within hepatocytes and, eventually, bile duct cells, Kupffer cells, and endothelial cells and extracellularly within fibrous tissue.

- With time the liver develops fibrosis and some degree of hepatocyte necrosis and regenerative nodule formation *(cirrhosis).*

- Key etiologic lesion in hereditary, primary hemochromatosis appears to be a defect in small bowel mucosal cells such that they absorb an excessive portion of iron presented to them in the food stream.

- *In hemochromatosis, excess iron, which is bundled up in the iron storage protein hemosiderin, accumulates in many body tissues, not just the liver; other affected organs include pancreas, skin, joints, heart, pituitary gland, and gonads.*

- The vast majority of hereditary hemochromatosis patients are males (at least 80%), with disease manifestations appearing in the fourth or fifth decade of life.

- 70% of patients exhibit the human leukocyte antigen (HLA)-A3.

- *"Classic" clinical triad for hereditary hemochromatosis* (Fig. 20.3)

- Pigmented micronodular cirrhosis (brown-orange-colored liver)

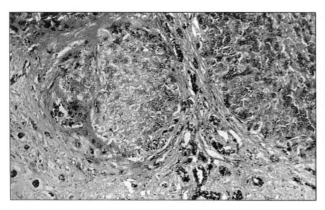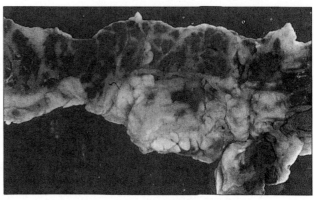

Fig. 20.3 A, Special staining reveals iron deposition in a patient with hemochromatosis; iron is deposited within hepatocytes and bile duct cells. **B,** Gross photograph of pancreas from a hemochromatosis patient demonstrates the characteristic appearance of tissue affected by this disease. *(From Stevens A, Lowe J:* Pathology, *London, 1995, Times Mirror International.)*

- Skin pigmentation (increased iron stimulates skin to make more melanin)
- Diabetes mellitus caused by pancreatic damage from hemosiderin deposition
  - *Major sequelae of hereditary hemochromatosis*

    - Cirrhosis and liver failure
    - Heart failure
    - 200 × increased risk for subsequently developing hepatocellular carcinoma (as compared to normal cohorts)
    - *Lab abnormalities helpful in making correct diagnosis*
    - Elevated serum iron and total iron binding capacity
    - Elevated serum ferritin level (another iron-rich protein found in the blood)
    - Quantitation of iron in liver biopsy specimens (levels of iron often greater than 10,000 μg/g dry liver tissue)

- *Treatment*—phlebotomy (to lower total body iron stores) and a cationic chelator (such as deferoxamine); genetic-counseling

SECONDARY HEMOCHROMATOSIS (FORMERLY CALLED *HEMOSIDEROSIS*)—Similar to hereditary hemochromatosis but is caused by *increased total iron ingestion* with a relatively normal ratio of absorbed to ingested iron

  - *Causes of secondary hemochromatosis*

    - Hemolytic anemias
    - Numerous transfusions of red blood cell mass

- *Note:* In secondary hemochromatosis, iron deposition usually commences in the Kupffer cells, but, over time, the histologic findings can be identical to those of hereditary hemochromatosis.

Other deposition disorders

WILSON'S DISEASE (HEPATOLENTICULAR DEGENERATION)

- Hereditary disorder (autosomal recessive, chromosome 13)
- Key lesion is a reduced level of serum ceruloplasmin, a copper binding protein, apparently caused by faulty hepatocyte secretion of copper-ceruloplasmin complexes into the sinusoid blood; interestingly,

intrahepatocyte ceruloplasmin content is actually increased in this disorder

- Copper is deposited in the liver, eyes, and brain; increased blood copper levels can also cause RBC hemolysis

  - *Clinical features of Wilson's disease usually not seen until adolescence or young adulthood*

- The liver is the first site of copper deposition; hepatic abnormalities vary from

  - Fatty metamorphosis (change) of hepatocytes with Mallory bodies (intracytoplasmic inclusions of cytoskeleton intermediate filaments)
  - Acute hepatitis with hepatocyte necrosis
  - Chronic hepatitis resembling hepatitis B virus
  - Fulminant hepatic necrosis (rare)
  - Cirrhosis

- *Note:* Look for increased liver copper content; can do special staining on liver biopsy specimen to demonstrate this or atomic absorption spectrophotometric quantitation of copper content on liver biopsy tissue.

- *Note:* Deposition of copper in Descemet's membrane of the peripheral cornea gives a characteristic *Kayser-Fleischer* ring.

  - *Diagnosis*

    - Family history
    - Clinical features
    - Low serum ceruloplasmin level
    - Elevated serum-free copper levels
    - Elevated copper in liver biopsy specimen (often greater than 250 µg/g of liver tissue)

  - *Treatment*—cationic chelation with penicillamine

ALPHA₁-ANTITRYPSIN DEFICIENCY (A1ATD)

- A group of disorders characterized by autosomal recessive inheritance and low functional levels of the enzyme alpha₁-antitrypsin, which is a major inhibitor of the protease known as *elastase*

- Over 70 different A1AT phenotypes; Pi-null (almost no AT1AT production), PiSZ, PiMZ, PiZZ, and PiFZ are associated with significant disease

  - *Key target organs of A1ATD*

    - Lung (development of emphysema)
    - Liver (development of cirrhosis)
    - In PiZZ, abnormal form of A1AT is produced in the liver; see impaired hepatic secretion of this molecule, which accumulates within hepatocytes and damages them

  - *Possible hepatic ramifications of A1ATD*

    - Hepatitis
    - Cirrhosis
    - Liver failure
    - Increased incidence of hepatocellular carcinoma in PiZZ variant

- *Note:* Histologically, one should look for the presence of periodic acid-Schiff stain (PAS) positive, diastase-resistant globules within the cytoplasm of hepatocytes.

GLYCOGEN STORAGE DISORDERS

- This is a group of disorders characterized by hepatomegaly, cardiomegaly, hypoglycemia, muscle weakness, central nervous system degeneration, and growth failure.

- There are multiple types, some of which may be associated with liver disease (steatosis, fibrosis, and, rarely, cirrhosis).

HEREDITARY TYROSINEMIA

- Autosomal recessive inheritance
- Caused by deficit in activity of the enzyme fumarylacetoacetate hydrolase, the last enzyme necessary to degrade tyrosine
- Accumulation of the metabolites fumarylacetoacetate and maleylacetoacetate in various cells (including liver cells), thereby causing cellular damage
- In the liver, may see steatosis, cholestasis, fibrosis, and cirrhosis

— *Hepatitis*

- Literally means inflammation of the liver, usually by viruses but, potentially, by any number of noxious stimuli (including fungi, bacteria, protozoans, complex parasites, drugs, and autoimmune disorders)

- By convention, the term *viral hepatitis* is reserved for those types of hepatitis caused by the following viral agents: hepatitis A, B, C, D, and E (even though other viruses [e.g., cytomegalovirus, herpes simplex, yellow fever virus, and Epstein-Barr virus, to name just a few] can and do cause hepatitis)

  - *Symptoms and signs of hepatitis, including viral hepatitis*

    - Fever
    - Jaundice
    - Anorexia (loss of appetite)
    - Weight loss
    - Malaise
    - Dark urine
    - Nausea and vomiting
    - Light-colored stools

  - *General facts regarding viral hepatitis*

    - Hepatitis A, C, D, E are all RNA viruses; hepatitis B is a DNA virus.
    - Hepatitis A and E have a feco-oral transmission, and, assuming survival from the acute event (which is the overwhelming rule), there is no risk of chronic disease, carrier state, or subsequent development of cirrhosis.
    - Hepatitis B, C, and D are all capable of causing chronic disease-carrier states and cirrhosis.
    - Currently, the leading cause of chronic liver disease worldwide is hepatitis C (formerly called non-A, non-B hepatitis).

— *Specifics of "viral hepatitis"*
Hepatitis A (infectious hepatitis)

* Feco-oral spread; outbreaks often traced to food handlers guilty of poor hygiene at work

* Incubation period 15 to 45 days; almost always a benign, self-limited process (although deaths from acute fulminant hepatitis A have been recorded); no chronic disease or carrier state if patient survives acute episode

Hepatitis B (serum hepatitis)

* Transmission often by exposure to infected blood (especially among injection drug users sharing needles); may be sexually transmitted as well

* 1 to 6 month incubation period

RELEVANT TERMINOLOGY FOR HEPATITIS B

* Complete hepatitis B virus is called the Dane Particle

* Dane particle consists of

    * B surface antigen

    * HB core antigen (HBcAg)

    * DNA

    * DNA polymerase

    * E antigen (HBeAg)

    * *Note:* HBs antigen is found free in the blood about 6 weeks after hepatitis B infection event; HBeAg is also found in blood and indicates active infection as well as a state of high infectivity to others.

DIAGNOSIS OF HEPATITIS B—PRIMARILY ACCOMPLISHED THROUGH SEROLOGIC (BLOOD) TESTING

* HBsAg and HBeAg are the main antigens found in blood and are seen early after infection.

* Anti-HBe antibody appears after this and indicates the infection is subsiding.

* Anti-HBs antibody rises last (after HBs antigen has been cleared from the blood).

* *Note:* Persistence of HBs antigen for more than 6 months indicates chronic disease.

* *Note:* Anti-HBs antibody will remain for life.

POSSIBLE OUTCOMES OF HEPATITIS B INFECTION

* Acute disease and normal recovery
* Fulminant hepatitis with necrosis and high mortality rate
* Chronic carrier state
* Chronic hepatitis state
* Cirrhosis
* Hepatocellular carcinoma

Hepatitis C

* Most common cause of viral hepatitis in the United States today; transmission same as for hepatitis B

- Accounts for 75% to 95% of transfusion-acquired viral hepatitis
- Incubation—2 to 26 weeks
- When contrasted to hepatitis B, the acute episode of hepatitis C is milder and fulminant hepatitis is rarer but the chronic disease potential for hepatitis C is much higher; up to 50% of hepatitis C victims suffer from chronic liver disease
- Increased risk of hepatocellular carcinoma also seen in chronic hepatitis C patients

Hepatitis D (delta agent)

- This "incomplete" RNA virus absolutely requires coinfection/superinfection with hepatitis B virus.
- Transmission is same as for hepatitis B virus.
- There is a 30- to 50-day incubation period.
- Fulminant hepatitis is more common with hepatitis D virus than is case for hepatitis B virus infection alone.

Hepatitis E

- Causes disease with feco-oral transmission—similar to hepatitis A; incubation period 6 weeks
- No chronic disease state if patient survives *acute* infection event (which the vast majority do)

Hepatitis F and hepatitis G

- These are newly described forms of viral hepatitis that we currently know little about.
- There are probably a number of additional viral hepatitis agents that we have not yet recognized.

— *Alcoholic liver disease (ALD)*

- A clinical and pathologic *spectrum* varying from fatty metamorphosis (steatosis); steatohepatitis (previously called *alcoholic hepatitis* but its histologic features may be seen in other, non–alcohol-related situations such as Wilson's disease, complicating the use of certain drugs, diabetes and obese patients), outright cirrhosis; hepatic failure; and superimposed hepatocellular carcinoma
- Pathogenesis of ALD is most likely caused by the harmful ef-effects of acetaldehyde, a metabolite of ethanol (ethyl alcohol); acetaldehyde hinders intracellular cytoskeleton microtubule formation and fatty acid oxidation; the latter results in intrahepatocyte accumulation of lipid (fatty change or steatosis); acetaldehyde also interferes with mitochondrial function; furthermore, induction of the cytochrome P-450 enzyme system may lead to enhanced metabolism of other drugs to toxic compounds

Steatosis (fatty change or fatty metamorphosis)

- Earliest morphologic expression of ALD; reversible and typically asymptomatic
- Histologically, intrahepatocyte lipid accumulation—fatty change

Alcoholic steatohepatitis (previously known as alcoholic hepatitis)

- Usually seen as a sequela of a major alcohol ingestion event (binge)

- Histologically, one sees

  - Hepatocyte necrosis
  - Intracytoplasmic hyaline material (Mallory bodies, or aggregates of cytoskeleton material known as ubiquitin—*not* specific for ALD)
  - Neutrophils reacting to dying and dead hepatocytes
  - Early centrilobular fibrosis

Cirrhosis

- First micronodular, then macronodular
- Histologically, broad bands of fibrous connective tissue (irreversibly deposited) delineating the borders for numerous nodules composed of regenerating hepatocytes

  - *Possible clinical outcomes of alcoholic cirrhosis*

    - Stable; good prognosis may be seen in those who stop imbibing alcohol
    - Hepatic failure with coma and death
    - Superimposed infection (cirrhosis predisposes to this)
    - Gastrointestinal tract bleeds (mainly from esophageal varices but also from ulcers of stomach and duodenum and from hemorrhoids)
    - Hepatorenal syndrome
    - Hepatocellular carcinoma
    - Bleeding from coagulation protein deficiencies

Biliary cirrhosis

- Result of long-standing biliary tract obstruction that eventually leads to liver cell necrosis, scarring (fibrosis), and regenerative nodule formation (cirrhosis)
- Three major types of biliary cirrhosis include primary biliary cirrhosis, secondary biliary cirrhosis, and sclerosing cholangitis

PRIMARY BILIARY CIRRHOSIS (PBC)

- An autoimmune disorder seen most often in females (80% to 90% of cases) over 50 years of age
- Key histologic lesion—nonsuppurative, granulomatous inflammatory process with destruction of medium-sized intrahepatic bile ducts; eventually these ducts disappear and cirrhosis occurs
- *Note:* A key aid in helping to make this diagnosis is the presence of antimitochondrial antibody in the serum of greater than 90% of PBC patients.

SECONDARY BILIARY CIRRHOSIS

- A number of clinical scenarios may result in long-standing extrahepatic biliary tract obstruction and, if not corrected, outright cirrhosis.
- These include stricture, cancers, calculi and any number of externally compressive lesions.
- Biliary tree ducts become impacted with bile, which may become infected and severely inflamed (cholangitis), thereby resulting in scarring.

- Cirrhosis occurs only if the inciting situation is not remedied.

PRIMARY SCLEROSING CHOLANGITIS (PSC)

- Another disease with a likely autoimmune genesis, as 60% of PSC victims also have underlying inflammatory bowel disease, most commonly ulcerative colitis

- Male gender predominance; occurs mainly in 25- to 40-year-old age group

- Disease process centers on both intra- and extrahepatic bile ducts; affects these in a "skiplike," random distribution, causing segmental stricture formation and associated nearby dilation; see a rather characteristic "beaded" appearance of biliary tract on radiographic evaluation

- Histologically, cholestasis with associated chronic inflammatory cells and a concentric fibrosis ("onion skin" type) around the bile ducts; in addition, small portal tract bile ducts eventually replaced by scar (fibrous) tissue; over time, these patients develop cholestatic jaundice and, later, cirrhosis

Postnecrotic cirrhosis (PNC)

- In postnecrotic cirrhosis, the initial stimulus for the cirrhosis is preceding hepatic necrosis, most often caused by hepatitis B virus or hepatitis C virus infection.

- Certain medications and toxins are also associated with PNC.

- Some cases are cryptogenic (idiopathic).

- Grossly, one typically sees macronodular cirrhosis.

- There is a markedly increased risk for later development of hepatocellular carcinoma.

Vascular disorders

HEART DISEASE/HYPOPERFUSION RELATED

- *Chronic passive congestion* (gives a gross hepatic appearance of a "nutmeg pattern")

- Seen in right sided heart failure, particularly tricuspid valve insufficiency

- A commonly encountered situation in clinical practice

- Histologically, sinusoidal congestion caused by increased pressure in hepatic vein-central vein system; results in centrilobular hepatocyte atrophy

- *Centrilobular hemorrhagic necrosis*

  - Seen in severe left sided heart failure, shock, and other hypoperfusion states

  - Histologically, ischemic necrosis of centrilobular hepatocytes with red blood cells forced into the lobules

- *Note:* Each of the above may lead to centrilobular fibrosis and, eventually, "cardiac" cirrhosis.

HEPATIC INFARCTION

- Rare event because the liver is protected by a dual blood supply

- May be caused by hepatic artery obstruction from

  - Vasculitis (such as polyarteritis nodosa)

  - Thrombosis

- Embolism
- Neoplasia

BUDD-CHIARI SYNDROME

- Occlusion of the main hepatic vein and/or inferior vena cava
- Neoplasms (especially renal cell carcinoma and hepatocellular carcinoma)
- Infectious (e.g., amoebic abscesses)
- Thrombotic disorders (e.g., polycythemia rubra vera, myelodysplastic syndrome)
- Membranous webs (seen especially in Asians)
- Clinically, an enlarged, tender liver with ascites, portal hypertension, and weight gain
- Histologically, look for severe centrilobular hepatocyte congestion and necrosis

PORTAL VEIN THROMBOSIS

- Consequences—signs and symptoms of portal hypertension
- Portal vein thrombosis associated with underlying

  - Cirrhosis
  - Neoplastic invasion of portal vein
  - Pancreatitis
  - Postsurgical states
  - Peritoneal sepsis

- *Note:* Banti's syndrome is a type of idiopathic (non-surgery-related) portal vein thrombosis caused by relatively low-grade chronic portal vein occlusion.

VENOOCCLUSIVE DISEASE

- An increasingly common entity in the United States
- Caused by endothelial cell damage induced by

  - Chemotherapy and radiotherapy induction in bone marrow transplant patients; up to 50% of such patients suffer from venoocclusive disease
  - Jamaican bush tea (not a popular drink in most of the United States)

- Histologically, look for central vein endothelial cell damage and eventual replacement by collagen with vessel lumenal compromise

Peliosis hepatitis

- Uncommon lesion
- Associated with use of anabolic steroids, synthetic estrogen, and immunosuppressive therapy; seen in patients with AIDS; some cases caused by *Bartonella* bacterial organisms (*B. henselae* and *B. quintana*)
- Histologically, look for damage to sinusoidal endothelial cells and gradual sinusoidal dilation

Pregnancy-associated hepatic disease

PREECLAMPSIA-ECLAMPSIA

- Really a part of the "hemolysis, elevated liver enzymes, and low platelets (HELLP)" syndrome

- Histologically, fibrin deposited in periportal sinusoids with hemorrhage into the space of Disse; areas of hemorrhage may coalesce to form a hematoma that, if large enough, may rupture

ACUTE FATTY LIVER OF PREGNANCY

- This is a *spectrum* of disease, ranging from asymptomatic to hepatic failure and, sometimes, death.
- Clinically, this occurs during the latter half of pregnancy and is heralded by nausea, vomiting, jaundice, bleeding, and coma.
- Histologically, there is microvescicular steatosis (fatty change).

INTRAHEPATIC CHOLESTASIS OF PREGNANCY

- This is seen during the third trimester, at which time patients note pruritus.
- Histologically, one sees mild cholestasis (bile stasis) without hepatocyte necrosis; this is related to estrogen milieu of late pregnancy.

Drug and toxin-induced liver disease

- ¼ of all fulminant hepatitis cases in the United States are caused by therapeutic drugs.
  - *Two major groups of drug-induced liver disease*
    - Predictable, expected, typically dose related
    - Unpredictable, idiosynchratic
  - *Mechanisms of drug-induced liver damage*
    - Direct cytotoxicity of drug
    - Liver conversion of drug to toxic metabolite(s)
    - Immune mechanism
- *Note:* Drug-induced hepatic damage may be indistinguishable from viral hepatitis (including possible acute, fulminant, and chronic disease manifestations); in addition, drugs can cause cholestasis and/or granulomatous hepatitis. Always check for history of drug/medication/toxin exposure in the evaluation of liver disease.

Autoimmune chronic hepatitis

- Associated with other autoimmune disorders, including thyroiditis, arthritis, vasculitis, Sjögren's syndrome
- Affects mainly young women
- No evidence for viral hepatitis on serologic evaluation
- Look for frequent occurrence of serum antinuclear antibodies and antismooth muscle antibody
- Predisposition toward this problem seen in HLA-B8, HLA DRW3 individuals
- Histologically, look for loss of hepatocytes, especially around the portal areas, with a prominent plasma cell component

HEPATIC INVOLVEMENT BY SYSTEMIC DISEASE

- Amyloidosis (amyloid may be deposited in the liver)
- Sarcoidosis (up to 85% of sarcoidosis patients have noncaseating granulomata on liver biopsy)

- Extramedullary hematopoiesis (seen in myeloproliferative disorders)
- Cardiac failure (see preceding)
- Diabetes mellitus (see fatty liver and glycogen accumulation and sometimes steatohepatitis)

REYE'S SYNDROME

- Seen primarily in children, although may occur in adults
- Clinically, usually follows a viral infection and the use of aspirin
- A fulminant disease that often presents with encephalopathy but no jaundice
- Histologically, key lesion is microvescicular steatosis (fatty change); ultrastructurally, this syndrome is apparently caused by mitochondrial damage and significant perturbation of hepatocyte lipid metabolism
- Fatty change also may be seen in kidneys
- Cerebral edema usually a prominent feature

- **Space occupying lesions (masses) of the liver**

    — *Nonneoplastic "tumors"*

    - *Cysts*

        - *Manifestation of polycystic kidney disease*—multiple hepatic cysts may be seen (these are lined by columnar or cuboidal epithelium)
        - *Solitary (nonparasitic) cysts* (lined by cuboidal, columnar, or squamous epithelium)

    - *Inflammatory lesions*

        - *Pyogenic abscess*—usually caused by biliary tree disease, intraabdominal sepsis, blunt trauma, spread from adjacent organs, or spread via bloodstream from extraabdominal source
        - *Amoebic abscess*—usually single (70% of time) but may be multiple; contents resemble "anchovy paste"; causative organism—*Entamoeba histolytica*; look for trophozoite organisms (protozoan)
        - Hydatid cysts—caused by the parasite Echinococcus

    — *Benign "tumors"*

    - *Adenoma*—mainly seen in females of reproductive age, especially those taking oral contraceptives

        - Forms a mass, up to 20 cm in greatest dimension
        - Histologically, what appears to be normal liver except no portal tracts or bile ducts are present within the lesion
        - May rupture and/or bleed

    - *Bile duct adenoma*

        - A very common lesion that some consider to be a hamartoma
        - Histologically, look for an abnormal proliferation of bile ducts within a collagenous stroma

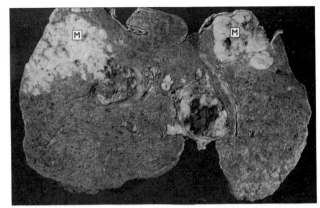
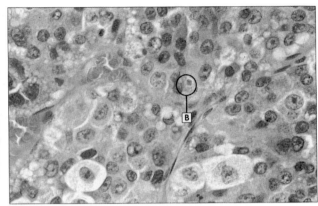

Fig. 20.4 A, Hepatocellular carcinoma may present with a single lesion or multiple masses *(M).* **B,** Hepatocellular carcinoma usually occurs in a previously cirrhotic liver and consists of atypical malignant hepatocytes that often produce bile *(B).* (*From Stevens A, Lowe J:* Pathology, *London, 1995, Times Mirror International.*)

- *Hemangioma*

  - Common liver lesion; *most common benign "tumor" of the liver*
  - Usually seen just beneath hepatic capsule and appears as a dark, spongy mass composed of benign blood vessels in a fibrous tissue milieu

- *Bile duct cystadenoma*

  - Seen mainly in women in their fourth to fifth decade of life
  - Cystic lesion lined by mucin-secreting, cuboidal-columnar epithelium
  - May recur if incompletely excised

— ***Malignant neoplasms involving the liver***

  - *Metastatic cancer—overwhelmingly, metastatic cancer (most often carcinoma) is the most common type of cancer to involve the liver.*

    - Most common primary sites for liver metastases are lung, breast, colon, and stomach.
    - Other cancers that commonly metastasize to liver are malignant lymphoma and leukemia.

  - *Hepatocellular carcinoma (HCC or hepatoma)* (Fig. 20.4)

    - *Most common primary malignant neoplasm of the liver (but far less common than are other cancers metastatic to liver)*
    - Accounts for 80% to 90% of all *primary* liver cancer
    - Predisposing factors for development of hepatocellular carcinoma include chronic hepatitis B infection; hepatic cirrhosis and hepatocarcinogens (such as aflatoxin, produced by the fungus *Aspergillus flavus*) in foods
    - Hepatocellular carcinoma is especially common in Asia and Africa, probably caused by high incidence of hepatitis B viral infection and environmental mycotoxins in the food supply
    - Grossly, may present as a single mass, multiple masses, or diffusely infiltrative lesions; the lesions are usually yellow-

white and commonly punctuated by necrosis and hemorrhage; typically, there is a cirrhotic background

- Histologically, a spectrum of differentiation, ranging from almost normal-appearing hepatocytes to lesions with bizarre cells and a primitive histologic configuration
- Approximately 50% of HCC patients have elevated serum alpha fetoprotein levels; alpha fetoprotein antigen often detectable by immunohistochemical evaluation of actual HCC tissue
- *Death from HCC is the rule and it usually occurs in less than 1 year*
- *Exception to this is the fibrolamellar variant of HCC, which tends to affect mainly young adults and has a much better prognosis (histologically, one sees dense fibrous tissue bands containing malignant cells having a pseudoglandular arrangement)*

- *Cholangiocarcinoma*

  - Accounts for 15% of all primary liver cancer
  - Predisposing factors—history of primary sclerosing cholangitis or liver fluke infection (*Clonorchis sinensis*)
  - Grossly, these lesions may be single, multiple, or diffusely infiltrative
  - Histologically—usually a reasonably well-differentiated adenocarcinoma in a markedly fibrotic (desmoplastic) stroma
  - Prognosis—poor, with death occurring in less than a year for most patients

- *Angiosarcoma*

  - Highly malignant cancer
  - Rare, unless patient has previous exposure to thorotrast (a radioactive contrast material used widely until the late 1950s); vinyl chloride monomer (used to make a plastic material commonly known as PVC); arsenic (commonly found in insecticides); and anabolic steroids
  - Histologically, vascular channels lined by malignant endothelial cells
  - A highly aggressive cancer with early metastases to lungs, pleura, spleen, and lymph nodes

- *Hepatoblastoma* (a cancer of childhood)

  - Most cases occur during first two years of life.
  - Often this is seen in association with congenital anomalies (hemihypertrophy, absence of portal vein, familial adenomatosis coli).
  - Male to female ratio is 2:1.
  - One looks for high serum alpha-fetoprotein levels in these patients.
  - Hemorrhage and necrosis are often seen within the lesion, which most often involves the right hepatic lobe.

- Histologically, one sees cells displaying a range of maturation within a mesenchymal matrix.
- This is a highly aggressive cancer that may rupture, cause liver failure, or metastasize to lymph nodes, lung, brain, bone, and heart.

GALLBLADDER AND EXTRAHEPATIC BILIARY TRACT

GALLBLADDER

- A clinically important organ (though nonessential for life) because of the high prevalance of calculous disease and inflammatory complications; over 600,000 cholecystectomies performed annually in the United States

  - *Background facts*

    - The gallbladder stores bile but is not an essential organ, as cholecystectomized patients do not suffer from malabsorption.
    - In contradistinction to the remainder of the gastrointestinal tract, the gallbladder wall does *not* have a muscularis mucosae or a submucosa.

- **Histologic "Game Plan" of the Gallbladder** *Inner lining* is mucosa, which is covered by a single layer of columnar cells. *Beyond this is a fibromuscular layer,* and external to this is a serosa containing fat, vessels, and nerves. Outpouchings of gallbladder mucosa may herniate through the muscle wall (Rokitansky-Aschoff sinuses).

- **Cholelithiasis (Gallstones)**

  - In developed countries, 10% to 20% of the population harbor one or more gallstones.

  - The vast majority of patients with gallstones (at least 80%) are asymptomatic and will remain free of any gallbladder problems or complications throughout their lifetimes.

    - Gallstones can be divided into two major types

      - *Cholesterol stones* account for the vast majority (80% of stones in the United States)—largely composed of crystalline cholesterol monohydrate
      - *Pigment stones*—mostly bilirubin stones and associated with chronic hemolysis states

    - *Risk factors*

      - Female gender
      - Obesity
      - Age greater than 40 years
      - Drugs-hormones that increase cholesterol excretion or decrease bile salt levels

- Clinical features of cholelithiasis

  - *Keep in mind that the vast majority of patients with gallstones will have no symptoms or problems from them.*
  - Asymptomatic patients convert to symptomatic patients at a rate of 1% to 3% per year.

- **Symptomatic cholelithiasis**
  - Biliary pain
  - Bloating
  - Nausea
  - Intolerance to fatty foods
- **Possible outcomes for cholelithiasis**
  - No problems—asymptomatic (vast majority of patients)
  - Cholecystitis (acute and/or chronic)
  - Perforation
  - Empyema (gallbladder filled with pus)
  - Cholangitis (inflammation of biliary tract)
  - Obstruction of common bile duct—more likely to occur with small calculi and calculous "gravel" than from larger stones
    - Erosion of stone into nearby loop of small bowel—gallstone ileus
    - Hydrops (mucocele)—mucosal resorption of lipids in an obstructed *noninflammed* gallbladder will leave an accumulation of clear mucinous fluid contents known as mucocele.
  - Gallstone associated pancreatitis
  - Possibly carcinoma development (this is still somewhat controversial)

Acute Calculous Cholecystitis

- Occurs in substrate of gallstones, most often precipitated by stone compression or occlusion of gallbladder vessel and/or cystic duct
- Acute calculous cholecystitis may appear suddenly and manifest as an acute surgical emergency
- *Clinically one sees*

  - Right upper quadrant or epigastric pain
  - Fever and elevated white blood cell count
  - Tachycardia
  - Diaphoresis (sweating)
  - Nausea and vomiting
  - Tender abdomen to palpation
  - If jaundiced, think about common bile duct obstruction by calculus
  - Mechanism of pathogenesis—bile stasis caused by obstruction to bile outflow; this results in phospholipase-activated hydrolysis of bile lecithin to lysolecithin, which is toxic to gallbladder mucosa, further damage to the gallbladder wall caused by the detergent properties of bile

- *Note:* These events do *not* involve bacterial infection, although such an event often subsequently occurs.
- Grossly, the gallbladder involved by acute cholecystitis is enlarged and reddened; gallbladder lumen filled with stones, fibrin, and sometimes pus; when pus is essentially the only content, one has gallbladder empyema; in particularly severe situations, the gallbladder wall becomes necrotic—*gangrenous cholecystitis*
- Histologically, look for edema, neutrophils, hemorrhage, and necrosis
- **Possible complications of acute cholecystitis**
  - Secondary bacterial infection, with subsequent cholangitis and possibly even sepsis

- Perforation or rupture of gallbladder with abscess-diffuse peritonitis
- Gallbladder/small bowel fistula
- Worsening of other medical problems, especially heart, lung, and renal related

■ Acute Acalculous Cholecystitis

- Between 5% and 12% of gallbladders removed for the clinical diagnosis of acute cholecystitis contain no calculi.
- This process is felt to be a result of impaired vascular supply to the gallbladder and occurs in the following clinical substrates.

  - Multisystem organ failure
  - Severe burns
  - Postoperative state
  - Postpartum state
  - Prolonged hyperalimentation
  - After severe trauma
  - Keep in mind that the cystic artery is an end artery, and the gallbladder is *not* endowed with a collateral circulation.

- Histologically, the appearance of acute acalculous cholecystitis is the same as that for acute calculous cholecystitis; *however, gangrene and perforation are much more often seen in acute acalculous cholecystitis.*

■ Chronic Cholecystitis

- This may be seen in context of repeated episodes of acute cholecystitis or in apparent absence of such preceding acute cholecystitis.
- It affects similar patient population as acute cholecystitis profile.
- In contradistinction to acute calculous cholecystitis, obstruction of bile outflow is not necessary in the genesis of chronic cholecystitis.
- Symptoms and signs for chronic cholecystitis are similar to those seen in acute cholecystitis.
- Histologically, one sees a variable picture; usually gallbladder wall thickening caused by chronic inflammation (lymphocytes, plasma cells, and monocytes) and fibrosis are seen. Sometimes, there is dystrophic calcification (that is calcification within previously damaged tissue) in the gallbladder wall giving a hard, so-called *porcelain gallbladder.* The porcelain gallbladder has a decidedly increased risk of developing an associated cancer. A chronically obstructed gallbladder may contain nothing but *clear secretions (hydrops gallbladder).*

■ Neoplasms of the Gallbladder

- The two major ones are adenomas and adenocarcinoma.
- ● Adenoma

  - A benign epithelial neoplasm arising from the gallbladder mucosa; is similar to adenomas that arise in the large bowel
  - *Key point:* about 10% of these show at least focal malignant change

- ● Carcinoma

  - Most frequently seen in women over 60 years of age but not a very common type of cancer
  - Usually discovered too late to allow for resectability

• 60% to 90% of these patients have gallstones, but etiologic role of stones is controversial

• *Histologically, 95% of primary gallbladder carcinoma is adenocarcinoma;* most of these have spread locally into the liver and nearby lymph nodes

• 5-year survival for gallbladder carcinoma is dismal (less than 5%)

■ Miscellaneous Gallbladder Lesions

● Cholesterolosis

• Accumulations of lipid-laden material within macrophages of gallbladder mucosa; this imparts to the mucosal surface a gross appearance of minute yellow flecks—"strawberry gallbladder"

• No clinical significance

● Inflammatory polyps

• Mucosal projections covered by columnar epithelial cells

• Cores of fibrous tissue infiltrated by chronic inflammatory cells and lipid-laden macrophages

● Adenomyosis

• Can create a sessile fundic mass; consists of muscularis hyperplasia with intramural hyperplastic diverticula or crypts

● Assorted congenital anomalies

• Agenesis

• Duplication

• Bilobed gallbladder

• Folded fundus—gallbladder fundus is folded inward, creating a "phrygion cap"

● Extrahepatic bile ducts

— *Extrahepatic biliary atresia (EHBA)*

• EHBA is complete obstruction to bile flow caused by destruction or absence of all or part of the extrahepatic bile ducts.

• This entity constitutes the most common cause of death from liver disease in early childhood.

• Liver transplantation is required in 50% to 60% of patients because of hepatic failure caused by secondary biliary cirrhosis.

• Histologically, most victims of EHBA start off life with a complete extrahepatic biliary tree; however, in the weeks after birth, these ducts are destroyed by an inflammatory process of uncertain etiology. Eventually, cirrhosis also occurs.

— *Choledochal cysts*

• Congenital dilations of the common bile duct

• Recognized mostly in the first decade of life; most cases seen in females (F:M ratio is 3:1)

• *Significance of these lesions*

• Stone formation sites

• Stenosis and stricture

• Pancreatitis

- Obstructive biliary complications
- Increased risk of bile duct carcinoma

— *Choledocholithiasis*

- Presence of calculi within the biliary tree
- Seen in about 10% of patients with cholelithiasis
- *Note:* Both *cholesterol and pigmented stones can form de novo ("from scratch") in the common bile duct and anywhere else in the biliary tree.*
- *However, most instances of choledocholithiasis in this country are caused by calculi formed in the gallbladder and passed into the biliary tree*
- Clinically, calculous disease of the biliary tract may be asymptomatic or be associated with signs and symptoms of

  - Obstruction
  - Pancreatitis
  - Cholangitis
  - Hepatic abscess
  - Secondary biliary cirrhosis
  - Acute calculous cholecystitis

— *Cholangitis*

- Cholangitis is a bacterial infection of the bile ducts; usually this is associated with obstruction caused by choledocholithiasis (other associated causes include indwelling medical devices [stents, catheters], neoplasms, strictures, parasitic infection, and obstruction associated with acute pancreatitis).
- Most instances of cholangitis are caused by gram-negative bacilli, especially *Escherichia coli, Klebsiella* and *Enterobacter* organisms. Also seen are *Clostridium* and *Bacteroides* organisms and group D streptococci.
- Clinically, one sees fever, chills, abdominal pain, and jaundice.
- Histologically, look for neutrophils infiltrating the bile duct walls and spilling into their lumens.
- In severe cases, pus may fill the bile ducts and distend them *(suppurative cholangitis).* Such a clinical scenario is particularly likely to ascend up into the intrahepatic bile ducts and cause hepatic abscesses; sepsis often further complicates this clinical picture.

— *Neoplasms of the extrahepatic biliary tract*

Adenoma

- Benign epithelial lesions arising from the mucosa, often seen around ampulla of Vater

Carcinoma

- An uncommon lesion; most examples are adenocarcinoma
- Generally, a disease of older adults, slightly more common in males
- Increased risk for biliary tract carcinoma

  - Choledochal cysts
  - Ulcerative colitis
  - Infection with parasite *Clonorchis sinensis*
  - Infection with the protozoan *Giardia lamblia*

- *Histologically, almost always adenocarcinoma* associated with a brisk fibroblastic stroma

Klatskin's tumors

- Arise from the common bile duct between the cystic duct and the confluence of right and left hepatic ducts at the liver hilus; are slow growing and have marked associated fibrosis
- Clinically, lesions usually present with obstructive jaundice preceded by weight loss, nausea and vomiting, and light-colored stools
- Prognosis for extrahepatic biliary tree cancer is poor, with mean survival of 6 to 18 months

EXOCRINE PANCREAS

BACKGROUND FACTS

- The adult pancreas weighs 60 to 140 g and has a length of about 15 cm; grossly, the pancreas is pink-tan colored and lobulated and lies posteriorly in the upper abdomen (retroperitoneal).
- The main pancreatic duct (duct of Wirsung) empties directly into the duodenum in only ⅓ of normals and joins the common bile duct (just before the ampulla of Vater) in ⅔ of the normal population.
- Eighty percent to 85% of the pancreatic mass is devoted to exocrine function and consists of acini (small glands) featuring cuboidal-columnar cells radially deployed about the gland lumen *(site of digestive enzyme production);* a system of ever larger caliber ducts drains these secretions into the duct of Wirsung and, eventually, the duodenum.
- *Key pancreatic enzymes are trypsin, chymotrypsin, elastase, amylases, lipases, aminopeptidases, and phospholipases.*
- Pancreatic exocrine function is regulated by hormonal and neural factors; among the hormones that regulate the exocrine pancreas, secretin and cholecystokinin (both produced in the duodenum) are the most important.
- *Note:* Enzymatic autodigestion of the pancreas is prevented by several mechanisms. Most pancreatic enzymes are produced as inactive zymogens (proenzymes), except for lipase and amylase.

  - These proenzymes are packaged in membrane-bound granules.
  - Proenzyme activation requires activated trypsin (inactive trypsinogen becomes trypsin by the action of duodenum-produced enterokinase).
  - Pancreatic acini and their secretions contain protective trypsin inhibitors.
  - Acinar cells are quite resilient to the effects of trypsin, chymotrypsin, and phospholipase A_2.
  - Lysosomal hydrolases are available to degrade zymogen granules when acinar secretion is blocked.

CLINICALLY SIGNIFICANT DISORDERS OF THE EXOCRINE PANCREAS

- Congenital abnormalities (including cystic fibrosis)
- Inflammation and its sequelae
- "Tumors" (nonneoplastic and neoplastic)

■ **Congenital Disorders of the Exocrine Pancreas**

● Variations in anatomy (usually not clinically significant)

- *Agenesis*—complete absence of pancreas is incompatible with life
- *Hypoplasia* of exocrine units
- *Annular pancreas*—head of the pancreas may completely surround the duodenum and cause duodenal obstruction
- *Pancreatic divisum*—failure of two pancreatic anlagen (embryonic precursors) to fuse normally; this predisposes to pancreatitis
- *Ectopic pancreatic tissue*—may be seen in about 2% of the population; most often encountered in stomach, duodenum, jejunum, Meckel's diverticulum, and ileum; *foci may become inflamed and bleed*

● Cystic fibrosis (CF or mucoviscidosis)

- CF is a genuinely systemic disease that is seen in 1 of 200 live births.
- *CF is the most common lethal inherited disorder of Caucasians, being uncommon in African Americans and Asians.*
- Autosomal recessive inheritance (heterozygotes are asymptomatic), its gene is located on chromosome 7.
- Key defect in CF is *faulty epithelial cell chloride transport; one sees loss of sodium chloride in exocrine glandular secretions. Indeed, all mucous-secreting and exocrine glands throughout the body are affected in CF.*
- Pancreatic involvement in CF is seen in 85% to 90% of patients.

  - *Mild pancreatic involvement*—inspissation of mucus within small pancreatic ducts without significant effect
  - *Severe pancreatic involvement*—total obstruction of pancreatic ducts by mucus plugs; results in loss of exocrine gland tissue and replacement by a fibrous tissue/scarring process; eventually, one sees exocrine (and possibly also endocrine) insufficiency

■ **Pancreatitis**

- A spectrum from both clinical and histologic perspectives; may vary considerably in duration and severity.

● Acute pancreatitis

- An acute inflammatory process of the pancreas heralded by abdominal pain and elevated pancreatic enzymes (especially amylase and lipase) in the blood
  - Most often seen in middle-aged to old-aged patients
  - Two predisposing conditions underlie 80% of all acute pancreatitis—*biliary tract disease (usually calculi) and alcoholism*
  - Other associated-predisposing conditions—Table 20.2
  - Histologically, pancreatic edema, with neutrophilic inflammatory cells and varying degress of tissue necrosis (Fig. 20.5)

● Acute hemorrhagic pancreatitis

  - An aggressive subtype of acute pancreatitis
  - Also known as necrotizing pancreatitis
  - Histologically, edema and neutrophil infiltrates and extensive tissue necrosis (including fat necrosis and hemorrhage)

Table 20.2 *Predisposing Factors in Acute Pancreatitis*

CAUSE	EXAMPLE
Mechanical obstruction of pancreatic ducts	Gallstones
	Trauma
	Postoperative
Metabolic-toxic causes	Alcohol
	Drugs (e.g., thiazide diuretics, azathioprine)
	Hypercalcemia
	Hyperlipoproteinemia
Vascular-poor perfusion	Atherosclerosis
	Hypothermia
Infections	Mumps

Modified from Stevens A, Lowe J: *Pathology,* London, 1995, Times Mirror International.

- Accounts for about 5% of all acute pancreatitis
- *Note:* In both acute pancreatitis and acute hemorrhagic pancreatitis, key processes are lipolysis, proteolysis, and hemorrhage that occur as a result of pancreatic enzymes released from damaged acinar cells; these enzymes act to autodigest the pancreatic parenchyma.
- *Note:* Severe acute pancreatitis and acute hemorrhagic pancreatitis are characterized by a number of possible systemic complications, including DIC, adult respiratory distress syndrome (ARDS), widespread fat necrosis, hemolysis, shock, and acute renal tubular necrosis.
- In patients who survive their bout(s) of acute pancreatitis, possible intermediate to long-range complications include pancreatic abscess formation, pseudocyst formation, and duodenal obstruction

● **Chronic pancreatitis (more aptly called "chronic relapsing pancreatitis")**

- Usually seen as progressive pancreatic damage caused by recurrent episodes of clinically silent or low grade episodes of acute pancreatitis.
- Grossly, this process results in a hard gland with focal calcifications and pancreatic calculi
- Histologically, variable fibrosis (often irregularly distributed) with loss of acinar cells and varying degrees of pancreatic duct obstruction; interestingly, islet of Langerhans tends to be more resilient than acinar cells and are often preserved even when the acinar cells are largely absent
- A chronic inflammatory cell infiltrate featuring lymphocytes and plasma cells
- *Possible complications of chronic pancreatitis*

    - Endocrine and exocrine insufficiency (e.g., diabetes, malabsorption)
    - Pseudocyst formation
    - Possibly an increased risk for development of carcinoma

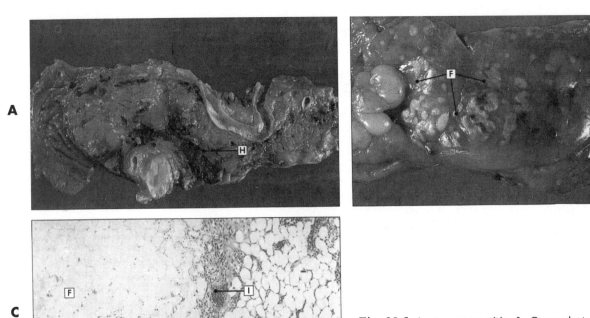

Fig. 20.5 Acute pancreatitis. **A,** Gross photograph of pancreas with edema and hemorrhage *(H)* characteristic of acute pancreatits. **B,** White spots *(F)* correspond to areas of fat necrosis. **C,** Photomicrograph of fat necrosis showing necrotic fat *(F)* and nearby inflammatory cells *(I)*. (*From Stevens A, Lowe J:* Pathology, *London, 1995, Times Mirror International.*)

■ **"Tumors" of the Pancreas**

● Nonneoplastic, false cysts

    • *Note:* A true cyst must have an epithelial lining.

— *Pseudocysts*

    • Discrete collections of pancreatic secretions (sometimes containing hemorrhagic/inflammatory debris) contained by a rind of chronically inflamed fibrous tissue; there is no epithelial lining

    • Most pseudocysts follow bouts of pancreatitis (acute or chronic), but may also represent a complication of traumatic injury

    • Clinically, form an often large mass that must be distinguished from pancreatic neoplasia

    • May become secondarily infected and even rupture

— *Sterile pancreatic abscess*

    • A collection of material that represents liquefactive necrosis of severely damaged pancreatic tissue; there is no epithelial lining

● True cysts of the pancreas

— *Congenital (types)*

    • Limited to pancreas—caused by abnormal pancreatic duct development

    • In association with cysts seen elsewhere, such as in polycystic kidney disease or von Hippel-Lindau disease

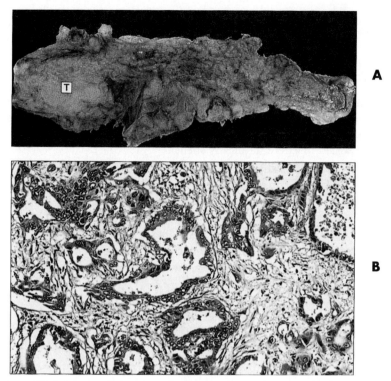

Fig. 20.6 Pancreatic head carcinoma. **A,** Gross photograph of pancreas with mass *(T)* representing carcinoma. **B,** Photomicrograph of pancreatic adenocarcinoma featuring malignant glands in a dense fibrous stroma. *(From Stevens A, Lowe J:* Pathology, *London, 1995, Times Mirror International.)*

- Histologically, the preceding entities show a cyst lined by cuboidal or very flattened epithelium

● **Benign neoplastic cysts of the pancreas**

- Usually seen in body-tail of pancreas

  - *Mucinous cystic tumors*—mucinous cystadenoma
  - *Serous cystic tumors*—microcystic adenoma
  - *Solid-cystic tumors*

● **Malignant cystic neoplasms of the pancreas**

- These are *not* commonly encountered lesions.

  - *Mucinous cystadenocarcinoma*
  - *Serous cystadenocarcinoma*

● **Malignant—non-cystic pancreatic neoplasms**

- *Carcinoma* is far and away the most common type of primary *exocrine* pancreatic cancer.

- The vast majority (99%) of these are adenocarcinoma arising from pancreatic ductal epithelium; only 1% of these lesions arise from pancreatic acinar cells.

- Demographically, these cancers typically occur in people over 50 years of age; there are about 30,000 new cases of pancreatic adenocarcinoma per year in the United States.

- Risk factors include cigarette smoking, high meat and/or fat diet, previous partial gastrectomy, and (perhaps) previous pancreatitis.
- Distribution of ductal adenocarcinoma within pancreas is 60% head, 10% body, 10% tail, and 20% diffuse involvement.
- *Note:* Pancreatic head lesions cause obstructive symptoms involving the common bile duct, ampulla of Vater, and duodenum; these patients often present with jaundice. In contradistinction, carcinomas arising in the body and tail tend not to cause symptoms or signs until they are well advanced in extent (clinically silent).
- Histologically, pancreatic duct adenocarcinoma is characterized by poorly formed tubular structures and infiltrating nests and columns of malignant cells embedded in a fibrotic (desmoplastic) stroma; the carcinoma cells have a tendency to track along nerve tissue (Fig. 20.6).
- *Prognosis* for pancreatic carcinoma is *dismal* with 5-year survival of less than 5% when taking into account all patients with this disease.

MULTIPLE CHOICE
REVIEW QUESTIONS

1. Icterus (jaundice) first appears when the total serum bilirubin level exceeds which of the following?

   a. 1.5 mg/dl
   b. 2.5 mg/dl
   c. 3.5 mg/dl
   d. 5.0 mg/dl
   e. 10 mg/dl

2. Which of the following viral infections is transmitted primarily by the feco-oral route?

   a. Hepatitis E
   b. Hepatitis B
   c. Hepatitis C
   d. Hepatitis D
   e. Human immunodeficiency virus

3. The most common type of gallstone encountered in the United States is which of the following?

   a. Pigmented stones
   b. Urate stones
   c. Cholesterol stones
   d. Cystine stones
   e. Magnesium ammonium stones

4. Which of the following statements regarding the gallbladder is *false?*

   a. It lacks a muscularis mucosa.
   b. It lacks a submucosa.
   c. It is essential for life.
   d. About 10% to 20% of the American population harbors calculi there.

5. Which of the following statements is *false* of bilirubin conjugated to glucuronic acid residues?

   a. It is water soluble.
   b. It is excreted into bile.
   c. It binds weakly to albumin.
   d. It is also known as direct bilirubin.
   e. Its high levels cause kernicterus in premature infants.

Chapter 21

Skin

The skin, which is a large, dynamic, and complex organ, provides a protective coat for the body. An active participant in the immune system, especially with regard to antigen processing, the skin also is an important contributor to vitamin D metabolism, an important regulator of body temperature, an important participant in body water homeostasis, and a mediator of multiple sensory functions.

Dermatopathology is a very complex speciality, and this review is intentionally brief. The reader is directed to one of the several excellent reference dermatopathology works for a more complete discussion. The boxed glossary at the end of the chapter is also a useful resource.

- Histologic game plan of the skin

  - Ectoderm gives rise to the skin's epithelial structures, while mesoderm gives rise to the mesenchymal components of the dermis (Fig. 21.1).

■ Inflammatory/Infectious Disorders of the Skin

- The skin is exposed to more potentially harmful agents than any other organ.

- Therefore, it is not surprising that skin exhibits a relatively large number of inflammatory and neoplastic lesions, some (but *not* all) of which have reasonably characteristic and specific histologic features.

- Provisos in skin pathology

  - Even though there is a large collection of reasonably specific histologic reaction patterns to certain harmful agents and stimuli, there are many more noxious agents than specific responses to meet them. *Therefore, in many cases, the histologic findings are not sufficiently specific to allow for categorization of exact lesional etiology.*

    - *The cause of many skin lesions is not currently known.*

    - *The history of nomenclature for dermatologic lesions is quite archaic and is based much more upon the in vivo (clinical) appearance of the lesion on the patient rather than its histologic attributes under a microscope.*

    - Many lesions that we associate as primarily skin disorders may also involve mucosal membranes, especially oral, vaginal, and conjunctival.

    - *Dermatitis* refers to inflammatory lesions of the skin and may involve dermis, epidermis, or both.

    - *Nonspecific dermatitis* is referred to as eczema and may have many etiologies.

    - *Note:* The etiology for nonspecific dermatitis usually can only be inferred from the lesion's in vivo characteristics and clinical history rather than any discriminant histologic features.

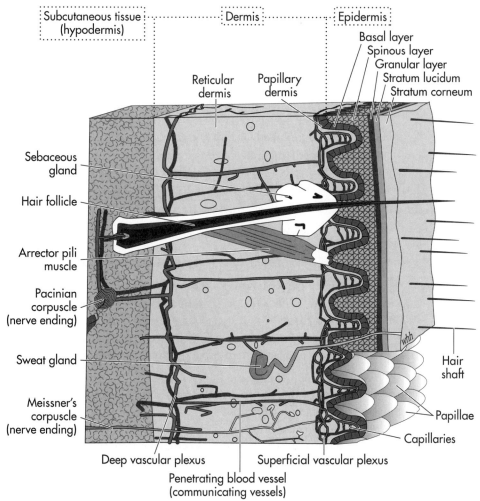

Fig. 21.1 Schematic representation of normal skin.

- **Nonspecific dermatitis**

    - *Atopic*—associated with a history of allergies, asthma (atopy), hay fever

    - *Gravitational*—affects the lower extremities preferentially, especially in patients with varicose veins and deficient venous drainage

    - *Irritant contact dermatitis*—caused by skin contact with strong detergent and alkalis

    - *Allergic contact dermatitis*—usually a skin reaction to metals (especially nickel) but also dyes, rubber (latex), and ingredients in certain cosmetics

    - *Seborrheic dermatitis*—reddened and inflamed skin covered by a thick waxy or white scaly material; among infants, is usually seen in the scalp (cradle cap), but in adults the face is a preferred site; skin creases in obese persons may also harbor seborrheic dermatitis

- **Relatively specific dermatitis with reasonably characteristic histologic-clinical features**

    - *Note:* This is merely a sampling, and the reader is directed to reference works for a more complete discussion.

— *Lichen planus*

   • Common inflammatory disorder that typically presents as raised, purplish red papules on the forearm, wrist, ankle and other sites; when these lesions resolve, they leave an area of hyperpigmented skin

      • Histologically, one sees degeneration of basal layer keratinocytes and melanocytes with occasional dead keratinocytes, which are called Civatte bodies
      • The epidermal rete ridges are typically saw-tooth shaped, and there is a dense upper dermal inflammatory cell infiltrate largely composed of lymphocytes (Fig. 21.2).

— *Psoriasis*

   • Psoriasis is a chronic disease that waxes and wanes over time (Fig. 21.3).
   • It is characterized by red plaques covered by a thick white scale.
   • It is seen mainly in knees, elbows, trunk, and scalp.
   • When the scale is removed, these lesions often show small areas of hemorrhage.
   • Histologically, one sees hyperkeratosis, parakeratosis, and acanthosis with enlarged rete ridges having a "test-tube" shape.

      • Neutrophils infiltrate the epidermis and upper dermis, and some of these neutrophils form Munro microabscesses within the stratum corneum.
      • Furthermore, there is markedly increased basal layer mitotic activity in the epidermis as compared to normal.
      • *Maturation time for epidermis is normally 28 days but is hastened to 3 to 5 days in psoriasis.*

   • *Note:* Other conditions may have skin lesions with at least some of the histologic and/or clinical features of psoriasis (psoriasiform dermatitis).

— *Pityriasis rosea*

   • This is a common skin inflammatory disorder, particularly of young patients.
   • Clinically, one sees a red patch surrounded by a whitish scale. The first such lesion (herald lesion) is usually the largest.
   • Histologically, the white scale is seen to be caused by parakeratosis; there is a chronic inflammatory cell infiltrate in the dermis.

● Infectious disorders of the skin

   • Most commonly caused by viruses but may be caused by fungi, bacteria, or parasites

— *Viral infection*

   • *Herpes simplex types 1 and 2* (nongenital and genital herpes, respectively)

      • One sees painful, blistering lesions of the skin and mucous membranes.

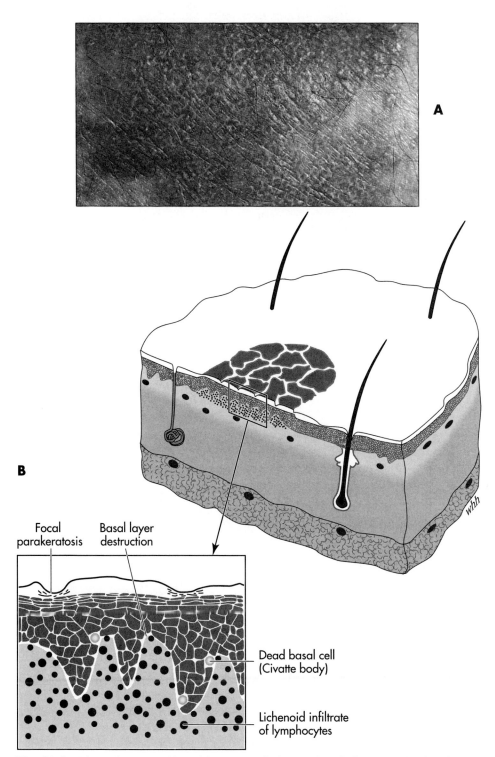

Focal
parakeratosis

Basal layer
destruction

Dead basal cell
(Civatte body)

Lichenoid infiltrate
of lymphocytes

B

A

Fig. 21.2 Lichen planus. **A,** Clinical features include raised, red plaques with white lines.
B, Schematic depicts the histologic changes. (*Modified from Stevens A, Lowe J:* Pathology, *London, 1995, Times Mirror International.*)

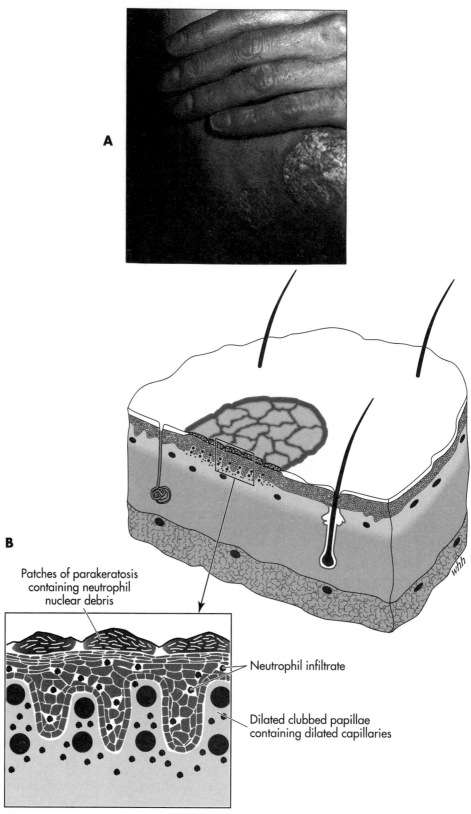

Fig. 21.3 Psoriasis. **A,** Clinical features include red patches covered by a thick, white scale. **B,** Schematic depicts the histopathologic changes. (*Modified from Stevens A, Lowe J:* Pathology, *London, 1995, Times Mirror International.*)

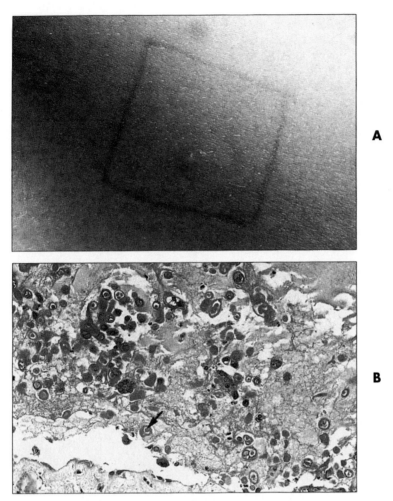

Fig. 21.4 Herpes virus. **A,** Clinical photograph of a herpes vesicle in a patient with chicken pox. **B,** Photomicrograph of skin involvement by chicken pox; note necrosis of epidermal keratinocytos and intranuclear viral inclusions (*arrow*). (*From Stevens A, Lowe J:* Pathology, *London, 1995, Times Mirror International.*)

- Histologically, there is epidermal necrosis with vesicle formation. Keratinocytes infected with the virus show cytopathic effects such as enlargement, multinucleation, and eosinophilic intranuclear inclusions (Fig. 21.4).

- *Herpes varicella-zoster virus*
  - Causes chickenpox in children and, in older adults, may reactivate from dormancy within dorsal root ganglia to cause "shingles"
  - Histology—identical to herpes simplex

- *Human papilloma virus (HPV)*
  - HPV is a wart virus, of which there are now over 70 known types (Fig. 21.5).
  - Histologically, one sees acanthosis and often a frondlike, papillary growth pattern. In the genital and perianal areas, this

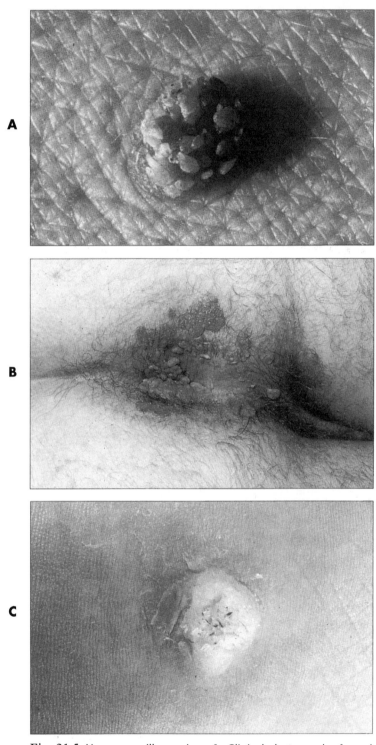

Fig. 21.5 Human papilloma virus. **A,** Clinical photograph of usual "wart". **B,** Clinical photograph of perineal condyloma acuminatum. **C,** Clinical photograph of plantar "wart" (verruca). (*From Stevens A, Lowe J: Pathology, London, 1995, Times Mirror International.*)

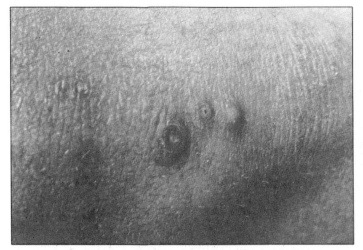
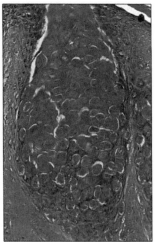

Fig. 21.6 Molluscum contagiosum. **A,** Clinical photograph depicts dome like nodules, each having a keratin filled central region. **B,** Photomicrograph of skin depicting the red-purple intracytoplasmic inclusions of molluscum. (*From Stevens A, Lowe J: Pathology, London, 1995, Times Mirror International.*)

type of virus produces the luxuriantly papillomatous (cauliflower-like) growth known as condyloma acuminatum.

- *Molluscum contagiosum*

    - Caused by a member of the pox virus family (double-stranded DNA) (Fig. 21.6)
    - Clinically, seen mostly in children and young adults on trunk and face and consists of pale raised, domelike lesions
    - Histologically, infected epidermal cells are literally packed with eosinophilic, intracytoplasmic viral inclusions

- *Generalized viremia*

    - Such as seen in measles and rubella
    - Gives a transient erythematous rash, almost never biopsied

— *Fungal infection*

- Superficial (epidermal) fungal infections (dermatophytoses) are *commonly seen in American clinical practice.*
- Commonly implicated are species of the *Trichophyton, Epidermophyton,* and *Microsporum* genera.
- Histologically, one observes that these fungal organisms are usually *limited to the stratum corneum (keratin layer)* and elicit either no or a limited inflammatory cell response.

— *Bacterial infections*

- Most bacterial infections of the skin are caused by staphylococcal and streptococcal organisms.

Impetigo

- Impetigo may be caused by both *Staphylococcus* and *Streptococcus* species.
    - Clinically, one sees the appearance of large epidermal blisters

that are filled with clear fluid or pus; eventually, these blisters crust over with a characteristic golden-yellow appearance.

Staphylococcal scalded skin syndrome (SSSS)

- Clinically, SSSS generally affects infants and small children.
- This condition is a cutaneous manifestation of what is *usually an extracutaneous staphylococcal infection* (centered often in conjunctiva, nose, throat) resulting in the elaboration of a toxin that causes epidermal necrosis and blistering; this toxin is called *"exfoliatin."*

Staphylococcus aureus folliculitis

- Results in pustules within the necks of hair follicles

Staphylococcus aureus boil (furuncle)

- Results from severe, deep folliculitis such that a relatively large collection of pus accumulates to form an intradermal abscess

Erysipelas

- A spreading infection of deep dermis and superficial subcutis caused by *Streptococcus* species, mainly occurring on the face

Cellulitis

- Similar to erysipelas but involves deeper tissue (mainly deep subcutis, fascia, and sometimes muscle); a variety of organisms can cause cellulitis, but *Staphylococcus* and *Streptococcus* species are particularly important and common ones.

Tuberculosis

- Chronic skin infection with this organism produces a lesion known as lupus vulgaris.
- Histologically, one sees a dermal-based, giant cell granulomatous process with destruction of collagen and skin appendages.

Leprosy (Hansen's disease)

- Leprosy is caused by the bacterium *Mycobacterium leprae.*
- Although uncommon in the United States, this disease is still a scourge in other, less developed, parts of the world.
- Histologically, one may see one of two basic types of skin involvement.

  - In *lepromatous leprosy* the dermis is distended by histiocytes stuffed with the acid-fast bacilli, *Mycobacterium leprae* organisms, thereby causing the formation of skin nodules and plaques.
  - In *tuberculoid leprosy,* numerous small granuloma are found throughout the dermis, especially around nerves; the latter may result in nerve damage.
  - In tuberculoid leprosy, the *Mycobacterium leprae* are not easily found, in contradistinction to the case for lepromatous leprosy.

Leishmania

- Caused by *Leishmania tropica* and *L. donovani,* transmitted via bite of the sandfly
  - Initially—the organism is introduced to the dermis, where it

incites a histiocytic response; organisms can be identified within these histiocytes

- Subsequently—a brisk lymphocytic and plasma cell response appears, forming a skin nodule that frequently ulcerates

Scabies

- The mite *Acarus scabiei* is the most common cutaneous parasitic infection in the United States.

- Clinically, one sees a very pruritic (itchy), red, raised, scaly skin lesion. Sometimes, lesions exhibit linear red tracks caused by mites burrowing through the epidermis, thereby eliciting an inflammatory response in the subjacent dermis.

- Histologically, one can often see the actual mite organism; characteristically, this infection initiates a brisk *eosinophil-rich inflammatory cell response in the dermis.*

- **Bullous disorders**

  - There are many types, only two of which will be mentioned here.

  — *Pemphigus vulgaris*

    - Most common type of the pemphigus family (80%)

      - Autoimmune condition mediated by autoantibody (IgG) to intercellular junctions of keratinocytes (adherens junctions)
      - May affect mucosal structures and skin
      - Produces fragile blisters that rupture and result in painful erosions
      - Positive Nikolsky's sign (grossly "normal" skin blisters when it is rubbed; not specific for pemphigus)
      - Histologically, suprabasal bulla formation (intraepidermal bulla) with a scant number of basal layer cells still attached to the dermis ("tombstones")

  — *Bullous pemphigoid*

    - Usually seen in older people
    - See large, tense bullae mainly on thighs, arms, abdomen
    - Key lesion—autoantibody to epidermal basement membrane, usually complement-binding IgG
    - Histologically, look for subepidermal blister (cleavage occurs at eipdermal-dermal junction); blister often filled with eosinophils and serum protein
    - An increased rate of other autoimmune disorders is seen in bullous pemphigoid patients

Skin "Tumors"

- These mass lesions most commonly arise from keratinocytes or melanocytes but may arise from any cells of the epidermis, skin appendages, or dermal mesenchymal tissues.

- **Lesions arising from epidermal squamous cells (keratinocytes)**

  — *Benign lesions*

    - *Cutaneous horn* is a hard protruding mass of keratin covering an area of abnormal skin.

- This is a lesion that overlies some other abnormality such as seborrheic keratosis, wart, or an underlying malignant or premalignant lesion.

- *Seborrheic keratoses* are common lesions, especially in older patients.

  - There are usually multiple lesions.
  - They are raised grey-brown masses that have a "stuck on" appearance.
  - Histologically, one sees a proliferation of keratinocytes (resembling those of the basal layer and are referred to as basaloid cells) accompanied by horny cysts (small cystic spaces filled with keratin material).

- *Keratoacanthoma* is commonly seen on the face of older individuals.

  - Growth progression is from slightly raised, red papule to a large dome-shaped nodule with a central keratin-filled crater exhibiting firm, overhanging edges.
  - These lesions, in contradistinction to squamous cell carcinoma, arise rapidly and most will spontaneously regress after several months.
  - Histologically, one sees a central keratin-filled crater; the lesion consists of proliferating keratinocytes extending into the dermis, and, in some cases, histologic differentiation from squamous cell carcinoma may not be possible.

- *Acrochordon* (skin tag or soft fibroma) is a very *common* lesion.

  - Some have a clinical appearance similar to a papilloma, while others are small nodules and still others are soft, baglike, pedunculated lesions.
  - Histologically, these resemble seborrheic keratosis; one sees papillomatosis, acanthosis, and hyperkeratosis.
  - These are *not* premalignant.

- *Pseudoepitheliomatous hyperplasia* (Pseudocarcinomatous hyperplasia) refers to a benign, *reactive* proliferation of epidermal keratinocytes that may clinically produce raised lesions.

  - Typically it is seen as a reaction to chronic inflammatory stimulus, including fungal infection, burn injury site, trauma sites, bedsore (stasis ulcer) sites, and in association with a nearby granular cell tumor.
  - Histologically, one sees an irregular epidermal keratinocyte proliferation (acanthosis) that may mimic squamous cell carcinoma. However, the cytologic/histologic features of malignancy are absent.

- *Solar keratosis* (actinic keratosis) is a benign condition but is generally considered to be a potentially premalignant lesion.

  - It presents clinically as raised plaquelike lesions, often associated with a scaly (hyperkeratotic) surface, usually found on sun-exposed skin.

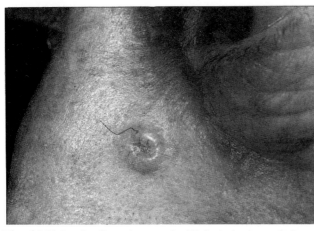 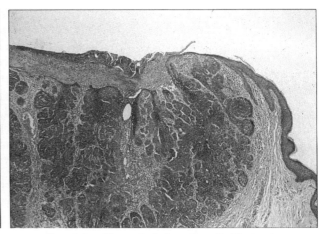

Fig. 21.7 Basal cell carcinoma. **A,** Clinical photograph features a small nodule with central ulceration. **B,** Photomicrograph. *(From Stevens A, Lowe J:* Pathology, *London, 1995, Times Mirror International.)*

- Histologically, one sees epidermal thickness changes *(sometimes atrophic and, in other cases, acanthotic), as well as varying degrees of abnormal keratinocyte differentiation (dysplasia or altered cell maturation). In the dermis, there is usually collagen degeneration known as solar elastosis wherein the collagen fibers appear to be broken down and have a basophilic (lilac-light blue) hue on routine microsections.*

- *Note:* Not all actinic keratosis will progress to squamous cell carcinoma if left untreated; however, some definitely will, and this may take years to happen.

— *Malignant lesions arising from epidermal keratinocytes*

- *Basal cell carcinoma (basal cell epithelioma)* is the *most common primary cancer of the skin* (Fig. 21.7).

  - This is usually seen on sun-exposed areas, and its development is predisposed to occur by sun exposure.

  - These are *indolent cancers* that may recur locally if not completely excised, but *metastases are exceedingly rare.*

  - Clinically, they usually appear as raised nodules, often with central ulceration.

  - Histologically, one sees collections of small, round, dark cells arising from the lower epidermis and invading into dermis; the cells are arranged into nests and characteristically show *peripheral palisading* of neoplastic cells radially about the edges of these nests. Also seen is *retraction of the neoplastic* cell groups from surrounding dermal collagen *(tumor retraction artifact).*

  - Treatment is complete excision.

- *Squamous cell carcinoma in situ (Bowen's disease)* is a lesion that occurs mainly on sun-exposed skin but, unlike solar keratoses, may also arise in non–sun-exposed areas.

  - Clinically, these present as either flat or raised, red-brown plaques sometimes accompanied by ulceration and keratin scale formation.

- Histologically, one sees full thickness epidermal keratinocyte dysplasia with atypical cells, occasional multinucleated cells, and increased mitotic activity. However, the epidermal basement membrane is intact and not transgressed by these atypical cells.

- Some, but not all, squamous cell carcinoma in situ lesions will, if left untreated, progress to invasive squamous cell carcinoma. The rate for transformation to invasive cancer is much higher for squamous cell carcinoma in situ than it is for solar keratosis.

- *Invasive squamous cell carcinoma* clinically presents as a raised, often irregularly nodular mass sometimes associated with ulceration.

  - Most of these are at least locally invasive. In addition, this skin cancer (unlike basal cell carcinoma) has a decided potential for metastases, initially to regional lymph nodes but, occasionally, to other sites.

  - Histologically, one sees malignant squamous cells invading dermis, often producing keratin (sometimes producing round structures known as keratin pearls). Not all squamous cell carcinomas produce keratin, however.

  - *Note:* A well-differentiated variant of squamous cell carcinoma has a cauliflower-like clinical appearance and is known as *verrucous carcinoma.* These lesions are particularly common on vulvar skin in elderly women and extend locally with infrequent metastases.

  - Treatment for squamous cell carcinoma is complete excision and follow-up monitoring for subsequent recurrent disease-metastases.

  - *Note: Xeroderma pigmentosum* predisposes toward squamous cell carcinoma at an early age (first decade of life) and is the result of an abnormality in a DNA repair enzyme. These patients also suffer from an increased incidence of basal cell carcinomas, fibrosarcomas, and melanomas of the skin.

- **Lesions arising from epidermal melanocytes**
  - *Benign lesions*
    - *Freckles* (ephelides)

      - These *common* lesions are flat and brown and are seen in sun-exposed skin.
      - They are *not* premalignant
      - Histologically, one sees a normal number of basal epidermal melanocytes, but there is an increased amount of melanin pigment in these cells.

    - *Lentigo simplex*

      - Flat brown lesions
      - Histologically, one sees an increased number of basal layer melanocytes and increased amounts of melanin pigment per melanocyte and the presence of upper dermal melanophages.

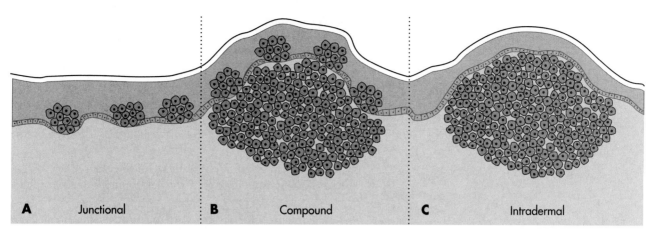

Fig. 21.8 Schematic showing the major types of benign melanocytic nevi. **A,** Junctional melanocytic nevus features clusters of melanocytes at the epidermal-dermal junction. **B,** Compound melanocytic nevus with both epidermal-dermal junction and intradermal proliferation of melanocytes. **C,** Intradermal melanocytic nevus formed by clusters of benign intradermal melanocytes. *(From Stevens A, Lowe J:* Pathology, *London, 1995, Times Mirror International.)*

- *Melanocytic nevi* (Fig. 21.8)

  - Common vernacular for these lesions is "moles."
  - These are *common* and appear as flat or raised brown lesions that may be found anywhere on the skin.

- *Melanocytic nevi—come in 5 major types*

  - *Junctional*—proliferation of benign melanocytes in lowermost epidermis, right at the epidermal-dermal junction
  - *Compound*—proliferation of benign melanocytes in the lower epidermis (as above for junctional type) *plus* the upper dermis
  - *Intradermal*—proliferation of benign melanocytes confined to dermis and not involving the lower epidermis
  - *Blue nevus*—proliferation of benign, spindle cell melanocytes in the *deep dermis*
  - *Spitz nevus (juvenile nevus)*—is seen mainly in children and young adults; presents clinically as a raised, reddish brown nodule; histologically, these benign lesions may have a somewhat worrisome appearance because the benign melanocytes may have alarming degrees of atypia and nuclear pleomorphism (variability)
  - *Note:* Except for intradermal melanocytic nevi, these lesions usually appear in children and/or during the adolescent years; intradermal nevi usually appear during adulthood.
  - *Note:* The vast majority of the above nevi are entirely innocuous and will not transform to malignant melanoma. The junctional component of junctional-compound melanocytic nevi is the most at risk for transforming into malignant melanoma, but, considering the number of such nevi seen in clinical practice, this is an uncommon event.

- *Dysplastic melanocytic nevi*

  - These are a type of atypical melanocytic lesion often characterized by multiple irregularly pigmented and shaped lesions that show varying degrees of histologic abnormality. Some of these lesions (if allowed to remain on the patient) will progress to malignant melanoma, and, in that sense, they should be considered as potentially premalignant lesions.

- *Histologically,* one sees cytologic and architectural abnormalities with increased mitotic activity and nuclear variability; these changes are not yet advanced enough to classify as cancer, however.

- *Treatment* is excision of clinically suspicious lesions and careful follow-up monitoring for the development of other such lesions.

- *Note:* Some patients present with multiple dysplastic melanocytic nevi and have a family history of such lesions (*dysplastic-nevus syndrome*).

— *Malignant lesions arising from epidermal melanocytes (malignant melanoma)*

- These cancers are increasing in frequency; their occurrence is related to ultraviolet (UV) light exposure, and fair skinned individuals are at particular risk, especially if they are "sun worshippers." Cutaneous melanomas are uncommon in people of color.

Malignant melanoma in situ

- In this situation, one sees malignant melanocytes, at least focally, extending through the entire epidermal thickness. However, the epidermal basement membrane is not crossed by these malignant cells, so there is no dermal invasion.

- Histologically, one sees atypical melanocytes with nuclear variability and increased mitotic activity.

Invasive malignant melanoma

- In this situation, one sees invasion of subjacent dermis (and sometimes subcutis) by malignant melanoma cells.

TWO MAJOR TYPES OF INVASIVE MALIGNANT MELANOMA

- *Invasive superficial spreading malignant melanoma* accounts for 75% of all skin *malignant melanoma.*

- *Nodular malignant melanoma* presents as a raised brown lesion; melanoma cells tend to grow in a so-called vertical growth fashion into subjacent dermis.

- Histologically, in both types, one sees invasion of dermis (and sometimes subcutis) by malignant melanocytes featuring cytoatypia, nuclear variability, and mitotic activity as manifested by mitotic figures. Variable cancer cell pigmentation is seen.

■ Determination of Prognosis for Cutaneous Melanomas

- *The single most important prognostic factor in cutaneous malignant melanomas is the depth of melanoma invasion.*

- The most accepted and commonly utilized way to measure this invasion thickness is the Breslow System; in this system, one determines the distance from the deepest point of melanoma penetration to the granular cell layer of the overlying epidermis, expressed in mm.

- **Breslow system**
  - Invasion less than 0.76 mm constitutes the lowest risk for melanoma metastases.
  - Invasion thickness between 0.76 and 1.5 mm has moderate risk for subsequent metastases.
  - Invasion thickness of greater than 1.5 indicates highest risk for subsequent metastases.

- **When melanoma spreads in the body, it does so by**
  - Lymphatics to regional nodes draining the primary site
  - Intradermal lymphatic spread to set up cutaneous satellite melanoma deposits
  - Hematogenously, *with a special tropism for liver metastasis* and, less commonly, lung and brain.

- **Treatment of melanoma**
  - *Surgical*—complete excision with uninvolved margins
  - *Chemotherapy*—for metastatic disease, but this treatment is not currently very effective

■ Other Miscellaneous Lesions Involving the Epidermis

- **Langerhans' cell histiocytosis (Langerhans' cell proliferation or histiocytosis X)**
  - This is a *spectrum of proliferation of Langerhans' cells,* which are a type of antigen processing immune system cell normally found in the epidermis.
  — *Letterer-Siwe disease*
    - Seen in infants
    - Often present as a yellow, scaly skin rash that resembles seborrheic dermatitis
    - Behaves in a *malignant* fashion, with spread of abnormal Langerhans' cells throughout the body (including to liver, spleen, bone)
  — *Hand-Schüller-Christian (HSC) disease*
    - Seen in children
    - Accumulation of Langerhans' cells in bone (resulting in osteolytic lesions), lung (giving rise to pulmonary infiltrates), and sometimes lymph nodes
    - *Classic HSC disease* (seen in only about 10% of cases)—diabetes insipidus, osteolytic bony lesions, and exophthalmos
  — *Eosinophilic granuloma*
    - *Least severe disorder* of the Langerhans' cell histiocytosis spectrum
      - Seen mainly in older children and adults
      - Usually solitary, but sometimes multiple lesions are seen
      - *Usually involves bone,* but may also involve skin

- **Merkel cell tumors**
  - This neoplasm is a *rare,* highly malignant cancer arising from intraepidermal Merkel cells (a type of neuroendocrine cell, normally found in epidermis, whose main function appears to be to act as a mechanoreceptor).

- Merkel cell tumors occur mainly in the head, neck, and arms of older people.
- Histologically, one sees a primitive, small, round, cell tumor morphologically very *similar* to small cell anaplastic carcinoma of the lung.

● Mycosis fungoides

- Despite its name this lesion, has *nothing to do with fungal infection.*
- Rather, the disease is a *primary T cell lymphoma of the skin* that may remain localized to skin for years.
- However, eventually, mycosis fungoides generally spreads to involve lymph nodes and visceral organs (including liver, spleen, and bone marrow), at which point it has a rather fulminant course.

- Histologically, one sees epidermal and upper dermal infiltration by atypical lymphoid cells possessing hyperchromatic (dark), highly convoluted nuclei; sometimes, one sees intraepidermal aggregates of these cells (*Pautrier's abscess*). Furthermore, these malignant T lymphocytes may gain access to the bloodstream, where they are referred to as *Sézary cells.*
- Treatment includes radiotherapy and, in advanced disease, chemotherapy.

● Other malignant lymphomas involving skin

- B-cell lymphoma of the skin usually involves the skin secondarily and represents a metastatic process (although it may represent a primary process).
- Clinically, one sees one or more raised, red-purple nodules, most often in the head and neck region.

■ **Tumor-producing Lesions Arising from Skin Adnexal Structures**

● Benign cystic lesions that produce a mass effect

— *Epidermal inclusion cysts*

- These very *common* lesions are most often seen on the face, neck, and upper trunk in young and middle-aged adults.
- Probably they derive from hair follicles.
- Histologically, one sees a cyst lined by keratinizing stratified squamous epithelium (epidermis). The cyst is composed of internally sloughed keratin debris.

— *Dermoid cyst*

- Less common than epidermal inclusion cyst but otherwise similar
- Histologically, skin adnexal structures (hair, sebaceous glands, eccrine glands) are formed in the *wall* of the cyst

— *Pilar cysts*

- Most often seen on the scalp of elderly patients
- Histologically, a cyst lined by stratified squamous epithelium

● Additional adnexal derived mass producing lesions

- These are not described in detail because such an endeavor is beyond the scope of this book.

  - Trichoepithelioma
  - Trichofolliculoma

- Pilomatricoma
- Sebaceous hyperplasia
- Sebaceous adenoma
- Sebaceous carcinoma (see Chapter 29, neoplasia section)
- Syringoma
- Eccrine poroma
- Clear cell acanthoma
- Eccrine adenocarcinoma
- Cylindroma
- Apocrine carcinoma

■ "Tumor"-producing Dermal Lesions

● Fibroblastic, neural, smooth muscle, and fatty proliferations

— *Keloid (dermal scar)*

- Commonly seen in clinical practice, and constitutes the most common non-neoplastic proliferation seen in the dermis
- Not a true neoplasm, but rather a brisk hyperplasia of collagen-producing fibroblasts
- Appear as firm, raised lesions covered by an intact epidermis; grow slowly and harden over time
- African-American women particularly prone to develop these keloid formations following some sort of traumatic antecedent event; a common site involves the earlobes as a consequence of ear piercing.

— *Fibromatoses*

- These are diffuse proliferations of fibroblasts and histiocytes that can occur at a number of body sites (including visceral).
- This group of disorders features a *histologically benign* proliferation that can invade locally and, in some cases, recur after excision.
- Most common site for this is the palms (palmar fibromatosis [Dupuytren's contracture]). There is a high incidence of palmar fibromatosis in alcoholics.

— *Benign fibrous histiocytoma (dermatofibroma)*

- Seen on the extremities of young to middle-aged adults, where it usually appears as a raised, brown nodule covered by epidermis
- Histologically, a relatively discrete proliferation of myofibroblasts (a cell having features of smooth muscle, fibroblast differentiation) and an admixture of histiocytes

— *Dermatofibrosarcoma protuberans*

- A malignant version of the dermatofibroma just described
- An irregular dermal lesion that behaves as a cancer and can even metastasize
- Histologically, a cellular lesion composed of atypical versions of the cells seen in dermatofibroma

— *Malignant fibrous histiocytoma*

- Most of these arise in deep tissues of the buttocks and thigh.
- However, some arise within subcutaneous fat and may present as a deep skin neoplasm.

- Histologically, one sees a cellular proliferation of atypical, fibroblast-like cells admixed with histiocytes. Necrosis, hemorrhage, and mitotic activity are often prominent.

— *Neural lesions*

- *Neurofibroma and neurolemmomas (schwannoma)* are benign proliferations of Schwann cells that may also arise at visceral organ sites.

    - Typically, one sees *numerous* skin neurofibromas in von Recklinghausen's disease (neurofibromatosis).
    - Histologically, in both neurofibroma and neurolemmomas, one sees a proliferation of benign spindle cells embedded in a delicate, neural ground substance.

- *Neurofibrosarcoma* is an uncommon malignant version of neurofibroma.

    - It is most often seen in patients with von Recklinghausen's disease.

— *Smooth muscle lesions*

- *Leiomyoma* is a benign smooth muscle neoplasm that, in the skin, may arise from blood vessel walls and erector pili muscles.

    - Histologically, one sees a proliferation of spindle cells having cigar-shaped nuclei. Necrosis, atypia, and significantly increased mitotic activity are *not* seen. (Malignant versions of this neoplasm are rare in the skin and are called *leiomyosarcoma*).

● Blood vessel proliferation

- Most are seen in the dermis.
- Some are true neoplasms, while others represent a reparative, reactive process.

— *Pyogenic granuloma*

- This is a total misnomer because this lesion does not feature pus or granuloma formation.
- Really, this represents a type of exuberant granulation tissue, and there is often antecedent trauma.
    - Clinically, these are red, raised masses that frequently ulcerate.
    - They are most commonly located on the head and neck and in buccal and gingival mucosal sites.
- *Histologically,* one sees highly vascular granulation tissue with numerous small blood vessels embedded in an inflammatory cell-rich stroma.

— *Capillary and cavernous hemangiomas*

- These are benign blood vessel proliferations lacking an associated stromal inflammatory cell response.
- *Histologically,* capillary hemangiomas consist of uniformly small-caliber vessels, whereas cavernous hemangiomas have larger caliber vascular channels.

— *Glomus tumors*

 • Reddish (sometimes blue) nodules most often seen in fingertips; often painful

— *Angiosarcoma*

 • A highly malignant neoplasm that can be seen in many locations of the body, including skin.

 • Cutaneous angiosarcomas are usually seen in the head and neck regions of elderly patients.

 • Clinically, these lesions are purplish-red patches, plaques, or nodules that often ulcerate.

 • Histologically, one sees blood vessel channels formed by malignant endothelial cells.

— *Kaposi's sarcoma*

 • This is a malignant neoplasm that has assumed great clinical importance with the emergence of the aquired immunodeficiency syndrome (AIDS) epidemic.

 • Prior to the recognition of AIDS in 1981, most Kaposi's sarcomas were seen in older men of Mediterranean extraction; these lesions usually occurred on the legs. Although they sometimes metastasized, this was *not* the usual course, and they behaved in a relatively indolent manner.

 • In patients with AIDS, these lesions are seen in a much younger population, and they are often multiple; they may involve visceral sites and tend to behave in *an aggressive* manner, often with widespread metastases.

 • Clinically, cutaneous Kaposi's sarcoma appears as red-purple plaques that often enlarge to form red-purple nodules.

 • Histologically, one sees a vascular proliferation with slitlike blood channels formed by malignant cells that are most likely endothelial in lineage.

GLOSSARY
General Terms Pertaining to Skin Pathology

Acantholysis—separation of epidermal cells consequent to dissolution of intercellular "cement" substance; seen (among others) in
- Viral infections
- Pemphigus vulgaris
- Darier's disease
- Solar keratosis
- Adenoid squamous cell carcinoma

Acanthosis—increased epidermal thickness consequent to an increased stratum spinosum; again, this is a *nonspecific finding* among the dermatoses

Actinic—relating to the chemically active rays of the electromagnetic spectrum; often used to describe the effects of sun on skin

Apoptosis—programmed cell death; in the skin, refers to individual keratinocyte cell death

Atypical cell—this definition is genuinely fraught with subjectivity; in general, atypical cells have varying degrees of the following characteristics
- An increased N:C ratio
- Nuclear hyperchromasia
- Giant forms or multinucleation
- Abnormal mitotic figures (e.g., tripolar)

Bulla—a fluid-filled space (may be subepidermal or intraepidermal); greater than 5 mm in diameter

Civatte body—a dead keratinocyte, usually seen in basal layer; often found in lichen planus

Desmosome—a specialized adhesion plate found between epithelial cells, especially those of the epidermis

Dyskeratosis—individual cell keratinization at the level of the stratum spinosum; seen (among others) in
- Bowen's disease
- Darier's disease
- Actinic keratosis

Dysplasia—deranged (altered), disorderly cell maturation; in the case of skin, this usually refers to epidermal keratinocytes or melanocytes

Edema—accumulation of excessive amounts of watery fluid in cells, tissues, or serous cavities

Hyperkeratosis—an abnormally thickened stratum corneum; this is a nonspecific abnormality seen in *numerous* dermatoses

(*Note:* On occasion, the thickened stratum corneum will assume a columnlike configuration (cutaneous horn); *a cutaneous horn does not exist alone and essentially always overlies some type of benign or malignant process, so be sure to include evaluable epidermis and dermis in your biopsy.*)

Continued.

GLOSSARY—continued

Keratinocytes—epidermal squamous cells, connected by intercellular bridges (desmosomes)

Melanophages—dermal histiocytes that have ingested melanin lost from cells of the epidermis

Macule—a flat, discolored skin lesion having a diameter less than 1 cm

Nodule—a palpable, raised, solid lesion greater than 1 cm in diameter

Papule—a raised, solid skin lesion having a diameter of less than 1 cm

Papilloma—a mass-forming proliferation of skin showing acanthosis and hyperkeratosis

Patch—a flat, discolored skin lesion having a diameter greater than 1 cm

Petechia—a small hemorrhage in the skin (pinpoint size)

Parakeratosis—Retention of nuclei in the stratum corneum; this is a nonspecific finding, being indicative of an increased epidermal proliferation rate

Polarity—refers to the arrangement of epithelial cells within a given epithelium; when loss of polarity occurs, the surface cells look similar or identical to the basal (germinative) cells consequent to abnormal (usually, lack of) cell maturation

Rete ridges—the projections of epidermal cells into the subjacent dermis

Spongiosis—accumulation of fluid between cells of the epidermis (keratinocytes)

Telangiectasis—refers to abnormally dilated small blood vessels (capillaries, venules, arterioles) that result in small red lesions of skin and mucous membranes

Tumor—literally means mass or swelling; commonly used as a synonym for neoplasia, but that is not an appropriate use of the word

Ulcer—loss of epidermis and at least part of dermis (generally less than 5 mm in diameter)

Vesicle—tiny blisters that form within the epidermis (less than 5 mm in diameter)

MULTIPLE CHOICE
REVIEW QUESTIONS

1. Munro microabscesses are classically seen in which of the following?

   a. Psoriasis
   b. Lichen planus
   c. Herpes simplex, type 2
   d. Mycosis fungoides
   e. Seborrheic dermatitis

2. In normal skin, the epidermal maturation time is approximately one month. In psoriasis, it is which of the following?

   a. 1 to 2 days
   b. 3 to 5 days
   c. 10 to 15 days
   d. 40 days
   e. 50 days

3. The effects of staphylococcal scalded skin syndrome are mediated by which of the following?

   a. Granuloma formation
   b. Abscess formation in the skin
   c. Viral infection
   d. A toxin

4. The most important prognostic factor in cutaneous melanomas is which of the following?

   a. Melanoma cell type
   b. Melanoma cell mitotic index
   c. Depth of melanoma invasion
   d. Associated solar damage

5. The *least* severe component of the Langerhans' cell histiocytosis spectrum is which of the following?

   a. Hand-Schüller Christian disease
   b. Letterer-Siwe disease
   c. Eosinophilic granuloma
   d. Lymphoma
   e. Melanoma

Chapter 22

Kidney and Urinary Tract

■ **Definitions**

● Azotemia

- Elevation of blood urea nitrogen (BUN) and creatinine
- Caused by decreased glomerular filtration rate

● Hematuria—blood in urine

● Proteinuria—protein in urine

● Oliguria-anuria—reduced or absent urine output

● Acute renal failure—acute onset of azotemia with oliguria or anuria

● Chronic renal failure

- Prolonged azotemia
- Associated clinical manifestations

  - Fluid-electrolyte—dehydration, edema, hyperkalemia, acidosis
  - Calcium-bone—hyperphosphatemia and hypocalcemia, secondary hyperparathryroidism, renal osteodystrophy
  - Hematologic—anemia, bleeding
  - Cardiovascular—hypertension, congestive heart failure, pericarditis
  - Gastrointestinal—nausea and vomiting, esophagitis, gastritis and stress ulcers, colitis
  - Neuromuscular—myopathy, peripheral neuropathy, encephalopathy

■ **Congenital Anomalies**

● Epidemiogy and etiology

- Found in 10% of newborns
- Account for 20% of chronic renal failure in children
- Not known to be genetic

● Unilateral agenesis

- Compensatory enlargement of other kidney
- Subsequent glomerulosclerosis of other kidney and renal failure

● Hypoplasia

- Less than six lobes and pyramids
- No scars
- Usually unilateral

- Ectopic
  - Within or just above pelvis
  - Tortuous or kinked ureters predispose to infection
- Horseshoe kidney
  - Fusion of lower (90%) or upper (10%) poles

■ **Cystic Diseases**

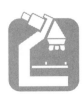

- Cystic dysplasia
  - Abnormality in metanephric differentiation
  - Morphology
    - Usually unilateral enlargement
    - Cysts up to 2 cm lined by flattened epithelium
    - Intervening cartilage, undifferentiated mesenchyme, immature collecting ducts
  - Usually associated with obstruction in pelvis or ureters
  - Clinical course
    - If unilateral, excise abnormal kidney
    - Bilateral, renal failure

- Adult polycystic kidney disease

  — *Epidemiology*
    - Prevalence—1/1000
    - Accounts for 10% chronic renal failure

  — *Etiology*
    - Autosomal dominant
    - 90% of cases are caused by mutations in APKD1 on chromosome 16

  — *Renal morphology*
    - Gross
      - Bilateral enlargement (up to 4 kg)
      - Cysts up to 4 cm without apparent intervening parenchyma

    - Histology
      - Functional nephrons between cysts
      - Cysts arise from tubules throughout nephron and have variable epithelial lining

  — *Associated abnormalities*
    - Hepatic cysts
    - Pancreatic cysts
    - Berry aneurysms of circle of Willis

  — *Clinical features*
    - Symptoms can develop in childhood or as late as 80s
    - Flank mass

- Abdominal pain
- Hematuria
- Renal failure
- Subarachnoid hemorrhage from ruptured berry aneurysms
- **Childhood polycystic kidney disease**
  - Autosomal recessive
  - Kidneys enlarged by dilated collecting ducts oriented at right angles to cortex, filling it and the medulla
  - Associated anomalies
    - Liver cysts and proliferating bile ducts often with congenital hepatic fibrosis
- **Nephrolithiasis-uremic medullary cystic disease complex**
  - Types
    - Sporadic (20%)
    - Autosomal recessive juvenile nephrolithiasis (50%)
    - Autosomal recessive renal-retinal dysplasia (15%)
    - Autosomal dominant, adult onset (15%)
  - Renal morphology
    - Small medullary cysts, often at corticomedullary junction
    - Atrophy of cortical tubules
    - Interstitial fibrosis

■ Glomerular Diseases

- Can be primary or secondary to a systemic disorder
- **Acute poststreptococcal (proliferative) glomerulonephritis**
  - — *Etiology*
    - Group A beta hemolytic streptococci
      - Greater than 90% caused by strains 12, 4, or 1

  - — *Pathogenesis*
    - Immune complexes involving microbial antigens
      - Uncertain if circulating immune complexes or if antigens are planted

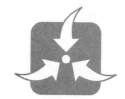

  - — *Renal morphology*
    - Histology
      - Diffuse (all glomeruli involved) hypercellularity
      - Proliferation of endothelial, mesangial, epithelial cells
      - Infiltration by neutrophils (Fig. 22.1)

    - Immunofluorescence
      - Granular IgG, IgM, C3
    - Electron microscopy
      - Subepithelial deposits ("humps")

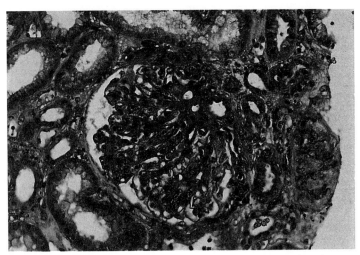

Fig. 22.1 Post-streptococcal glomerulonephritis. Note the glomerular hypercellularity primarily caused by neutrophilic infiltration. (*Damjanov I, Linder J:* Anderson's pathology, *ed 10, vol 2, St Louis, 1996, Mosby.*)

— *Laboratory manifestations*

- Low serum complement
- Antibodies to antistreptococcal exoenzyme (ASO)

— *Clinical features and course*

- Acute nephritis (hematuria, mild to moderate proteinuria, oliguria, hypertension) 1 to 4 weeks after streptococcal infection of throat or skin
  - 95% of children recover
  - 60% of adult sporadic cases recover
  - Other outcomes
    - Rapidly progressive glomerulonephritis
    - Delayed but eventual resolution
    - Chronic renal failure

● **Other forms of postinfectious glomerulonephritis**

— *Acute proliferative glomerulonephritis*—not caused by streptococcal infection
Etiology

- Bacterial infections
  - Pneumococcal pneumonia
  - Meningococcemia
- Viruses
  - Hepatitis B
  - Mumps
  - Varicella
  - Epstein-Barr virus

- Parasites

  - Malaria

  - Toxoplasmosis

Morphology

- Same as poststreptococcal glomerulonephritis

● **Rapidly progressive glomerulonephritis (RPGN)**

— *Acute nephritis*—with renal failure and accumulation of cellular "crescents" in Bowman's space

Etiology

- Idiopathic

  - Accounts for 50% of cases of RPGN

  - No antecedent infection or systemic disease known to cause RPGN

- Postinfectious, complicating acute proliferative GN (preceding)

- Systemic diseases (see following)

  - Systemic lupus erythematosis (SLE)
  - Goodpasture's syndrome
  - Polyarteritis nodosa and other vasculitides
  - Wegener's granulomatosis
  - Henoch-Schönlein purpura
  - Essential cryoglubulinemia

Morphology

HISTOLOGY (COMMON TO ALL FORMS OF RPGN)

- Crescents

  - Proliferation of parietal epithelium

  - Migration of monocytes and macrophages into Bowman's space

  - Eventual obliteration of Bowman's space

IMMUNOFLUORESCENCE AND ULTRASTRUCTURE IN IDIOPATHIC RPGN

- About 50%, negative immunofluorescence with minimal or no immune complexes

- About 25%, granular immunofluorescence pattern associated with immune complexes

- About 25%, linear immunofluorescence pattern (similar to Goodpasture's syndrome)

Laboratory and clinical features of idiopathic RPGN

- Antineutrophil cytoplasmic antibodies usually present in patients with negative immunofluorescence

- Most patients develop chronic renal failure

● **Nephrotic syndrome (nephrosis)**

- Definition—heavy proteinuria (greater than 3.5 g/1.73m^2 body surface/day), hypoalbuminemia, edema, hyperlipidemia, lipiduria, tendency to infection and thrombosis

  - Proteinuria can be selective or nonselective

- Primary (95% in children; 60% in adults)

  - Membranous nephropathy most common cause in adults (40%)
  - Minimal change disease (lipoid nephrosis) most common cause in children (65%)

- Secondary to systemic diseases

  - Diabetes mellitus (DM)
  - SLE
  - Amyloidosis
  - Malignancies
  - Infections (human immunodeficiency virus [HIV], hepatitis B, syphillis, malaria)
  - Drugs (gold, penicillamine, heroin)

- **Membranous nephropathy (membranous glomerulonephritis)**

  - Most common cause of nephrotic syndrome caused by primary glomerular disease in adults (about 40% of cases)
  - Etiology

    - 85% primary
    - 15% secondary to systemic disorders (DM, SLE)

  - Pathogenesis

    - Immune complex (circulating or in situ formation)

  - Morphology

    - Diffuse thickening of capillary walls
    - Basement membrane material (spikes) project between deposits (Fig. 22.2)
    - Immunofluorescence—granular pattern IgG, C3 (Fig. 22.3)
    - Ultrastructure—subepithelial dense deposits

  - Clinical course

    - Can begin as non-nephrotic range proteinuria
    - Full-blown nephrotic syndrome
    - As many as 40% progress to chronic renal failure within 20 years (some as rapidly as 2 years)

- **Minimal change disease**

  - Accounts for about 65% of cases of nephrotic syndrome in children
  - Etiology and pathogenesis unknown
  - Morphology

    - Histology—normal
    - Immunofluorescence—negative
    - Ultrastructure—uniform diffuse effacement of visceral epithelial foot processes

  - Clinical features and course

    - Maintain normal renal function and blood pressure

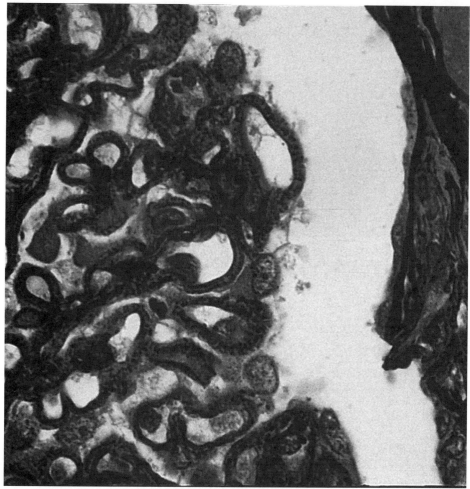

Fig. 22.2 Membranous nephropathy. Glomerulus with spikes of basement membrane material adjacent to subepithelial deposits. *(Damjanov I, Linder J: Anderson's pathology, ed 10, vol 2, St Louis, 1996, Mosby.)*

- Most children successfully treated with a single course of corticosteroids
- Some become steroid dependent, requiring long-term therapy
- Adults respond more slowly

● **Focal segmental sclerosis**

- Ten percent of childhood nephrotic syndrome, 15% of adult idiopathic nephrotic syndrome

— *Etiologic categories*

- Idiopathic
- Concurrent with another primary glomerular disease
- Associated with loss of renal mass (nephrectomy, unilateral agenesis, reflux, analgesic abuse)
- Secondary to known agents (HIV)

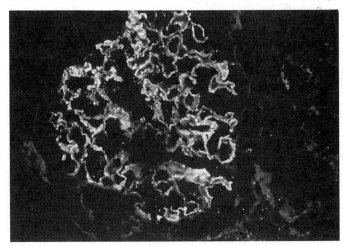

Fig. 22.3 Membranous nephropathy. The glomerulus shows granular capillary wall IgG. (*Damjanov I, Linder J:* Anderson's pathology, *ed 10, vol 2, St Louis, 1996, Mosby.*)

— *Morphology*

Histology

- Focal—some glomeruli; segmental—only part of involved glomerulus affected

  - Increased mesangial matrix, hyalinosis

  - Some totally sclerotic glomeruli (global sclerosis) that increase in number with time

  - Arteriolar hyalinization and tubular atrophy

Immunofluorescence

- IgM, C3 in hyalinized areas

Ultrastructure

- Nonsclerotic areas show effacement of epithelial foot processes and detachment of epithelial cells, denuding basement membrane

— *Clinical features and outcome*

- Higher incidence of hematuria, reduced glomerular filtration than in minimal change disease
- Nonselective proteinuria
- Poor response to glucocorticoids
- 20% have rapid course (malignant sclerosis) with renal failure within 2 years
- 50% have chronic renal failure by 10 years

● **Membranoproliferative (mesangiocapillary) glomerulonephritis**

- Five to ten percent of cases of idiopathic (NS)

— *Pathogenesis*

- Type I—immune complex
- Type II—alternate complement pathway (low serum C3)

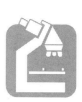

— *Morphology*

Histology (common to both types I and II)

- Mesangial proliferation
- Double contour capillary wall

Type I

- Immunofluorescence—granular

  - Immunoglobulins
  - Early complement components (C1q and C4)

- Ultrastructure—subendothelial deposits

Type II

- Immunofluorescence—C3
- Ultrastructure

  - Ribbonlike deposits in basement membrane
  - Subepithelial humps

— *Clinical features*

- Glucocorticoids sometimes slow progress
- 50% develop chronic renal failure within 10 years
- High recurrence rate after transplantation, especially in type II

- **IgA nephropathy (Berger's disease)**
  - Probably most common cause of mild glomerular dysfunction
  - Defined by presence of mesangial IgA

— *Etiology and pathogenesis*

- Primary cases

  - Possible genetic abnormality of IgA1—increased serum IgA1, circulating and glomerular IgA1 immune complexes
  - Activation of alternate complement pathway

- Secondary cases

  - Celiac disease (intestinal mucosal abnormality)
  - Hepatobiliary disease (decreased clearance of IgA)

— *Morphology*

- Histology variable (normal, focal segmental sclerosis, diffuse mesangial proliferation, crescents)
- Immunofluorescence

  - Mesangial IgA is key feature (Fig. 22.4)
  - Sometimes C3, properdin, IgG, or IgM

— *Clinical course*

- Usually affects children and young adults
- Hematuria following mucosal infection of gastrointestinal tract or urinary tract
- Hematuria subsides and recurs
- 50% develop chronic renal failure in 20 years

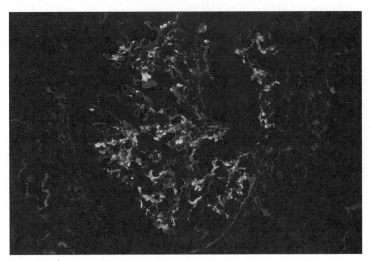

Fig. 22.4 IgA nephropathy. The glomerulus shows granular mesangial IgA. (*Damjanov I, Linder J:* Anderson's pathology, *ed 10, vol 2, St Louis, 1996, Mosby.*)

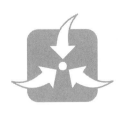

● **Focal proliferative and necrotizing glomerulonephritis**

- Proliferation in some glomeruli (focal), often involving only part of the glomerulus (segmental)
- Etiology

  - Component of IgA nephropathy
  - Primary (not known to be related to other primary glomerular disease or systemic disease)
  - Early manifestation of systemic disorder that involves glomeruli

- Morphology
- Clinical course

  - Usually mild hematuria
  - Sometimes nephrotic syndrome

● **Systemic diseases involving with prominent glomerular involvement**

— *Amyloidosis (see Amyloidosis chapter)*

— *Diabetes mellitus (see Endocrine Diseases chapter)*

— *Systemic lupus erythematosus (see Immunity chapter)*

- Symptomatic renal involvement occurs in about 70% of patients
- Pathogenesis—DNA-anti-DNA immune complex deposition in glomeruli
- Morphologic categories and clinical features

  - Class I—Rare; normal by light microscopy, immunofluorescence, and electron microscopy
  - Class II—Mesangial lupus glomerulonephritis presents in about 25% of patients; characterized by slight increase in mesangial matrix, and immunoglobulin and complement within the mesangium; minimal clinical features (mild hematuria or protinuria)

- Class III—Focal proliferative glomerulonephritis present in about 20%; mesangial and endothelial proliferation, neutrophils, and sometimes necrosis in some glomeruli are present; immunoglobulin and complement found in mesangium and capillaries; more severe hematuria than class II (one third have renal failure)
- Class IV—Diffuse proliferative glomerulonephritis occurs in 35% to 40% of patients; endothelial and mesangial, and sometimes epithelial proliferation found in most glomeruli; immunoglobulin and complement found in mesangium and capillaries; subendothelial immune complexes can form "wire loops"; sometimes associated with immune complexes in the tubules; one or more serious clinical features (gross hematuria, nephrotic syndrome, and moderate to severe renal failure) usually present
- Class V—Membranous glomerulonephritis present in about 15% of patients; morphologically similar to idiopathic membranous glomerulonephritis; immune complexes are subepithelial; nephrotic syndrome usually present

— *Henoch-Schönlein purpura*

- Multisystem disease involving skin, kidneys, gastrointestinal tract, joints
- Most common in children 3 to 8 years, but occurs in adults

Etiology and pathogenesis

- ⅓ atopic
- Onset often follows upper respiratory tract infection
- Morphologically similar to IgA nephropathy

Morphology

- Renal histology

  - Variable and nonspecific
  - Mesangial proliferation of varying degrees, sometimes crescents

- Renal immunofluorescence similar to IgA nephropathy

  - Mesangial IgA
  - Sometimes IgG, C3

- Small vessel necrotizing vasculitis with IgA deposition in skin, gastrointestinal tract (rare in kidney)

Clinical course

- Renal

  - Variable, usually good prognosis in children
  - Recurrent hematuria
  - Proteinuria, sometimes nephrotic syndrome
  - Renal failure in patients with crescents

- Purpuric skin lesions
- Abnormal pain, vomiting, intestinal bleeding

— *Bacterial endocarditis*

- Pathogenesis

    - Immune complexes, including bacterial antigens

- Morphology

    - Focal necrotizing, diffuse glomerulonephritis, crescents

— *Goodpasture's syndrome*

- Acute nephritis (usually RPGN) and pulmonary hemorrhage
- Pathogenesis

    - Antibodies to Goodpasture's antigen (non-collagenous portion of $\alpha 3$ chain of type IV collagen) present in basement membranes of glomeruli and pulmonary alveoli

- Morphology

    - Glomerular crescents consisting of proliferated parietal epithelium, mononuclear cells infiltrating Bowman's space, fibrin
    - Immunofluorescence—IgG in linear pattern on glomerular and pulmonary alveolar basement membranes

- Laboratory and clinical features

    - Antibodies detected in serum
    - Dramatic improvement after plasma exchange
    - Some patients develop chronic renal failure
    - Other causes of pulmonary hemorrhage and RPGN—Wegener's granulomatosis, systemic vasculitides

— *Alport's syndrome*

- Etiology

    - Inherited
    - Most common is X-linked caused by mutation in gene $\alpha 5$ chain of collagen type IV

- Clinical features

    - GN, deafness, lens dislocation, cataracts, corneal dystrophy

● **Chronic glomerulonephritis**

- End stage of several types of glomerular diseases

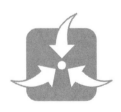

— *Etiology*

- 20% have no antecedent glomerular disease
- Likelihood of progression to chronic glomerulonephritis

    - Rapidly progressive GN—90%
    - Focal glomerulosclerosis—50% to 80%
    - Membranoproliferative GN—50%
    - Membranous nephropathy—40%
    - IgA nephropathy—30% to 50%
    - Poststreptococcal GN—1% to 2%

— *Morphology*

Gross

- Kidneys symmetrically shrunken, diffusely granular

Histology

- Most glomeruli totally hyalinized
- Evidence of antecedent disease—may or may not be present
- Vascular changes of hypertension
- Tubular atrophy
- Interstitial fibrosis and lymphocytes
- Dialysis-related changes

    - Arterial intimal smooth muscle proliferation
    - Tubular and interstitial deposition of calcium oxalate
    - Increased numbers of renal neoplasms

Extrarenal manifestations of uremia and hypertension

- Uremic pericarditis
- Diffuse alveolar damage (uremic pneumonitis)
- Secondary hyperparathryroidism and renal osteodystrophy
- Left ventricular hypertrophy

Clinical features

- Chronic renal failure
- Hypertension
- Dialysis associated

■ **Tubulointerstitial Diseases**

● Acute tubular necrosis (ATN)

— *Etiology*

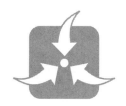

- Ischemic ATN

    - Shock following trauma/burns, transfusion, crush injury, reactions, sepsis
    - Cardiogenic shock
    - Hemorrhage

- Nephrotoxic ATN

    - Drugs (gentamycin, cephalosporins, contrast medium, cyclosporin)
    - Mercury, arsenic, lead
    - Ethylene glycol, methyl alcohol

— *Pathogenesis*

- Tubular injury causes arteriolar constriction (possible mediated by angiotensin)
- Tubular obstruction by casts
- Back leak of tubular fluids
- Changes in glomerular filtration

— *Morphology*

- Ischemic ATN

- Patchy necrosis in straight segments of proximal tubules, ascending limbs of Henle's loops
- Nephrotoxic ATN
  - Extensive necrosis, mostly in proximal tubules
- Features common to both
  - Casts in distal tubules and collecting system
  - Recovery phase shows flat tubular epithelium, mitoses (indicating regeneration)

— *Clinical features*
- Initiating phase related to cause
- Maintenance phase—oliguria, renal failure, and hyperkalemia
- Recovery—polyuria, hypokalemia, vulnerability to infection
- Prognosis related to cause and type
  - Poor for patients with shock
  - Good for patients with nephrotoxicity

● **Urinary tract infection (UTI) and pyelonephritis**
- UTI—involves kidney (pyelonephritis) or urinary bladder (cystitis)

— *Etiology and pathogenesis*
- Risk factors for UTI
  - Female (shorter urethra, effects of hormones on bladder mucosa)
  - Catheterization
  - Diabetes mellitus
  - Immunosuppression
  - Pregnancy
  - Obstruction (prostatic enlargement, neoplasms, congenital anomalies, stones)
- Pyelonephritis usually caused by ascending infection
  - Usually caused by *Escherichia coli, Proteus* and *Enterobacter* organisms
  - Vesicoureteral reflux is major contributor; usually caused by congenital incompetence of vesicoureteral valve

- Blood-borne infections (often from endocarditis) account for minority cases

— *Morphology*
Acute pyelonephritis
- Early, patchy interstitial acute inflammation
Subsequent involvement of tubules (Fig. 22.5)
  - Tubular epithelial necrosis
  - Neutrophils within tubules
- Abscesses
- Papillary necrosis

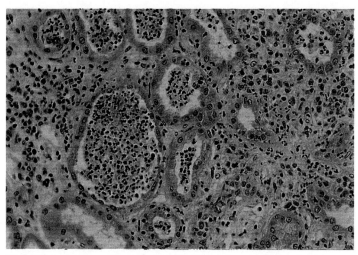

Fig. 22.5 Acute pyelonephritis. Neutrophils are present within tubules and intersititum. (*Damjanov I, Linder J:* Anderson's pathology, *ed 10, vol 2, St Louis, 1996, Mosby.*)

- Especially in patients with diabetes mellitus or obstruction
- Necrosis of distal tips of some or all papillae in one or both kidneys
- Inflammation restricted to junction between necrotic and nonnecrotic tissue

- Perinephric abscesses

  - Extension of inflammation through the renal capsule

- Pyelonephrosis

  - Exudate unable to drain because of obstruction
  - Fills pelvis and calyces

Chronic pyelonephritis

GROSS

- Corticomedullary scars overlie blunt, dilated deformed calcyes

HISTOLOGY

- Dilated tubules filled with eosinophilic material (thyroidization)
- Interstitial fibrosis and chronic inflammation
- Obliterative endarteritis of arcuate and interlobular arteries in scarred areas
- Hyaline arteriolosclerosis, if hypertension develops
- Glomeruli

  - Often normal
  - Sometimes changes caused by ischemia (fibrosis)
  - Uncommonly, focal segmental sclerosis

XANTHOGRANULOMATOUS PYELONEPHRITIS (RARE VARIANT)

- Large yellow-orange masses in pelvis composed of acute and chronic inflammation with many foamy macrophages

- Often caused by *Proteus* organisms
— *Clinical features*
    - Asymptomatic bacturia
    - Dysuria, increased frequency
    - Flank pain and fever in pyelonephritis
    - Recurrent infections and chronic pyelonphritis with obstruction
    - Reflux nephropathy
        - Begins in childhood
        - Infection superimposed on congenital reflux
    - Chronic pyelonephritis—can cause chronic renal failure
        - Accounts for 10% to 12% of all cases

- **Acute interstitial nephritis**
    - Etiology—many types of drugs
        - Methcillin, ampicillin
        - Thiazides
        - Nonsteroidal antiinflammatory agents
        - Cimetidine
    - Morphology (Fig. 22.6)
        - Edema
        - Patchy tubular necrosis
        - Interstitial infiltration with neutrophils, eosinophils, lymphocytes, plasma cells, macrophages, and sometimes granuloma
    - Clinical features
        - Begins 2 to 40 days after exposure to drug
        - Skin rash, fever, eosinophilia, sterile pyuria, hematuria, albuminuria, azotemia
        - Usually recovery after withdrawl of drug

- **Analgesic abuse**
    - Etiology
        - Consumption of phenacetin containing analgesic mixtures
    - Morphology
        - Papillary necrosis and chronic tubulointerstitial inflammation
    - Clinical features
        - Polyuria, headache, anemia, gastrointestinal symptoms, pyruia, UTI, hypertension
        - Drug withdrawal can stabilize renal function
        - Can develop chronic renal failure
        - Increased risk of transitional cell carcinoma of pelvis

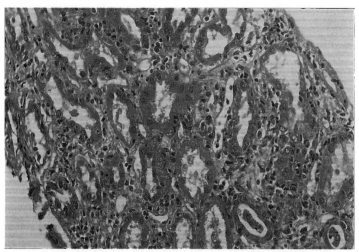

Fig. 22.6 Acute interstitial nephritis. Interstitial edema, mononuclear inflammmatory cells within interstitium and tubules, and focal necrosis of tubular epithelial cells are present. (*Damjanov I, Linder J:* Anderson's pathology, *ed 10, vol 2, St Louis, 1996, Mosby.*)

● Miscellaneous tubulointerstitial disorders

— *Urate nephropathy*

- Gout—chronic renal failure
- Chemotherapy for leukemia, lymphoma—acute renal failure

— *Hypercalcemia*

- Deposition in kidney (nephrocalcinosis) or stones (nephrolithiasis)
- Can cause renal failure

— *Multiple myeloma*

- Pathogenesis

- Light chains (toxic to tubular epthelium) combine with Tamm-Horsfall protein forming obstructive casts

- Dehydration, infection, hypercalcemia, nephrotoxic drugs can precipitate acute renal failure
- 50% develop acute or chronic renal failure

■ **Diseases of Blood Vessels**

● Benign nephrosclerosis

- Renal abnormalities in persons with benign hypertension
- Morphology

- Small kidneys with finely granular surface
- Hyaline arteriolosclerosis (hyaline thickening of arterioles)
- Fibroelastic hyperplasia of muscular arteries
- Diffuse atrophy of nephrons

- Clinical features

- Mild proteinuria not uncommon

- About 5% develop chronic renal failure, usually after developing malignant hypertension

- ● **Malignant nephrosclerosis**
  - Kidney disease associated with accelerated (malignant) hypertension
  - Epidemiology
    - Usually superimposed on preexisting benign hypertension
    - Occurs in 1% to 5% of hypertensives
    - Black males at greatest risk
  - Pathogenesis
    - Elevated renin, angiotensin, aldosterone

  - Morphology
    - Necrotizing arteriolitis (fibrinoid necrosis of arterioles)
    - Hyperplastic arteriolitis ("onion-skinning")
    - Necrotizing glomerulitis
    - ± Thrombotic microangiopathy

  - Clinical features
    - Diastolic blood pressure >130 mm Hg
    - Proteinuria, hematuria, encephalopathy, papilledema, cardiovascular abnormalities, renal failure
    - 50% 5-year survival

- ● **Renal artery stenosis**
  - Accounts for 2% to 5% of hypertension
  - Etiology and pathogenesis

    - 70% caused by atheroma at origin of renal artery
    - 30% caused by fibromuscular dysplasia
    - Pathogenesis of hypertension—renin secretion by involved kidney
  - Clinical course
    - Hypertension curable if affected kidney removed before arteriolosclerosis develops in opposite kidney

- ● **Microangiopathies**
  - Postulated pathogenic mechanisms
    - Intravscular coagulation
    - Endothelial damage
  - Common morphologic features
    - Thrombosis in interlobular arteries, afferent arterioles, glomeruli
    - Necrosis of vascular walls
  - Common clinical features
    - Microangiopathic hemolytic anemia
    - Thrombocytopenia
    - Renal failure

- Childhood hemolytic uremic syndrome

    - 75% infected with verotoxin producing *Escherichia coli*
    - Acute renal failure after prodomal flulike illness

- Adult hemolytic uremic syndrome

    - Associated with infections (*Shigella* organisms, typhoid fever, *E. coli* septicemia, viruses)
    - Pregnancy or postpartum
    - Secondary to renal vascular diseases (SLE, scleroderma, malignant hypertension) or drugs (cyclosporin, mitomycin)
    - Hereditary

- Thrombotic thrombocytopenic purpura

    - Central nervous system (CNS) manifestations prominent, renal failure in only 50%

■ **Urinary Tract Obstruction**
- **Causes**
    - Congential anomalies
    - Stones
    - Prostatic hyperplasia
    - Neoplasms
    - Inflammation and fibrosis
    - Pregnancy
    - Neurogenic bladder

- **Morphology—hydronephrosis**
    - Gross

        - Dilation of pelvis and calyces

    - Histology

        - Tubular atrophy and interstitial fibrosis

- **Clinical features**
    - Unilateral obstruction—can be clinically silent
    - Bilateral parietal obstruction decreased concentrating ability, stones, hypertension

■ **Stones (Nephrolithiasis)**
- **Etiology**
    - 75%—calcium oxalate (± calcium phosphate)

        - 60%—associated with hypercalcemia and hypercalciuria
        - 25%—no known association
        - Others—hyperoxaluria or hyperuricosuria

    - 15%—magnesium ammonium phosphate (struvite or "triple" stones)

        - Associated with *Proteus* organism infection

    - 6%—uric acid
    - 1% to 2%—cystine

- **Pathogenesis**
  - Increased concentrations of stone constituents
  - Changes in urine pH
  - Low urine volume
  - Bacteria

■ Renal Neoplasms

- **Benign neoplasms**
  - Cortical adenoma
    - Found in 7% to 20% of autopsies
    - Composed of epithelial cells often forming tubules
    - Histologically identical to renal cell carcinoma
    - Smaller than 3 cm
  - Oncocytoma
    - Neoplasm composed of eosinophilic epithelial cells (with many mitochondria)

- **Renal cell carcinoma (RCC)**
  - — *Epidemiologic aspects*
    - 3% adult cancers
    - 90% renal malignancies
  - — *Risk factors*
    - Male sex (3:1)
    - Middle age (sixth to seventh decades)
    - Cigarette smoking
    - Von Hippel-Lindau (VHL) disease
      - $\frac{2}{3}$ deveolp RCC, sometime bilateral
      - VHL gene—a tumor suppressor on 3p

  - — *Morphology*
    - Gross
      - >3 cm
      - Grey to yellow with focal hemorrhage, necrosis, cysts
      - Often invade renal vein to inferior vena cava (Fig. 22.7)
    - Histology
      - Clear (glycogen or lipid) or granular (mitochondria-rich) cells
      - Mild to moderate cytologic variation
      - Anaplastic sarcomatoid pattern
      - Sometimes more than one pattern in same type (Fig. 22.8)

  - — *Clinical features*
    - Hematuria (90%), flank pain and mass, fever, amyloidosis, paraneoplastic syndromes (Cushing's syndrome, polycythemia, hypercalcemia, virilization or feminization)
    - Prognosis based on tumor size and extent of spread

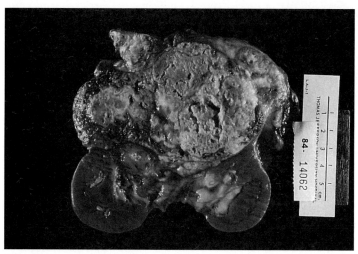

Fig. 22.7 Renal cell carcinoma. Note the round mass with hemorrhagic and necrotic surface. (*Damjanov I, Linder J:* Anderson's pathology, *ed 10, vol 2, St Louis, 1996, Mosby.*)

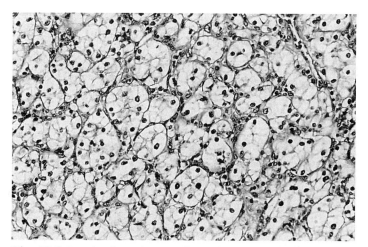

Fig. 22.8 Renal cell carcinoma. The malignant cells with small round nuclei and clear cytoplasm are arranged in tubule-like structures set off by a delicate vascularized stroma. (*Damjanov I, Linder J:* Anderson's pathology, *ed 10, vol 2, St Louis, 1996, Mosby.*)

- 25% have metatstasis at time of diagnosis
- 5-year survival, 45%; 70% if no metastasis

● **Transitional cell carcinoma (TCC) of the renal pelvis**

- About 10% renal malignancies in adults
- Morphology

  - Varies from well-differentiated papillary TCC to anaplastic, invasive
  - 50% multiple, sometimes with bladder tumors

- Clinical features

  - Obstruction (often early)
  - 70% 5-year survival with superficial lesions to 10% with deeply invasive ones

- **Wilms' tumor (nephroblastoma)**
  - Childhood malignancy derived from nephrogenic remants
  - 85% of pediatric renal neoplasms
  - — *Pathogenesis*
    Precursor lesion—nephroblastosis
    WAGR (Wilms' tumor, aniridia, genitourinary abnormalities or gonadoblastoma, and mental retardation) syndrome
    - Wilms' tumor (⅓), aniridia, genital abnormalities, mental retardation
      - Deletion of tumor suppressor gene WT-1 (11p13)
      - DNA-binding protein necessary for normal renal development
    Denys-Drash syndrome
    - Gonadal dysgenesis, renal failure, majority develop Wilms' tumor
    - Mutations in WT-1 affecting DNA binding
    Beckwith-Wiedemann syndrome
    - Enlarged viscera, hemihypertrophy, renal medullary cysts, enlarged adrenocortical cells
    - Loss of maternal allele in WT-2 (11p15.5)

  - — *Morphology*
    Gross
    - Large, soft, grey (brainlike) renal mass
    Histology
    - Triphasic
      - Blastema—small, round blue cells
      - Stroma—loose fibroblastic or myxoid
      - Epithelium—usually forms tubule-like structures
    - Anaplasia in about 5%
      - Large hyperchromatic nuclei
      - Multipolar mitoses

  - — *Clinical features*
    - Usually present with abdominal mass
    - Typical age 2 to 5 years
    - Without treatment, 5-year survival 10% to 40%
    - Presently, with chemotherapy and radiation >90% long-term survival
    - Anaplasia—predicts poor response to therapy
- **Lower Urinary Tract (Ureters, Urinary Bladder, and Urethra)**
  - **Ureters**
    - — *Causes of obstruction of ureters*
      Intrinsic
      - Strictures
        - Congenital
        - Acquired

- Stones
- Neoplasms
- Blood clots
- Neurogenic

Extrinsic

- Pregnancy
- Inflammation
- Endometriosis
- Neoplasms

● **Urinary Bladder**

— *Diverticulum*

- Outpouching of bladder wall
- Can also be acquired or congenital
- Predispose to urine stasis, infection, stones

— *Exstrophy*

- Congenital defect in anterior abdomen—allows bladder to communicate with body surface
- Predisposes to chronic infection, adenocarcinoma (rare)

— *Cystitis*

Etiology

- Most caused by gram-negative bacteria—*E. coli, Proteus, Klebsiella,* and *Enterobacter* organisms
- Others infectious—*Mycobacteria, Candida,* and *Cryptococcus* organisms in immunosuppressed, schistosomiasis (Egypt), adenovirus, chlamydia, mycoplasma
- Others— radiation, busulfan, cyclophosphamide

Clinical features

- Frequency, pain and/or on urination, abdominal pain

Ulcerative interstitial cystitis (Hunner's ulcer)

- Localized ulceration and fibrosis of all layers

Malakoplakia

- Morphology

  - Soft, yellow, raised mucosal plaques up to 4 cm
  - Foamy macrophages with periodic acid Schiff (PAS)-positive granules and Michaelis-Gutmann bodies (targetoid intracellular structures derived from partly digested bacteria) and lymphocytes
  - Similar sturctures in other organs (colon, lungs, bones, kidneys)

— *Bladder Carcinoma*

- 90% transitional cell (TCC), 5% squamous cell, 5% mixed

Epidemiology and etiology

- 3:1 male predominance
- Most cases occur in persons 50 to 80 years old

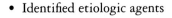

- Identified etiologic agents
  - Industrial exposure to arylamines
  - Cigarette smoking
  - Analgesic abuse
  - Cyclophosphamide
  - *Schistosoma haematobium* (squamous cell carcinoma)

Pathogenesis of TCC

- Low-grade lesions, 9q deletions
- Invasive lesions, 17p deletions (involving p53)
- Multiple and recurrent lesions are clonal
  - Neoplastic cells "seed" urothelium

Morphology of TCC

- Many lesions are multicentric

PATTERNS

- Papillary or flat
  - Papillary—polypoid lesions attached to stalk
  - Flat—plaquelike thickening of wall
- Noninvasive or invasive
  - Noninvasive—increased thickness of wall, does not breach basement membrane

HISTOLOGIC GRADES

- Grade I
  - Closely resembles normal urothelium
  - Greater than 7 cells thick
- Grade II
  - Recognizable as urothelial
  - Loss of polarity
  - More variation in cell size, shape, degree of chromasia than in grade I
- Grade III
  - Difficult to recognize as being urothelial
  - Changes of grade II even more marked in grade III

— *Clinical features and course*
  - Present with painless hematuria, frequency, urgency, dysuria
  - Recurrence rate high
    - About 60% of grade I lesions
    - About 90% grade II or III
  - Prognosis—varies with grade and invasiveness
    - >90% 10-year survival for noninvasive grade I
    - 30% 10-year survival for grade III

- Urethra
  - Urethritis
    - Causes—*Neisseria gonorrhoeae, E. coli,* and other gram-negative enterics, mycoplasma, chlamydia

MULTIPLE CHOICE REVIEW QUESTIONS

1. A previously healthy 25-year-old suffered extensive crush injury and burns in an industrial accident. The hospital course was marked by hypotension, oliguria, and elevation of blood urea nitrogen and creatinine. Death occurred on the third hospitalization day. At autopsy the kidney would most likely show which of the following?

    a. Crescents in most glomeruli
    b. Pus within tubules and abscesses in the interstitium
    c. Multiple infarctions
    d. Multiple foci of tubular necrosis and casts in tubules
    e. Fibrinoid necrosis of the arterioles and hyperplastic arterolosclerosis

2. A four-year-old develops nephrotic syndrome. The most probable outcome is which of the following?

    a. Therapy with the appropriate antibiotic will cure the disease.
    b. Therapy with synthetic glucocorticoids will control the disease.
    c. The patient will require life-long immune suppression.
    d. Despite therapy, the patient will develop chronic glomerulonephritis within five years.
    e. Despite therapy, the patient will develop systemic lupus erythematosus (SLE) within five years.

3. Antiglomerular basement membrane antibodies are most likely to play a role in the development of which of the following?

    a. Membranous nephropathy
    b. Goodpasture's syndrome
    c. Minimal change disease (lipoid neophrosis)
    d. Nodular glomerulosclerosis
    e. Post-streptococcal glomerulonephritis

4. Which of the following is most likely to cause acute pyelonephritis?

    a. *Escherichia coli*
    b. Group A beta hemolytic *Streptococcus*
    c. *Mycobacterium tuberculosis*
    d. *Schistosomiasis hematobium*
    e. *Neisseria gonorrhoeae*

5. Most renal stones are composed of which of the following?

    a. Calcium oxalate/calcium phosphate
    b. Magnesium ammonium phosphate
    c. Uric acid
    d. Cystine
    e. Unknown

Chapter 23

Bone, Joint, and Soft Tissue Disorders

■ **Developmental and Genetic Disorders of Bone**

● Achondroplasia

- Most common cause of disproportionate short stature
- Autosomal dominant (AD), but 80% are the result of new mutations to the fibroblast growth factor 3 receptor
- Enchondral bone-forming growth plates defective, but morphologic abnormalities are poorly characterized
- Appositional growth and intramembranous bone formation—occurs normally
- Produces proportionally short but thickened long bones with a normal calvarium and other membranous bones

● Osteogenesis imperfecta

- Mutations in the collagen type 1 genes that account for 90% of the osteoid matrix
- Varying phenotypes, with most severe defects showing AD inheritance and less severe AD or autosomal recessive (AR) patterns; double heterozygotes for different defects can occur
- Pathology—net result is osteopenia or too little bone, with thin cortices and trabeculae, resulting in fragile, easily broken bones
- Other tissues rich in type 1 collagen, including joints, ears, skin, eyes, (often translucent blue sclera) and teeth—also affected

● Osteopetrosis (marble bone's disease)

- Inherited osteoclast defect (AR and AD), giving rise to osteosclerosis or thickened but brittle bones
- Pathology—thickening of cortex and filling in of medullary cavity by disorganized overgrowth of bone lacking the ability to remodel
- Bone marrow transplantation—can cure, as osteoclast is derived from the hematopoietic stem cell

■ **Metabolic Bone Disease**

● Osteoporosis

- Reduction in bone mass or osteopenia, resulting in weakened bones predisposed to fracture
- Caused by an imbalance between the physiologic continuous remodeling activities of bone formation and bone resorption
- Diffuse or localized (i.e., immobilization of limb) forms

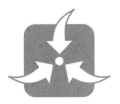

- Diffuse may be

  - Primary—has well-known risk factors, but no specific etiologies are known
  - Secondary—has specific causes and mechanisms

- Primary risk factors—genetic factors (mostly genetic variation in vitamin D receptors), sex, race, body weight, low calcium intake, sedentary lifestyle, smoking, excessive alcohol consumption, sex steroid deficiency

- Secondary causes—endocrine (diabetes mellitus, hyperparathyroidism, hyperthyroidism, Cushing's syndrome, acromegaly), drugs (anticonvulsants, glucocorticoids), immobilization, hepatic disease, mastocytosis, gastrointestinal disease, malignant tumors, starvation, hemochromatosis

- Primary osteoporosis—most important because it is common and the fractures result in costly medical care

- Factors favoring bone deposition and maintenance—young age, physical activity, diet, hormonal state (presence of estrogens and androgens)

- Factors favoring bone loss—age over third decade (time of peak skeletal mass), Caucasian, immobilization, postmenopausal state

- Pathology—trabeculae become thinned, lose interconnections, suffer microfractures, then generalized collapse; the cortex thins from endosteal and periosteal resorption, and the haversian channels widen

● **Rickets and osteomalacia**

- Characterized by defective mineralization of osteoid matrix
- In children—this primarily affects the epiphyseal growth plate, causing rickets
- In adults—because the growth plates are closed, sites of osteoid from bone remodeling are affected, causing osteomalacia (soft bones)
- In children lack of vitamin D—the etiology of classic rickets
- Abnormal vitamin D metabolism or renal phosphate loss—common causes osteomalacia in adults

— *Pathology*

  - Rickets

    - Bony deformities—largely from bending and bowing of the soft, thickened, poorly mineralized, epiphyseal plates
    - Produces short stature, soft skull (craniotabes or deformable skull bones), frontal bone bossing, flaring of ribs, nodular swelling of the costochondral junction (rachitic rosary) in ribs, kyphosis, swelling of wrists, elbows, and knees with genu varum

  - Osteomalacia

    - Produces delayed mineralization, visible as thickened osteoid seams, bone pain, muscle weakness, and fatigue

● **Hyperparathyroidism**

- Excess parathyroid hormone (PTH) mobilizes calcium from the skeleton

- Parathyroid adenoma (90%), hyperplasia of all four glands (10%), or rarely parathyroid carcinoma

- Resulting bone disease called *osteitis fibrosa cystic*
- Pathology

    - Microscopically—prominent, deep Howship's lacuna (sites of resorption), increased vascularity and fibrosis of marrow space and cystic degeneration (osteitis fibrosa cystica)
    - Brown tumors of bone—masses of hemosiderin-laden macrophages (brown colored), multinucleate giant cells and granulation tissue form in response to secondary hemorrhage and microfractures in areas weakened by resorption

    - Radiology—mottled bone cortex, loss of lamina dura of teeth and lytic areas from brown tumors
    - Clinically—"stones (renal Ca stones), bones (aches and pains of microfractures), moans (hypercalcemic psychosis), and groans (gastrointestinal effects of hypercalcemia)"

- **Renal osteodystrophy**

    - Occurs in patients with chronic renal failure and dialysis
    - Renal failure—causes hyperphosphatemia (from decreased excretion) and hypocalcemia (failure of renal hydroxylation of vitamin D) resulting in secondary hyperparathyroidism
    - Pathology—changes are a mix of osteomalacia and osteitis fibrosa cystica, with unexplained osteosclerosis in some patients
    - Chronic acidosis and aluminum deposition may contribute to changes

Fractures

- Most common bone lesion
- Classifications—complete vs. incomplete (greenstick or partial break), simple (closed) vs. compound (open, through skin), comminuted (bone fragments) vs. noncomminuted, displaced (ends out of alignment) vs. undisplaced, pathologic (at the site of a disease process, such as metastatic tumor), stress (caused by a period of sudden increased activity causing repetitive localized stress [i.e., marching stress fractures of the metatarsals])

- **Stages of fracture healing**

    - Inflammatory phase (week 1)

        - *Hematoma*—from torn vessels, fills gap between break and surrounds injured tissue, *inflammatory-coagulation repair response* occurs on the fibrin scaffold
        - *Organization*—invading fibroblasts and vessels produce collagen replacing the fibrin clot, known as a soft callus or precallus

    - Reparative phase (2 to 3 weeks)

        - Starting from the outside edges—osteoblasts begin to deposit matrix and early mineralization forms woven bone
        - Cartilage formation also occurs in organizing tissue
        - Repair tissue (soft callus)—maximal in simple fractures, and the site is stabilized but not strong enough for any stress

    - Bony callus formation (4 weeks)

        - Progressive mineralization from subperiostium and intramedullary area and endochondral mineralization of the cartilage

- Fracture site—bridged by mineralized tissue becoming more stable and able to accept limited stress

- Remodeling stage (4 weeks onward)

    - In response to gradually increased load bearing the woven bone remodels, callus shrinks in unstressed areas, medullary cavity reforms, and fracture site may eventually be undetectable

- Inadequate immobilization, infection, nutritional or systemic diseases—may alter the repair sequence, producing delayed union, non-union, or pseudoarthrosis

■ Inflammatory Disorders

● Osteomyelitis

— *Pyogenic osteomyelitis*

- Bacterial infections commonly via occult bacteremia
- Sites of involvement—reflect local increased vascularity

    - Neonates—epiphysis, metaphysis
    - Children—metaphysis
    - Adults—epiphysis, subchondral

- Organisms—up to 50% culture negative, *Staphylococcus aureus* most frequent in culture positive cases; *Escherichia coli, Pseudomonas* and *Klebsiella* organisms, and other urinary pathogens occur in the setting of antecedent urinary tract infection; *Haemophilus influenzae* and group B streptococci common in neonates and *Salmonella* organisms in patients with sickle cell disease

- Pathology

    - Acute—acute inflammatory reaction and osteonecrosis; in children, process may track to subperiostium and cause sequestrum (nonviable bony pieces caused by vascular insufficiency) or soft tissue abscesses and draining cutaneous sinuses from periosteal rupture; in adults and neonates, joint extension and septic arthritis more common

    - Subacute and chronic—chronic inflammatory cells and fibrosis; involucrum—a sequestrum incorporated in the repair-invoked fibrosis and new bone formation

- Infection—may persist despite surgical drainage or antibiotic therapy

- Complications—secondary amyloidosis, fracture, squamous cell carcinoma of sinus tract, and rarely sarcoma of bone

— *Tuberculous osteomyelitis*

- Spine-favored site (Pott's disease)

■ Paget's Disease of Bone (Osteitis Deformans)

- A chronic idiopathic disorder of one or more bones resulting in pain, deformities, and osteolytic-osteoblastic lesions
- Predominantly Caucasians over 40 years old
- Commonly detected by alkaline phosphatase measurement or x-ray films, but most cases are asymptomatic

- Possibly the result of a slow virus infection of osteoblasts by a paramyxovirus

- Polyostotic (80% of cases) and monostotic forms with axial skeleton and femur most common sites

    - Pathology

        - Cycles of uncoordinated bone resorption (osteoclastic activity), bone deposition (osteoblastic activity), and inactivity results in weakened, thickened, irregularly shaped pieces of lamellar bone with a jigsawlike or mosaic appearance and prominent cement lines

        - Osteoclasts—may achieve giant size with excessive nuclei

    - Bone enlargement—causes deformities (especially cranial enlargement, leonine facies, kyphosis, bowing of long bones) and cranial nerve entrapment; rarely highly vascular bone causes high output cardiac failure

    - Predisposed to fractures and tumors—giant cell tumor and bone sarcomas in the polyostotic form (1%)

■ Osteonecrosis (Avascular Necrosis)

- Bone and bone marrow death, characteristically of the femoral head, in the absence of infection

- Thought caused by *ischemia,* but this is only definite with trauma, infection, vasculitis, sickle cell disease, radiation, thrombotic disorders, nitrogen embolus, and other disorders

- An *idiopathic mechanism*—associated with steroids (immunosuppresants), alcohol abuse, pregnancy, hyperlipidemia, and hyperuricemia

- Increase in medullary pressure also postulated as a mechanism

- Pathology (Fig. 23.1)

    - Infarction evokes an inflammatory response that rims the area consisting of a fibrotic inner zone and an hyperemic outer zone.

    - A granulation tissue repair response extends into the infarction, gradually replacing the dead bone along the scaffold of the old bone (creeping substitution).

    - Small infarcts may repair completely.

    - For larger infarcts, stress produces fracture, impaction, and collapse of the underlying femoral head bone and separation from the overlying subchondral plate.

    - Instability and deformity of the joint surface results in degenerative joint disease.

■ Bone Tumors (Fig. 23.2)

- Classified by the tissue they resemble or by unique histologic-clinical features when there is no normal tissue counterpart

- Tumors caused by metastatic carcinomas and multiple myeloma—far more frequent than the most common osteogenic tumor, osteogenic sarcoma

- ● Metastasis

    - Adults—carcinoma of lung, breast carcinoma, prostatic carcinoma, renal cell carcinoma, and thyroid carcinoma.

    - Children—neuroblastoma, Wilms' tumor, osteosarcoma, Ewing's sarcoma, and rhabdomyosarcoma

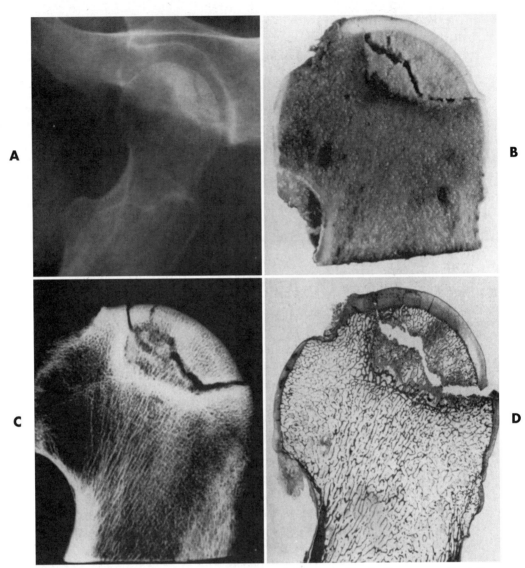

Fig. 23.1 Avascular necrosis of the femoral head. The x-ray film findings are on the left (**A, C**) with the corresponding gross specimen (**B**) and whole mount microscopic findings (**D**). Note the fracture and bone necrosis and repair reaction. (*Rosai J:* Ackerman's surgical pathology, *St Louis, 1989, Mosby.*)

- Vertebrae—most common site, followed by other areas of active bone marrow hematopoiesis

● Osteoma

- Benign hamartoma of slow-growing woven and lamellar bone (resembling reactive bone), forming an irregular, rounded mass on the cortical surface
  - Solitary or with Gardner's syndrome (multiple intestinal polyposis)
  - Often craniofacial and of cosmetic or local significance only

● Osteoid osteoma, osteoblastoma

- Common, benign, 1 to 2 cm-sized, tumors in the cortex of femur or tibia

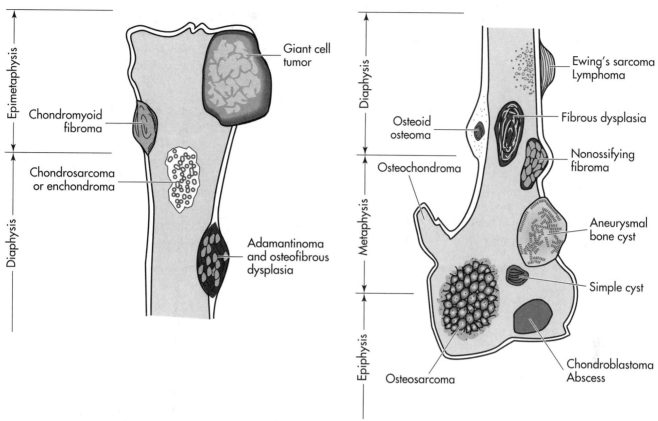

Fig. 23.2 Sites of common bone tumors. *Left,* proximal tibia; *right,* distal femur. (*Modified from Madewell JE, Ragsdale ED, Sweet DE: Radiol Clin North Am 19:715, 1981.*)

- 5-to 25-year-old males with severe *nocturnal pain,* relieved by aspirin (high prostaglandin production)
- Pathology

  - Reddish to pink center (nidus), surrounded by reactive sclerotic bone

  - Center composed of irregular osteoid trabeculae, with osteoblasts and osteoclasts and woven bone trabeculae

- Radiology—nidus appears variably lytic sometimes with a calcified center giving a targetlike appearance
- Treatment—complete surgical removal
- *Osteoblastoma*—similar histologically to osteoid osteoma, but most frequently involves the spine, is larger, and not as painful

● **Osteosarcoma**

  - Highly malignant, mesenchymal tumor-producing osteoid and neoplastic bone

  - Most common primary malignant tumor of bone origin, 20% of bone tumors

  - Occurs in adolescent males at metaphyseal sites around knee and in patients over 40 years with Paget's disease or previous local irradiation

- Rb gene mutations—found in familial cases, and p53 mutations in both Li-Fraumeni syndrome and some sporadic osteosarcoma

- Radiology—evidence of bone destruction and neoplastic bone formation (sunburst pattern); elevation of periosteum with new bone formation forms a triangle (Codman's triangle) between cortex and periosteal bone

  - Pathology (Fig. 23.3)

    - Highly variable gross and microscopic appearance caused by varying amount of bone, stroma, cartilage, and vessels, giving rise to many histologic subtypes

    - Always has malignant osteoblasts forming osteoid and neoplastic woven bone

    - Neoplastic chondrocytes, cartilage, and tumor giant cells frequent

    - Commonly spreads to lung via blood stream

  - Surgical resection of primary and chemotherapy treatment—has improved survival in the range of 65% to 75% for conventional osteosarcoma

● **Osteochondroma (exostosis)**

- Cartilage-capped bony process derived from lateral outgrowth of the epiphysis

  - Sporadic or autosomal dominant, males, long bones

  - Pathology—mushroomlike stalk of bone capped by hyaline cartilage, resembling a growth plate that undergoes endochondral bone formation

● **Chondroma (enchondroma)**

  - Benign tumors (or hamartomas) of near normal-appearing hyaline cartilage arising from displaced cartilage of the epiphyseal plate

  - All ages at metaphysis of short tubular bones, especially hands and feet

  - Enchondromatosis (Ollier's disease)

    - Multiple, asymmetric, and deforming enchondroma

    - May be more cellular and the chondrocytes atypical vs. solitary chondroma

    - May undergo a change to chondrosarcoma

  - Maffucci's syndrome

    - Enchondromas with soft tissue hemangiomas

    - Higher frequency of chondrosarcoma, ovarian carcinoma, and gliomas of brain

● **Chondroblastoma**

  - Rare, benign tumors most frequent in teenage males at knee epiphyseal sites

  - Pathology—cellular sheets of round cells with distinct cytoplasmic borders and large nuclei, surrounded by an immature variably calcified hyaline matrix; osteoclast giant cells may be present

    - Radiology—a lace or chicken-wire appearance

    - Causes joint pain, and may recur after curettage

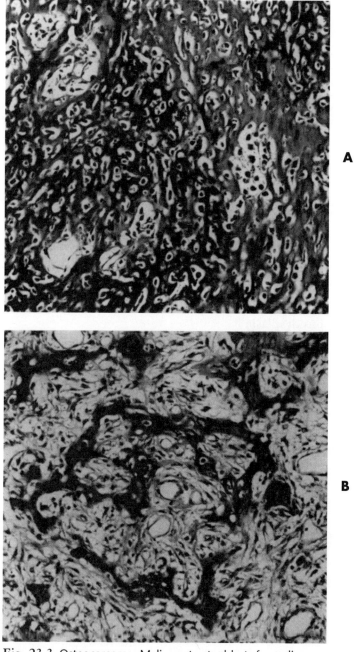

Fig. 23.3 Osteocarcoma. Malignant osteoblasts form disorganized thin **(A)** and thick **(B)** bone trabeculae. (*Rosai J:* Ackerman's surgical pathology, *St Louis, 1989, Mosby.*)

- Chondrosarcoma
  - Malignant cartilaginous tumor
  - Second most common malignant primary bone tumor
  - Arises de novo or in multiple enchondromatosis and osteochondroma

- Males, peak incidence 40 to 60 years old
- Commonly central skeleton
- Radiologically—expansile lytic mass with focal calcification
- Pathology—grossly lobulated and glistening masses

  - Composed of abnormal chondrocytes in hyaline matrix
  - Histologic grading—low grade is common with good survival vs. high grade (cellular, pleomorphic cells with prominent nucleoli and frequent mitosis) with a poor prognosis

● Nonossifying fibroma (fibrous cortical defect)

- Common benign lesion of childhood at the metaphysis of long bones
- 25% to 50% under 10 years old
- Most regress spontaneously with sclerosis
- Large defects—may cause pain or fracture
- Radiology—central lucent zone with sclerotic margins
- Pathology—bland spindle cells in storiform (spokelike or pinwheel) arrangement with giant cells and foamy macrophages

● Fibrous dysplasia

- Developmental disorder
- Monostotic and polyostotic
- Monostotic—common, in any bone, presenting as an incidental finding or with a pathologic fracture between the ages of 10 and 30 years old
- 5% have the McCune-Albright syndrome of polyostotic fibrous dysplasia, skin pigmentation (café-au-lait spots), and endocrine dysfunction (precocious puberty in females)
- Radiology—deformed enlarged bone with ground-glass lucency and sharp margins
- Pathology—loose fibrous tissue with "Chinese letter" woven bone spicules that lack osteoblastic rimming
- Rarely may transform to sarcoma

● Giant cell tumor

- Common benign tumor arising most often in females, 20 to 40 years old at the junction of metaphysis and epiphysis in long bones
- Pathology

  - Circumscribed, soft, red-brown, focally hemorrhagic
  - Composed of an admixture of multinucleated, osteoclast type of giant cells (osteoclastoma) and round mononuclear cells with high nuclear/cytoplasm ratio in a richly vascular stroma

- Can be locally aggressive and frequently recur with curettage (50%)

● Ewing's sarcoma

- One of the pediatric "small blue cell" malignancies (that includes lymphoma, rhabdomyosarcoma, and neuroblastoma)
- Third most common malignant primary tumor of bone
- Cytogenetically (t11;22 translocation involving EWS gene and FLI-1

gene) and phenotypically linked to primitive neuroectodermal tumors (PNET)

- Males, less than 20 years old, long bones
- Radiology—"onion skin" appearance caused by formation of layers of reactive periosteal bone
- Pathology—soft, grey-white, expansile medullary cavity masses composed of small, monomorphous cells with scanty clear (glycogen-rich) cytoplasm; evidence of neural differentiation may be seen in PNET
- Survival—about 60% for localized disease with chemoradiotherapy or chemosurgical treatment

● **Simple bone cyst**

- Common lesion of unknown etiology in children and adolescents
- Usually diagnosed after trauma or pathologic fracture
- Develop at or beneath the epiphyseal growth plate, then enlarges and migrates with diaphyseal growth
- Pathology—a thin, fibrous, connective tissue wall filled with pink fluid that has high levels of prostaglandins
- Most heal following instillation of methylprednisolone

■ Joints

● **Osteoarthritis (OA)**

- Degenerative joint disease
- Noninflammatory progressive degeneration of articular cartilage with new bone formation at the joint surfaces and margins
- Most common cause of arthritis
- May result from an intrinsic abnormality in the cartilage or bone under conditions of normal use or arise in normal cartilage and bone under conditions of abnormal use
- Primary (idiopathic) and secondary types

- Secondary—inherited or acquired disorders that impair the well-being of the joint cartilage, underlying bone, and synovium through direct effects on these tissues or by causing increased wear and tear because of generalized or focal excessive load bearing
- Common joints are distal interphalangeal (DIP) and proximal interphalangeal (PIP) of hands, cervical and lumbar spine, and knee and hip joints
- Pathology (Fig. 23.4)

  - Repetitive damage and repair results in similar degenerative joint changes in both primary and secondary types
  - Early changes—fibrillation (cracks in joint surface cartilage), loss of cartilage matrix with basophilic change, chondrocytes death, and proliferation of remaining chondrocytes to form clusters
  - Intermediate changes—subchondral bone cysts from exposure to synovial fluid pressure, fibrous repair tissue arising from subcartilaginous bone fills cartilage cracks, synovitis caused by fragments of cartilage in the joint space

  - Late changes—loss of articular cartilage and exposure of bone, eburnation (ivory-like thickening and polishing) of bone surface,

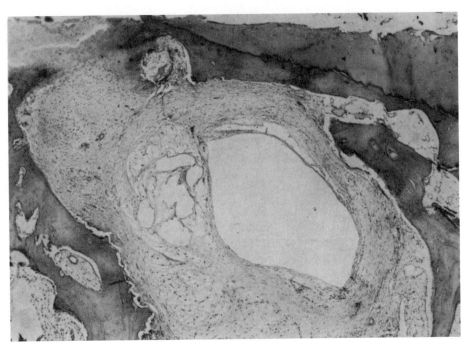

Fig. 23.4 Osteoarthritis. The cartilage is lost, the bone thickened, and there is a cyst present. (*Rosai J:* Ackerman's surgical pathology, *St Louis, 1989, Mosby.*)

underlying bony sclerosis and focal osteonecrosis, osteophyte formation (lateral growths of bone and cartilage)

- Heberden's nodes—osteophytes at the DIP

• Primary OA—occurs in middle to old age, and a generalized form in females is associated with human leukocyte antigen (HLA) B8

• Secondary causes—hemophilic arthropathy, hemochromatosis, Wilson's disease, ochronotic arthropathy, acromegalic, hyperparathyroidism, aseptic necrosis, Legg-Calvé-Perthe's disease, slipped capital, femoral epiphysis, trauma, joint deformity, and laxity

● **Rheumatoid arthritis (RA)**

• An autoimmune idiopathic systemic inflammatory disorder

• The predominant manifestation—chronic, nonsuppurative, destructive synovitis leading to loss of articular cartilage and fusion of the joints

- All ages, peak in 30- to 50-year-old females
- Classically insidious onset of symmetrical arthritis involving the hands in the PIP and metacarpal phalangeal (MCP) joints
- HLA DR4 linked
- Postulated to have an infectious viral trigger that initiates the synovitis; currently Epstein-Barr virus (EBV) suspected

• Rheumatoid factor (RF)—an antiimmunoglobulin antibody (usually IgM) with specificity for the Fc portion of IgG, present in 80% of cases

• RF—does not cause the synovitis, as it is absent in some patients with RA and may be seen in other disorders or healthy individuals

- RF immune complexes do cause the extraarticular manifestations
— *Pathology*
    - All rheumatoid lesions—characterized by lymphoid hyperplasia and fibrinoid vasculitis
    - In the synovium, causes hypertrophic villous synovitis

        - Rheumatoid pannus—the characteristic joint lesion consisting of a dense synovial lymphocytic infiltrate with plasma cells and macrophages in a hypervascular edematous stroma (Fig. 23.5)
        - Pannus—envelopes the cartilage surface, destroying it, and erodes into the juxtaarticular bone
        - Fibrin—covers portions of the synovial membrane, and fibrinoid necrosis of the synovium may organize and fragment into small "rice" bodies floating in the joint space
        - Neutrophils—prominent on the synovial surface and in the joint fluid
        - Loss of bone from the lateral joint surfaces—leads to instability of the joint and deformities, including the classic ulnar deviation of the MCP joints and the swan-neck deformity of the PIP joints of the hands as the result of their fixed subluxation
        - With joint destruction, fibrous fusion occurs (ankylosis)

    - Rheumatoid nodules—occur anywhere, but are common in subcutaneous tissue of forearm, elbows, and other pressure sites

        - Nodules consist of central fibrinoid necrosis surrounded by epithelioid histiocytes, lymphocytes, and plasma cells in a granuloma-like arrangement

    - Other affected tissues—tendon sheaths, bursae, blood vessels, pericardium, pleura, lungs, lymphoid tissue, and heart that may exhibit rheumatoid nodules, fibrinoid vasculitis, pulmonary fibrosis, chronic pericarditis, reactive follicular lymphoid hyperplasia, and hypersplenism
    - Diagnosis of rheumatoid arthritis—based on the presence of a number of clinical, pathologic, laboratory, and radiologic features (standardized as criteria)
        - Diagnosis—imprecise, and there is no specific test

- Spondyloarthropathies
    - A group of related arthropathies characterized by the absence of rheumatoid factor, a high prevalence of HLA B27 and sacroiliitis
    - Bacterial infections of the gastrointestinal and genitourinary tract—frequent antecedent events
    - Includes ankylosing spondylosis, Reiter's syndrome, psoriatic arthritis, and enteropathic arthritis
    - Many develop ankylosis of spine
    - Pathology—synovitis of joints without pannus formation and inflammation of ligaments at their insertion to bone
    - **Ankylosing spondylosis**

        - Late adolescents, males

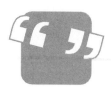

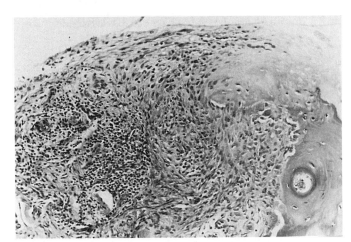

Fig. 23.5 Rheumatoid pannus. Only a small amount of articular cartilage remains amid the granulation tissuelike, destructive pannus. (*Damjanov I, Linder J:* Anderson's pathology, *ed 10, vol 2, St Louis, 1996, Mosby.*)

- Associated with inflammatory intestinal disorders
- Frequent ankylosis of the hip joints, in addition to the spine

- **Reiter's syndrome**

  - Males
  - Originally described after bacillary dysentery
  - Consists of nongonococcal urethritis, conjunctivitis, small joint arthritis, and a skin rash on the palms and soles identical to pustular psoriasis

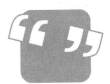

- **Gout**

  - Recurrent acute arthritis caused by formation of monosodium urate crystals in and around joints often accompanied by hyperuricemia.

  - Gout also results in urate nephropathy and crystal deposition at other sites (tophi).

  - Most cases are *primary* with an unknown but presumed defect in urate metabolism in either the purine synthesis or salvage pathway with a few primary cases caused by a known enzyme deficiency (i.e., hypoxanthine-guanine phosphoribosyl transferase).

    - *Secondary* causes include

      - Increased purine synthesis—malignancies with a high cell turnover such as leukemia
      - Increased uric acid production—ethanol, obesity, and diet
      - Decreased urinary excretion—renal disease, thiazide diuretics, or lead poisoning

  - Idiopathic primary gout is seen in males over 30 years with hyperuricemia (5% of adult males have hyperuricemia, but only 2% or 3% of this group develop gout) and a familial predisposition.

    - Deposition of uric acid crystals causes an acute inflammatory reaction.
    - Disease course is of exacerbations and quiescent periods.
    - Pathology (Fig. 23.6)

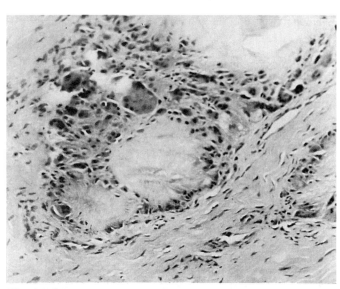

Fig. 23.6 Gout. A tophus consists of giant cells and granulation tissue surrounding a protein matrix that originally held urate crystals. (The crystals dissolve during the preparation of the tissue to make the microscopic slides.) (*Damjanov I, Linder J:* Anderson's pathology, *ed 10, vol 2, St Louis, 1996, Mosby.*)

- Acute arthritis—neutrophilic infiltrates in tissue and joint fluid (joint aspiration for crystal identification diagnostically useful with uric acid crystals appearing slender and needlelike rods exhibiting negative birefringence within neutrophils)
- Chronic (tophaceous) arthritis—widespread joint deposits of urates, hyperplastic synovium with pannus formation and joint destruction similar to rheumatoid arthritis
- Tophi—pathognomonic of gout; consist of urate crystal masses surrounded by chronic inflammation, fibrosis, and foreign body giant cells; common sites are achilles tendon, olecranon, volar forearm, adjacent to joints, and ear helix
- Gouty nephropathy—urate deposition in the renal medullary interstitium and intratubularly, renal stone formation and secondary complications such as pyelonephritis and renal failure

- Good control can be attained with drugs but untreated involves increasingly more sites, causing greater destruction, and renal complications may lead to death.

- **Calcium pyrophosphate deposition disease**
  - Pseudogout or chondrocalcinosis
  - A common crystal arthropathy, analogous to gout except crystals are composed of calcium pyrophosphate
  - Idiopathic—elderly, associated with osteoarthritis
  - Secondary—hemochromatosis, previous joint damage, ochronosis, acromegaly, hyperparathyroidism, Wilson's disease
  - Pathology—white chalky crystal deposition, can resemble tophus

    - Crystals show weak positive birefringence and incite acute synovial inflammation.

- Knee most common joint
- **Ganglion cysts**
  - Common rubbery, mobile, subcutaneous nodules, associated with synovium at joint or tendons
  - Frequent around the wrist
  - Pathology—cysts filled with translucent, gelatinous, myxoid material and surrounded by a fibrous capsule that lacks a cell lining
  - May be caused by myxoid degeneration of the connective tissue, with no direct connection to synovium or possibly synovial herniation
- **Pigmented villonodular synovitis**
  - Benign tumor of synovium
  - Young adults
  - Presents as monarticular arthritis, usually at the knee
  - Exophytic and locally invasive
  - Pathology—composed of bland mononuclear cells, multinucleate giant cells, and hemosiderin-laden macrophages (hence, pigmented)
  - May recur and invade and destroy bone
  - Localized nodular tenosynovitis (giant cell tumor of tendon sheath)—same process at tendon synovial membrane in young to middle-aged women, usually in the hand

Soft Tissue Tumors

- Neoplastic proliferations of all nonskeletal connective tissue except bone marrow, central nervous system (CNS) glial tissue, pleura, peritoneum, and lymphoid tissue
- Classified by their resemblance to a normal mature or embryonic mesenchymal tissue (Table 23.1)
- Benign tumors, notably lipomas, not only the most common soft tissue tumors, but one of the most common tumors
- Sarcoma—malignant soft tissue tumors that may metastasize typically by venous routes to the lung, liver, and bone
- Sarcoma—uncommon (1% of all cancers) and occur at all ages
- Sarcoma—more likely to be deep in soft tissues, large, rapidly growing (infiltrating edges), vascular, and focally necrotic than their benign counterparts
- Histologic grading—prognostically important for some sarcoma

Fibrous Tumors

- **Fibroma**
  - A tumor composed of mature collagen and fibroblasts
  - Location—neck, tendon sheath, and as solitary or localized fibrous tumor of soft tissue
- **Fasciitis**
  - Benign, likely reactive proliferation of fibroblasts
  - Possibly caused by trauma
  - Nodular type—occurs on the forearm, trunk, and back of adults
  - Mimics sarcoma (sometimes called pseudosarcomatous fasciitis) by rapid growth, hypercellularity, high mitotic rate

Table 23.1 *Classification of Soft Tissue Tumors*

Fibrous
Benign
  Fibroma
  Fasciitis
    Nodular
    Proliferative
  Fibromatosis
    Superficial
    Deep
  Other
Malignant
  Fibrosarcoma

Fibrohistiocytic
Benign
  Fibrous histiocytoma (dermatofi-
    broma)
  Xanthoma
Intermediate
  Dermatofibrosarcoma protuberans
Malignant
  Malignant fibrous histiocytoma

Lipomatous
Benign
  Lipoma
Malignant
  Well-differentiated liposarcoma
  Myxoid liposarcoma
  Round cell liposarcoma
  Pleomorphic liposarcoma
  Dedifferentiated

Smooth Muscle
Benign
  Leiomyoma
Malignant
  Leiomyosarcoma

Skeletal Muscle
Malignant
  Rhabdomyosarcoma

Endothelial Tumors
Benign
  Hemangioma
  Pyogenic granuloma
Intermediate
  Hemangioendothelioma
Malignant
  Malignant angiosarcoma
  Kaposi's sarcoma

Perivascular
Benign hemangiopericytoma
Glomus tumor
Malignant hemangiopericytoma

Synovial Tumors
Benign
  Tenosynovial giant cell tumor
Malignant
  Synovial sarcoma

Neural Tumors
Benign
  Neuroma
  Neurofibroma
  Schwannoma (neurilemoma)
  Granular cell tumor
Malignant
  Malignant peripheral nerve sheath
    tumor
  Clear cell sarcoma
  Neuroblastoma

Paraganglionic Tumors
Benign paraganglioma
Malignant paraganglioma

Cartilage and Bone
Benign
  Myositis ossificans
Malignant
  Extraskeletal chondrosarcoma
  Extraskeletal osteosarcoma

Miscellaneous Tumors
Benign
  Tumoral calcinosis
  Myxoma
Malignant
  Epithelioid sarcoma
  Alveolar soft-part sarcoma

- Pathology—composed of polymorphic spindle fibroblastic cells and fresh collagen, resembling exuberant granulation tissue
- Similar lesions arising on muscular fascia and within muscle—called proliferative fasciitis and proliferative myositis

- **Fibromatosis**
  - Superficial—palmar (Dupuytren's contracture), plantar, and penile
    - Pathology—masses of dense collagen and fascicles of fibroblasts causing contracture of the fascia to which they are attached
    - Most often palmar in elderly males; associated with alcoholism, diabetes, epilepsy, and human immunodeficiency virus (HIV)
  - Deep—desmoid tumor
    - Firm, white, poorly demarcated masses, most frequently at rectus abdominis muscular aponeurosis in young females
    - Pathology—mixture of monomorphous bland fibroblasts dispersed in a dense collagen background with infiltrating margins
    - Common local recurrence
    - Occurs as a component of Gardner's syndrome

- **Fibrosarcoma**
  - An uncommon sarcoma arising at any site, but most frequently a mass in the lower extremities
  - Rarely arises in a previously irradiated location or causes hypoglycemia
  - Pathology
    - Low grade—short fascicles of uniform spindle cells having elongated nuclei and scanty cytoplasm (herringbone pattern) may resemble some of the reactive and benign conditions outlined previously
    - High grade—anaplastic pleomorphic hypercellular tumors, diagnosed after special studies exclude other undifferentiated sarcoma

■ Fibrohistiocytic Tumors

- **Benign fibrous histiocytoma (dermatofibroma)**
  - Common dermal tumor of young to middle-aged adults
  - Painless, firm, red-brown, mobile cutaneous nodule
  - Pathology—bland dermal spindle cells in a storiform (pinwheel) pattern

- **Xanthoma**
  - Soft tissue or dermal lesion composed of lipid-laden macrophages and often associated with hyperlipidemia

- **Dermatofibrosarcoma protuberans**
  - A low-grade malignancy of young adults arising as an enlarging cutaneous mass of the chest wall or trunk
  - Pathology—spindle fibroblast cells with a regular storiform pattern that invades the subcutaneous fat
  - High local recurrence rate, but only very rarely metastasizes

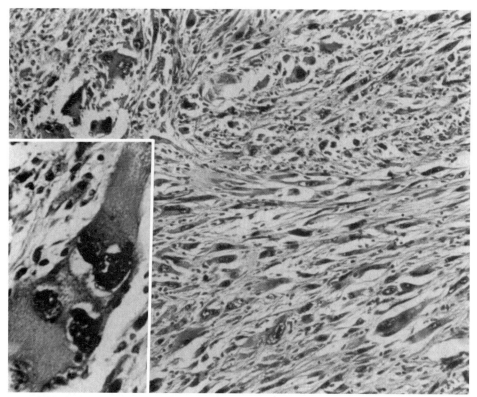

Fig. 23.7 Malignant fibrous histiocytoma. Highly malignant, hyperchromatic cells and pleomorphic giant cells form this undifferentiated sarcoma. (*Rosai J:* Ackerman's surgical pathology, *St Louis, 1989, Mosby.*)

● **Malignant fibrous histiocytoma (MFH)**

- Most common adult sarcoma
- Appear to have primitive fibroblast or mesenchymal cell differentiation (histiocytoma is a misnomer as there are not real histiocytes)
- Large masses at deep muscle or fascia sites
- Pathology (Fig. 23.7)

    - Pleomorphic-storiform—most common pattern, composed of spindle cells in storiform bundles or polygonal cells in sheets with some pleomorphic multinucleate tumor giant cell
    - Atypical fibroxanthoma—arising in sun-exposed skin, this neoplasm resembles the pleomorphic-storiform type, but it is in a superficial location and has a very good prognosis with local treatment
    - Myxoid malignant fibrous histiocytoma—has myxoid areas in over 50% of the tumor, less aggressive than pleomorphic-storiform
    - Giant cell type—clinically similar to pleomorphic-storiform, but contains numerous osteoclast-like giant cells
    - Inflammatory—uncommon subtype in retroperitoneum of adults; contains abundant xanthoma cells and granulocytes

- High cytologic grade, deep location, and large size poor prognostic indicators
- Local recurrence or metastasis in about 25% to 50% of cases

■ **Fat Cell Tumors**

● Lipoma

- • Benign tumors of encapsulated, near-normal-appearing adipose tissue
- • Most common soft tissue tumor
- • Soft, mobile, subcutaneous
- • Many variants with distinct morphologic and clinical features, such as angiolipoma—a tender, small, subcutaneous nodule in a young adult that consists of adipocytes and dilated capillaries, some containing thrombi

● Liposarcoma

- • Second most common adult sarcoma
- • Virtually never seen in children
- • Thigh or retroperitoneal in deep soft tissue, as opposed to superficial, subcutaneous location of lipoma
  - • Pathology
    - • Must have *lipoblasts* (cells with lipid vacuoles that deform the nucleus, mimicking the appearance of fetal fat cells)
  - • Myxoid
    - • Most common type, t12;16 a characteristic translocation
    - • Composed of a network of fine branching capillaries with tumor cells suspended in a mucopolysaccharide-rich (myxoid) matrix
  - • Well differentiated
    - • Similar to lipoma but has malignant lipoblasts
    - • Recurs but seldom metastasizes, can achieve huge size (100 lb range) in the abdomen
    - • May progress to a high-grade *dedifferentiated liposarcoma*
  - • Round cell
    - • Appears to be the high-grade counterpart of myxoid liposarcoma, analogous to the relationship of dedifferentiated and well differentiated
    - • Consists of sheets of uniform, poorly differentiated, round cells
  - • Pleomorphic
    - • Rare, resembles MFH except for the presence of lipoblasts
  - • Well-differentiated and myxoid types are low-grade tumors, while round cell, pleomorphic, and dedifferentiated types are high-grade sarcomas

■ **Smooth Muscle**

● Leiomyoma

- • Benign, smooth muscle tumors
- • Excluding uterine and gastrointestinal tract are uncommon
- • Characteristic skin presentation—a painful superficial lesion
- • Pathology—1 to 2 cm, intersecting smooth muscle cells with blunt end, cigar-shaped nuclei, no or rare mitosis

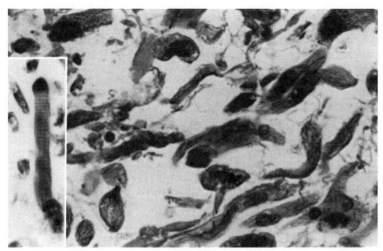

Fig. 23.8 Rhabdomyosarcoma. Some of the large malignant cells have cytoplasmic elongations with cross striations: evidence of muscle differentiation. (*Rosai J:* Ackerman's surgical pathology, *St Louis, 1989, Mosby.*)

● Leiomyosarcoma

- Histologically similar to leiomyoma, but has increased mitosis and nuclear pleomorphism
- Mitotic rate—most important indicator of malignancy
- Can recur and metastasize with tumors from deeper sites, having a poorer outcome

■ **Skeletal Muscle**

● Rhabdomyosarcoma

- Commonest sarcoma of childhood and adolescence
- Sites—head and neck, genitourinary tract, retroperitoneum
- All have striated muscle differentiation—cross striations by routine microscopy, muscle filaments (actin-desmin) on electron microscopy, or with immunohistochemistry (Fig. 23.8)
  - Embryonal type

    - Most common subtype
    - Infants and young children
    - Pathology—cellular tumor varying from relatively undifferentiated mononuclear cells to rhabdomyoblasts with abundant eosinophilic cytoplasm
    - Most—have cytogenetic finding of delllp with +2, 8 and/or 20

  - Alveolar type

    - Adolescents, most unfavorable type
    - Pathology—mononuclear cells similar to embryonal type arranged around spaces resembling lung alveoli
    - 80% have t2;13 or 1;13 involving the FKHR gene on chromosome 13

- Botryoid type (sarcoma botryoides)

  - Pathology—grows as a polypoid, lobulated mass into a cavity, resembles a "bunch of grapes," myxoid stroma with scattered, undifferentiated, malignant cells and rhabdomyoblasts showing cytoplasmic elongations and cross striations (strap cells)
  - Frequently at urogenital sites
  - Infants, fairly good prognosis with multi-agent chemotherapy

- Pleomorphic type

  - Rare sarcoma of elderly in deep muscle
  - Pathology—large eosinophilic cells, multinuclear tumor giant cells, resembles MFH but electron microscopy or immunohistochemistry identifies muscle differentiation

- Rhabdomyosarcomas—aggressive tumors, but respond to combined surgery, radiotherapy, chemotherapy

■ **Vascular Tumors**

● **Hemangiomas**

- Common benign tumors of vascular origin, usually arising in subcutaneous tissue and skin
  - May be nevi (congenital), hamartomas, reactive or true neoplasms
  - Many clinical and microscopic variants
  - *Capillary hemangioma*—composed of capillary-like vascular channels lined by endothelial cells, is seen at all ages and commonly in the skin
  - *Angiomatosis*—a large hemangioma involving a body segment or multiple tissue planes in the same region
  - *Lymphangiomas*—similar to hemangiomas but arise from lymphatic channels

● **Pyogenic granuloma**

- Common benign lesions of skin or oral mucosa appearing as bulging red nodules, often with surface ulceration associated with trauma
- Pathology—likely reactive proliferation of sprouting capillaries surrounding a parent vessel, imparting a lobular appearance that resembles exuberant granulation tissue

● **Hemangioendothelioma**

- Arise from the wall of a vessel in adults
- Pathology—composed of cells with abundant cytoplasm resembling histiocytes in a varying fibromyxoid stroma; characteristically cells have intracellular vascular lumens that can contain erythrocytes
  - Up to one third behave in a malignant fashion with metastasis

● Angiosarcoma

- Rare adult sarcomas
- Often aggressive, arising in four typical settings

  - *Cutaneous* in head and neck of elderly
  - *Lymphedema associated* in areas of chronic lymphedema (Stewart-Treves syndrome refers to angiosarcoma arising in lymphedematous areas postmastectomy)

- *Angiosarcoma of breast* often very well-differentiated, occurring in premenopausal women in the fourth and fifth decades
- *Angiosarcoma of deep tissue*

  - Pathology—well-differentiated tumors consist of anastomosing channels lined by atypical endothelial cells difficult to separate from hemangiomas, while poorly differentiated angiosarcomas may be diagnosed only through vessel differentiation on electron microscopy or immunohistochemistry

- Kaposi's sarcoma

  - Spindle cell sarcoma of vascular origin frequently arising in the skin
  - An indolent, sporadic form—occurs in elderly males, but now most common in HIV-positive homosexual males associated with a herpes type virus
    - Pathology—composed of vascular slits surrounded by atypical spindle cells associated with extravasated erythrocytes

Perivascular Tumors

- Glomus tumor

  - Small painful nodules of nail beds and subcutis of extremities in adults, recapitulates the arteriovenous channels regulating blood flow to the distal extremities
  - Derived from vascular smooth muscle
  - Pathology—composed of uniform round and polygonal cells in sheets and cords with distinct cell borders caused by encircling basement membrane and a variable stroma of vessels, mast cells, and myxoid background

- Hemangiopericytoma

  - Rare tumors of deep soft tissue in middle-aged adults
  - Pathology—consists of dilated vascular channels surrounded by spindle cells in a fibrous stroma that has the appearance of an expansion of the perivascular tissue
  - May recur locally and rarely metastasize

Synovial Tumors

- Tenosynovial giant cell tumors

  - Commonly arise in adult women as a small nodule of the finger
  - Pathology—composed of uniform, bland, polygonal cells with cytoplasm resembling histiocytes mixed with xanthoma cells, hemosiderin-laden histiocytes, and multinucleated giant cells

- Synovial sarcoma

  - Resembles synovium morphologically but now grouped with tumors of unknown origin in the World Health Organization classification of soft tissue tumors, as there is no real evidence of synovial differentiation
  - 20 to 40 years old
  - Usually arises in the region of a large joint (knee), uncommonly within the joint
  - Radiology—may have calcifications

- Pathology—biphasic appearance with cellular spindle cell stroma and epithelioid gland-forming areas
- tX;18(p11;q11)
- Highly malignant with 50% 5-year survival

■ Neural Tumors

● Benign

— *Neuroma*

- *Traumatic neuroma* is a regenerative hyperplastic growth of peripheral nerve at a previous incision site or amputation site.
- *Morton's neuroma* occurs between the third and fourth toes as the result of trauma to the plantar digital nerve by repeated compression in which the nerve shows surrounding fibrosis.

— *Neurofibroma*

- Benign tumor of peripheral nerves composed of Schwann cells, fibroblasts, and perineural cells
- Usually dermal nodules or polypoid skin lesions
- Pathology—unencapsulated proliferation of slender spindle cells intermingled with collagen fibers; may have a diffuse subcutaneous pattern or involve a nerve as multiple nodules, like a string of beads (plexiform neurofibroma)
- Both patterns—may occur in type 1 neurofibromatosis, but the plexiform type is virtually diagnostic

— *Schwannoma (neurilemoma)*

- Benign tumor of Schwann cells
- Young and middle-aged adults, often as a deep lesion (the most common benign deep soft tissue lesion)
- Bilateral acoustic nerve schwannomas are pathognomonic of neurofibromatosis type 2
- Pathology—circumscribed tumors composed of cellular areas (Antoni A) and myxoid areas (Antoni B); cellular areas are composed of spindle cells that may palisade around acellular matrix areas (Verocay bodies)

— *Granular cell tumors*

- Small tumors often in oral cavity or subcutaneously in middle-aged females
- Pathology—grossly yellow; microscopically composed of large cells with abundant eosinophilic granular cytoplasm and small bland nuclei
- Almost all are benign and are derived from Schwann cells

● Malignant

— *Malignant peripheral nerve sheath tumor (malignant schwannoma)*

- Uncommon sarcoma arising in patients with neurofibromatosis type 1 within a preexisting neurofibroma
- Pathology—resemble fibrosarcoma

— *Clear cell sarcoma*

   • Rare melanocytic tumor occurring in young female adults along tendons and aponeurosis, especially the feet

   • Pathology—composed of large clusters of tumor cells separated by septa into compartments; the tumor cells are usually polygonal with vesicular nuclei and a prominent basophilic nucleolus

   • Shows melanocytic differentiation (electron microscopy and immunohistochemistry) and sometimes melanin production

   • t(12;22) (q13;q12)—a characteristic cytogenetic change, but this is not seen in cutaneous melanoma

   • While often clinically slow growing, metastasis—occurs in half the cases with about a 50% 5-year survival

■ **Cartilage and Bone**

● Benign

— *Myositis ossificans*

   • Pseudoneoplasm likely caused by trauma; frequent in athletic young adults

   • Pathology—a central core composed of a mixture of fibroblasts, giant cells, and immature connective tissue surrounding trabecular bone

● Malignant

   • Malignant osteosarcoma and chondrosarcoma of soft tissue resemble those arising in primary sites.

■ **Miscellaneous Soft Tissue Tumors**

● Benign

— *Tumoral calcinosis*

   • Amorphous, periarticular, soft tissue calcification surrounded by a giant cell reaction occurring frequently in the hands and feet

   • A rare primary disorder, but more common in renal failure and other setting of hypercalcemia

— *Myxoma*

   • Intramuscular tumor composed of loose myxoid stroma with scanty stellate cells

   • Must be differentiated from sarcomas with myxoid areas

   • Similar lesions in cutaneous and perineural locations

● Malignant

— *Epithelioid sarcoma*

   • Rare sarcoma of finger, hand, and ankle area in young adults (30 to 35 years old) that may be ulcerated

   • Histologic origin unclear

   • Pathology

      • Appear as deceptively benign polygonal cells with eosinophilic cytoplasm and complex nuclear outlines

- Central necrosis and extensive infiltration microscopically
- Metastasis in 50% with a 50% 10-year survival

— *Alveolar soft part sarcoma*
- Rare sarcoma of children and adolescents
- Site—deep thigh common
- Origin—may be skeletal muscle
- Pathology

  - Nests of uniform polygonal cell with small nuclei and abundant cytoplasm that may contain periodic acid-Schiff (PAS) stain positive crystals that are surrounded by fibrovascular septa
  - Central spaces caused by degeneration of cells in the middle of the nests give a lung alveolar appearance

- Clinical course—slow but relentless, showing late recurrences and metastasis

Multiple Choice
Review Questions

1. A 15-year-old male presents with complaints of severe pain in proximal tibia that awakens him at night. This has been relieved with aspirin. A small lesion is identified on x-ray film with sclerotic margins and a central lytic area. Surgical removal is performed. The most likely histologic findings are which of the following?

   a. Malignant osteoblasts forming osteoid and bone
   b. Normal appearing cartilage
   c. A nidus of woven bone trabeculae in osteoid
   d. Metastatic adenocarcinoma of the lung
   e. Mitotically active cells with atypia in a hyaline matrix

2. A 70-year-old male has a pathologic fracture of the femur. The lesion appears lytic on x-ray film with a circumscribed punched-out appearance. The curetting from surgical pinning of the fracture site are most likely to show which of the following?

   a. Diminished and thinned trabecular bone fragments (consistent with osteoporosis)
   b. Sheets of atypical plasma cells
   c. Metastatic prostatic adenocarcinoma
   d. Malignant cells forming osteoid and bone
   e. Thickened trabeculae with a mosaic tile pattern

3. The bony trabeculae of osteoporosis typically show which of the following?

   a. A decrease in number
   b. Expanded osteoid
   c. A mosaic tile appearance
   d. Thinning with prominent osteoblastic rimming
   e. Prominent osteoclastic activity

4. The most common sarcoma of childhood is which of the following?

   a. Malignant fibrous histiocytoma
   b. Synovial sarcoma
   c. Ewing's sarcoma
   d. Rhabdomyosarcoma
   e. Clear cell sarcoma

5. Fracture repair may show formation of all *except* which of the following?

   a. A "brown tumor" (reparative granuloma)
   b. Organizing hematoma
   c. Woven bone
   d. Fibroblastic callus
   e. Osteonecrosis and osteoclastic resorption

Chapter 24

Peripheral Nervous System and Muscle

DISEASES OF PERIPHERAL NERVES—OVERVIEW

- Peripheral nerves (PN) are composed of nerve fibers and Schwann cells and their myelin sheaths, all supported by connective tissue cells and blood vessels.
- Motor nerve fibers are axons derived from lower motor neurons of the brain stem and spinal cord.
- Sensory nerve fibers are functional dendrites (since the nerve impulses travel **toward** their cell bodies located in ganglia or brain stem).
- Myelinated and unmyelinated nerve fibers are usually mixed within a PN. If unmyelinated, groups of fibers are enveloped by the cytoplasm of a Schwann cell. If myelinated, a single Schwann cell provides **one** segment of myelin along the length of a single fiber, and its cytoplasm and nucleus are in close proximity to the fiber.
- Peripheral nerves may be mixed (i.e., have both sensory and motor fibers).
- The junction between two myelin segments (node of Ranvier) is bridged by a layer of basement lamina, which covers all Schwann cells (even those of a schwannoma), and passes from one Schwann cell to the next.
- Connective tissue surrounds individual nerve fibers (endoneurium), groups of nerve fibers (perineurium), and the entire nerve (epineurium).
- Peripheral nerves have the ability at least partially to regenerate after damage. Fibers slowly extend from the proximal cut or damaged ends (growth cones), guided by preexisting Schwannian and endoneurial sheaths and may reestablish connections with muscle or other organs, with eventual recovery of at least partial function.
- Dissolution of the myelin along a nerve fiber (demyelination) occurs when the fiber within is no longer viable (the entire myelin sheath degenerates). **Segmental** demyelination (degeneration of one or more individual myelin segments on a single nerve fiber) may occur along an intact axon caused by disease of the Schwann cells or direct damage to the myelin itself (e.g., an autoimmune attack directed against myelin antigens); the nerve fiber within shows no primary abnormality.

DISEASES OF PERIPHERAL NERVES

■ Noninfectious Inflammatory Diseases

- Guillain-Barré syndrome (acute inflammatory demyelinating polyradiculopathy, Landry's ascending paralysis)
  - Incidence is 1 to 2 cases per 100,000 persons in the United States.
  - Often this is preceded by an acute illness, usually viral, often resem-

404

bling influenza. A cluster of cases followed government-recommended flu inoculations during the Reagan Administration.

- Ascending paralysis begins in the distal limbs and rapidly progresses to affect proximal muscles. Facial muscles are often involved.

- Muscle reflexes are lost; sensation also may be affected. Respiratory paralysis may necessitate mechanical ventilation.

- Mononuclear inflammatory cell infiltration of nerve roots, spinal root ganglia, and nerves is characteristic and may be severe.

- Segmental demyelination occurs, but axonal damage is also common.

- An infectious agent usually cannot be identified.

- The most likely etiology is an autoimmune attack directed against peripheral nerve myelin. A laboratory model (experimental allergic neuritis), induced by injecting experimental animals with peripheral myelin, closely mimics the morphology of the human disease.

- Recovery of function is often good but may be slow.

- Chronic inflammatory demyelinating polyradiculopathy

  - This is a subacute or chronic disease resembling the acute ("one-shot") syndrome described above.

  - Relapses and remissions occur over a prolonged period.

  - Both motor and sensory deficits may occur.

■ **Infectious Diseases**

- Varicella-zoster neuropathy

  - After chickenpox, latent virus often remains in sensory ganglia (virus can often be detected in the fifth cranial nerve ganglion of adults who have had chickenpox as children).

  - Reactivation later in life results in a painful vesicular eruption (shingles) following the course of cutaneous nerves in sensory dermatomes.

  - Mononuclear inflammation and neuronal destruction in ganglia, focal necrosis, and hemorrhage may occur. Nerves show nerve fiber damage secondary to neuronal cell destruction.

- Leprosy

  - Leprosy is caused by infection with *Mycobacterium leprae*.

  - In lepromatous leprosy, active growth and spread of the bacteria occurs. Schwann cells, and other cells and organs, are invaded by the mycobacteria. Segmental demyelination, remyelination, or loss of both axons and their myelin sheaths occur. Reactive fibrosis with thickening of the nerves sheaths is prominent.

  - In tuberculoid leprosy, granulomatous inflammation, often in the dermis and often disfiguring, occurs as a result of a typical cell-mediated immune granulomatous response. Eventually fibrosis causes damage in and around the cutaneous nerves. Anesthesia results and may be severe.

- Diphtheritic neuropathy

  - This is caused by exotoxin secreted by *Corynebacterium diphtheriae* that damages peripheral nerves.

  - Sensory ganglia are usually affected first, with segmental demyelination of the adjacent sensory and motor fibers.

■ Metabolic Neuropathies

- Neuropathy of adult-onset diabetes mellitus

  - This may be primarily sensory, distal in the limbs, and bilaterally symmetric (the most common type); but mixed sensory-motor, autonomic, focal, multifocal, asymmetric, or a mixture of all these type may occur.
  - Patients often develop decreased sensation in the distal limbs, which predisposes to trauma. In diabetes, because of microvascular insufficiency and poor healing, even minor trauma may lead to the development of ulceration and infection and eventual loss of digits or entire limbs.
  - Primary axonal degeneration and segmental demyelination occur, with loss of small myelinated and unmyelinated nerve fibers.
  - Endoneurial vascular thickening and basement laminar thickening and reduplication, similar to diabetic vascular changes in the kidney, occur.
  - Autonomic dysfunction is also common.

- Neuropathy of uremia

  - A majority of patients with renal failure and uremia develop peripheral neuropathy, typically symmetric and distal in the extremities.
  - Abnormal sensations in the limbs (dysesthesias), depressed deep muscle reflexes, and cramping are common.
  - Axonal degeneration and fiber loss occur.
  - Regeneration with recovery of function may occur following dialysis or transplantation.

- Metabolic neuropathies caused by vitamin deficiencies

  - Thiamine deficiency may be associated with axonal degeneration (neuropathic beriberi).
  - Similar axonal degenerations occur in deficiencies of vitamins B_6, B_{12}, and E.

■ Toxic Neuropathies

- Exposure to many metallic and organic compounds, toxins elaborated by infectious agents, or drugs may result in peripheral neuropathy, most often because of nerve fiber degeneration.

  - Arsenic acute poisoning is associated with severe cerebral edema. Chronic intoxication often results in peripheral axonal degeneration, both sensory and motor; the sensory deficiency is usually more severe.
  - Lead poisoning in children, relatively common in inner cities, usually results in encephalopathy with cerebral edema, seizures, and mental retardation. Lead intoxication in adults usually results in motor neuropathy resulting in weakness. Upper limbs are more affected than lower; extensors of the wrists usually are the most affected (resulting in "wrist drop"). Sensory deficit is usually absent. Motor nerve fiber degeneration is present, but neuronal perikarya and Schwann cells may also be directly affected.
  - Vinca alkaloids, used in cancer chemotherapy, may cause axonal degeneration and mixed sensory-motor neuropathy because of interference with assembly of microtubules within neurons and neuronal processes.

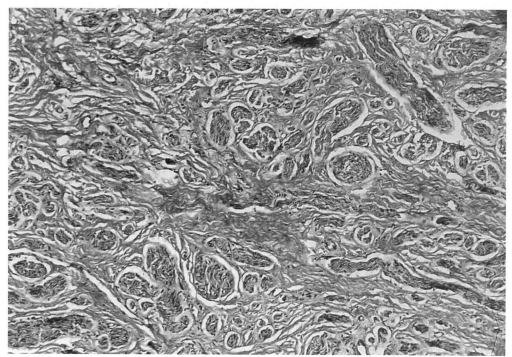

Fig. 24.1 Traumatic neuroma. Numerous, small, irregular nerve bundles, outgrowths from a severed peripheral nerve, are surrounded by fibrous connective tissue.

- Organic phosphorus compounds, often used in pesticides, fuel additives, and in the plastics industry may cause severe, acute sensory-motor neuropathy after a 1- to 3-week latent period. Many cases following accidental food contamination have been reported. Degeneration of long axons in both central and peripheral nervous systems occurs.

■ Traumatic Neuropathies

- Nerves are often injured during trauma. Lacerations, avulsions because of pulling on limbs (common in children), and crush or compression injuries all occur. Nerve fibers degenerate distally from the point of injury, with subsequent loss of myelin. Regeneration may occur.

- Unregulated axonal growth following injury may result in a mass of tangled axons (traumatic or amputation neuroma) surrounded by Schwann cells, perineurial cells, and connective tissue and fibroblasts. These tumors (Fig. 24.1) may be extremely painful and require surgical removal.

- Entrapment-compression injuries occur at anatomic sites such as the ulnar nerve at the elbow, peroneal nerve at the knee, radial nerve in the upper arm and are often seen in the homeless following prolonged positioning of the arm over the back of a park bench ("Saturday night palsy") or in the foot following compression of interdigital nerves by poorly fitting shoes.

- The most common of these injuries is entrapment of the median nerve at the wrist by the transverse carpal ligament (carpal tunnel syndrome), now increasingly common in computer operators but also seen during pregnancy, in degenerative joint disease, renal dialysis patients, systemic amyloidosis, or hypothyroidism. Females are more commonly affected than males.

■ **Hereditary Neuropathies**

● Most affect both motor and sensory functions—termed the hereditary motor and sensory neuropathies (HMSN), types I, II, III, and IV

  • HMSN I

    • Charcot-Marie-Tooth disease (CMT HMSN I—hypertrophic form), often called "peroneal muscular atrophy," is a disease of childhood or early adult onset, transmitted as an autosomal dominant trait. Calf weakness and atrophy and orthopedic abnormalities (e.g., pes cavus) are often present. The distal lower limb atrophy with preservation of the muscles of the upper leg resembles an "inverted champagne bottle." Episodes of demyelination-remyelination occur, with loss of large axons. Clinically palpable nerve enlargement is caused by concentric proliferation of Schwann cells ("onion bulb" formation). Gene abnormalities on chromosome 17, 1, or X may give rise to clinically similar phenotypes.

  • HMSN II

    • Charcot-Marie-Tooth disease (CMT HMSN II—neuronal form) is less frequent than CMT HMSN I, with onset at a slightly later age. Nerve enlargement is not present. A slowly progressive distal loss of axons occurs.

  • HMSN III

    • Dejerine-Sottas disease (infantile hypertrophic neuropathy) is inherited as an autosomal recessive disease. Delayed motor skill development, distal weakness, weakness of the trunk, and atrophy, not limited to the legs, become evident in early childhood. Reflexes are usually depressed. Striking, palpable nerve enlargement is caused by "onion bulb" formation; axonal loss develops later.

  • HMSN IV

    • Refsum's disease is pigmentary retinopathy combined with neuropathy and cerebellar ataxia, inherited as an autosomal recessive trait. The underlying cause is reduced peroxisomal α-oxidation of phytanic acid. Onion bulb formation on peripheral nerves is prominent as is atrophy of the inferior olivary nuclei of the medulla and the olivocerebellar tracts in the central nervous system. Elevated phytanic acid levels distinguish this disease from the other forms of HMSN.

    • Other forms of HMSN IV include **giant axonal neuropathy,** a childhood disease inherited as an autosomal recessive trait, characterized by the accumulation of neurofilaments within axons.

● Other hereditary neuropathies—affect sensory and autonomic functions, termed the hereditary and autonomic neuropathies (HSAN)

● Hereditary amyloid neuropathies with amyloid deposition, usually derived from transthyretin, result from mutation on chromosome 18q

■ **Neuropathies Resulting from Ischemia**

  • Nerve injury may result from large or small vessel disease, including atherosclerosis, which may involve an entire limb. One or more nerves may be focally damaged as a result of small vessel insufficiency.

■ **Neuropathies in Neoplastic Processes**

- Nerves may be entrapped or compressed by neoplasms, invaded by metastatic malignancies, or compromised by products elaborated by malignancies (paraneoplastic syndromes).

- Peripheral neuropathy, especially of the facial nerve, is sometimes present in patients with sarcoidosis.

■ **Neoplasms of Peripheral Nerves**

- Schwannomas and neurofibromas are relatively common neoplasms (see Central Nervous System chapter).

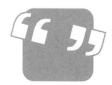

  - Malignant peripheral nerve-sheath neoplasms usually originate from peripheral mixed motor-sensory nerves rather than from cranial nerves or spinal nerve roots. Many are associated with neurofibromatosis (NF), type 1 (von Recklinghausen's disease).

- Neurofibromatosis—type 1 (NF1)

  - A relatively common (1 per 4000 people) neurocutaneous syndrome in which tumors are formed. Autosomal-dominant transmission in families is responsible for approximately 50% of cases; the remainder represent de novo mutations. The tumors formed include neurofibromas that may affect any organ, schwannomas, optic nerve gliomas, meningiomas, pheochromocytomas, hamartomas of the iris (Lisch nodules), and pigmented macules of the skin (café-au-lait spots). The cutaneous neurofibromas may be extremely numerous and disfiguring.

  - Similar tumors may also occur sporadically.

  - The plexiform neurofibroma seems to be unique to NF1; in this tumor, each fascicle of a peripheral nerve is expanded into a complicated mass. Adjacent nerves may be incorporated into the tumor.

  - The responsible gene is located on chromosome 17q and impairs the function of neurofibromin, a growth-regulating protein.

  - Up to 5% of NF1 cases will develop malignant nerve-sheath neoplasms.

- Neurofibromatosis—type 2 (NF2)

  - This is a distinct syndrome, less common than NF1.
  - Bilateral eighth cranial nerve schwannomas are pathognomonic. Skin tumors may or may not occur.
  - Lisch nodules are not formed, but café-au-lait spots are present.
  - Patients are *not* at risk for developing malignant nerve-sheath tumors.
  - The responsible gene has been mapped to chromosome 22.

DISEASES OF MUSCLE—OVERVIEW

- Reduction in size of muscle fibers (atrophy) may be caused by

  - Disuse (e.g., prolonged bed rest), starvation, aging, or vascular disease
  - Loss of innervation ("neurogenic atrophy") caused by disease or death of lower motor neurons or their axons (e.g., in amyotrophic lateral sclerosis)

- Hypertrophy

  - Enlargement of muscle fibers occurs in athletes and in *congenital fiber type disproportion,* a genetic disease with type 1 fiber atrophy but type 2 fiber enlargement, often associated with small stature and bony abnormalities. In some stages of certain muscular dystrophies, individual fibers may also become transiently enlarged.

- Necrosis

  - Muscle fiber necrosis occurs in ischemia, traumatic muscle injury, infections, autoimmune disorders directed against muscle or muscle vasculature, toxic or drug reactions, in muscular dystrophies, and other conditions.

- Regeneration

  - Skeletal muscle fibers may regenerate to a limited extent following injury or disease.

Muscle in Denervation

- A motor axon provides an essential trophic influence on the muscle fibers that it innervates. Disruption of innervation results in shrinkage of the muscle fiber (atrophy). Denervation may result from

  - Disease or destruction of anterior horn cells (e.g., amyotrophic lateral sclerosis, Werdnig-Hoffmann disease, acute anterior poliomyelitis).
  - Injury or disease of the motor axon (e.g., trauma, motor neuropathy).

- A single motor axon usually innervates a group of muscle cells, randomly interspersed with muscle cells innervated by other axons. The anterior horn cell, its axon, and all the muscle fibers that it innervates must be considered as a unit—*the motor unit.*

  - Acute denervation of the scattered muscle cells supplied by the axon of the motor unit usually results in shrinkage and angulation of those muscle fibers, when seen in cross sections.
  - Acutely denervated fibers may be reinnervated by sprouting from adjacent viable axons. Thus, more muscle fibers are innervated by fewer axons.
  - As more and more axons become inoperative, groups of shrunken fibers become apparent (Fig. 24.2), all fibers in the group having been innervated by a single axon and exhibiting the characteristics, on enzymatic histostaining, determined by that axon.
  - "Target fibers" exhibiting a central zone of disrupted fibrils, a surrounding intermediate transitional zone, and a peripheral zone of normal architecture are characteristic of denervated muscle fibers, although not always seen.
  - In Werdnig-Hoffmann disease (infantile spinal muscular atrophy), the atrophic fibers appear rounded rather than angular.

The Muscular Dystrophies

- A group of inherited, intrinsic disorders of muscle, some beginning during the earliest years of life but some with delayed onset. All are characterized by weakness and muscle fiber loss.

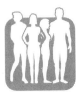

- **Duchenne muscular dystrophy (pseudohypertrophic muscular dystrophy)**

  - The most common of the dystrophies, its incidence is approximately 1:10,000 males (an X-linked disorder).
  - Onset is in childhood, usually before the age of 5 years; weakness and disability progress steadily to death during the third decade.

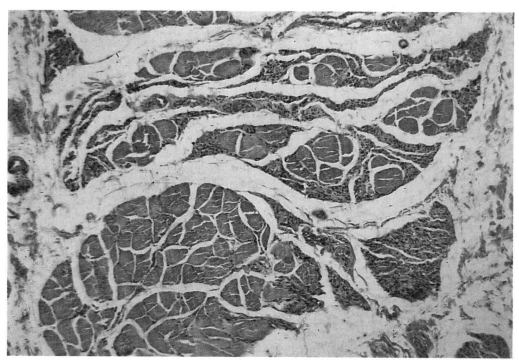

Fig. 24.2 Muscle atrophy. Groups of muscle fibers of normal size are admixed with groups of shrunken nerve fibers. The nuclei of the atrophic, collapsed fibers are crowded together, suggesting an inflammatory reaction at low-power examination, but no inflammation is present.

• Early weakness is usually most pronounced in the pelvic girdle muscles and then spreads to other muscle groups. *Gower's sign* (placing the hand on the knee to use the arm to assist standing) may be the earliest clinical sign of weakness.

• "Pseudohypertrophy" or enlargement of the calf, because of early increase in fiber size (but later because of replacement of muscle by adipose and connective tissue) is characteristic.

• Death often results from cardiac failure (heart muscle is also involved), pulmonary insufficiency, or intercurrent infection.

• Microscopically, as in all the dystrophies, there is variation in fiber size, with both shrinkage and enlargement, internalization of sarcolemmal nuclei, muscle fiber necrosis, phagocytosis, and regeneration. Replacement of lost fibers by adipose and fibrous tissue is more pronounced than in the other dystrophies. Eventually, few muscle fibers remain. Interstitial fibrosis and scarring of the myocardium may resemble old infarction.

• The genetic defect is localized to the dystrophin gene on chromosome Xp21, whose product is necessary for the integrity of the muscle membrane, especially during contraction.

● **Becker's muscular dystrophy**

• An X-linked muscular dystrophy, similar to Duchenne muscular dystrophy, but less common, of later onset, less severe, and generally more slowly progressive.

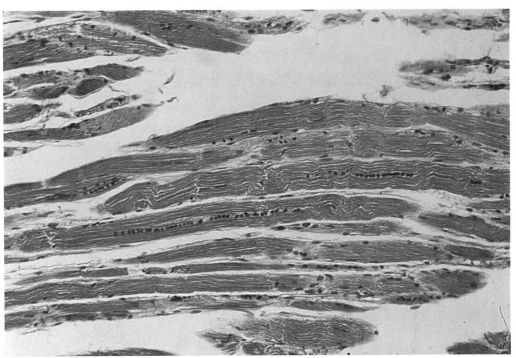

Fig. 24.3 Myotonic dystrophy. Long chains of internalized sarcolemmal nuclei can be seen, to some extent, in all the muscular dystrophy, but they are most prominent in myotonic dystrophy. Fibers of irregular size, foci of fiber degeneration, and fibrous connective tissue replacement are also present.

● **Myotonic disorders**

- Myotonia is sustained, involuntary muscular contraction (inability of muscles to relax promptly after contraction).
- Dystrophic and nondystrophic myotonic disorders occur.
- Myotonic muscular dystrophy is

  - Transmitted as a mendelian-dominant trait with variable penetrance; age of onset is variable but often begins in childhood.
  - Facial muscles, particularly the muscles of mastication (temporalis and masseters) and elevators of the eyelids, are involved.
  - Cataracts develop early.
  - Frontal balding, gonadal atrophy, cardiomyopathy, smooth muscle involvement, and an abnormal glucose tolerance test are also present.
  - Mental retardation or dementia is present in some cases.
  - Microscopically, there are changes similar to Duchenne muscular dystrophy, but proliferation of sarcolemmal nuclei in chains is striking (Fig. 24.3), as is the number of internalized muscle nuclei.
  - Ring fibers (one dystrophic fiber wrapped around another like a napkin ring around a napkin) is a distinctive feature. A mass of muscle cytoplasm (sarcoplasmic mass) may project from the ring.
  - The genetic defect is located on the long arm of chromosome 19.
  - Table 24.1 lists the muscular dystrophies.

Table 24.1 *The Muscular Dystrophies*

DISEASE	INHERITANCE	COMMENTS
Duchenne, Becker muscular dystrophy	X-linked	Pseudohypertrophy, especially of calf muscles; cardiac involvement in Duchenne type
Fascioscapulohumeral muscular dystrophy	Autosomal dominant	Weakness and dystrophic degeneration of face, neck, and shoulder girdle muscles. Onset usually between 10 to 30 years of age. Gene defect at 4q35
Oculopharyngeal muscular dystrophy	Autosomal dominant	Ptosis, extraocular muscle weakness, and weakness of muscles of swallowing
Limb-girdle muscular dystrophy	Autosomal recessive; also sporadic cases	Weakness of proximal muscle of upper and lower limbs. Prognosis variable but usually slowly progressive. Onset between 10 to 30 years
Myotonic muscular dystrophy	Autosomal dominant, penetrance variable	Myotonia, cataracts, frontal balding, gonadal atrophy, muscular weakness, and wasting; involvement of the muscles of mastication. Ring fibers distinctive. Age at onset variable

- Myotonia congenita (Thomsen's disease)

    - Not a muscular dystrophy

    - Onset from childhood to adolescence

    - Transmitted as a dominant or recessive trait in different families

    - Myotonia pits agonist against antagonist muscles during movement with muscle hypertrophy resulting

    - Usually compatible with a normal life span, although muscular weakness may occur late

    - Diphenyl hydantoin (Dilantin) often alleviates the myotonia and permits normal activity

■ **Congenital Myopathies**

- These are a group of congenital muscle diseases with similar clinical features—including early onset, muscle weakness, poor muscle tone, and static or slow progression—distinguished by morphologic differences in the affected muscles. Especially early onset may result in a "floppy baby," but other diseases, such as Werdnig-Hoffmann disease (see Central Nervous System chapter), also result in congenital hypotonia.

- Central core disease is a myopathy of infants usually inherited as an autosomal dominant trait. Motor development is retarded. Proximal type 1 fibers are affected, with central areas (cores) with deficiency of oxidative enzyme activity and sometimes with disorganization of myofibrils and abnormalities of the sarcotubular system. There is only slow progression, if any.

- Nemaline (rod) myopathy is inherited as a mendelian-dominant or mendelian-recessive disease in different families and more common in women. An elongated face, high-arched palate, projecting chin, and other skeletal abnormalities (e.g., pes cavus) are often present. Small rodlike or threadlike bodies are present within the sarcoplasm, diffusely or focally. By electron microscopy, they are continuous with the Z bands, possibly proliferations of Z band material.

- Centronuclear myopathy may be inherited as a dominant, recessive or X-linked disease. Most fibers contain a central nucleus often surrounded by a halo of poorly stained sarcoplasm. Extraocular and facial muscles are often involved early, with slow progressive weakness of the limb muscles.

■ Inborn Errors of Metabolism Associated with Myopathies

- Myopathies may occur in metabolic diseases, especially those associated with glycogen and lipid metabolism.

  - Deficiency of acid maltase, a lysosomal enzyme that cleaves alpha-glycosidic linkages, results in the accumulation of glycogen systemically (Pompe's disease) and in muscle. Weakness and retarded motor development, tongue enlargement, and cardiac enlargement resulting in heart failure caused by massive accumulation of glycogen are prominent.

  - Other glycogen storage diseases are also associated with myopathies, including debranching enzyme deficiency, branching enzyme deficiency, and myophosphorylase deficiency.

  - Abnormalities that interfere with the metabolisms of long-chain fatty acids, a major energy source of muscle, are associated with myopathies. Carnitine (which facilitates transport of these acids across the mitochondrial membrane) deficiency results in the accumulation of lipid droplets within muscle cells and progressive weakness and muscle pain. A systemic form of the abnormality may result in hepatic and cerebral dysfunction mimicking Reye's syndrome.

  - Carnitine palmitoyl transferase deficiency is associated with myoglobinuria as a result of episodes of rhabdomyolysis (widespread necrosis of individual muscle fibers), especially after exercise or exposure to cold.

  - Neuronal ceroid lipofuscinosis (Batten disease) is accumulation of lipoid pigments in the brain and other organs; clinically, there are mental retardation, visual impairment, and seizures. Infantile, late infantile, juvenile, and adult forms have been described. The diagnosis is often made by the identification of these pigments in muscle biopsies.

■ Mitochondrial Myopathies

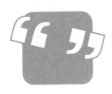

- Functional or structural abnormalities of muscle mitochondria result in a group of disorders usually presenting in early adulthood rather than in childhood, with weakness, usually of proximal muscles of the extremities and of the external eye muscles. Neurologic symptoms, cardiomyopathy, and lactic acidosis may be present. Groups of abnormal mitochondria cluster under the sarcolemmal membrane giving the muscle cell an irregular contour and staining pattern—"ragged red fibers." Ultrastructurally, the mitochondria often show complicated crystal like inclusions.

  - Kearns-Sayre syndrome is progressive weakness of extraocular muscles, pigmentary degeneration of the retina, cerebellar ataxia, and heart block, with death sometimes resulting from cardiac conduction defects. Deficiencies of mitochondrial DNA and cytochrome-*c* oxidase activity have been identified.

■ Toxic and Drug-related Myopathies

- Muscle abnormalities in thyroid disease

  - Thyrotoxicosis may be associated with proximal and extraocular muscle weakness. Occasionally, episodes of severe weakness accompanied by hypokalemia may occur. Muscle fiber necrosis and regeneration and interstitial mononuclear inflammatory infiltrates are present.

  - Hypothyroidism may be associated with muscle pain or cramps and slowing of deep muscle ("deep tendon") reflexes. Muscle fiber atrophy, internalization of sarcolemmal nuclei, and mucopolysaccharide accumulation in connective tissue are often present.

- Muscle abnormalities in alcoholism

  - Alcoholic binges may be followed by rhabdomyolysis and myoglobinuria, sometimes resulting in renal failure.

- Drug-related myopathies

  - Exogenous (therapeutic) or endogenous (e.g., Cushing's syndrome) steroids may induce severe myopathy, with atrophy of type 2 fibers but sparing of type 1 fibers.

  - Chloroquine, an antimalarial drug also used in the treatment of collagen-vascular diseases, may produce vacuoles within muscles cells (vacuolar myopathy) with resulting weakness. Resolution may occur after discontinuance of the drug.

  - Colchicine, after prolonged therapy for gout, may produce a myopathy with scattered fiber necrosis or vacuolization. Nerve fiber degeneration may also occur.

■ Diseases of the Neuromuscular Junction

- The neuromuscular junction

  - This consists of the presynaptic terminal end of the motor axon, a narrow gap of intercellular space (the synaptic cleft), and the postsynaptic region of the muscle. Acetylcholine, released from the presynaptic terminal of the axon crosses the synaptic cleft and triggers receptors on the postsynaptic motor end plate membrane of the muscle. The acetylcholine is rapidly inactivated by acetylcholinesterase at the postsynaptic motor end plate, readying the muscle for another cycle.

- Myasthenia gravis

  - This is an autoimmune disease characterized by fluctuating weakness, often first noted in the extraocular muscles, causing ptosis and diplopia; dysphagia and dysarthria are also often present. Limb muscles are also involved. The weakness and easy fatigability often increase as the day progresses.

  - Disease incidence is 3:100,000 and is more common in young adult females.

  - A transient, often startling, improvement in strength after the administration of the anticholinesterase agent, Tensilon, is characteristic.

  - Circulating autoimmune antibodies against the acetylcholine receptor protein on the motor and plate, blocking neuromuscular excitation, is the underlying cause, eventually resulting in complement-dependent damage to the end plate.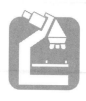

  - Thymic hyperplasia or thymoma is found in the majority of patients, and most have a salutory response to thymectomy.

  - Muscle biopsies are frequently nondiagnostic and may reveal mild-to-moderate type 2 fiber atrophy. Lymphocytic infiltrates of mild degree are often present throughout the muscle but are probably nonspecific.

- Lambert-Eaton myasthenic syndrome (LEMS)

  - LEMS is an autoimmune disorder of neuromuscular transmission, but, unlike myasthenia gravis, proximal limb muscles are most involved.

- Autonomic dysfunction is often present.
- LEMS is often associated with neoplasia (as a paraneoplastic syndrome), especially with small cell carcinoma of the lung; 40% of cases apparently have no neoplastic process detectable.
- Fewer synaptic vesicles are released by each action potential, although each vesicle contains a normal amount of acetylcholine. Gamma globulin from patients with LEMS, injected into mice, transfers the abnormality.

- Botulism

  - *Clostridium botulinum* toxin disrupts presynaptic neuromuscular transmission, and only small amounts may cause profound paralysis and death. The toxin may be formed in improperly canned foods or in infected deep wounds where the anaerobic environment favors growth of the bacteria. Traces of toxin in honey have been suggested as a cause of sudden infant death syndrome (SIDS).

■ Inflammatory Diseases of Muscle

● Inflammation in muscle

- This may be infectious or related to cellular immunity. Most patients have weakness, muscle pain, often fever; the muscle creatine kinase is usually elevated. Infiltrates may be neutrophilic, mixed, or mononuclear, depending upon the etiology and time course of the disease.

● Bacterial myositis

- This may be diffuse or focal (abscess).
- Most infections are hematogenous in origin but may be facilitated by closed trauma to the muscle.
- Weakness, muscle pain, fever, and generalized malaise are common clinical manifestations.

● Viral myositis

- Many viruses may cause myositis, including hepatitis B, coxsackievirus, echovirus, adenovirus, human immunodeficiency virus (HIV) and human T-cell leukemia/lymphoma virus-1 (HTLV-1).

- Resolution may be spontaneous, but massive destruction of muscle cells (rhabdomyolysis) may result in myoglobinuria, renal failure, and death.

- In acquired immunodeficiency syndrome (AIDS), an immune attack directed against blood vessels results in red cell leakage, hemosiderin deposition in muscle. Direct HIV myositis has been reported.

● Parasitic infection of muscle

- Toxoplasmosis infection of muscle occurs in AIDS and other immunodeficient states.

- Trichinosis (Fig. 24.4) is relatively common, acquired by eating inadequately cooked pork infected with *Trichinella spiralis* larvae. Eosinophilia and intense mononuclear inflammation in muscle may be present, but, if sections do not include the parasites, diagnosis may be difficult.

- Cysticercosis *(Taenia solium)* is rare in natives of the United States who have not traveled abroad but is more common in immigrants. Larvae may encyst any organ, including the brain. Death of the organisms, sometimes precipitated by treatment, causes an intense inflammatory reaction.

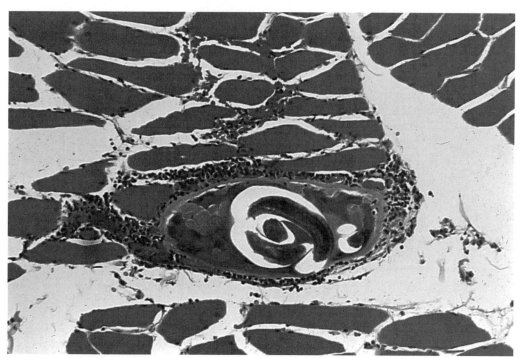

Fig. 24.4 Trichinosis. A larva of a *Trichinella spiralis* is encysted in skeletal muscle, surrounded by an abundant inflammatory reaction. Higher-power microscopic examination shows that numerous eosinophils are present.

● Myopathies with autoimmune injury

• Inflammatory diseases of muscle with injury mediated by autoimmune mechanisms include polymyositis, dermatomyositis, and inclusion body myositis.

— *Polymyositis*

• Incidence is 5 to 10:1,000,000 and is more common in African-Americans and in women. Age of onset is usually in the fourth to fifth decade of life.

• Generalized weakness develops relatively acutely (weeks); proximal muscles are often most involved. Remissions and exacerbations are usual.

• Muscle pain, fever, malaise, and dysphagia often are present.

• Erythrocyte sedimentation rate and muscle serum creatine kinase levels rise early.

• Antinuclear antibodies are present in a majority of cases.

• Cell-mediated immunity is probably responsible for the tissue damage.

• Mature lymphocytes, mostly CD8 T cells, invade muscle interstitium and surround necrotic muscle fibers (Fig. 24.5) and, to a lesser extent, blood vessels. Many macrophages are also present; eosinophils are not involved.

• Regenerating fibers appear, but regeneration is incomplete.

• Chronic interstitial pulmonary disease develops in a majority of patients.

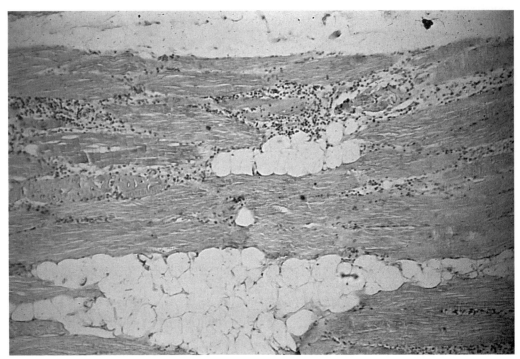

Fig. 24.5 Polymyositis. Abundant lymphocytic infiltration between muscle fascicles and into individual, degenerating muscle fibers is present.

- Malignant neoplasms are sometimes present, especially those with onset in the sixth decade of life and older; lung, breast, and gastrointestinal tract are most commonly involved.

— *Dermatomyositis*

- This is more common in women (F:M is 3:2).

- Muscle changes are similar to polymyositis, but the disease usually starts with a skin rash, often in a "butterfly" distribution on the face, with severe periorbital edema. The rash usually extends to the neck, shoulders, and extremities, including the digits.

- Subcutaneous nodular calcification develops with overlying ulcerations.

- Generalized vasculitis, especially in cases of childhood onset, may result in gastrointestinal ulceration and hemorrhage and neuritis.

- Interstitial infiltrates, more prominent around blood vessels are composed of CD8 T cells in the majority, but CD4 and B lymphocytes are also common.

- In muscle, capillaries are damaged most severely at the periphery of muscle fascicles, resulting in atrophy of muscle cells most prominent at the periphery of the fascicle.

- Humoral, rather than cellular, immunity is primarily involved, with IgG, IgM, and complement, especially C3, deposits in intramuscular vessels and other vessels, and also immune complex deposits.

- As in polymyositis, malignancies are often present.

— *Inclusion Body Myositis*

● This is most common in males in the sixth to eighth decades of life.

● Painless weakness is only slowly progressive and most pronounced distally in the extremities.

● Lymphocytic infiltrates in muscle and muscle fiber necrosis are present in less than half the cases.

● Rimmed vacuoles in muscle cells, seen on frozen sections, are lined by granules, composed of whorls of membranous profiles by electron microscopy. Rare filaments, possibly composed of mumps virus or β-amyloid are also present.

MULTIPLE CHOICE
REVIEW QUESTIONS

1. In Guillain-Barré syndrome (acute inflammatory demyelinating polyradiculopathy), the inflammation is caused by which of the following?

   a. A conventional virus infection of the axon
   b. A slow-virus infection (prion disease) of the axon
   c. A slow-virus infection (prion disease) of the spinal cord
   d. An autoimmune delayed hypersensitivity attack directed against the axon
   e. An autoimmune delayed hypersensitivity attack directed against myelin

2. Which of the following is *true* of varicella-zoster neuropathy (shingles)?

   a. It is caused by a latent virus that undergoes reactivation.
   b. It always accompanies childhood chicken pox.
   c. It only occurs in adults who have never had chicken pox and are therefore highly susceptible.
   d. It typically causes deep muscle pain and weakness of the extremities.
   e. It causes "glove-and-stocking" numbness of the distal extremities.

3. The most common compression-entrapment neuropathy is which of the following?

   a. Compression of the interdigital nerves in the foot
   b. Compression of the peroneal nerve at the knee
   c. Compression of the radial nerve at the wrist
   d. Compression of the ulnar nerve at the elbow
   e. Compression of the sciatic nerve exiting the pelvis

4. Necrosis of muscle fibers may occur in all *except* which of the following?

   a. Duchenne muscular dystrophy
   b. Vascular occlusion of a local blood vessel
   c. Staphylococcal myositis
   d. Amyotrophic lateral sclerosis
   e. Polymyositis

5. Myasthenia gravis is characterized by all *except* which of the following?

   a. Deficiency in the amount of released acetylcholine at the terminal axon
   b. Associated thymic hyperplasia or thymoma
   c. Reduction of weakness after administration of anticholinesterase drugs
   d. Circulating antibodies against acetylcholine
   e. Motor end-plate damage

Chapter 25

Central Nervous System

■ **Overview**

● **The central nervous system (CNS)**

• Contains specialized cells and tissues (Table 25.1), some having particular susceptibilities (selective vulnerability) to deficiencies of nutrients (e.g., O_2, glucose) or attack by physical, chemical, or microbiologic agents

• Is highly organized, anatomically and functionally; damage to a particular set of cells or area will produce a stereotyped set of signs and symptoms regardless of the etiology

• Is contained within a rigid, bony case ("closed box") after the cranial sutures have set, which does not allow for expansion of the contents; localized swelling may result in compression of brain substance or shifts ("herniations") of portions of the brain into, through, or around natural barriers (Table 25.2)

• Generally manifests little fibroblastic activity as a consequence of disease and healing (with certain few exceptions); therefore resolution of disease processes is different from that seen in other organs

■ **Anoxia and Cerebrovascular Disease**

• Glucose—the major oxidizable substrate of the CNS. Oxygen and glucose reach the parenchymal cells via the blood stream. Some CNS cells, especially neurons, are extremely sensitive to oxygen and/or glucose deprivation, even for a short time; loss only of sensitive cells to complete necrosis of all parenchymal elements (infarcts) may result.

• Deprivation of necessary nutrients, at the cellular level may be a consequence of

• Insufficiency of nutrients in freely flowing blood (e.g., hypoxemia in partial asphyxia or hypoglycemia in insulin shock) *or*

• Inability of blood to reach the cells because of vascular disease or obstruction

• The effects of hypoxemia on the CNS are frequently indistinguishable from the effects of hypoglycemia.

● **Hypoxemia or hypoglycemia**

• Tissue changes depend on the relative sensitivities of the various cells.

• Neurons generally are the most sensitive, followed by the oligodendrogliocytes.

• Astrocytes are relatively resistant to hypoxia-hypoglycemia; ependyma and choroid plexus cells are quite resistant.

Table 25.1   *Cells and Tissues of, and Adjacent to, the Central Nervous System (CNS)*

CELL OR TISSUE	COMMENTS
Neurons	Are not replaced after loss; neuronal processes (dendrites and axons) in the CNS regenerate poorly or not at all; peripheral nerve axons may regenerate fully or partially
Ectodermal glia Astrocytes	React to CNS abnormalities by proliferation; produce glial fibrillary acidic protein (GFAP) fibers; may be phagocytic; the cell of origin of the majority of primary CNS neoplasms
Oligodendroglia	Manufacture and maintain CNS myelin
Ependyma	Ventricular lining cell; in the spinal cord found at the location of the central canal (usually not patent in adulthood)
Choriod plexus	Produces cerebrospinal fluid
Microglia	Controversial; may be bone marrow-derived antigen processing or phagocytic cells; probably participate in the formation of Alzheimer's senile plaques; are active in some infectious diseases (e.g., syphilis)
Dura (pachymeninx)	Mostly collagen; dural venous sinuses (draining veins) present within splits in the dura. Outer portion is endosteum of cranium
Leptomeninges (pia and arachnoid)	Closely applied to the CNS surface; carry pial (surface) blood vessels; cerebrospinal fluid carried in subarachnoid space; arachnoid cells proliferate to form meningiomas; a site of common CNS infection (leptomeningitis)
Cranial nerves and myelin sheaths	Olfactory tracts and optic nerves: are fiber tracts of brain (oligodendroglial myelin) Proximal portions of cranial neves III-XII: oligodendroglial myelin Distal portions of cranial nerves III-XII (including portions still intracranial) and peripheral nerves: Schwannian myelin
Pineal body	Outside CNS parenchyma, posterior to collicular plate of midbrain; may produce a variety of hormones
Pituitary gland	In pituitary fossa (sella turcica), covered by a dural membrane (diaphragma sella)
Bone	Forms a rigid case ("closed box") for the brain after sutures have set in early childhood; cranial cavity is divided into anterior, middle, and posterior cranial fossae
Blood vessels	4 feeding high-pressure arteries (2 internal carotid and 2 vertebral arteries), 2 low-pressure draining veins (internal jugular veins)
Lymph vessels	None in central nervous system
Other cells and tissues	Adipose tissue, melanocytes, often present

- The following are relative sensitivities to hypoxemia or hypoglycemia of subgroups of neurons:

  - Sommer's sector (CA1) neurons in Ammon's horn of the hippocampus are the most sensitive.

  - This is followed by (in order of decreasing sensitivity) Purkinje cells of the cerebellum, small neurons of the basal ganglia especially in the outer portions of the caudate and putamen (corpus striatum), neurons of the neocortex (phylogenetically more recently developed areas), and neurons of the paleocortex (phylogenetically older areas).

  - **Limited degrees** of oxygen-glucose deprivation at the tissue level may therefore cause **limited** cell loss only (of particularly sensitive cells, usually specific groups of neurons, without total infarction).

- Cerebrovascular disease—the effects on the CNS of insufficient blood flow at the tissue level because of diseased, occluded, or ruptured blood vessels

---

Table 25.2 *Important Sites of Herniation of the Brain and Common Consequences*

HERNIATION	CONSEQUENCES
Cingulate gyrus (subfalcine herniation): herniation of the cingulate gyrus beneath the lower free edge of the falx cerebri	Infarction of the cingulate gyrus; infarction of the midline cerebral gyri caused by compression of branches of the anterior cerebral artery against the lower falcine edge
Uncus (transtentorial): herniation of medial temporal lobe (uncus) and/or hippocampus through the incisura of the tentorium cerebelli	Dilation of the ipsilateral pupil (compression of nerve III against the tentorial edge); ipsilateral occipital lobe, thalamic infarction (compression of the posterior cerebral artery against the tentorial edge); ipsilateral hemiparesis (compression of the contralateral cerebral peduncle by the tentorial edge, a "false" localizing sign often called "Kernohan's notch"); contralateral hemiparesis (compression of the ipsilateral cerebral peduncle); depressed levels of consciousness, coma, death (compression of the midbrain and brain stem reticular activating system)
Cerebellar tonsil(s): herniation of the inferior cerebellum into the spinal canal through the foramen magnum)	Cardiorespiratory arrest, death (compression of medulla)
Herniation of brain through a meningeal and calvarial defect	Increased intracranial pressure causes brain to extrude through the defect forming an external mushroomlike mass ("cerebral fungus")

- Atherosclerosis—intimal disease of the elastic and larger muscular arteries, similar to that seen in vessels elsewhere

    - Initial dilation (ectasia) and tortuosity eventually give way to narrowing and occlusion from thrombus or hemorrhage into a plaque; 80% to 90% narrowing is required to significantly impair flow.

- Arteriolar sclerosis (arteriolosclerosis)—disease of the media of smaller arteries and arterioles—medial degeneration, lipohyalinosis, fibrinoid necrosis; often related to systemic hypertension

● **Occlusion of blood vessels** Results in infarction (encephalomalacia, softening are synonyms)—usually anemic or white infarction—in the field of supply of the occluded vessel

    — *The CNS responds with*

        - Edema (early); may make the area of damage seem larger than the area of true damage because of pressure and interference of function of adjacent viable parenchyma; may take 7 days or more to resolve

        - Cellular responses

            - Infiltration by neutrophils—approximately the first 8 to 24 hours only (acute response to necrosis)

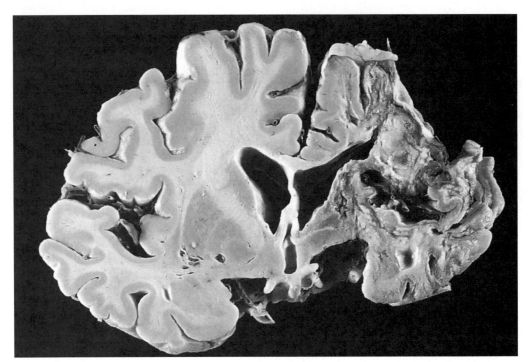

Fig. 25.1 A large, partially resolved anemic infarct is present in the right cerebral hemisphere. Remaining necrotic tissue will eventually be removed by macrophages. The right sylvian fissure and lateral ventricle are slightly enlarged and distorted by the enormous loss of brain substance.

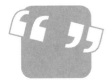

- Macrophage (histiocytic—gitter cell) response—starts after 48 hours); macrophages phagocytize necrotic debris, including myelin breakdown products; hemosiderin-laden macrophages are present if the infarct is hemorrhagic
- Astrogliosis (gliosis)—proliferation of astrocytes in the surrounding area starts after 48 hours with appearance of plump, reactive "gemistocytic" astrocytes; after about 7 days, the astrocytes begin to produce glial fibrillary acidic protein (GFAP) fibers

- Resolution—a cavity bordered by astrocytes, their processes, and GFAP fibers (gliosis) after all necrotic debris has been removed by macrophages (Fig. 25.1).
- Distant effects—demyelination and gliosis of tracts cut by the infarct

● Border-zone (watershed) infarction

- Occurs in areas at the junctions of fields of supply of two or three major vessels; these areas are supplied by the smallest terminal vessels and are particularly vulnerable to generalized reduction of blood flow (e.g., shock, cardiac arrest with resuscitation)

● Other common causes of vascular occlusion and infarction

- Embolization—often results in hemorrhagic (red) rather than anemic (white) infarction; infarcts of any etiology are often a mixture of anemic and hemorrhagic areas

- *Note:* Hemorrhagic infarction in the nervous system is usually a "reflow" phenomenon, when blood again flows through temporarily occluded vessels (e.g., breakup of an occlusive embolus) into an infarcted area, it leaks out of damaged vessels and infiltrates the infarcted tissue. ***Do not* confess hemorrhagic infarction with intracerebral hemorrhage.**

- Blood diseases (e.g., leukemic leukostatic plugging; sickle cell plugging)
- Iatrogenic (e.g., surgical occlusion, air embolism)
- Thrombosis because of intravascular or extravascular infection or vasculitis
- Fat emboli following long bone fracture (grossly appears as myriads of petechial hemorrhages especially in the white matter)

- **Intracerebral hemorrhage (hematoma)**

  - A solid mass of blood from a ruptured intraparenchymal artery that pushes the brain substance aside; *do not* confuse hemorrhage (hematoma) with hemorrhagic infarction
    - Causes include

      - Hypertension (**the most common historical correlate**)—predisposes to arteriolar sclerosis, including segmental dilations (Charcot-Bouchard aneurysms) leading to rupture, most commonly in the basal ganglia and thalamus
      - Vascular anomalies—arterial, capillary, venous, mixed, and cavernous
      - Inflammation—infectious or noninfectious vasculitis
      - Neoplasms (especially metastatic choriocarcinoma, melanoma, bronchogenic and renal cell carcinomas)
      - Trauma
      - Clotting disturbances
      - Aneurysm rupture (atherosclerotic or "congenital" aneurysms of the circle of Willis)—with a high-pressure jet of blood directed into the parenchyma
      - Cerebral amyloid angiopathy (β-amyloid deposition in the walls of leptomeningeal and superficial cortical arteries) *in the absence of systemic amyloidosis*

    - Effects

      - The hematoma—acts as a suddenly occurring mass (Fig. 25.2); rapid rise of intracranial pressure may lead to herniations
      - Edema in the surrounding parenchyma
      - Dissection of the hematoma into the cerebrospinal fluid space—external subarachnoid space (rarely) or ventricular system (commonly)
      - Herniations
      - Secondary (Duret) hemorrhages—midbrain and pons (never the medulla) and middle cerebellar peduncle; related to sudden increase in pressure above the tentorium

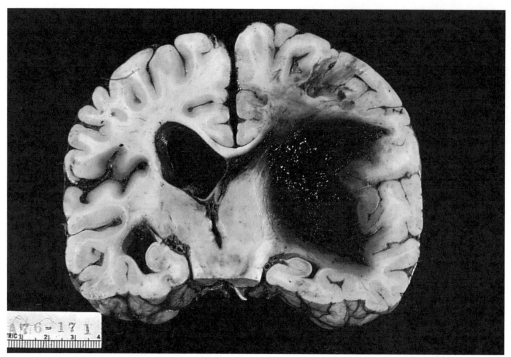

Fig. 25.2 The circle of Willis is viewed from above (the brain side). A large "berry" aneurysm is located at the junction of the right internal carotid artery stump and the posterior communicating artery, one of the most common locations for a "congenital" aneurysm. Note the absence of atherosclerotic plaques in this 25-year-old female. The aneurysm had ruptured, causing devastating subarachnoid hemorrhage.

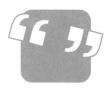

- Resolution—similar to the resolution of ischemic infarction, with removal of necrotic tissue by macrophages; astrogliosis in the adjacent parenchyma

● **Aneurysms**

- Atherosclerotic aneurysms—similar to atherosclerotic aneurysms elsewhere

- "Congenital" aneurysms—not found at birth; probably caused by a congenital or acquired weakness of the arterial wall, which leads to aneurysm formation under the steady pounding of the pulse

    - Always found at the branch points of the arteries of the circle of Willis, most frequently at the internal carotid-posterior communicating artery junctions (Fig. 25.3) and at the anterior communicating artery-anterior cerebral artery junctions (but also elsewhere on the circle, including the middle cerebral artery trifurcation and rostral tip of the basilar artery); often they are multiple

    - *Note:* The term "berry" aneurysm, frequently applied to the "congenital" aneurysm, is a morphologically descriptive term. An atherosclerotic aneurysm, if it looks like a "berry," may also be called a "berry."

    - Rupture—results in subarachnoid hemorrhage (or intraparenchymal hemorrhage, if the jet of blood from the rupture is directed into the substance of the brain); may obstruct the flow and reab-

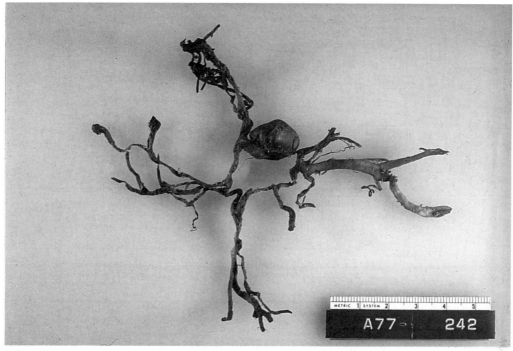

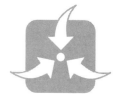

Fig. 25.3 A large, recent intracerebral hemorrhage is centered in the right posterior basal ganglia-thalamic region. Note the general enlargement of the right cerebral hemisphere, partially caused by the mass of the hemorrhage and partially caused by edema. A small amount of blood is present in the right lateral ventricle because of early dissection of the hemorrhage into the ventricle at a more anterior site, not shown in this photograph.

sorption of cerebrospinal fluid and increase intracranial pressure; morbidity and mortality high

- Mycotic (septic) aneurysms—because of infection of the vessel wall
- Dissections (rare)

● **Vascular anomalies (malformations)**

- Arterial, venous, capillary (telangiectases) mixed, cavernous, and anomalies with unidentifiable vessel types all occur, with or without arteriovenous connections.

  - May bleed, act as mass lesions, form irritative foci triggering seizures, or be clinically silent

■ **Infectious Diseases**

● **Noninfectious causes of inflammation**

- Infarction; radiation injury; toxins; chemical injury; neoplasms
- Any process where necrosis present

● **Responses of the CNS to infectious agents—limited and stereotyped (Table 25.3)**

● **Origins of CNS infection**

- Most are secondary to infections outside the CNS and reach the CNS

  - Via the blood stream
  - By direct extension from adjacent structures

Table 25.3   *Patterns of Inflammation in Central Nervous System Infection*

Type of Inflammation	Typical Infections
Acute (suppurative)	Acute bacterial infection*; other acute infections if necrosis is present
Chronic (mononuclear)	Fungal and viral infections; tertiary neurosyphilis; toxoplasmosis; autoimmunue processes
Granulomatous	Mycobacterial, some fungal infections; parasitic worm, larvae, and ova infestations; tertiary neurosyphilis (granulomatous arteritis, gumma)
No inflammation	Slow virus infections (prion diseases)

*Polymorphonuclear inflammation is pure only in the earliest stages of infection.
Chronic inflammatory cells join the inflammatory exudate within hours.

Table 25.4   *Sites (Compartments) of Central Nervous System Infections**

Site	Comments
Bone	Osteomyelitis or paranasal sinus infections may spread inward to involve dura, leptomeninges, cranial nerves, vessels, CNS parenchyma
Cranial epidural space	The outer dural layer is the endosteum of the cranial bones; the cranial epidural space is a potential space but is limited by the tight attachment of the dura to the bones
Spinal epidural space	A large, open space, filled with adipose tissue and fluid, an excellent culture medium for infectious agents; spinal epidural infections enlarge and spread rapidly, compressing the spinal cord
Dura	Pachymeningitis (infection of the dura)
Subdural space	Subdural abscess (empyema)
Subarachnoid space	Leptomeningitis (infection in cerebrospinal spinal fluid space)
CNS parenchyma	Cerebritis, encephalitis (diffuse inflammation of the brain); myelitis (inflammation of the spinal cord)
Vessels and nerves	Infectious vasculitis, neuritis

Note: Infection in one compartment is not necessarily exclusive and often involves, or spreads to, other compartments.
CNS, Central nervous system.

- Along vessels and nerves entering and leaving the CNS
- By direct introduction of infectious agents through congenital bony defects (e.g., spina bifida), trauma, or surgery

● Infections—occur in various structures or spaces (compartments) of, or adjacent to, the nervous system (Table 25.4)

● Suppurative infections

— *Acute purulent cerebrospinal leptomeningitis (meningitis)—most common CNS infection*

- The most common organism varies with age (Table 25.5).
- The brain and spinal cord are swollen and congested.
- Subarachnoid exudate—pus—extends from sulci over the con-

Table 25.5 *Most Common Microorganisms in Acute Bacterial Leptomeningitis*

AGE OF PATIENT	ORGANISM
Neonatal period	Coliforms and Group B Streptococci
Infancy and early childhood	*Streptococcus pneumoniae**
Middle childhood—adulthood	*Streptococcus pneumoniae; Neisseria meningitidus;* especially during spring and fall epidemics
Older adults and the aged	*Streptococcus pneumoniae*

*Because of the now widely used inoculation against *Haemophilus influenzae B, Streptococcus pneumoniae* has replaced *H. influenzae,* previously the most common organism by far, as the most common organism in acute bacterial meningitis during the childhood period. Staphylococci, streptococci, and gram-negative bacilli are common at any age.

vexities and crowns of the gyri, distending the subarachnoid space, often obscuring the leptomeningeal blood vessels. After 2 to 3 days, lymphocytes, plasma cells, and macrophages appear.

- The ependyma and choroid plexuses may be infected. Meningitis may begin as choroid plexus infection (blood borne) and spread outward from the ventricles.

- Even if the infection is controlled and cured, the leptomeninges may heal with slow fibrosis leading to obstructive hydrocephalus because of obstruction of cerebrospinal fluid (CSF) circulation and resorption.

- Waterhouse-Friderichsen syndrome involves bacteremia (usually meningococcemia) with **adrenal hemorrhage** (adrenal apoplexy), disseminated intravascular coagulation, and purpura and skin sloughing.

- Involvement of the parenchyma includes abscess or generalized cerebritis—a relatively rare complication.

- Vessels and nerves may be infected in the subarachnoid space, resulting in infarction and cranial nerve deficits (common complications).

- Death occurs from irritation of the brain, swelling, herniations, infarcts, hemorrhages, and disruption of cerebral function.

- The CSF in acute leptomeningitis exhibits the following:

  - Polymorphonuclear cells—greater than 1 neutrophil/mm^3 *by the usual counting methods* is abnormal

  - Elevated protein

  - Decreased glucose (usually about ⅔ of the blood glucose); therefore, a **blood** glucose level is essential at the time of lumbar puncture

  - Neutrophils, not bacteria—mainly responsible for the decreased CSF glucose levels

— *Cerebral or spinal cord parenchymal abscess*

- Etiology—infected emboli or extension of infection from adjacent structures (e.g., mastoiditis following otitis media)

- May be multiple
- Often at grey-white matter junctions
- Central liquefactive necrosis with acute inflammation and surrounding edema in the initial stages
- Resolution—formation of the pyogenic membrane—the developing wall of the abscess—formed by glial cells and processes and true granulation tissue, including fibroblasts and collagen (exception to the rule that fibroblasts usually do not take part in CNS processes)

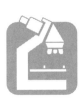

— *Epidural abscess*

- Cranial epidural abscess is limited from spreading by the tight attachment of the endosteal dura to the cranial bones.
- Spinal epidural abscess forms in a space that contains loose fibroadipose tissue and fluid, an excellent culture medium; the abscess expands rapidly, producing mechanical pressure on the spinal cord and infective vasculitis with spinal cord infarcts. Prompt surgical decompression and antibiotic therapy are essential to prevent paralysis.

— *Subdural empyema (abscess)*

- Infection may erode into the subarachnoid space causing leptomeningitis.
- Infection may track back along the emissary veins (infective thrombophlebitis) to the brain, causing cerebritis or brain abscess.

● Granulomatous CNS disease

— *Tuberculous meningitis*

- Often this is a disease of children, acquired from a close relative. Also common in acquired immunodeficiency syndrome (AIDS) and other immunodeficient patients, drug addicts, and immigrants from certain parts of the world.
- CNS infection is secondary to disease elsewhere, usually the lungs.
- Blood-borne mycobacteria lodge in the parenchyma, forming miliary granulomas. One or more of these granulomas may rupture into the CSF space where the bacteria multiply rapidly, forming granulomas.
- The heavy inflammatory exudate settles to the base of the brain and percolates up over the convexities of the cerebral hemispheres.
- Granulomas grow larger by coalescence of adjacent smaller granulomas.
- Drug treatment may not be effective because of the emergence of drug-resistant strains.
- Healing is accompanied by progressive fibrosis of the leptomeninges obstructing CSF circulation, resulting in slowly developing obstructive hydrocephalus.
- Endarteritis, endothelial cell proliferation, thromboses, and adventitial fibrosis of meningeal blood vessels may result in parenchymal ischemia.
- Tuberculoma is a large granuloma that may mimic a neoplasm.

— *Other granulomatous infections*

- Include nocardia, fungi, toxoplasma, and parasitic worms, larvae, and ova

— *Sarcoidosis*

- Although probably not infectious, resembles tuberculosis

— *Syphilis (lues)—"the great imitator"*

- Primary lesion—the **chancre** or venereal sore; resolves spontaneously
- Secondary stage—occurs 2 to 10 weeks after the chancre, with rash, fever, lymphadenopathy, headache; resolves spontaneously
- Both primary and secondary stages—may be accompanied by mild leptomeningitis with cerebrospinal fluid pleocytosis

Tertiary stage—onset occurs years after secondary stage

MENINGOVASCULAR NEUROSYPHILIS

- Chronic mononuclear meningitis (lymphocytes, **plasma cells,** macrophages)
- Proliferative endarteritis (endarteritis obliterans) and granulomatous arteritis of leptomeningeal vessels

PARENCHYMATOUS TERTIARY NEUROSYPHILIS

- Tabes dorsalis (locomotor ataxia)

  - Destruction of sensory neurons in the posterior root ganglia or their afferent sensory axons between the posterior root ganglia and the cord results in demyelination and nerve fiber loss in the posterior columns. Only fibers that will enter the ipsilateral posterior column of the cord are affected.
  - Patients show loss of position and vibratory sense and loss of two-point discrimination, most pronounced in the lower extremities.
  - Romberg's sign—falling if the eyes are closed, when the patient has no proprioceptive clues to position in space.
  - Tabetic gait—a slapping gait because of loss of position sense in the legs; traumatic arthritis of the knee joints (Charcot joints) eventually results.

- General paralysis of the insane (GPI)

  - Neuronal loss and disorganization of the frontal cortex ("wind-blown cortex"); fibrosis of the frontal leptomeninges
  - Mononuclear perivascular inflammation in the cortex and mononuclear leptomeningitis with numerous plasma cells in the exudate
  - Rod cells (microglia) with elongated nuclei in the frontal cortex
  - Spirochetes present
  - *Note:* Spirochetes *cannot* be demonstrated in meningovascular syphilis or tabes dorsalis.

GUMMA (SYPHILITIC GRANULOMA)

- The only unique lesion of syphilis; may occur in any tissue or organ

● **Other bacterial and rickettsial infections involving the nervous system**

- Actinomycosis (*Actinomyces bovis* or *A. israelii*), a filamentous bacterium; abscesses contain sulfur granules—yellow colonies of the organisms

- Rickettsial diseases—Rocky Mountain spotted fever *(Rickettsia rickettsii)* and epidemic typhus *(R. prowazekii)* typically show necrosis of small vessels, swollen endothelial cells, and glial nodules (glial shrubs) within the neutrophil

- Lyme disease *(Borrelia burgdorferi))*—now common in the eastern United States, spread by the deer tick

● **Parasites**

- Schistosomes—frequently cause granulomatous lesions when CNS involved

- *Taenia solium (Cysticercus cellulosae)*—pork tapeworm larvae encyst in brain or meninges with little inflammatory reaction until larvae die; then intense inflammatory and granulomatous reaction occurs

- Malaria—falciparum is the only variety of CNS malaria; organisms infect red blood cells, causing plugging of cerebral capillaries, tissue ischemia, and infarction

- Amebiasis *(Naegleria* species)—free-living amoeba found in fresh water ponds, lakes, and, occasionally, swimming pools; organism enters through nose, uses olfactory nerves to reach CNS, and causes acute, severe (and almost always fatal) meningitis

- Toxoplasmosis *(Toxoplasma gondii)*—common in cat feces; humans acquire organisms in utero (transplacental congenital infection) or from environment, especially if immunosuppressed; congenital infection—severe, with mental retardation, granulomatous or subacute inflammatory CNS lesions, intracerebral calcifications, and hydrocephalus; acquired infection—usually mild in nonimmunosuppressed individuals, but chorioretinitis leading to blindness may occur; now one of the most common and most severe infections, and a leading killer, in AIDS

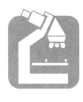

● **Conventional virus infections**

- Table 25.6 lists viruses that cause CNS disease. This list is not inclusive.

- In general, acute viral meningitis and/or encephalomyelitis shows the following:

  - Congestion, hemorrhage, swelling, focal necrosis of the parenchyma

  - Leptomeningeal and intraparenchymal perivascular mononuclear inflammatory infiltrates (perivascular cuffing)

  - Death of neurons with phagocytosis of the dead cells by mononuclear or polymorphonuclear inflammatory cells (neuronophagia—literally "eating of neurons") with tissue necrosis and edema—may be focal or widespread

  - Glial nodules (glial shrubs or Babes' nodes)—mononuclear inflammatory and glial cells, including macrophages and microglia, collect at sites of neuronal destruction

  - Demyelination and astrogliosis of the affected areas—result if the patient survives

  - Some DNA viruses (e.g., herpes, cytomegalovirus, adenovirus, papovaviruses and **measles virus in subacute sclerosing panen-**

Table 25.6	*Viruses That Infect the Nervous System*		

TYPE	VIRUS	DISEASE	INCLUSION
RNA			
	Arboviruses, (arthropod-borne) including togavirus, flavivirus, bunyavirus	Encephalitis*	None
	Enteroviruses including picorna, coxsackie, echo viruses	Encephalitis*	None
	Polio virus	Poliomyelitis	
	Rhabdovirus	Rabies	Intracytoplasmic—"Negri body"
	Retroviruses (HTLV-I and HIV)	T cell leukemia-lymphoma & AIDS	None
	Arenavirus	Lymphocytic choriomeningitis	None
	Paramyxovirus (measles virus)	Subacute sclerosing panencephalitis	Cowdry type A intranuclear
DNA			
	Herpesviruses	Encephalitis	Cowdry type A intranuclear; CMV also has intracytoplasmic inclusions
	Papova (JC virus)	Progressive multifocal leukoencephalopathy	Cowdry type A intranuclear
	Adenovirus	Encephalitis	Cowdry type A intranuclear

Note: Where encephalitis is noted, leptomeningitis, myelitis, and neuritis may also occur.
HTLV, Human T cell lymphotropic virus; *HIV,* human immunodeficiency virus; *CMV,* cytomegalovirus.

cephalitis are associated with prominent *intranuclear* inclusion bodies, usually eosinophilic, surrounded by a halo (Cowdry type A inclusions).

• Some viruses (herpes simplex 1 and 2, varicella-zoster, cytomegalovirus [CMV]) may occur as latent infections and cause acute manifestations when activated.

— *Specific viral infections*

• Poliomyelitis is an RNA gastrointestinal virus infection. It may produce a nonspecific encephalomyelitis, but some strains are tropic and lethal to large motor neurons of the spinal cord and brain stem motor and reticular formation neurons (bulbar polio) resulting in respiratory paralysis and neurogenic (denervation) muscular atrophy.

   • The epidemiology of poliomyelitis is similar to that of multiple sclerosis (i.e., these diseases are rare in the tropics and become more prevalent as the distance from the equator increases).

   • Some victims of polio in early life develop postpolio syndrome years later, with progressive disability, weakness, and muscle wasting, clinically similar to amyotrophic lateral sclerosis.

• Rabies is an RNA virus carried in the saliva of animals (such as dogs, cats, skunks, raccoons, rabbits, foxes, and bats).

   • Virus is inoculated into the skin by a bite or inhalation (bat guano dust); it travels up the nerves to reach the spinal cord or brain resulting in severe mononuclear encephalomyeli-

tis, delirium, headache, spasms of pharyngeal muscles, and profuse salivation precipitated by attempts to eat and drink. Coma, respiratory paralysis, and death ensue.

- Characteristic intracytoplasmic inclusion bodies (Negri bodies) form in larger neurons, particularly the pyramidal neurons of Ammon's horn and cerebellar Purkinje cells.

- Herpes simplex type 1 (HSV-1) most often causes hemorrhagic and necrotic meningoencephalitis, usually of the mesial temporal lobes and other portions of the limbic system.

- Herpes simplex type 2 (HSV-2) causes mononuclear meningitis in adults and severe necrotizing encephalitis of infants.

- CMV is an intrauterine infection that often causes necrotizing and calcifying periventricular encephalitis, multifocal parenchymal focal necrosis, and calcifications resulting in prematurity or stillbirth. Both intranuclear and intracytoplasmic inclusions occur. CMV also causes encephalitis in AIDS and other immunodeficient patients.

- Varicella-zoster virus remains latent in the trigeminal and other ganglia and reactivates as painful vesicles along the course of cutaneous nerves (shingles), cranial vasculitis, or meningoencephalomyelitis.

- Adenovirus may produce severe encephalitis with prominent intranuclear inclusion bodies.

- Human immunodeficiency virus (HIV-1) directly infects the CNS, gaining entry via macrophages. It causes encephalomyelitis, often associated with dementia or psychosis (AIDS-dementia complex), leukoencephalopathy with multinucleated giant cells, spongy white-matter degeneration of the spinal cord (vacuolar myelopathy), and, in children, microcephaly, leukoencephalopathy, and calcifications of the basal ganglia and white matter.

    - Various opportunistic infections, often multiple, are common in AIDS, including tuberculosis (TB), toxoplasmosis, CMV, cryptococcosis, and aspergillosis.
    - CNS lymphoma (usually large cell, cleaved, or uncleaved) complicates approximately 5% of cases.

- ● "Slow" virus diseases—diseases caused by

    - Conventional viruses acting in a chronic, delayed, or unusual manner
    - An abnormal form of a normal extracellular protein (prion protein), causing invariably fatal CNS diseases, with long incubation periods, but without cellular inflammatory or antibody responses

    — *"Slow" virus diseases caused by conventional viruses*

        - Progressive multifocal leukoencephalopathy (PML)

            - Usually caused by the JC or BK strain of the papovavirus group
            - Affects patients with immune compromise or paralysis

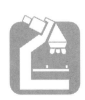

            - Demarcated, softened, areas of white-matter degeneration, bizarre, neoplastic-like astrocytes, and enlarged oligodendroglial nuclei with intranuclear viral inclusions characteristic; inflammation usually minimal

        - Subacute sclerosing panencephalitis (SSPE)

- Caused by persistence of measles virus in the CNS
- Children and young adults affected—all have had measles, usually severe, and carry high antimeasles antibody titers in blood and spinal fluid
- Onset—occurs years after acute measles, with personality changes, intellectual deterioration, involuntary movements; coma and death 6 months to 2 years after clinical onset
- Brain—atrophic with severe perivascular mononuclear inflammation, neuronal loss, demyelination, and astrogliosis
- **Intranuclear** (*Note:* measles virus is an RNA virus) Inclusion bodies composed of smooth, tubular nucleocapsids found in CNS cells

— *Unconventional slow-virus diseases*

- Characteristics of the unconventional slow-virus agent

  - The primary infectious particle (prion) is made of a stable, abnormal form of a normal extracellular protein (prion protein).
  - No nucleic acid is present in the prion.
  - One or more amino acid substitutions (because of mutations of the prion protein gene on chromosome 20 or posttranslational abnormalities of the prion protein) changes the globular prion protein to a β-pleated sheet, which is infectious and highly stable, causing fatal diseases in animals (e.g., scrapie, bovine scrapie, transmissible mink encephalopathy) and in humans (e.g., Creutzfeld-Jakob disease (CJD), Gerstmann-Sträussler-Scheinker disease (GSS), and fatal familial insomnia (FFI). (Kuru, in the Fore people of the eastern New Guinea highlands, transmitted by cannibalism, is now probably eradicated.)
  - Normal prion protein molecules use the infectious protein molecule as a "template," converting to the abnormal form, and thus apparently "replicating" without benefit of nucleic acids.

- Characteristics of unconventional slow virus diseases

  - They have long, asymptomatic incubation periods (possibly up to 20 years).
  - Clinical disease is subacute and progressive, lasting months to years, with dementia, always ending fatally.
  - Lesions are restricted to the CNS, although infectious material is recoverable from many other tissues and body fluids.
  - They are transmissible under certain conditions to a limited range of experimental animals—and to other humans.
  - Microscopically, clear areas within grey matter cell processes (especially postsynaptic dendrites) appear like holes in a sponge—hence "spongiform encephalopathies." Accompanying astrogliosis is severe.
  - Deposits of prion protein amyloid may be present.
  - Fever, inflammation, antibody response, and spinal fluid changes **do not occur.**

- Mechanisms of human transmission include corneal and dural transplantation, improper sterilization of cortical electrodes, hereditary transmission in GSS and FFI, contaminated human pituitary growth hormone derived from human autopsy-harvested human pituitary glands and ingestion of infected brains (Kuru). Person-to-person contact does *not* transmit these diseases.

● **Fungal diseases**

- CNS infections are usually secondary to infection elsewhere, often the lung or nasal sinuses. Immunoincompetence is an important risk factor; diabetes mellitus is also a risk factor. Many fungi have a geographic predilection.

— *Aspergillosis (Aspergillus niger* or *A. fumigatus)*

- This is a filamentous, branching mycelil fungus; new branches make an acute angle with the main trunk.
- CNS lesions include abscesses with acute inflammation, chronic granulomas, vascular invasion with thromboses and infarcts, and chronic active meningitis. Abscesses may contain masses of mycelia (fungus balls).

— *Candidiasis (Candida albicans* and others)*

- These are common organisms in the mouth, intestinal tract, and vagina in normal persons; organisms may have filamentous or yeastlike forms.
- CNS lesions include disseminated small abscesses or meningitis, especially in infants.

— *Phycomycosis, zygomycosis, mucormycosis*

- Several species of these fungi cause infection of lungs, ears, nervous system, and intestinal tract, with necrotizing lesions and suppuration. These are especially common in patients with uncontrolled diabetes mellitus, leukemia, or other debilitating diseases, especially when immunodeficiency is present.
- Branching, nonseptate filaments, much larger and broader than aspergillus, are attached to the main trunk of the mycelium at nearly right angles.
- Often these grow intravascularly, causing thromboses and infarction.

— *Histoplasmosis*

- *Histoplasma capsulatum,* a 1 to 4 micron in diameter, oval, yeastlike fungus, common in the dropping of birds (chickens, pigeons, starlings) and bats only rarely causes CNS disease, usually granulomatous meningitis; lesions may mimic TB. The immunoincompetent are at risk.

— *Cryptococcosis (torulosis)*

- *Cryptococcus neoformans,* a budding yeastlike fungus with a thick, mucopolysaccharide capsule is intensely antigenic and is found in soil and bird droppings. The CNS and lungs are most often affected.
- CNS lesions include chronic mild-to-severe mononuclear men-

ingitis or granulomatous meningitis. Cystic spaces in the parenchyma, teeming with organisms but virtually free of inflammation, are characteristic.

— *North American blastomycosis*

   • *Blastomyces dermatitidis,* a budding yeastlike organism, occasionally causes granulomatous meningitis. Lung and skin lesions are more common and severe. The organisms reproduce with single buds.

— *Coccidioidomycosis*

   • *Coccidioides immitis,* a round fungus with a thick, refractile wall, inhabits the soil of the dry regions of the American Southwest, San Joaquin Valley of California (Valley Fever), and other desert regions. Inhaled with the dust, the spores develop and cause pulmonary and disseminated disease.

   • Granulomatous meningitis is the most common CNS lesion.

   • It reproduces by endosporulation.

■ Neoplasms

● Primary intraparenchymal or intraventricular neoplasms (gliomas and tumors of primitive neuronal origin)

   • They are usually infiltrative and unencapsulated (because of the paucity of fibroblastic activity in the CNS); therefore, most are ultimately fatal.

   • They may occur in areas inaccessible to surgery (e.g., basal ganglia, brain stem).

   • They rarely metastasize outside the CNS but may spread throughout the spinal fluid space.

   • They may originate in multiple areas simultaneously (multicentric origin) or in a wide field of simultaneous neoplastic transformation (e.g., gliomatosis cerebri).

   • They may transform, in a relatively short period of time, from well differentiated and slow growing to malignant.

   • Because of the enclosed environment of the CNS (the "closed box"), any enlarging neoplasm will eventually cause increased CSF pressure and shifts of cranial contents (herniations).

   • They constitute approximately 9% of all neoplasms and in children are the second most common site of neoplasia (after the hematopoietic system).

   • Most intraparenchymal neoplasms of adults arise above the tentorium cerebelli; most childhood intraparenchymal neoplasms arise below.

● Glial neoplasms

   • These are neoplasms arising from astrocytes, oligodendrogliocytes, ependymal cells and choroid plexus cells. (*Note:* A neoplasm arising from microglia is not recognized.)

   • Table 25.7 shows a classification of glial neoplasms.

   • Table 25.8 lists the incidence of glial neoplasms and neoplasms of neuronal origin.

   • In children, the incidence of primary glial and neuronal neoplasms is different than in adults (Table 25.9).

   • Many grading schemes have been proposed, with variable prognostic

Table 25.7 *A Classification of Common Glial Neoplasms*

GROUP	NEOPLASMS
Astrocytic Origin	
Benign	Fibrillary and protoplasmic astrocytomas, pilocytic astrocytoma, subependymal giant cell astrocytoma
Malignant	Gemistocytic astrocytoma, anaplastic astrocytoma, glioblastoma multiforme
Oligodendrogliocyte Origin	
Benign	Oligodendroglioma
Malignant	Anaplastic oligodendroglioma
Ependymal Cell Origin	
Benign	Ependymoma, cellular ependymoma, papillary ependymoma, myxopapillary ependymoma, subependymoma
Malignant	Anaplastic ependymoma
Choroid Plexus Origin	
Benign	Papilloma of the choroid plexus
Malignant	"Carcinoma" (malignant papilloma)
Mixed Glial Cell Origin	
Benign	Oligoastrocytoma
Malignant	Anaplastic oligoastrocytoma (occasionally other cell types are present)
Diffuse (Malignant)	Gliomatosis cerebri

Table 25.8 *Incidence of Primary Glial and Neuronal CNS Neoplasms (All Ages)*

NEOPLASM	INCIDENCE (%)
Glioblastoma multiforme (Astrocytoma—grade IV)	55
Astrocytomas (all other grades)	20.5
Ependymomas	6
Oligodendrogliomas	5
Choroid plexus papillomas	2
Colloid cysts of the third ventricle	2
Others	3.5
Neoplasms of neuronal origin: primitive neuroectodermal tumors—medulloblastomas, neuroblastomas, etc.	6

CNS, Central nervous system.

ability. Generally, grades I and II are "benign," while grades III and IV are "malignant." The degree of cellularity and anaplasia increases from grades I to IV.

• In considering benign vs. malignant glial neoplasms, because of the inability of the CNS to encapsulate neoplasms and because of the rarity of

Table 25.9 *Incidence of Primary Glial and Neuronal Neoplasms in Children*

Neoplasm	Incidence
Astrocytomas (all grades and sites)	48%
Ependymomas	8%
Neoplasms of neuronal origin: primitive neuroectodermal tumors—medulloblastomas, neuroblastomas, etc.	44%

metastases from primary CNS neoplasms, these terms do not have the same meaning as these terms applied to neoplasms of other organs.

- Benign—fewer cells per microscopic field, higher differentiation (the cells resemble their non-neoplastic counterparts), less pleomorphism, **presumption of slower growth**
- Malignant—higher cellularity, significant anaplasia and pleomorphism, mitoses, **presumption of rapid growth**
- However, even benign neoplasms—if not completely eradicated (as they often are not) will kill, eventually

— *Benign astrocytoma (grades I and II)*

- Fibrillary astrocytoma—cell processes form an interlacing loose network; usually GFAP is expressed; mitoses not present

- Protoplasmic astrocytoma—rare; small cells show little GFAP expression

- Pilocytic astrocytoma—slow growing, moderately circumscribed, densely fibrillar, often located near the midline of the cerebral hemispheres and brain stem; many microcysts in the stroma may coalesce into larger cysts; carrot-shaped, eosinophilic, Rosenthal fibers within astrocytic processes (also seen in areas of dense, non-neoplastic gliosis) are characteristic; usually a tumor of children

- Subependymal giant cell astrocytoma—masses of large astrocyte-like cells (some possibly of neuronal origin) in the walls of the lateral ventricles in patients with tuberous sclerosis project into the ventricular lumens like candle drippings ("gutterings"); mitotic activity negligible; calcifications common; grow slowly, if at all, and sometimes are totally resectable; occasionally may transform to true astrocytomas

— *Malignant astrocytoma*

- Gemistocytic astrocytoma—cells resemble gemistocytic astrocytes with copious pink cytoplasm in a loose fibrillar background; mitoses usually not present; although cytologically benign, these tumors tend to convert to malignant astrocytoma and are considered malignant

- Anaplastic astrocytoma (grade III)—higher cellularity and pleomorphism than benign astrocytomas; moderate nuclear atypia and mitotic activity

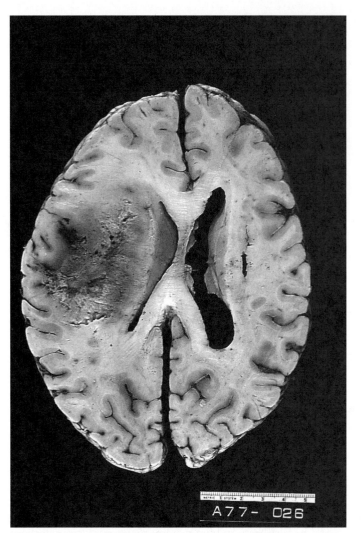

Fig. 25.4 The brain has been sectioned horizontally in the plane of the computed tomography (CT) scan. The frontal poles are above, the occipital poles below. A glioblastoma multiforme occupies almost the entire midlateral portion of the left cerebral hemisphere. Note the enlargement of the left hemisphere and the compression of the lateral ventricle ("mass effect") in the region of the tumor. Solid neoplastic and softened, necrotic tissue and small hemorrhages are apparent on the cut surface of the tumor.

- Glioblastoma multiforme (grade IV astrocytoma)—rapidly growing, highly anaplastic (Fig. 25.4), but mitoses may be surprisingly scanty

  - Generally occurs after the age of 45 years, grows rapidly, spreads to the opposite hemisphere via the commissures
  - Pseudopalisading, areas of necrosis bordered by small, dark tumor cells, an important diagnostic feature
  - May contain bizarre tumor giant cells
  - Areas of more differentiated neoplastic astrocytes often admixed

- Capillary proliferation with endothelial cell proliferation and swelling, in the tumor and surrounding parenchyma, common (also seen with other malignant neoplasms including metastases)
- Prognosis poor
- Occasionally is admixed with (fibro)sarcoma (gliosarcoma)

— *Oligodendrogliomas*

- Benign

  - Slowly growing
  - Composed of small, dark, round or oval nuclei "floating" in clear cytoplasm, an artifactitious appearance of oligodendrogliocytes
  - Delicate blood vessels—divide the tumor into pseudolobules
  - Calcifications common and often seen on plain radiographs
  - Sudden, often fatal, hemorrhage—may occur without warning

- Malignant

  - Rapidly growing
  - High cellularity, pleomorphism, and mitotic activity, and often capillary proliferation and focal necrosis
  - May be morphologically similar to glioblastoma; however, prognosis may be slightly better.

— *Ependymomas*

- Benign

  - Slowly growing, minimally invasive; related to the ventricular walls and central canal region of the spinal cord
  - Moderately cellular; cells have bland, relatively uniform round, or oval nuclei without mitotic activity
  - Neoplastic cells—often form rings (pseudorosettes) around blood vessels; nuclei stand well back from the vessel wall leaving a nucleus-free zone composed of the tapering processes of the tumor cells; GFAP may be present in the pseudorosettes
  - Small rings of tumor cells—may form canal-like structures (ependymal canals), a diagnostic feature
  - Neoplastic ependymal cells—often have cilia
  - If tumor well demarcated and accessible to surgery, prognosis good
  - Cellular ependymoma—a variant with sheets of uniform neoplastic ependymal cells, no mitotic activity, and no perivascular pseudorosettes; behavior similar to the above
  - Papillary ependymoma—a variant, with papillary structures similar to a papilloma of the choroid plexus
  - Myxopapillary ependymoma—ependymomas are most common neoplasm of spinal cord; this benign variant occurs in cauda equina-filum terminal, conus medullaris region of the

cord; the tumor cells form a perivascular papillary pattern in a mucinous stroma around blood vessels

- Subependymoma—a slow-growing tumor of adults, often in the fourth ventricle; ependymal cells and astrocytes form a nodular mass in a fibrillary stroma, often with calcifications; tumor rarely causes symptoms and is often an incidental finding at autopsy

  - Malignant

    - Anaplastic ependymoma—highly cellular, with nuclear atypia, high mitotic activity, and capillary and endothelial cell proliferation; necrosis often present; metastasizes (seeds) via the CSF

— *Choroid plexus neoplasms*

- Benign papilloma is an intraventricular tumor, histologically appearing similar to normal choroid plexus.

  - Small foci of necrosis—may be present without ominous significance

  - Forms a bulky intraventricular mass and may obstruct outflow of CSF

- Malignant papilloma (carcinoma of the choroid plexus)

  - Highly anaplastic; resembles metastatic papillary adenocarcinoma; often a tumor of children

  - May seed extensively via the CSF

- Colloid cyst of the third ventricle forms a benign cyst arising in association with the choroid plexus of the third ventricle.

  - The cyst is lined by one or more layers of columnar or flattened cells and is filled with gelatinous "colloid."

  - It may act as a "ball-valve," obstructing CSF outflow through a foramen of Monro or into the cerebral aqueduct. Usually it is surgically removable and curable.

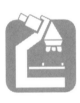

— *Mixed gliomas*

- Gliomas with roughly equal mixtures of multiple neoplastic glial cell type, usually neoplastic astrocytic and oligodendroglial cells, either admixed or in separate areas; occasionally areas of ependymoma present; may be benign or malignant

— *Gliomatosis cerebri*

- Diffuse infiltration of malignant neoplastic glial cells throughout a wide area of the cerebral hemispheres, including more than one lobe; brain stem, cerebellum, and spinal cord may also be involved

● Neuronal and mixed neuronal and glial tumors

— *Primitive neuroectodermal tumors (PNETS)*

- Malignant tumors of early life with small cells, often with a mixture of other cell types, including neurons, glial cells, muscle cells, and melanocytes (multipotential stem cell origin); usually located in the cerebellum

— *Medulloblastoma (a PNET)*

• This is a malignant midline cerebellar tumor of childhood and of young adults with small cells, dark nuclei, a variable number of mitoses, and occasional areas of necrosis.

• Neuroblastic (Homer Wright) rosettes (small circlets of cells with only scanty fibrillar material at the center) are diagnostic.

• Most of these tumors express neuronal markers.

• Extension into the fourth ventricle frequently causes obstruction to CSF outflow.

• Invasion of neighboring brain structures and the leptomeninges is common, as is spread throughout the CSF pathway with establishment of tumor nodules at distant sites.

• Response to radiotherapy is often good (the entire neuraxis must be irradiated).

• It may originate from primitive neuronal and glial cells of the external granular layer of the cerebellum.

— *Desmoplastic medulloblastoma (a PNET)*

• Similar to the medulloblastoma, but usually occurs later in life (late teen period through adulthood), often in the lateral cerebellar hemispheres; may have a slightly better prognosis than midline medulloblastomas

• Dense reticulin-fiber meshworks interspersed with islands of pale medulloblastoma cells, free of reticulin fibers characteristic

— *Other variants of medulloblastomas*

• Tumors with neuronal, astrocytic, melanotic, and muscle elements; all malignant

— *Gangliocytoma*

• A benign, slowly growing tumor of childhood and early adulthood

• Often occurs in the temporal lobes, but may appear at any site

• Neoplastic mature-appearing neurons supported by a stoma of nonneoplastic glial cells

— *Ganglioglioma*

• This tumor is similar to the above, but may be cystic

• Neoplastic neurons admixed with neoplastic glial cells that are the determinant of the rate of growth and prognosis; most of these tumors grow slowly and are benign.

— *Neuroblastoma (a PNET)*

• A highly cellular, malignant neuroblastic tumor, similar to neuroblastomas of other organs, with neuroblastic (Homer Wright) rosette formation

• Rare in childhood, extremely rare in adulthood; may occur at any CNS location, including the spinal cord

● Pineal tumors

— *Pineocytoma*

• This is a rare, differentiated tumor of pineal parenchymal cells.

• Rosettes resembling large neuroblastic rosettes are common.

• The tumor mass may compress adjacent structures, including the tectum of the midbrain, causing loss of upward gaze (Parinaud's syndrome) and obstructive hydrocephalus because of compression of the cerebral aqueduct and anterior fourth ventricle.

— *Pineoblastoma*

• A highly cellular, malignant tumor resembling a medulloblastoma (PNET), including neuroblastic rosette formation

— *Pineal germinoma*

• The most common tumor in the pineal body

• Of germ cell origin, identical to the testicular and ovarian germinomas

• Large, polygonal, neoplastic germ cells admixed with a variable population of lymphocytes

• Similar neoplasms also found at other (midline) sites in the CNS (third ventricle, base of brain) and throughout the body along the germ cell migratory pathway

● **Meningiomas**

• Common (up to 15% of all intracranial tumors and 25% of intraspinal tumors), usually benign, neoplasms arising from arachnoid cells

• Often attached to dura, but also originate at other sites, including ventricular lumens, originating from "rests" of arachnoid cells in the choroid plexuses

• Many histologic subtypes; most benign and, if totally removed, curable

• Common and diagnostic—whorls of meningothelial cells with round, vesicular nuclei or laminated, calcified psammoma bodies

• Some meningiomas fibrous in character; others quite vascular (angiomatous meningiomas); some may exhibit metaplasia with areas of cartilage, bone, or lipoid cells

• Occasional meningiomas exhibit aggressive and invasive characteristics or metastasize to distant organs and must be considered malignant in spite of unimpressive histologic features; other meningiomas are frankly anaplastic

• Invasion of bone, including erosion through both tables of the calvaria, **not** a sign of malignancy

• Meningiomas above the foramen magnum—slightly more common in women than men; spinal cord meningiomas at least 9 times more common in women

● **Nerve tumors**

— *Schwannoma (neurinoma, neurilemoma, "acoustic neuroma")*

• A benign tumor arising from the Schwann cells of the distal but still intracranial portions of cranial nerves III to XII and peripheral nerves

• Most common on cranial nerve VIII and spinal dorsal roots; bilateral cranial nerve VIII schwannomas—pathognomonic of neurofibromatosis type II

- Interlacing bundles of elongated cells (Antoni A tissue) with true palisading (parallel lines of nuclei bordering a nucleus-free area containing the processes of the cells and collagen, but no necrosis)—interspersed with loose, lipid-containing cells (Antoni B tissue)
    - Hemosiderin-containing macrophages often present as a result of small hemorrhages

— *Neurofibroma*

- Composed of a loose mixture of Schwann cells, fibroblasts, perineurial cells, and trapped, nonneoplastic axons; nuclei elongated and wavy; background often myxoid or mucinous; mast cells commonly present
- May occur as a solitary tumor or as part of neurofibromatosis where numerous tumors originate from skin and spinal nerves
    - Malignant transformation may occur (neurogenic sarcoma)

● **Hemangioblastoma**

- A highly vascular tumor, usually of the cerebellum, sometimes growing as a cyst with a "mural nodule" on the wall of the cyst
- Numerous capillary-sized blood vessels—interspersed with cells with hyperchromatic nuclei and lipid- or glycogen-containing cytoplasm
- May elaborate erythropoietin or hemorrhage catastrophically
- Histologically—resembles renal cell carcinoma, clear cell type

● **Pituitary adenomas**

- Arise from the cells of the anterior pituitary (adenohypophysis)
- May (or may not) elaborate one or more pituitary hormones
- Cause upward pressure toward the base of the brain; bitemporal hemianopia from midline pressure on the optic chiasm—a common presenting sign
    - Rarely, malignant transformation may occur

● **Craniopharyngioma**

- This is a benign, cystic, epidermoid or squamous tumor in the region of the infundibular stalk, sella turcica, or third ventricle.
- Bitemporal hemianopia may be an early sign because of pressure on the optic chiasm.
- The cysts often contain cholesterol, squamous pearls, and "machine-oil" squamous debris.
- The tumor originates from remnants of Rathke's pouch, a posterior outpouching of the embryonic stomatodeum, which differentiates into the anterior pituitary gland.

● **Chordoma**

- Originates from remnants of the notochord
- Usually occurs at either end of the spinal axis (clivus or sacrum), but occasionally at any vertebral level
- Masses of foamy physaliferous cells in a mucoid matrix—diagnostic; occasionally appear similar to low-grade chondrosarcoma (chondroid chordoma)
- Its behavior (benign or aggressive) not readily predicted from the microscopic appearance

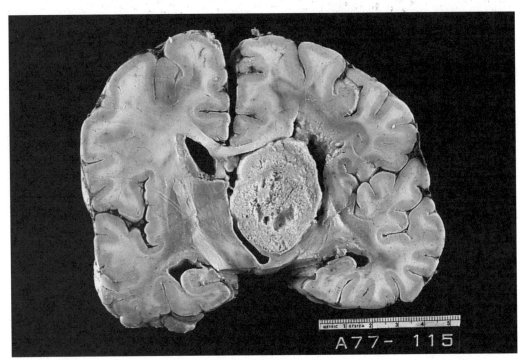

Fig. 25.5 A large, rounded, well-circumscribed, but not encapsulated, mass of metastatic bronchogenic carcinoma is centered in the right thalamus. The tumor is mainly intraparenchymal but encroaches into the right lateral ventricle.

● **Lymphomas**

   • In the nervous system, may occur as part of generalized lymphoid disease or be limited to the nervous system; usually non-Hodgkin's lymphomas, they resemble lymphomas in other organs

   • Occur sporadically or (now commonly) in AIDS and other diseases with immunosuppression

   • A perivascular pattern of infiltrating large-cell, cleaved or noncleaved lymphoma—often called a "microglioma," but is unrelated to microglial cells

● **Metastatic tumors**

   • Accounting for approximately 25% of all CNS tumors, they may be secondary to almost any malignancy outside the CNS; but breast, lung, and kidney and melanoma are the most common sites of origin.

   • They are often spherical, well circumscribed but not encapsulated (Fig. 25.5).

   • Some (particularly choriocarcinoma, melanoma, bronchogenic carcinoma) may hemorrhage massively.

   • Metastases have no blood-brain barrier.

● **Others**

   • Numerous other primary neoplasms occur in the CNS, including lipomas, osteomas, chondromas, angiomas. Their behavior is similar to their counterparts at other sites.

■ Demyelinating Diseases

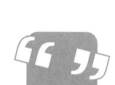

- Myelin, a complex, highly antigenic substance derived from the membranes of myelin-forming cells (oligodendrogliocytes or Schwann cells) may be damaged by infections, toxins, and autoimmune, genetic, and metabolic abnormalities. The presence of an axon is necessary for the formation of myelin, and destruction of the axon results in dissolution of the myelin sheath.

    - Infectious diseases that destroy oligodendrogliocytes or Schwann cells (e.g., progressive multifocal leukoencephalopathy), secondary axonal loss (e.g., infarcts with Wallerian degeneration), neuronal degenerations (e.g., amyotrophic lateral sclerosis), and others are not considered demyelinating diseases, even though loss of myelin may be extensive.

- Demyelinating diseases involve myelin primarily, generally sparing the axons within the sheaths.

    - Myelinoclastic diseases—presumably normal myelin undergoes dissolution because of a delayed cellular immune attack against the myelin; the "trigger" usually unknown but thought to involve an immunologic cross-reaction between myelin antigens and infectious or environmental agent(s).

    - Leukodystrophies—a group of genetically determined diseases in which myelin is abnormally formed (or not formed at all), with extensive demyelination, usually with axonal loss, but with sparing of the myelin of the subcortical cortico-cortical association fibers (U fibers).

● Myelinoclastic diseases

- Acute disseminated encephalomyelitis (ADE)—also known as postinfectious or postvaccinal encephalomyelitis

    - ADE occurs days-to-weeks after an attack of a childhood viral disease or vaccination (such as measles, mumps, chicken pox). The trigger is probably a cross-reaction between myelin and viral antigens. There is disseminated perivenous and pericapillary inflammation with destruction of myelin by mononuclear inflammatory cells. Usually ADE is not fatal, but there is often residual neurologic deficit. It is a "one-shot" disease that does not recur.

    - ADE is the human counterpart of experimental allergic encephalomyelitis (EAE), a laboratory disease induced by the injection of myelin or myelin basic protein, with or without an immunologic adjuvant to speed the reaction.

- Multiple sclerosis (MS)—disseminated sclerosis (disseminated in time, disseminated in space)

    - MS is a disease of young adults (rarely the onset is before puberty) with exacerbations and remissions. Any area of the CNS may be involved; cerebellum, brain stem, or spinal cord are often involved preferentially.

    - Acute MS resembles ADE or EAE with perivenous inflammation and demyelination. In MS, however, adjacent areas of demyelination coalesce into larger plaques with dense demyelination, relatively sharp borders, reactive astrogliosis, and preservation of axons.

    - Plaques are often periventricular (Fig. 25.6), especially at the

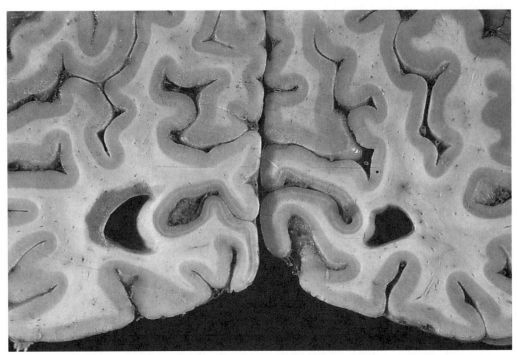

Fig. 25.6 A dark, sharply demarcated multiple sclerosis plaque is present adjacent to the lateral wall of the occipital horn of the left lateral ventricle. Plaques are commonly found adjacent to the walls or at the lateral angles of ventricles.

angles of the lateral ventricles, and may be relatively bilaterally symmetric.

- Anatomic boundaries (i.e., tract boundaries, cortical-white matter junctions, or deep gray nuclei) may be involved (myelin is also present in grey matter areas).

- The optic nerves (optic nerves are fiber tracts of the brain with central myelin) may be involved (acute retrobulbar neuritis) with rapid onset of painless blindness; the retina and optic nerve head appear normal.

- Recurrent attacks occur without apparent reason or warning. Severe neurologic deficit eventually results, but there may be limited return of function after an attack. However, after only one or a few attacks, some patients remain disease free.

- Cause, prevention, and cure are unknown; however, clinical trials are currently underway using β-interferon and various corticosteroids as therapeutic agents in acute attacks and show some promise.

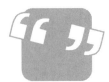

- Acute hemorrhagic leukoencephalitis—a rare, acute, and usually fatal necrotizing, inflammatory, and hemorrhagic demyelinating disease occurring shortly after a minor illness, often a viral upper respiratory infection; edema fluid, acute and chronic inflammatory cells, and fibrin infiltrate perivenous areas and the surrounding parenchyma; this condition is the human counterpart of "hyperacute EAE," a laboratory disease induced by the injection of myelin with two adjuvants.

- **Leukodystrophies (dysmyelinating diseases)**

  - Metachromatic leukodystrophy

    - This is the most common leukodystrophy; it is caused by a defect in sulfatide metabolism (deficiency of arylsulfatase A), a generalized metabolic abnormality caused by a mutation on chromosome 22q.

    - The sulfatide myelin breakdown product, found in both the CNS, peripheral nervous system (PNS), and other organs, is excreted by the kidneys; an office-performed test on urine is diagnostic.

  - Adrenoleukodystrophy

    - A sex-linked (males only) genetic defect (on Xq28) leads to extensive demyelination of the posterior portions of the brain and the accumulation of very long-chain fatty acids in the brain and adrenal cortex, often accompanied by adrenal hypofunction.

    - The demyelinated areas, usually in the posterior portions of the brain, have severe perivascular mononuclear inflammation, unusual for a leukodystrophy. The inflammation is probably immunologically mediated.

  - Krabbe's disease (globoid cell leukodystrophy)

    - A severe dysmyelinating disease without systemic manifestations, causing death in the early childhood period

    - A deficiency of galactocerebroside-β-galactocerebrosidase, caused by a defect on chromosome 14, results in the accumulation of a toxic product (psychosine)

    - Groups ("packets") of large singly nucleated or multinucleated cells accumulate in white matter areas and perivascularly; these cells stain with the periodic acid-Schiff (PAS) reaction

- **Other myelin disorders**

  - Central pontine myelinolysis

    - Demyelination with intramyelin sheath edema, axon loss, and gliosis located in the midline pons

    - Sometimes related to alcoholism, but probably caused by rapid changes in serum osmolality, especially sodium

  - Marchiafava-Bignami disease

    - Changes similar to central pontine myelinolysis, but lesions are in the midline corpus callosum

    - Thought to affect heavy drinkers of Italian red wine (possibly related to naturally occurring cyanide traces in the wine of certain regions)

■ Vitamin Deficiency and Toxic and Metabolic Diseases

- **Thiamine deficiency**

  - Wernicke's encephalopathy

    - This affects alcoholics or others with severe dietary insufficiency and may be fatal if not treated promptly with thiamine replacement.

- Petechial hemorrhages, endothelial swelling, and astrogliosis affect the mamillary bodies, walls of the third ventricle, periaqueductal grey matter, floor of the fourth ventricle, and thalamus.
- Cranial nerve signs, confusion, and ataxia are common clinical manifestations.

- Korsakoff's syndrome
  - Probably chronic (or "burned-out") Wernicke's encephalopathy
  - Atrophy of the same areas affected by Wernicke's encephalopathy, with neuronal loss, hemosiderin pigment deposition, and gliosis
  - Patients often manifest severe loss of recent memory, but construct a well-organized fiction to fill in the gaps in memory (confabulation)

● Vitamin B$_{12}$ deficiency

- Subacute combined degeneration of the spinal cord (posterolateral sclerosis)

  - Pernicious anemia may be also present.
  - Spongy (because of intramyelin sheath edema) demyelination and axonal loss in both the posterior columns (up-going sensory tracts) and posterolateral columns (down-going motor tracts), most severe in the thoracic spinal cord; this may also affect the optic nerves and peripheral nerves. Microscopically it resembles the vacuolar myelopathy of AIDS.
  - Vitamin B$_{12}$ treatment will arrest the myelopathy and the anemia. Folate will promptly reverse the anemia but not the myelopathy.
  - Vitamin B$_{12}$ deficiency may also be caused by infestation with the freshwater fish tapeworm *(Diphyllobothrium latum),* which absorbs the vitamin from the gut.

● Metabolic encephalopathies

- Various metabolic disturbances (e.g., uremia) may cause decreased mentation, including coma. Most cause no, or nonspecific, CNS abnormalities.
- In liver failure (hepatic encephalopathy), large bean-shaped vesicular nuclei (Alzheimer's type II astrocytes) appear in the globus pallidus, cerebellar dentate nuclei, and other areas, particularly when elevated blood ammonia levels are present.

● Storage diseases

- Genetic abnormalities with enzyme deficiencies result in the accumulation of an abnormal substance or intermediate metabolite within neurons and other CNS cells. Table 25.10 provides a summary of important storage diseases.

● **Many metal compounds, environmental pollutants, botanicals, drugs, and chemicals may damage the CNS in various ways. Important toxicities include**

- Lead—in adults causes motor neuropathy; in children, cerebral edema, seizures, and mental retardation
- Organic mercury salts—loss of cerebellar internal granular cells with severe cerebellar dysfunction (Minamata Bay disease)

Table 25.10 *Important Storage Diseases*		
DISEASE	**STORAGE PRODUCT**	**ENZYME DEFICIENCY**
Tay-Sachs	G_{M2} ganglioside	Hexosaminidase A
Gaucher's	Glucocerebroside	Glucocerebrosidase
Niemann-Pick	Sphingomyelin	Sphingomyelinase
G_{M1} Gangliosidosis	G_{M1} Gangliosides	G_{M1}-β-galactosidase A
Mucopolysaccharidoses	Mucopolysaccharides	Various
(Hurler's, Sanfilippo)	(glycosaminoglycans)	
Pompe's	Glycogen	α-1,4-glucosidase

Note: Numerous other diseases and subtypes have been described. Globoid leukodystrophy (Krabbe's disease), adrenoleukodystrophy and metachromatic leukodystrophy, described with the demyelinating diseases, are also characterized by a storage product.

- Arsenic—brain stem necrosis and hemorrhage; peripheral nerve axonal degeneration
- Methyl alcohol—cerebral edema, optic nerve atrophy, retinal ganglion cell loss
- Ethyl alcohol—Purkinje cell loss in cerebellum, peripheral neuropathy
- Amphetamines—cerebral vasculitis, hemorrhage
- Cocaine—cerebral edema; hemorrhage secondary to hypertension
- MPTP (1-methyl-4-phenyl-1,2,3,6-tetrahydropyridine)—loss of pigmented neurons of the brain stem, resulting in severe, irreversible parkinsonism
- Phenothiazines—destruction of neurons in the extrapyramidal system, resulting in movement disorders
- Antineoplastic drugs—cystic degeneration of the corpus callosum (Adriamycin); leukoencephalopathy (Methotrexate); axonal degeneration (Vincristine)

■ CNS Trauma

- Linear acceleration and deceleration, sudden rotational movements, crushing injuries to the skull or spinal column, penetrating wounds, and repeated impacts, as in boxing, all cause brain or spinal cord injuries including the following:

  - Lacerations or contusions of the brain or spinal cord; cerebral contusions typically at the tips of gyri where the brain strikes the adjacent bone
  - Blood vessel tears with resulting extradural, subdural, or parenchymal hemorrhages
  - Axonal tears (common in repeated blows to the head as in boxing) resulting in dementia pugilistica (punch drunkenness)
  - Bullet wounds (*Note:* Most of the damage occurs in vacuum cone in the wake of the bullet.); the higher the velocity of the projectile, the more damage

- Table 25.11 summarizes important lesions associated with trauma

Table 25.11	*Central Nervous System Trauma*	
SITE	LESION	COMPLICATIONS
Cranial vault or base of skull	Fracture	Communications with nasal sinuses or infected sites—*infection*
Lateral cranium	Tear of middle **meningeal** artery by the fracture line	Extradural hematoma (arterial bleeding) with cerebral compression and herniations
Subdural space	Arterial tears in subdural space	Compression of brain, increased intracranial pressure, herniations
Subdural space	Venous tears ("bridging veins") (much more common than acute arterial subdural hematoma)	Slow accumulation of blood, with organization of hematoma by granulation tissue at inner and outer surfaces forming a "bag" that may slowly enlarge because of capillary bleeding and fluid dilution
Brain	Contusions	Brain hits inner table of skull; exposed tips of gyri are traumatized—contusion hemorrhage and contusion necrosis

Note: "Coup" injury—cerebral injury beneath the point of impact. Often occurs when a moving object strikes a nonmoving head.
"Contra-coup" injury—cerebral injury 180° away from the point of impact. Often occurs when a moving (accelerating) head strikes a fixed object.

■ **Congenital Diseases, Malformations, and Anomalies**

● Kernicterus

• Jaundice in the newborn may affect the deep grey-matter nuclei of the brain (the "kernels") because of an undeveloped blood-brain barrier; neuronal loss may be severe.

• At 4 to 5 days of age in the term infant, the blood-brain barrier for bilirubin becomes established, and bilirubin is excluded.

● Cerebellar agenesis

• This is often associated with maldevelopment of other areas of the CNS and other organs.

● Meningocele—meningomyelocele—encephalocele

• These are external sacs with direct communication into the spinal canal or cranial subarachnoid space through bony defects.

• Spinal or cranial meninges (meningocele) or portions of spinal cord and meninges (meningomyelocele) herniate into the sac, usually with severe degenerative changes.

• Portions of brain and meninges (encephalocele) protrude through a cranial defect.

● Syringomyelia—syringobulbia

• Slits or cavities within the spinal cord (syringomyelia) or brain stem (syringobulbia) often involving both grey- and white-matter areas, usually lacking an ependymal lining

- Hydromyelia

  - Dilation of a patent central canal of the spinal cord; an ependymal lining is usually present.

- Phakomatoses

  - Hereditary neuroectodermal dysplastic diseases with malformations and tumors (phakomas) that often involve the skin, nervous system, or eyes

  - Tuberous sclerosis—mental retardation, seizures, and tumors of many organs, including skin, eyes, kidneys, bones, and brain. Bizarre astrocytes or neurons form hard tumors (tubers) of the cerebral cortex or white matter, sometimes in the walls of the ventricles (see neoplasms)

  - Sturge-Weber syndrome—flat, unilateral, cutaneous angiomas of the face, venous angiomas of the leptomeninges and brain, especially posteriorly in the cerebral hemispheres, and parallel arrays of calcifications in cortical layers II and III forming parallel lines ("tram tracks") on plain skull films

  - Neurofibromatosis, type 1 (NF1, von Recklinghausen's disease)—café-au-lait spots, pigmented nevi, subcutaneous and deep nerve-root neurofibromas, schwannomas, meningiomas, and optic nerve gliomas all may occur

  - Neurofibromatosis, type 2 (NF2)—a distinct syndrome, less common than NF1; bilateral eighth cranial nerve schwannomas virtually pathognomonic; skin tumors may or may not occur

- Others

  - Anencephaly—failure of brain development, meninges, cranial vault, and overlying skin; base of the skull covered only with a vascularized membrane

  - Cyclocephaly—single ventricle with a single median eye

  - Porencephaly—focal cavitation of the cerebral mantle with communication between the ventricle and the surface

  - Hydranencephaly—destructive process with cavitation communicating to the surface, but not incorporating ventricle

  - Arrhinencephaly (holoprosencephaly)—failure of formation of the olfactory bulbs and tracts, usually with other malformations, including failure of formation of the corpus callosum and septum pellucidum (single ventricle); often associated with trisomy 13 or 15

  - Lissencephaly (smooth brain)—absence of gyrus and sulcus formation

  - Microgyria-polymicrogyria—one or more small gyri, irregularly formed

  - Hydrocephalus—dilation of the ventricles; may be caused by hypersecretion of CSF or inadequate resorption of CSF; atrophy of brain results in compensatory ventricular enlargement (hydrocephalus ex vacuo) without increased intracranial pressure

  - Arnold-Chiari malformations—hydrocephalus associated with cerebellar malformations (elongated tonsils that herniate into the foramen magnum, and/or platybasia, or elongation of the pons and medulla that herniate into the foramen magnum)

    - Type I—herniated cerebellar tonsils in older children and adults, but with no (or little) displacement of the brain stem; probably represents only chronic herniation of the tonsils; usually asymptomatic

- Type II—herniation of the cerebellum (inferior vermis, sometimes tonsils and other portions) and lower brain stem through the foramen magnum; may be deformation of the medulla into an "S" curve
- Type III—cervical spina bifida with herniation of the cerebellum through the defect (encephalocele)

■ Degenerative Diseases

- Diseases that affect neurons or groups of neurons and nerve fiber tracts that are related ("systems"); idiopathic, progressive, and usually symmetric
- ● Diseases of the cerebral cortex
  - *Alzheimer's disease (AD)*
    - Dementia with gradual loss of recent memory, cognition and judgment, and defects in fine motor skills, language, and learning ability; plateaus are typical in the clinical decline
    - Definitive diagnosis—cannot be made without tissue confirmation; all features found to some degree in normal-aged brain
    - Variable cortical (gyral) atrophy, most prominent in frontal and temporal lobes; ventricular dilation (hydrocephalus ex vacuo) may be greater than expected from the degree of gyral atrophy
    - Selective loss of neurons in the frontal and temporal neocortices, hippocampus, amygdala, nucleus basalis of Meynert, and other areas
    - Surviving neurons—have degenerated dendritic spines with loss of synapses, possibly the anatomic substrate of the dementia
    - Diffuse deposits of nervous system-specific β-amyloid precursor protein—occurs early
    - Intraganglionic neurofibrillary tangles (NFT)—in neurons of the neocortex, hippocampus, amygdala, substantia nigra, locus ceruleus, and other brain stem nuclei; tangles—collections of 10 nm-paired filaments, one wrapped around the other in a right-handed spiral (paired helical filaments [PHF]) within the cytoplasm and processes of neurons; PHFs contain the proteins tau and ubiquitin; NFT also found in Down syndrome, dementia pugilistica (punch drunkenness), Parkinson-dementia complex of Guam, SSPE, and in otherwise normal-aged brains and may be a nonspecific response to cellular injury
    - Alzheimer's senile plaques—the most important and characteristic microscopic lesion; accumulate in association areas of the frontal temporal and parietal lobes, amygdala, hippocampus, and piriform cortex; at various stages in development, plaques contain dystrophic neuronal cell processes, astrocytes, PHF, microglia, extracellular β-amyloid precursor protein or fibrillary β-amyloid resulting from abnormal cleavage of the amyloid precursor protein; mature plaques have a central core of β-amyloid surrounded by a ring of degenerated dendrites containing PHF (Fig. 25.7); β-amyloid also usually present in blood vessel walls in the brain and leptomeninges
    - Granular-vacuolar degeneration—usually found only in hippocampal neurons; best seen with the standard hematoxylin-eosin stain; appear as clear intracytoplasmic vacuoles containing an eosinophilic granule; characteristic of AD, but of unknown significance

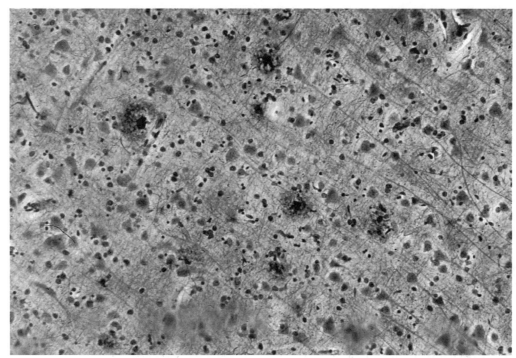

Fig. 25.7 Numerous Alzheimer's senile plaques are present in this section of frontal cortex from a 60-year-old demented male. Note the dense, black, argyrophilic β-amyloid cores surrounded by rings of dystrophic neuronal processes. Silver (Hirano) stain, 50 times magnification.

- AD—associated with multiple neurotransmitter and neuropeptide deficits

- Genetics—familial AD accounts for approximately 40% of cases; autosomal dominant inheritance pattern is the most common

- Evidence suggests that the gene for the low-density lipoprotein apolipoprotein E (ApoE), allele epsilon 4 on chromosome 19, is associated with AD (i.e., patients with AD carry this allele with significantly higher frequency); this protein binds β-amyloid, possibly increasing its neurotoxicity; allele epsilon 2 protective against AD

- Down syndrome (trisomy 21)—victims develop tissue and chemical abnormalities similar to AD

- Etiology unknown; all alterations of AD probably occur at a lower rate in aged brains; suggested etiologic factors—genetic defects, systemic metabolic defects, slow or latent viruses, environmental toxins (especially metals including aluminum), stress, or excess formation of excitatory and neurotoxic amino acids

— *Pick's disease*

- Rare, severe, presenile or senile dementia

- Frontal or temporal lobes or both usually affected; parietal and occipital lobes usually spared

- Gyral atrophy ("knife-edged" gyri), neuronal loss, and reactive astrogliosis severe

- The posterior ⅔ of the superior temporal gyrus often spared (is of normal size)

- Intracytoplasmic, nonviral inclusion bodies (Pick bodies) that stain positively with silver stains occasionally present in neurons, especially in hippocampus and amygdala

- Amyloid deposition, senile plaques, intraganglionic neurofibrillary tangles, and granular-vacuolar degeneration *not* present

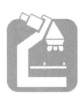

Diseases of the basal ganglia and brain stem nuclei

— *Huntington's disease (Chorea)*

- Hereditary (strict mendelian dominant) premature (starting between the ages of 25 and 45 years) degeneration of neurons, especially in the caudate nuclei, cerebral cortex, and other parts of the extrapyramidal system

- Clinically characterized by chorea (random purposeless movements of the limbs, head, face, tongue) followed by dementia, eventual coma, and death, with an average clinical course of 15 years

- Severe atrophy with neuronal loss and astrogliosis of the heads of the caudate nuclei, resulting in a concave profile of the lateral walls of the dilated lateral ventricles, characteristic; also severe atrophy and neuronal loss and gliosis of the cerebral cortex and extrapyramidal system

- Etiology—a mutation of a gene on the short arm of chromosome 4; most cases stem from a single source, but the mutation has apparently appeared in other families

— *Parkinsonism*

- Idiopathic Parkinson's disease (paralysis agitans)—a disease starting in middle age, progressive and disabling, with paucity of movement and expression, "cog-wheel rigidity," tremor at rest, and eventual intellectual impairment; death in 10 years on average

- Morphology—loss of neurons in the melanin-pigmented nuclei of the brain stem (substantia nigra, locus ceruleus, dorsal motor nucleus of the vagus nerve) and other portions of the extrapyramidal system

- Lewy bodies (concentric, hyaline, intracytoplasmic, nonviral inclusions)—develop in the remaining neurons of the pigmented nuclei (most easily found in the locus ceruleus) and elsewhere (idiopathic Parkinson's disease *only*)

- Parkinsonism—often associated with dementia and morphologic changes of AD (especially in the Parkinson-dementia complex of Guam)

- Other forms of parkinsonism—caused by drugs, especially phenothiazines and certain designer drugs including MPTP, carbon monoxide poisoning, and encephalitis, including von Economo's encephalitis

- von Economo's encephalitis—a severe "sleeping sickness" that affected influenza victims of the pandemic during World War I; first reported in 1915, last case seen in 1922, and the disease not reported since; in addition to lethargy or coma, the victims manifested "cog-wheel rigidity"; etiology never determined but probably a virus; many years later—survivors developed a parkinsonian syndrome differing in some respects from idiopathic Parkinson's disease

— *Progressive supranuclear palsy (PSP)*

• Parkinson's diseaselike syndrome with diminution or loss of vertical eye movements and dementia

• In addition to depigmentation of the substantia nigra, there is neuronal loss and gliosis in the globus pallidus, subthalamic nucleus, and tectum of the brain stem, including the superior colliculi

• Intraganglionic neurofibrillary tangles prominent but filaments differ from those in AD (PSP filaments—straight single filaments rather than the paired filaments of AD)

● **Brain stem and spinocerebellar degenerations**

• Multiple syndromes have been described, many carrying eponymic names. Heredity varies. Most, to some degree, clinically exhibit ataxia, incoordination of movements, tremor, sensory abnormalities, and abnormal muscle tone, depending upon which nuclei and which spinal cord tracts are affected and the degree of involvement of the cerebellar cortex and roof nuclei.

— *Olivopontocerebellar atrophy (OPCA)*

• Neuronal loss, most severe in the inferior olives and nuclei of the basis pontis and cerebellar Purkinje cell loss; basis pontis and cerebellum atrophic

— *Friedreich's ataxia*

• Autosomal recessive inheritance

• Begins during the teenage years; most die within 10 years

• Corticospinal tracts, spinocerebellar tracts, and dorsal columns—degenerate, with loss of neurons in Clark's column, dorsal root ganglia, cranial nerve nuclei (including CN VIII), and cerebellar dentate nuclei; loss of Purkinje cells, and optic nerve atrophy common

• Other organs also affected, most commonly the heart (hypertrophic cardiomyopathy or myocarditis)

● **Degenerative diseases of the motor system**

• The motor system involves only two neuron groups—the upper (cortical) motor neurons and lower motor neurons (brain stem cranial motor nerve nuclei neurons and spinal cord motor neurons). Three possible variations of motor system disease are possible (i.e., upper motor neuron disease only, lower motor neuron disease only, or combined upper and lower motor neuron disease).

— *Involvement of upper motor neurons only—primary lateral sclerosis of the spinal cord*

• Loss of cortical motor neurons results in axon (and therefore myelin) loss in the motor tracts (corticobulbar tracts in the brain stem and the pyramidal tracts of the brain stem and spinal cord).

• Muscles do not atrophy (because they are not denervated), but minor loss of muscle mass (disuse atrophy) may occur.

• Patients show pareses, hyperactive motor reflexes (deep tendon reflexes, clonus), and abnormal long motor tract signs (e.g., Babinski's sign).

— *Involvement of the lower motor neurons only—progressive spinal muscular atrophy*

* Degeneration of anterior horn cells and their axons resulting in atrophy of corresponding muscles (neurogenic atrophy)

* Patients—show weakness or paralysis, fasciculations, and fibrillations (which clinically can be observed only in the tongue), and depression of spinal reflexes, secondary to the lower motor neuron loss

* Muscular atrophy (neurogenic or denervation atrophy) in the muscles innervated by the degenerated anterior horn cells

* Werdnig-Hoffmann disease—infantile form of spinal muscular atrophy; anterior horn cells absent or die in the early childhood period; other neurons of the brain stem nuclei may also be involved; defective gene localized to chromosome 5q

— *Combined upper and lower motor neuron disease—amyotrophic lateral sclerosis (ALS, Lou Gehrig's disease)*

* Most cases are sporadic; about 10% are inherited (usually as an autosomal dominant).

* Etiology is in doubt (there may be multiple etiologies). In some inherited cases, mutations of a gene on chromosome 21 coding for superoxide dismutase, a scavenger of free radicals, have been found. Three professional football players on the same team during the same year were affected. The home field was fertilized the summer before with sewage sludge, leading to speculation that an environmental toxin was involved.

* ALS begins in adulthood and is invariably fatal, with fasciculations and fibrillations (of the tongue) and muscular atrophy beginning distally in the limbs and progressing centrally. The clinical picture depends upon the balance of upper and lower motor neuron loss at the time. Severe paralysis, breathing difficulty, and paralysis of the facial and oropharyngeal muscles eventually result in death, commonly within 2 years of the onset of symptoms, often from infection; but occasional cases show an extended clinical course. Sensation and mentation are unaffected.

* Cortical motor neuron loss is usually difficult to demonstrate. The pyramidal tracts in the brain stem and spinal cord show loss of axons and myelin with gliosis. Cranial nerve nuclei motor neuron and spinal cord anterior horn cell loss may be extensive, leading to atrophy of corresponding muscles.

MULTIPLE CHOICE REVIEW QUESTIONS

1. An old cerebral infarct is usually represented by which of the following?

    a. A cavity bordered by astrocytic cells and fibers
    b. A cavity with a thick, collagenous wall
    c. A dense mass of microglial fibers
    d. A mass of necrotic brain tissue surrounded by a wall of glial fibrillary acidic protein fibers
    e. A central mass of β-amyloid surrounded by a ring of dystrophic dendritic processes

2. The most common central nervous system infection in a 6-year-old, otherwise healthy, child in the United States is which of the following?

    a. Tuberculous meningitis
    b. Staphylococcal brain abscess
    c. Acute purulent cerebrospinal leptomeningitis caused by *Haemophilus influenzae* type B
    d. Acute purulent cerebrospinal leptomeningitis caused by *Streptococcus pneumoniae*
    e. *Aspergillus niger* abscess at the cortical–white matter interface

3. Which of the following is *true* of tuberculous meningitis?

    a. It never affects children.
    b. It always responds promptly to properly prescribed drug therapy.

    c. It may be an infection limited to the nervous system with no other organs involved.
    d. Patients may develop obstructive hydrocephalus many years later.
    e. It is usually fatal within days of the onset of symptoms.

4. An 8-year-old child is found to have papilledema and a neoplasm within the fourth ventricle, blocking the outflow of cerebrospinal fluid. It is most likely to be which of the following?

    a. A glioblastoma multiforme
    b. An ependymoma
    c. A colloid cyst
    d. A medulloblastoma
    e. A cystic astrocytoma

5. The most specific abnormality in Alzheimer's disease is which of the following?

    a. Senile plaque
    b. Cerebral amyloid angiopathy
    c. Neuronal loss and reactive astrogliosis
    d. Intraganglionic neurofibrillary tangle
    e. Hirano bodies

Chapter 26

Breast

The female breast is a modified sweat gland serving the specialized role of providing nourishment to an infant; as such, it is anatomically and physiologically fully developed *only* during the lactating state. The "game plan" for breast structure is basically one of ever smaller caliber ducts as one moves from the nipple surface into the breast substance (Fig. 26.1). The smallest duct structures are referred to as terminal ducts; these lead finally into ductules (also known as acini). The secretion from the acinar cells is human milk. Ultimate breast development and function depend upon multiple hormones, preeminently estrogen (stimulates ducts) and progesterone (stimulates acinar cells); other important hormones are prolactin, growth hormone, cortisol, parathyroid hormone, human placental lactogen, insulin, and (for milk let down) oxytocin.

■ Terminology Worth Remembering

- **Duct**—has inner epithelial and outer myoepithelial lining (the latter having contractile capability)
- **Lobule**—clusterlike collection of acinar cells (ductules) and their terminal duct
- **Stroma**—connective tissue (fibrocollagen and fat) in which lobules and ducts are found

BREAST DISEASES

Significant problems in the breast may be heralded by one or more of the following signs and symptoms:

- Mass (lump)
- Pain (may be associated with menstrual cycle)
- Swelling (diffuse)
- Nipple discharge (with or without blood)
- Breast skin changes (i.e., peau d'orange, eczematoid, ulceration)
- Red breast skin (diffuse)
- Nipple retraction
- Lymphedema

The most frequent presenting complaint of breast disease is a mass (detected by palpation or by mammography or both). Of these, the vast majority are benign. Among the benign lesions, the largest category is fibrocystic change (formerly called fibrocystic disease).

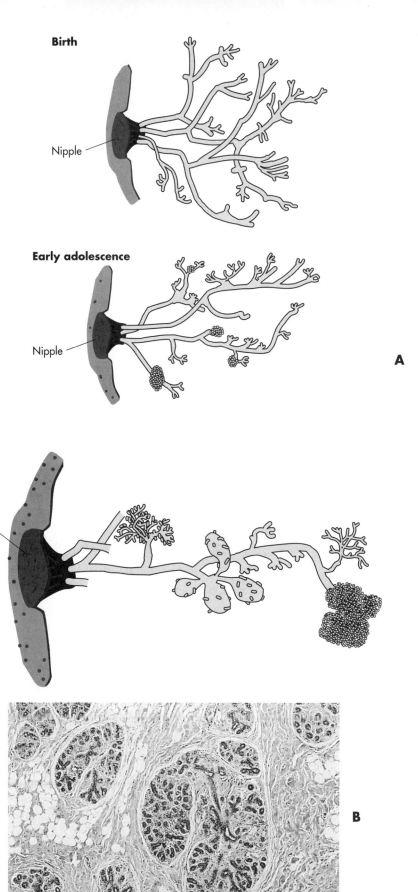

Fig. 26.1 A, Breast architecture at birth, adolescence, and adulthood. **B,** Photomicrograph depicting normal breast lobular architecture. *(From Damjanov I, Linder J:* Anderson's pathology. *ed 10, vol 2, St Louis, 1995, Mosby.)*

■ **Benign Lesions of the Female Breast**

● **Fibrocystic change**

- Common (up to 90% of women have some form of this); also formerly called "mammary dysplasia"
- Can see varying combinations of the following:

    - **Cysts and fibrosis**—often multifocal and bilateral; look for cysts, intralobular and interlobular fibrosis, and apocrine metaplasia
    - **Cysts and fibrosis with epithelial hyperplasia** (proliferation)
    - **Sclerosing adenosis**—may mimic carcinoma microscopically and clinically; look for proliferation of intralobular stroma and small ducts
    - **Cysts and fibrosis with atypical epithelial hyperplasia** (proliferation)—in extreme form, can be virtually impossible to separate microscopically from in situ carcinoma

- The importance of fibrocystic change is that at least some of these patients are at increased risk for subsequently developing breast carcinoma according to the following guidelines:

    - Those that are associated with no or minimally increased risk for developing invasive breast carcinoma—apocrine metaplasia, cysts, duct ectasia, fibrosis, hyperplasia (two to four cells in depth), and squamous metaplasia
    - Those that are at slightly increased risk (1.5 to 2 times)—moderate or florid hyperplasia, adenosis, and ductal papillomatosis
    - Those that are at significantly increased risk (5 times)—atypical epithelial hyperplasia, either ductal or lobular

● **Fibroadenoma**

- Most common benign neoplasm of female breast

    - Encapsulated, usually solitary and movable
    - Peak incidence: puberty, 20s 30s
    - May be large (up to 10 cm)
    - Stromal overgrowth with compressed, ductlike, epithelial-lined spaces

● **Intraductal papilloma**

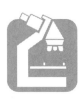

- Found in large duct structures
- Consists of benign neoplastic proliferation having a papillary configuration
- Often present with bloody nipple discharge and small subareolar mass

● **Phyllodes tumors**

- Previously called cystosarcoma phyllodes, but was a misnomer because they are *usually* benign, although some forms may behave in a malignant fashion
- Characterized by appearance similar to fibroadenoma, but with more pronounced stromal component

● **Other benign lesions**

- Fat necrosis—often seen after trauma; fat cells undergo necrosis with resultant scarring; may clinically mimic cancer

- Plasma cell mastitis—see sheets of plasma cells; may result in enlarged axillary lymph nodes that may clinically mimic cancer

- Chronic mastitis—infiltrate composed of lymphocytes, monocytes, and plasma cells

- Intramammary lymph node—not an uncommon benign "mass" in the breast

- Granulomatous mastitis—look for granuloma formation

- Acute mastitis and abscess—seen mainly in pregnant and/or lactating women; usually caused by *Staphylococcus aureus* or *Streptococcus* organisms

■ Breast Cancer

● Incidence of breast cancer (the vast majority of these are carcinomas)

- In 1995, there were approximately 185,000 newly diagnosed breast cancers in this country, and nearly 46,000 patients died of breast cancer.

- Breast cancer is the most common malignant neoplasm in females and the second most common cause of cancer death in females (following lung cancer).

- For every 100 breast cancers that occur in women, less than one occurs in men.

- The incidence and mortality are highest in North American and Northern European countries, intermediate in Southern European and South American countries, and lowest in many Asian and African countries.

- Death rate from breast carcinoma has held steady for decades; breast cancer accounts for 20% of cancer deaths in American women every year.

● Risk factors

— *Genetic predisposition (family history)*

- Women who have a first-degree relative (mother, sister, daughter) with breast cancer have a risk two to three times that of the general population.

- This risk is increased further if the relative was affected at an early age or had bilateral disease.

- Women whose families have cancer family syndromes (Li-Fraumeni syndrome, Cowden syndrome, Muir-Torre syndrome).

— *Radiation*

- An increased risk has been demonstrated in

  - Survivors of the atomic bombings of Hiroshima and Nagasaki

  - Women having multiple fluoroscopies in the course of pneumothorax treatment of tuberculosis

  - Children treated with radiotherapy for thymic enlargement

— *Hormonal factors*

- Early menarche, late menopause, and nulliparity increase the risk.

- Women who have a first full-term pregnancy before the age of 18 years have only one third the cancer risk of those whose first child is delayed until after the age of 30 years.

- Long-term treatment with estrogens for symptoms of menopause increases the risk.

- Castration, either by surgery or radiotherapy, substantially *reduces* a woman's breast cancer risk.

— *Certain types of fibrocystic change (see preceding discussion)*

● Histopathologic types of carcinoma

- *Most common location is the upper outer quadrant*

— *Carcinomas arising from mammary duct (nearly 90% of breast carcinomas)*

- Intraductal carcinoma (ductal carcinoma in situ)

- Incidence is 0.8% to 5% of all breast carcinomas and 15% to 20% of all breast cancers among patients undergoing mammographic screening.
- They may be found incidentally on breast biopsy specimens removed for clinically benign diseases, or by mammography, or present with nipple discharge, or a palpable mass.
- When discovered by mammography, they are usually small (less than 1 cm).
- The morphologic types include comedocarcinoma (characterized microscopically by central necrosis) and cribriform, solid, and papillary carcinomas. Any of these types may become, or be associated with, invasive carcinoma. Twenty-eight percent of patients treated with biopsy alone subsequently developed invasive carcinoma over a period of 15 years.

— *Invasive (infiltrating) carcinomas*

- Scirrhous carcinoma (infiltrating duct carcinoma, usual type)

- **This is the most common form of breast carcinoma, accounting for more than approximately 70% of all breast carcinomas.**
- It has a stony, hard consistency and foci of chalky, yellow streaks.
- Microscopically, the cancer cells are polygonal or round, infiltrating a stroma that is densely fibrotic (scirrhous).
- Ductlike structures (in varying numbers) are formed by these malignant epithelial cells (Fig. 26.2).

— *Medullary carcinoma*

- It is an infiltrating carcinoma with abundant lymphoid and plasmacytic infiltration around the neoplastic cell groups.
- The cancer cells are large and pleomorphic and form sheets and anastomosing cords.
- They are usually large and soft and bulge from the cut surface on gross examination.

— *Colloid carcinoma (mucinous)*

- Infiltrating duct carcinoma with abundant extracellular mucin

— *Tubular carcinoma*

- Essentially a well-differentiated infiltrating carcinoma with uniform tubules (lined by a single layer of neoplastic cells) embedded in abundant fibrous stroma

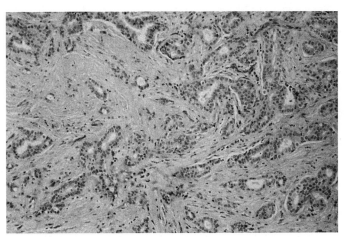

Fig. 26.2 Photomicrograph of infiltrating duct carcinoma.
(From Damjanov I, Linder J: Anderson's pathology, *ed 10, vol 2, St Louis, 1995, Mosby.)*

— *Papillary carcinoma*

- Usually intraductal; invasion may be characterized by disruption of the duct

— *Carcinoma arising from mammary lobules (nearly 10% of breast carcinomas)*

- In situ lobular carcinoma

  - Most patients in their 40s and 50s
  - Clinically and grossly often indistinguishable from fibrocystic changes
  - Arise from the acini (ductules) or terminal ducts
  - Microscopically characterized by distended lobules filled by loosely cohesive, uniform cancer cells that are smaller than cancer cells of ductal origin
  - 15% to 30% bilateral
  - ¼ of patients treated by local excision develop infiltrating carcinoma (ductal or lobular) in 10 years; 35% in 20 years

- Infiltrating lobular carcinoma

  - Grossly similar to scirrhous carcinoma
  - Microscopically characterized by threadlike strands of carcinoma cells, loosely dispersed throughout a fibrous matrix; strands usually one cell thick ("Indian file"; Fig. 26.3)

— *Paget's disease of the nipple*

- Begins as an "eruption" revealing a florid, intensely red, raw, and granular nipple surface
- May present 1 to 2 years before the underlying breast neoplasm is detected
- *Nearly always* associated with a demonstrable underlying carcinoma, either intraductal or infiltrating duct carcinoma of the same breast

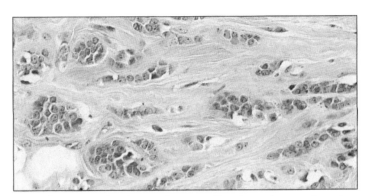

Fig. 26.3 Photomicrograph depicts infiltrating columns of carcinoma cells; single file groups are referred to as "Indian-file" invasion. *(From Stevens A, Lowe J:* Pathology, *London, 1995, Times Mirror International.)*

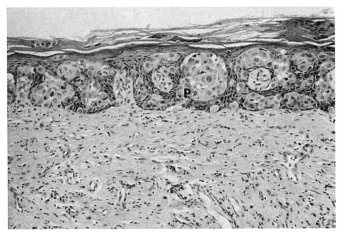

Fig. 26.4 Photomicrograph of Paget's disease reveals the epidermal clusters of Paget's cells with large nuclei and abundant pale staining cytoplasm *(P)*. *(From Damjanov I, Linder J:* Anderson's pathology, *ed 10, vol 2, St Louis, 1995, Mosby.)*

- • Paget cell—large, ovoid nucleus with prominent nucleolus and abundant pale-staining cytoplasm (Fig. 26.4)
- • May also occur in males with breast cancer

— *Miscellaneous types*

- • Quite uncommon, accounting for less than 1% of all breast carcinoma
- • Signet-ring cell carcinoma, metaplastic carcinoma, and others

● Biologic behavior

- • Local spread by direct infiltration into the breast parenchyma, along mammary ducts and by lymphatics in the breast
- • Regional spread to the lymph nodes; the most commonly involved groups are

  - • Axillary lymph nodes—up to 40% of patients with breast cancer have evidence of spread to axillary lymph nodes, and is the most common lymph node site to be involved by metastatic breast cancer

- Internal mammary lymph nodes— involvement more common for inner quadrant or central primaries than for outer quadrant lesions
- Supraclavicular lymph nodes—involved in 18% of patients who have axillary lymph node involvement

- Distant metastasis—lung, liver, bone, pleura, and skin are the most common sites; many other organs may also be involved; occasionally, patients may present with symptoms and/or signs of the metastasis as the first clinical manifestation of their underlying breast carcinoma

● **Factors that are important in determining the type of therapy**

- Status of the primary carcinoma

  - Fixation of cancer to the chest wall
  - Rapid growth of cancer with clinical signs of inflammation (the so-called inflammatory carcinoma)

- Bilateral involvement

  - It varies from 0.5% to 12.5% of breast cancers.
  - *Lobular carcinoma has the highest incidence (see preceding).*
  - The contralateral carcinomas can be either noninvasive or invasive.

- Multifocality (multicentricity) within the same breast

  - The incidence varies depending on the method of sampling, the definition, and the pathologic type of the first primary. It is estimated to be in the range of 25% to 50%. At least 5% to 10% of these multicentric carcinomas are invasive.
  - The multicentric carcinomas may be found outside the quadrant where the first primary is found.

- Type of cancer
- Estrogen receptor (ER) and progesterone receptor (PR) status
- Lymph node metastasis
- Distant metastasis

● **Factors that are important in determining prognosis**

- Extent of lymph node involvement
- Size of the primary carcinoma; favorable prognosis <2 cm in greatest dimension; unfavorable prognosis if larger
- Type of primary cancer; lobular in situ and intraductal carcinomas, especially the former, have the best prognosis; good prognosis—tubular and papillary types; intermediate prognosis—mucinous and medullary; poorest prognosis—(scirrhous) infiltrating ductal carcinoma and infiltrating lobular carcinoma
- Grade of cancer (well, moderately, or poorly differentiated)
- ER and PR status—ER-PR positive patients more likely to respond to hormonal manipulation than ER-PR negative patients; in general, breast carcinoma patients who respond to endocrine therapy have a longer disease-free interval and longer survival than those who do not
- DNA index and S-phase fraction using flow cytometry; (aneuploidy and elevated S-phase fraction are associated with poorer prognosis)

Table 26.1 *5-year Survival for Breast Carcinoma*

Local Disease	90%
Regional Disease	71%
Advanced	18%

From Damjanov I, Linder J: *Anderson's pathlogy,* ed 10, vol 2, St Louis, 1996, Mosby.

- Distant metastasis
- Lymphatic invasion
- Others—Her 2 neu onco-gene (a growth factor receptor); when over-expressed, associated with poorer prognosis. Another marker is P-53, a suppressor protein normally found in cells; mutated forms not functional and accumulate in some breast cancers; prognosis worse in these patients
- Table 26.1—shows the 5-year survival rates as a function of breast carcinoma stage at diagnosis
- *Note:* Approximately 60% of breast cancer patients present with disease limited to the breast; 30% have regional lymph node metastases, and 10% have distant metastases at presentation.

● **Other malignant neoplasms**

- *Note:* Though rare, other types of carcinoma (not listed here), sarcomas, lymphomas, and metastatic neoplasms may be seen in the breast.

■ **Male Breast Lesions** Only two lesions are meaningful for our discussion:

- *Gynecomastia*

  - Enlargement of the male breast caused by absolute or relative *estrogen* excess
  - Seen in association with hepatic cirrhosis, estrogen-producing neoplasms, estrogen therapy, physiologic states (i.e., puberty), certain medications (i.e., tricyclic antidepressants [TCAs], cimetidine, spironolactone, digitalis)
  - Histologically, gynecomastia characterized by varying degrees of epithelial and stromal proliferation

- *Carcinoma*

  - Less than 1% as often as is seen in female breast (1400 cases/year in United States)
  - Morphologically and biologically resembles carcinomas of female breast
  - Treatment similar to that for carcinoma of the female breast
  - Stage for stage felt to have similar prognosis as breast carcinoma in females

MULTIPLE CHOICE
REVIEW QUESTIONS

1. Which of the following organisms (which gains access to the breast through breaks in nipple skin) is most likely to cause acute mastitis?

    a. *Staphylococcus aureus*
    b. *Histoplasma capsulatum*
    c. *Proteus vulgaris*
    d. *Mycobacterium tuberculosis*
    e. *Mycobacterium avium-intracellulare*

2. Cancer at which of the following sites accounts for the most *cancer deaths* in American females?

    a. Breast
    b. Colon
    c. Ovary
    d. Lung
    e. Endometrial

3. Which of the following breast carcinomas has the best prognosis from the standpoint of histologic type alone?

    a. Intraductal carcinoma
    b. Tubular carcinoma
    c. Papillary carcinoma
    d. Medullary carcinoma
    e. Mucinous carcinoma

4. The classical presenting (clinical) complaint for a breast intraductal papilloma is which of the following?

    a. Bloody nipple discharge
    b. Peau d'orange skin changes
    c. Enlargement of ipsilateral (same side) axillary lymph nodes
    d. Eczematoid skin changes
    e. A red, firm, painful mass

5. All *except* which of the following items are possible histologic components of "fibrocystic change" in the female breast?

    a. Apocrine metaplasia
    b. Cysts (benign)
    c. Fibrosis
    d. Sclerosing adenosis
    e. Fat necrosis

Chapter 27

Gynecologic Pathology

■ **Inflammatory Processes**

● Sexually transmitted diseases (STDs)

• A rampant problem, STDs affect millions of Americans. Women may develop pelvic inflammatory disease (PID), which can cause **infertility** and is a predisposing factor for **ectopic pregnancy,** an important cause of maternal death.

• See the Infectious Disease chapter for a more complete discussion of STDs. Human papilloma virus will be discussed at this time, however.

— *Human papilloma virus (HPV)*

• HPV is a DNA "wart" virus (with over 70 known types) associated with characteristic histologic changes in squamous cells and raised, wartlike lesions in the perianal area, vulva, vagina, and cervix (condyloma acuminatum or venereal wart) (Fig. 27.1). Lesions in the cervix are usually flat and often associated with squamous dysplasia.

• **HPV 6 and 11 are the types most often associated with condyloma, whereas HPV 16, 18, 31, 33, 35, and 45 are most often identified in cases of dysplasia and squamous cell carcinoma (in situ and invasive) of the lower genital tract.**

• Histologically, HPV-infected cells have enlarged, hyperchromatic nulcei with irregular nuclear borders and perinuclear halos (koilocytes) (Fig. 27.2).

● Nonsexually transmitted infections

• **Candida albicans**—a common genital infection in females

• Tuberculosis—involves this area through hematogeneous spread

● Nonspecific cervicitis

• **Acute**—usually in postabortion or postpartum infection situations

• **Chronic**—in women of childbearing age; usually asymptomatic; variable infiltrates of lymphocytes and plasma cells; lymphoid follicles may be present (**follicular cervicitis**)

● Nonspecific vaginitis

● Nonspecific vulvitis and dermatologic disorders

• Remember that essentially any dermatopathy that affects nonvulvar skin may also affect vulvar skin.

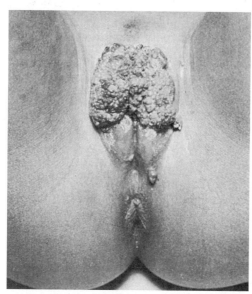

Fig. 27.1 Condyloma acuminatum. Clinical photograph features cauliflower like lesion of vulvar condyloma acuminatum. (*From Damjanov I, Linder J: Anderson's pathology, ed 10, vol 2, St Louis, 1996, Mosby.*)

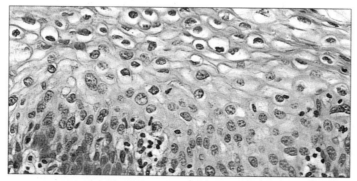

Fig. 27.2 Human papillomavirus (HPV) in uterine cervix. Photomicrograph depicts the presence of atypical HPV infected epithelial cells known as koilocytes. (*From Stevens A, Lowe J: Pathology, London, 1995, Times Mirror International.*)

■ Vulvar Lesions

● Benign conditions of the vulva

— *Cysts*

- Bartholin's duct cysts
- Epidermal inclusion cysts (common lesions)

— *Benign "tumors"*

- Squamous papilloma
- Condyloma acuminatum (caused by HPV, mostly types 6 and 11)
- Hidradenoma and other skin adnexal tumors
- Ectopic breast tissue

— *Vulvar dystrophies*

- Squamous hyperplasia (previously called hyperplastic dystrophy) has two types

  - No epithelial atypia
  - Dysplasia (atypia) of squamous epithelium

- Atrophic dystrophy (**also known as lichen sclerosis et atrophicus and is not a premalignant lesion**)

  - Histologically, one sees epidermal thinning and upper dermal fibrosis with chronic inflammation.

- Vulvar intraepithelial neoplasia (VIN) analagous to cervical intraepithelial neoplasia (CIN) of cervix (see following)

● **Malignant lesions of the vulva**

- *Note:* **The most common primary malignant neoplasm of the vulva is squamous cell carcinoma (95% of vulvar cancer).**
- Bowen's disease (squamous cell carcinoma in situ)—full thickness epidermal squamous cell maturational arrest (dysplasia), but epithelial basement membrane not transgressed by these abnormal cells so the lesion is in situ
- **Invasive squamous cell carcinoma**—often preceded by vulvar dysplasia

  - Condyloma acuminatum is associated with about 10% of invasive vulvar carcinomas (Fig. 27.3).

- Extramammary Paget's disease (about ⅓ of vulvar Paget's disease associated with an underlying carcinoma, usually adenocarcinoma)
- Malignant melanoma
- Bartholin's gland carcinoma

■ **Lesions of the Vagina**

● **Benign lesions of the vagina**

- Cysts

  - Gartner duct cysts
  - Epithelial inclusion cysts

- **Benign epithelial lesions,** such as papilloma, seborrheic keratosis, melanocytic nevi, and adenoma are relatively common.
- **Benign mesenchymal neoplasms,** such as fibroma, leiomyoma and lipoma, are rarely seen.

● **Malignant neoplasms of the vagina**

- Extension of squamous cell carcinoma from cervix and adenocarcinoma from endometrium are the most common cancers to involve the vagina.
- **Squamous cell carcinoma** is by far the most common **primary** malignant neoplasm of the vagina.
- Clear cell adenocarcinoma (see following)
- Sarcoma botryoides is a cancer of young girls (90% are less than 5 years old) with characteristic gross appearance (soft polypoid masses); **a subtype of embryonal rhabdomyosarcoma.**

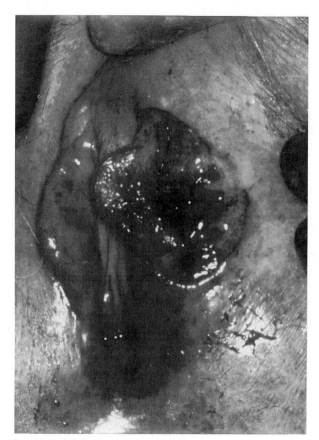

Fig. 27.3 Clinical photograph features an ulcerated and hemorrhagic squamous cell carcinoma of the vulva. (*From Damjanov I, Linder J:* Anderson's pathology, *ed 10, vol 2, St Louis, 1996, Mosby.*)

- In females, neoplasms may arise in vagina as well as urinary bladder; in males, they may be seen in urinary bladder.

◼ Uterine Cervix

● Benign lesions of the uterine cervix

- **Cervical polyps** (arise in endocervical canal, typically); are **common** lesions
- **Microglandular endocervical hyperplasia**—birth control pill-associated benign proliferation of endocervical glands
- **Condyloma acuminatum**—caused by HPV infection; may have cauliflower-like mass but is often flat

● Precancerous conditions and carcinoma of the uterine cervix

- Etiology and epidemiology

  - **Risk factors** include young age at first intercourse, sexual promiscuity, "high-risk" male sexual partners (i.e., those partners who are promiscuous or who have a history of penile condyloma), low socioeconomic groups, and lack of cervical Pap smear surveillance.
  - Dysplasia (altered cell maturation) and carcinoma of the cervix are associated with HPV infection in many cases.

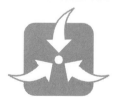

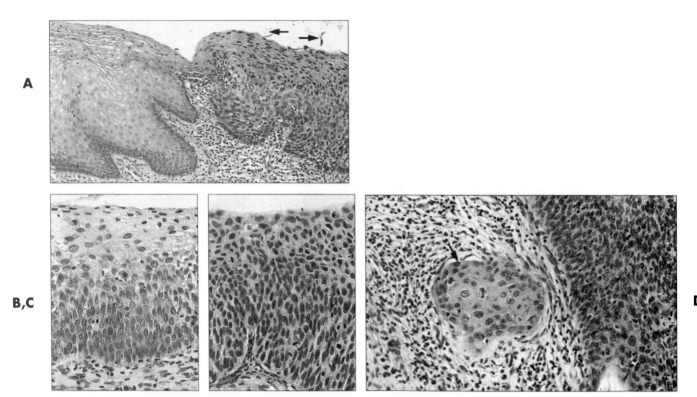

Fig. 27.4 Cervical intraepithelial neoplasm (CIN). **A,** Photomicrograph of normal squamous epithelium (left half of field) and severe, nearly full thickness dysplasia. Abnormal surface epithelial cells *(arrows)* are easily removed during Pap smear procedure. **B,** Photomicrograph of mild to moderate dysplasia (CIN-I to CIN-II). Surface cells feature good maturation but deeper cells exhibit disordered maturation (dysplasia). **C,** Photomicrograph showing moderate to severe cervical epithelial atypia CIN-II to CIN-III). **D,** Photomicrograph features early, microinvasive squamous cell carcinoma. *(From Stevens A, Lowe J:* Pathology, *London, 1995, Times Mirror International.)*

- HPV DNA is detected by hybridization techniques in 75% to 100% of patients with cervical dysplasia (a precancerous condition) and invasive carcinoma. The E-6 protein of HPV appears to accelerate the inactivation of an important human tumor-suppressor protein called p53.

- Although there is overlap in the HPV types present in various lesions, **HPV 6 and 11 (low-risk HPVs)** are found most frequently in condylomas, whereas **HPV 16, 18, 31, 33, 35, and 45 (high-risk HPVs)** are more often present in carcinomas.

— *CIN in cervical tissue biopsies* (Fig. 27.4)

  • **CIN-I** (mild dysplasia)—maturational abnormality involves the lower third of the cervical epithelium

  • **CIN-II** (moderate dysplasia)—maturational abnormality involves the lower two thirds of the cervical epithelium

  • **CIN-III** (severe dysplasia and carcinoma in situ)—dysplasia extends into the upper third of the cervical epithelium; full maturational arrest of the epithelium designated as carcinoma in situ (CIS) in which there is **no malignant invasion through mucosal basement membrane**

  • The Bethesda system of **cytology reporting** and its biologic relevance—**in the Bethesda system** (devised to introduce consistency in cytologic diagnostic terminology), **CIN-I is equal to SIL-LG (squamous intraepithelial lesion, low grade), while CIN-II and CIN-III are encompassed by SIL-HG (squamous intraepithelial lesion, high grade)**

- *Note:* 65,000 new cases of cervical squamous cell CIS were diagnosed in the United States in 1995.

- *Note:* Progression of CIN to invasive squamous cell carcinoma may occur; however, not all CIN (including CIN-III) eventually proceeds to invasive carcinoma, if left untreated. Some remain stable, and some actually revert to normal.

- Role of **colposcopy** and **Pap smear cytology**

    - Improved visualization of the cervix is provided by colposcopy.

    - **Corroboration of abnormal cervical-vaginal Pap smear results is done by colposcopically directed biopsy.**

- **Invasive squamous cell carcinoma**—constitutes over 90% of primary cervical carcinoma

    - There were an estimated 15,000 new cases and 5,000 deaths caused by this lesion in 1995.

    - The declining mortality caused by invasive cervical squamous cell carcinoma is largely credited to the widespread use and efficacy of cervical Pap smear screening.

    - **Histologically,** one sees four distinct types—keratinizing, large cell nonkeratinizing, small cell, and verrucous.

- **Natural history of invasive squamous cell carcinoma**—local tumor extension typically first involves the vagina, parametria, and lower uterine segment

    - Advanced lesions may extend into the rectum, urinary bladder, and pelvic side wall.

    - Ureteral obstruction may also occur, resulting in uremia and death.

    - **Regional lymph node involvement and distant metastases are typically later events.**

    - Distant metastases most often affect the lungs, bones, and liver.

    - **Clearly, detection of the preinvasive lesion is of the utmost importance in order to avoid the consequences of invasive malignancy.**

- **Field effect**

    - Patients with CIN or cervical carcinoma quite commonly will also have involvement of the vagina or vulva (other areas lined or covered by squamous epithelium) by dysplasia or carcinoma (**multifocal disease**).

- **Staging and prognosis** shown in Table 27.1

- **Therapy**—involves surgery and/or radiation therapy (stage dependent)

Table 27.1 *Staging and Prognosis*

STAGE	5-YEAR SURVIVAL
0—carcinoma in situ	Nearly 100%
Ia—microinvasion (clinically inapparent)	Nearly 100%
Ib—carcinoma limited to cervix	90%
II—carcinoma may involve upper two-thirds of vagina and parametrium	75%
III—carcinoma involves lower one-third of vagina and/or extends to the pelvic side wall	30%
IV—carcinoma extends beyond pelvis or involves rectal and/or bladder mucosa	10%

● Adenocarcinoma

  • Incidence—5% to 10% of cervical carcinoma; **possible relative increase in recent years**

  • **Adenocarcinoma in situ, the precursor lesion, increasingly recognized**

  • **Natural history**—mode of spread similar to squamous cell carcinoma; earlier involvement of pelvic lymph nodes makes prognosis somewhat worse

  • *Note:* Although glandular dysplasias and malignancies (adenocarcinoma) are diagnosable by cervicovaginal Pap smears, this technique is not as good at detecting said lesions as compared to detecting squamous lesions.

● Gynecologic disorders associated with exposure to diethylstilbestrol (DES) in utero

  • We are seeing fewer and fewer of these lesions because DES is no longer used in pregnant women to help prevent spontaneous abortions (miscarriages). Female offspring of DES-treated mothers may have

    • Genital malformations (cervical and vaginal)
    • Vaginal adenosis (a benign glandular change)
    • Clear-cell adenocarcinoma of cervix and vagina (but **not** endometrium or ovary)

■ **Diseases of the Uterus**

● Uterus—normal structure and function

  • Endometrium—inner uterine lining; undergoes cyclic changes in response to hormonal stimulation (follicle-stimulating hormone [FSH], luteinizing hormone [LH])

  • Myometrium—smooth muscle exhibiting a tremendous capacity for extensive anatomic and physiologic adaptation (especially during and after pregnancy)

- **Inflammatory diseases and polyps of the endometrium**
  - — *Acute endometritis*
    - Seen in postabortion or in full-term delivery scenarios and is caused by retention of placental tissue; potential for spread of infection and pelvic inflammatory disease
    - Implicated organisms principally group A hemolytic streptococci and staphylococci; not commonly seen in this era of legal abortion
  - — *Chronic endometritis*
    - **Nonspecific**
      - Usually self-limited; most instances believed caused by infectious agents
      - May be associated with use of an intrauterine device (IUD), which induces inflammatory changes and predisposes to secondary infection
      - Histologically, inflammatory infiltrate of lymphocytes, occasional neutrophils, and (**diagnostically**) **plasma cells**
    - **Tuberculosis**
      - Caseating granulomas present; acid fast bacilli may or may not be demonstrable with special stains; uncommon in United States; often associated with infertility caused by endometrial scarring (Asherman's syndrome)
  - — *Endometrial polyps*
    - Common—occur at any age, but **more common at menopause**; may be incidental finding in hysterectomy specimen or may actually cause abnormal uterine bleeding
    - Histologically, one sees fingerlike projections of endometrial tissue, often with fibrotic stroma and thick-walled vessels
    - Usually benign, **but may contain a focus of dysplasia** or, less commonly, carcinoma

- **Abnormal uterine bleeding (AUB)**
  - Definition
    - Abnormal bleeding originates in the uterus and may result from organic disease of endometrium or myometrium or in the absence of organic disease (dysfunctional uterine bleeding [DUB]). Causes are shown in Box 27.1.
  - **Anovulatory cycles—most common cause of DUB;** prolonged estrogenic stimulation and breakthrough bleeding; no secretory (or luteal) endometrial phase.
    - **Anovulatory cycles are most common at menarche (onset of menses) and perimenopausally, but they can occur throughout reproductive years.**
    - In most cases, the cause cannot be determined, but a number of endocrine and metabolic abnormalities affect ovulation.
    - **Chronic anovulatory cycling is associated with an increased risk for endometrial adenocarcinoma.**

Box 27.1

CAUSES OF ABNORMAL UTERINE BLEEDING

Pregnancy related
Spontaneous abortion
Endometritis
Leiomyomatous disease
Intrauterine device
Adenomyosis
Endometrial polyp
Endometrial hyperplasia
Endometrial cancer
Endocervical cancer
Myometrial cancer
Cervical cancer
Dysfunctional uterine bleeding
Exogenous hormones

● **Endometrial hyperplasia**

• **Etiology**—caused by relative or absolute hyperestrinism; associated with polycystic ovaries, chronic failure of ovulation, estrogen-producing ovarian lesions (e.g., granulosa cell tumors), and prolonged use of exogenous therapeutic estrogens

• **Simple hyperplasia without atypia** (formally called cystic hyperplasia)—diffuse proliferation of tubular glands, less than 1% of these patients develop adenocarcinoma

• **Complex hyperplasia without atypia** (formerly called adenomatous hyperplasia without atypia)—increased number of glands relative to stroma; back-to-back glands (crowded glands with little or no intervening stroma); slightly increased risk of eventual transition to endometrial adenocarcinoma

• **Complex hyperplasia with atypia** (formerly called adenomatous hyperplasia with atypia)—contains features of complex hyperplasia together with cytologic atypia (variation in nuclear size and shape, nuclear enlargement, loss of nuclear polarity, coarse chromatin clumping, prominent nucleoli, and hyperchromasia may be present); may be difficult to distinguish from well-differentiated endometrial adenocarcinoma and constitutes a significantly increased risk (30%) of eventual progression to endometrial adenocarcinoma

● **Benign myometrial lesions, adenomyosis, and endometriosis**

— *Leiomyoma ("fibroid")*

• Benign smooth muscle neoplasm; most common uterine neoplasm and **the most common benign neoplasm of women**

• Epidemiology—peak age 35 to 45 years; common (up to 40% of women have one or more of these)

• Clinical features—depend on size and location (e.g., submucosal tumors frequently cause abnormal uterine bleeding; pedunculated subserosal lesions may twist and infarct, causing symptoms of an acute abdomen; multiple and/or large leiomyomas may result in pelvic discomfort by mass effect; infertility is yet another possible complication)

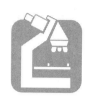

- Gross appearance—usually occur as multiple, well circumscribed, but unencapsulated firm, rubbery nodules with a characteristic whorled cut surface; usually in the uterine corpus but also may be found in the cervix, broad ligament, or elsewhere in the pelvis; large tumors may undergo degenerative changes such as hemorrhage, necrosis, and cyst formation; leiomyomas tend to "shell out" easily from the surrounding myometrium; histologically, proliferation of smooth muscle cells and intervening collagen-rich stroma

- Natural history—seem to be estrogen dependent, as evidenced by their rapid growth during pregnancy and their tendency to regress following menopause; **malignant change in a leiomyoma is extremely rare**

- Therapy—hysterectomy (if woman no longer desires her fertility); otherwise, newer medical treatment includes use of gonadotropin-releasing hormone agonists, which result in hypoestrogenism and shrinkage of leiomyoma tissue

— *Adenomyosis*

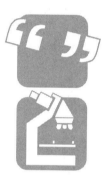

- Definition—endometrial glands and stroma deeply situated in the myometrium; occurs as a result of growth of the basal endometrial layer down into the myometrium; cyclic bleeding into the penetrating endometrial tissue is uncommon because the basal layer of the endometrium, from which the penetrations arise, is not functional

- Typically, symmetric enlargement of uterine corpus with thickened, fasciculated myometrium; small cystic spaces may be present; the histologic diagnosis rests on identification of buried endometrial stroma and glands one low-power field or more (2 to 3 mm) below the normal endomyometrial junction

- Clinical features—marked involvement may produce menorrhagia, dysmenorrhea, and pelvic pain

— *Endometriosis*

- Definition—ectopic endometrial glands and stroma, frequently in or on ovaries, uterine serosa, broad ligaments, fallopian tubes, and elsewhere

  - **In contrast to adenomyosis, endometriosis almost always contains functioning endometrium, which does undergo cyclic bleeding.**

  - *Note:* Endometriosis is most commonly seen to involve the ovaries but may literally be seen almost anywhere in the body.

- Blood collects in these foci; usually appear grossly as red-blue to yellow-brown nodules often associated with adhesions

  - In the ovaries, they may form large, blood-filled cysts that are referred to as "chocolate cysts" (when the blood ages, its appearance changes to a dark brown color).

  - Histologically, look for hemosiderin-laden macrophages, endometrial glands, and stroma.

- Clinical features—typically menorrhagia, dysmenorrhea, pelvic pain prior to the onset of menstruation, and infertility

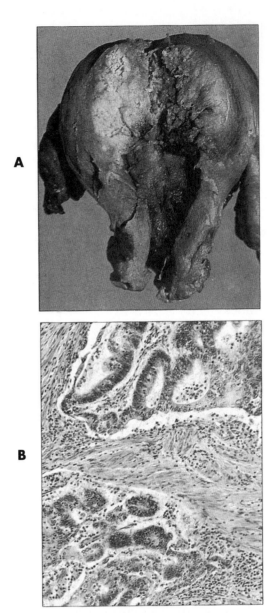

Fig. 27.5 **A,** Gross photograph of endometrial cavity filled with soft, friable cancer featuring necrosis and hemorrhage. **B,** Photomicrograph of endometrial adenocarcinoma. (*From Stevens A, Lowe J:* Pathology, *London, 1995, Times Mirror International.*)

- Long-standing, extensive disease may lead to widespread fibrosis and adherence of pelvic structures to one another ("frozen" pelvis).

- Etiology—three potential ones including regurgitation of menstrual tissue through the fallopian tubes, metaplasia of pelvic lining cells, lymphatic or vascular spread of endometrial tissue

● **Endometrial adenocarcinoma (Fig. 27.5)**

— *Incidence*   Estimated 30,000 new cases and 2,900 deaths in 1992

- **Endometrial carcinoma is the most common invasive cancer of the female genital tract and accounts for 11% of all malignancies in women.**

Box 27.2

RISK FACTORS FOR ENDOMETRIAL CARCINOMA

Infertility/nulliparity
Obesity
Hypertension
Diabetes mellitus
Hyperestrinism

— *Epidemiology*   Uncommon in women under 40, with a peak incidence in the 55- to 65-year age range.

   • Risk factors associated with endometrial carcinoma are shown in Box 27.2.

— *Diagnosis*   Endometrial biopsy sampling yields a high degree of diagnostic material.

   • Routine cervical Pap smears are *not* highly effective in screening for this disease (40% to 50% sensitivity).

   • However, endometrial cancers tend to cause irregular bleeding, permitting their diagnosis while still confined to the uterus, and, therefore, are curable by surgery and/or radiotherapy in the vast majority of patients.

— *Classification of endometrial carcinoma (vast majority are adenocarcinomas)*

   • **Favorable subtypes** tend to be low grade, have minimal or no myometrial invasion, are often associated with hyperplasia and hyperestrinism, and occur in pre- and perimenopausal women.

   • Endometrioid type—**most common type of endometrial adenocarcinoma**

   • Adenocarcinoma with squamous metaplasia (adenocanthoma); has same prognosis as the endometrioid type

   • **Unfavorable subtypes** tend to be deeply invasive and metastasize readily. They also tend to occur in an older age group than typical endometrial carcinoma and are rarely associated with hyperplasia.

   • **Adenosquamous carcinoma**—adenocarcinoma with ma-lignant **squamous** epithelial component

   • Clear-cell carcinoma—unlike cervical and vaginal clear cell carcinoma, is *not* associated with in utero (DES) exposure

   • **Papillary serous carcinoma**—resembles ovarian papillary serous carcinoma; has poorer prognosis

— *Therapy and prognosis*

   • Choice of surgery, radiation therapy, or chemotherapy is stage dependent.

   • Prognostic factors are shown in Table 27.2.

   • **Stage is the most important prognostic factor; 85% to 90% of all patients are stage I or stage II at time of diagnosis**

Table 27.2 *Staging System for Endometrial Adenocarcinoma*

STAGE	5-YEAR SURVIVAL
I Carcinoma confined to the uterine corpus	71%-89%
II Involvement of corpus and cervix	44%-72%
III Extension outside the uterus but confined to the pelvis	38%
IV Carcinoma either outside the true pelvis or involves the mucosa of the bladder and/or rectum	18%

- Grade—well-differentiated lesions (low grade) tend to be low stage and, therefore, have a better prognosis; there are architectural and nuclear grading schemes; well differentiated (grade 1) features easily recognizable glandular pattern; moderately differentiated (grade 2) features presence of well-formed glands mixed with solid sheets of malignant cells; poorly differentiated (grade 3) is characterized by solid sheets of cells with few recognizable glands; great degree of nuclear atypia and high mitotic activity usually seen in higher-grade lesions

- Depth of myometrial invasion—deeply invasive lesions have a higher incidence of lymph node metastases

- Vascular invasion—associated with an increased probability of recurrence

- Endometrial hyperplasia—if present, indicates a **favorable** prognosis

● Malignant mesenchymal neoplasms (sarcomas) arising in endometrium or myometrium

- *Note:* Sarcomas constitute 5% or less of all uterine cancers.

— *Leiomyosarcoma*

- Incidence—**uncommon;** usually arise de novo, but may **rarely** originate in preexisting leiomyoma

- Gross appearance—soft and typically hemorrhagic with necrosis; often infiltrates into the surrounding myometrium (in contrast to leiomyoma); histologically, may be well differentiated; microscopic criteria are cell density, nuclear atypia, and number of mitotic figures

  - **Mitotic activity is the most important diagnostic criterion; greater than 5 mitoses per 10 high dry power fields** with cytologic atypia allows for classification into malignant category.

  - Other helpful diagnostic features include **invasive borders,** large lesional size, extensive necrosis, and extension of leiomyosarcoma beyond the uterine corpus.

- Clinical features—average age 52 years; patients present with enlarging abdominal mass or vaginal bleeding

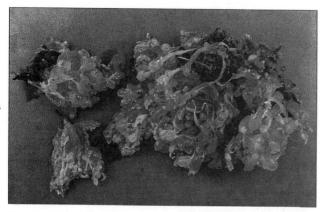 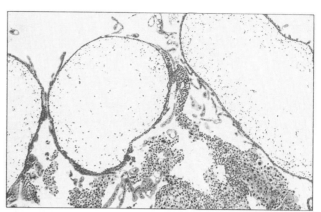

Fig. 27.6 A, Gross photograph of hydatidiform mole shows the characteristic vesicles ("white grapes"); no fetal parts or normal placental tissues are observed in this complete mole. **B,** Photomicrograph demonstrates enlarged, cystic vesicles with nearby proliferation of trophoblastic elements. (*From Stevens A, Lowe J:* Pathology, *London, 1995, Times Mirror International.*)

- Therapy and prognosis—total abdominal hysterectomy and bilateral salpingo-oophorectomy constitute the usual treatment; 20% to 25% 5-year survival

    - Pelvic recurrence and lung metastasis are often seen.

— *Endometrial stromal sarcoma*

    - A malignant neoplasm arising in stromal cells of endometrium; 50% 5-year survival with surgery

— *"Mixed" neoplasms*

- Adenofibroma—benign stromal and glandular components
- Adenosarcoma—malignant stroma with benign glandular component
- **Malignant mixed Müllerian tumors**—both stromal and glandular components malignant

    - **Homologous type (carcinosarcoma)**—one (or more) malignant mesenchymal elements arising from a mesenchymal element normally found in the uterus (e.g., malignant smooth muscle, malignant endometrial stromal cells)

    - **Heterologous type**—contains one (or more) malignant mesenchymal element not "native" to the uterus (e.g., malignant cartilage, malignant skeletal muscle, and malignant bone)

● Gestational trophoblastic neoplasia

- This is a spectrum of lesions showing proliferation of pregnancy-associated trophoblastic tissue with varying degrees of malignant potential. Essentially all elaborate human chorionic gonadotropin (HCG). HCG levels (especially the β subunit of HCG) are thus important diagnostically and also aid in assessing the patient's response to therapy. Women under 20 and over 40 years of age are most commonly affected.

— *Hydatidiform mole (H. Mole)*

- Cystic, hydropic swelling of chorionic villi with variable hyperplastic and atypical changes in trophoblastic elements; can be divided into two subtypes—"complete" and "partial" (Fig. 27.6)

- **A complete hydatidiform mole never contains an umbilical cord, embryo, or amniotic membranes.** The chorionic villi are abnormal, and the trophoblastic elements usually have a 46,XX karyotype.

- **The partial hydatidiform mole** contains an embryo, umbilical cord, and amniotic membranes; has some normal chorionic villi; **and is almost always cytogenetically triploid.**

- Clinically H. mole can be seen at any age, but risk increases in pregnancies involving women in their teens or those between the ages of 40 and 50 years. Incidence varies geographically (higher in Far East). In the United States, incidence is 1 to 1.5 per 2000 pregnancies.

- Patients present with abnormal uterine bleeding early in pregnancy (16 to 17 weeks). Passage of thin, watery fluid and **white, grapelike tissue fragments** is noted by patient. Uterus is larger than expected for gestational date. Typically, no fetus is seen or palpated, and fetal heart tones are absent.

- Lab shows elevated β-HCG levels in blood and urine.

- Pathogenesis begins at conception as a form of neoplasia.

- Gross appearance reveals a large uterus, filled with thin-walled, translucent cysts (white grapelike clusters).

- Histologically one looks for hydropic swelling of chorionic villi, absent or poor vascularization of villi, and varying degrees of trophoblastic proliferation.

- Treatment includes curettage of mole; hysterectomy, if indicated; and following patient with periodic serum HCG (β subunit) determinations.

- Prognosis is 80% benign behavior, 20% have complications; choriocarcinoma arises in 2% to 3% of patients.

— *Invasive mole*

- Invasive mole behaves in a manner that is intermediate between a benign mole and choriocarcinoma.

- This is a cellular invasive mole that destructively penetrates myometrium. Emboli of hydropic villi can involve distant sites (lung, brain); emboli can regress. This does not have any true metastatic potential.

- Clinically there is vaginal bleeding, enlarged uterus, and elevated serum HCG. This can lead to death secondary to rupture of uterus with hemorrhage and sepsis. In most cases, cure is possible by chemotherapy.

- Histologically, one sees retention of hydropic villi. Trophoblastic elements proliferate and exhibit cytoatypia.

— *Choriocarcinoma*

- Rare malignancy of trophoblastic cells; in United States, seen in one in 40,000 to 70,000 pregnancies

  - Aggressive cancer that often metastasizes early, **especially to the lungs**

  - Clinical—preceded by H. mole 50%; previous abortion 25%; remainder occur after an apparently normal pregnancy;

patient presents with irregular bloody-brown discharge; in contrast to H. mole, primary site typically not bulky; metastases often present at time of discovery; markedly elevated serum HCG titers usually seen

- Histologically, one sees malignant trophoblastic elements that do not form villi; rapid growth with myometrial invasion and penetration of blood vessels; fleshy lesion with a tendency toward extensive hemorrhage and necrosis; metastatic sites include lung, vagina, brain, liver, kidney; **metastases are hematogenous** and lymphatic invasion is uncommon; characteristically has two cell types—cytotrophoblasts and syncytiotrophoblasts

- Treatment—formerly nearly uniformly fatal; now, with chemotherapy, nearly 100% cures obtained in cases that have not spread beyond the pelvis, vagina, and lungs

■ Diseases of the Ovary and Fallopian Tube

- ● Nonneoplastic diseases of the ovary

  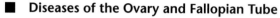
  — *Nonneoplastic cysts*

    - **Follicular and luteal cysts** are common in clinical practice; lined by granulosa-thecal or luteal cells, respectively, and contain fluid; sometimes may be filled with hemorrhagic debris.

        - Hemorrhagic luteal cysts may rupture, causing a true medical emergency.

    - **Polycystic ovaries (Stein-Leventhal syndrome)** affect young women.

        - In the classic Stein-Leventhal syndrome, patients have **secondary amenorrhea, obesity, hirsutism, infertility.**
        - Microscopic features are bilaterally enlarged ovaries, a thickened, white outer capsule, and multiple subcortical cysts.
        - Etiology is thought to be caused by an abnormal hypothalamic-pituitary axis.
        - Treatment is bilateral ovarian wedge resection.

- ● Ovarian neoplasms

    - **Ovarian cancer accounts for more deaths** (about 12,000) than cancers of the cervix and uterine corpus together.
    - The classification of ovarian tumors may be based upon the likely tissue of origin.

        - Neoplasms derived from surface (coelomic) epithelium (**most common site of origin for ovarian neoplasms)**
        - Neoplasms derived from germ cells
        - Neoplasms derived from gonadal stromal elements

    — *Common epithelial neoplasms*

        - Are the largest group of primary ovarian neoplasms

        - They arise from the multipotential, surface (coelomic) epithelium of ovary, which can differentiate to resemble epithelium of fallopian tube (serous lesions), endocervix (mucinous lesions), endometrium (endometrioid lesions), bladder (transitional cell or Brenner tumor), or into clear cells (clear-cell carcinoma).

- There are **both benign and malignant neoplasms within the common epithelial categories.**

- In addition, **any of the common epithelial neoplasms may fall into a "borderline" or low malignant potential category,** which has a better prognosis and requires less aggressive therapy than frank carcinoma.

- In general, common benign epithelial neoplasms are characterized by a **simple, bland, nonstratified lining, lack architectural complexity, and have no underlying stromal invasion.**

- Borderline epithelial neoplasms have cytologic atypia, stratified lining, and architectural complexity but still lack stromal invasion.

- Common epithelial malignant neoplasms have the same features as borderline lesions, with the addition of stromal invasion and greater cytoatypia.

Serous neoplasms

- **Most frequent ovarian neoplasms**—40% of epithelial neoplasms

- **Often bilateral**—(up to 70% of serous cystadenocarcinomas are bilateral, **and this malignancy has the highest rate of bilaterality of all ovarian neoplasms)**

- Occur at any age, but the majority of benign serous neoplasms occur during the reproductive years

  - Serous carcinomas occur most frequently in women over 40 years of age.

- Gross—commonly cystic and often papillary; **solid areas typically present when lesion is malignant**

  - Jutting into the cystic cavities are polypoid or papillary projections, which become more prominent in malignant lesions (papillary excrescences).

  - In general, **the more prominent the papillary excrescences and solid areas, the more likely the lesion is malignant.**

  - The cystic spaces are usually filled with **clear serous fluid.**

- Histologically—benign lesions (serous cystadenomas) have a single layer of cells resembling fallopian tube epithelium

  - Borderline lesions are characterized by complex, budding papillae covered by stratified epithelium with some degree of cytologic atypia.

  - Malignant neoplasms (serous carcinomas or serous cystadenocarcinomas) are similar to borderline neoplasms except that stromal invasion is present and there is usually more cytoatypia.

  - **Psammoma bodies** (concentrically laminated calcified bodies) **are commonly seen in serous neoplasms but are not** in and of themselves **malignant** (they are also seen in benign neoplasms as well as nonneoplastic reactive processes).

- Frank, clear cut, ovarian carcinoma—tends to spread contiguously within the pelvis and seeds the peritoneal cavity with malignant cells (malignant ascites)

  - Spread to regional lymph nodes is common and distant metastases are infrequent.

- Treatment—surgery, sometimes followed by radiation or chemotherapy

  - Five-year survival rate for borderline tumors is nearly 100% vs. frank carcinoma, which is less than 20%.
  - **Cancer stage is the most important prognostic factor.**

Mucinous neoplasms

- Most commonly occur in the fourth through sixth decades of life
- Less common than serous neoplasms (6% to 10% of common epithelial neoplasms) **and less commonly bilateral (25%)**
- Benign and borderline mucinous neoplasms much more common than frank mucinous carcinomas
- Gross—differ little from serous neoplasms except that their cystic contents are usually mucinous (thick, viscid material).

  - Mucinous neoplasms also tend to be larger and more often multiloculated.

- Histologically—epithelium of mucinous neoplasms consists of mucin-secreting cells similar to those of endocervical or colonic mucosa

  - Criteria for distinguishing benign from borderline and malignant mucinous neoplasms are similar to those for serous lesions.

- **Prognosis for mucinous carcinoma—better than for its serous counterpart; overall 5-year survival rate is 40%**

  - *Note:* Mucinous neoplasms (both benign and malignant) of the ovary may be associated with the formation of abundant free mucin (mucinous ascites) in the peritoneal cavity (**pseudomyxoma peritonei**).

Endometrioid neoplasms

- May arise in association with endometriosis (10% to 20% of cases)
- 30% are bilateral
- Most are frank carcinomas (i.e., benign and borderline forms are rare) and occur in older women
- Gross—usually indistinguishable from serous and mucinous lesions

  - These neoplasms may present as a mass projecting from the wall of an endometriotic cyst filled with chocolate-colored fluid.

- Histologically, resembles adenocarcinoma of endometrium; may also have foci of squamous differentiation (as is seen in endometrial adenoacanthoma)
- Prognosis—overall 5-year survival rate for all stages of endometrioid carcinoma is 55%; for stage I lesions it is 92%

Clear-cell neoplasms

- Uncommon; almost all are carcinomas
- Resemble clear-cell carcinomas of cervix, vagina, and endometrium
- Occur in older women and are *not* related to in utero DES exposure
- Prognosis—5-year survival rate is 41%

Transitional cell (Brenner) neoplasms

- Uncommon, age 40 to 70 years
- Vast majority (more than 95%) are **benign** and often an incidental finding
- May be associated with signs of hyperestrinism
- Gross—firm, solid, grey-white tumors with a whorled cut surface
- Histologically, nests of urothelial-like transitional cells in a fibrous stroma

  - The **extremely rare malignant Brenner neoplasms** characteristically have stromal invasion.

— **Germ cell neoplasms**

- Originate from primitive germ cells and collectively account for 15% to 20% of all ovarian neoplasms but only 2% of ovarian cancers

  - **Most are seen in children and young adults.**
  - **About 95% are mature cystic teratomas.**

Teratomas—contain elements representative of more than one germ cell layer (ectoderm, endoderm, mesoderm)

- Mature (benign) cystic teratomas (dermoid cysts)

  - Common benign neoplasm of ovary, usually marked by ectodermal differentiation (skin, hair, and teeth are commonly found within these lesions)
  - Usually unilateral
  - **Most common ovarian tumor of children and young adults**
  - Gross—unilocular cyst filled with hair and sebaceous material
  - Histologically, cysts lined by skin (including appendages); any other mature tissue may be present (such as bronchial, gastrointestinal [GI] tract, thyroid, central nervous system [CNS])
  - Malignant transformation of one of the tissue elements occurs in about 1% of dermoid cysts, usually taking the form of squamous cell carcinoma

- Torsion of the lesion may produce an acute abdomen

- Immature (malignant) teratomas

  - Occur in patients under 40 years of age with a significant number before puberty

  - Contain primitive embryonal tissue mixed with adult tissue (i.e., immature and mature tissue)

  - Prognosis generally poor (depends on nature and amount of immature tissue)

- Overall 5-year survival is 25% to 30%; better differentiated lesions confined to the ovary can be cured by excision

Endodermal sinus tumor (yolk sac tumor)

- Neoplasm of children and young adults
- Elevated levels of serum alpha-fetoprotein characteristically seen
- Histologically—this lesion recapitulates the yolk sac—see meshwork of cysts and channels lined by flattened, cuboidal, or low columnar cells; **Schiller-Duval bodies** (resemble glomeruli); **hyaline globules** containing alpha-fetoprotein
- Poor prognosis, although a few cases achieve long-term survival with current multiagent chemotherapeutic regimens

Embryonal carcinoma

- Rare in ovary
- Median age—15 years
- Poor prognosis

Choriocarcinoma

- Rare in ovary and usually occurs as part of a mixed germ cell neoplasm
- "Pure" choriocarcinoma is most often a metastasis from a trophoblastic neoplasm
- In its pure form, highly aggressive and usually lethal

Dysgerminoma

- 3% to 5% of malignant ovarian neoplasms
- Most in women under 30 years of age
- Well-defined associations with congenital malformations of the genitals and with Turner's syndrome described
- Gross—unilateral, lobulated, solid, and fleshy
- Histologically, **identical to seminoma of testis;** sheets of large, vesicular, clear cells separated by fibrous trabeculae that have a lymphocytic infiltrate and (occasionally) granulomas
- Radiosensitive (may have good cure rate even with metastases present); 5-year survival rate is 75% to 90%

— ***Gonadal stromal tumors***

- Composed of varying combinations of sex cord and stromal cells capable of differentiation in an "ovarian direction" (granulosa, theca cells), in a "testicular direction" (Sertoli and Leydig cells), or in a stromal direction to remain fibromatous

- Uncommon (8% of ovarian neoplasms) and most are benign (only 2% are malignant)
- May be hormonally active

Granulosa cell tumors

- Occur at all ages (most common in adult postmenopausal women)
- 5% or less bilateral
- **Most produce estrogen** (precocious puberty in children; endometrial hyperplasia and abnormal uterine bleeding in adults)

  - **Occasionally associated with adenocarcinoma of the endometrium**
  - Rarely, produce androgenic hormones

- Histologically, cells with distinct nuclear grooves growing in a variety of patterns—diffuse, follicular, trabecular, solid

  - Call-Exner bodies (acinus-like structures with central eosinophilic material, having a resemblance to an ovum) sometimes present

- Usually have a low malignant potential

Others

- Thecoma
- Fibroma
- Luteoma
- Sertoli-Leydig cell tumors

— *Metastatic tumors*

- Most common sources of metastatic tumor to ovary—the GI tract, breast, and nearby pelvic organs
- "Krukenberg tumor"—term used for bilateral ovarian involvement by metastatic adenocarcinoma having a "signet-ring" histologic appearance

  - **Stomach** is most common primary site for Krukenberg tumor, but may also orginate from elsewhere in the GI tract, the breast, and (rarely) other sites

- Malignant lymphoma (especially Burkitt's type, in children)

- Fallopian tubes

— *Nonneoplastic disorders*

  - **Inflammation of the fallopian tube is almost always part of PID**

    - **PID is the most common clinically significant primary tubal disease.**
    - PID is usually caused by bacterial infection (an ascending infection), often sexually transmitted; *Neisseria gonorrhoeae* accounts for 45% of cases and *Chlamydia trachomatis* for 20% of cases.
    - Nongonococcal organisms such as *Mycoplasma hominis,* coliforms, and (in the postpartum scenario) streptococci and

staphylococci are now major offenders. Also anaerobic bacteria may have a role in a substantial number of patients.

- Granulomatous salpingitis

  - Uncommon in United States
  - Tuberculous (TB) salpingitis most important; seen as complication of TB; spread is hematogenous (as a manifestation of miliary TB)

- Tubal sequelae and complications of PID

  - Tuboovarian abscess (pus material)
  - Hydrosalpinx (tube dilated and filled with watery fluid)
  - Infertility
  - Ectopic pregnancy (see following)

- Ectopic pregnancy

  - The implantation of the fertilized ovum in any site other than the normal uterine location is **ectopic pregnancy.**
  - **Fallopian tube** is the most common site for ectopic implantation of fertilized ovum. Other sites include ovaries, peritoneal cavity, and the intrauterine portion of the tube (**interstitial pregnancy).**
  - Ectopic tubal pregnancy results in tubal rupture in most instances and may cause an acute abdomen with emergent need for immediate medical attention.
  - Until rupture occurs, an ectopic pregnancy may be indistinguishable from a normal one, with cessation of menstruation and elevation of serum and urinary HCG. **However, absence of elevated HCG does not exclude the diagnosis.**
  - Tube shows presence of chorionic villi and/or fetal parts.
  - Endometrial curettings may show any pattern, but gestational hypersecretory endometrium and decidual changes in association with a tubal mass are suggestive of tubal pregnancy.
  - Etiology is usually chronic inflammatory changes within the tube, although intrauterine tumors and endometriosis may also hamper passage of the ovum. This is occasionally associated with an IUD. In about 50% of cases, no associated anatomic defects can be demonstrated.

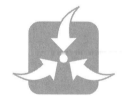

— *Benign neoplasms*

  - Rare, adenomatoid tumors (mesotheliomas) are small nodules that are the counterparts of those seen in the testes and epididymis and are usually of little clinical significance.

— *Malignant neoplasms*

  - Rare; when you encounter these, they are usually in postmenopausal women
  - Cancer almost always arises from the mucosal lining of the tubes (usually near the distal ends)

- **Virtually all primary tubal malignancies are adenocarcinomas**
- Symptoms—vaginal discharge, abnormal uterine bleeding, adnexal mass, pelvic pain
- Prognosis—poor

MULTIPLE CHOICE
REVIEW QUESTIONS

1. The most common *primary* malignancy of the *vagina* in women is which of the following?

    a. Adenocarcinoma
    b. Rhabdomyosarcoma
    c. Clear cell carcinoma
    d. Squamous cell carcinoma
    e. Malignant melanoma

2. A 35-year-old woman presents to you with substantial abnormal uterine bleeding and pelvic discomfort. You perform a pelvic examination and note an enlarged uterus with multiple large nodular masses. This patient most likely has which of the following lesions?

    a. Lipoma
    b. Leiomyomata
    c. Endometrial adencarcinoma
    d. Sarcoma botryoides

3. Which of the following represents the most common site of *metastatic* gestational choriocarcinoma?

    a. Periaortic lymph nodes
    b. Deep pelvic lymph nodes
    c. Kidney
    d. Liver
    e. Lung

4. The type of primary ovarian cancer with the highest rate of bilaterality is which of the following?

    a. Serous cystadenocarcinoma
    b. Mucinous cystadenocarcinoma
    c. Malignant Brenner tumor
    d. Clear cell carcinoma
    e. Endometrioid carcinoma

5. A 73-year-old woman presents to the emergency room with a watery vaginal discharge, pelvic pain and, by your examination, a left adnexal mass. Ultrasound evaluation reveals the presence of a large left fallopian tubal mass. Assuming that this is a primary neoplasm, which one of the following types of cancer is it most likely to be?

    a. Squamous cell carcinoma
    b. Malignant lymphoma
    c. Adenocarcinoma
    d. Rhabdomyosarcoma
    e. Fibrosarcoma

Chapter 28

Pathology of the Male Genital Tract (Penis, Testis, Prostate)

PENIS

■ Malformations

- **Hypospadias**—abnormal urethral opening(s) on the ventral surface of the penis
- **Epispadias**—abnormal urethral opening(s) on the dorsal surface of the penis
- *Note:* Both hypospadias and epispadias are often associated with other abnormalities of the genitourinary tract, including cryptorchidism.
- **Phimosis**—condition in which the orifice of the foreskin (prepuce) is too small to permit its normal retraction; may result from anomalous development or represent a sequela of postinflammatory scarring

  - The significance of phimosis is that it allows for the accumulation of secretions and debris under the foreskin, and this predisposes toward infection and, probably, cancer.

■ Infections

- Syphilis
- Gonorrhea
- Chancroid
- Fungi
- Lymphogranuloma venereum
- Herpes simplex
- Granuloma inguinale
- Staphylococci

■ "Tumors"

- ● Benign/Borderline

  - — *Condyloma acuminatum*

    - Etiologic agent is human papilloma virus (HPV), which is related to the common wart virus that causes verruca vulgaris
    - Sexually transmitted process
    - HPV—many different antigenic types (over 70); types 6 and 11 most clearly associated with condyloma acuminatum
    - **Gross**—single or multiple, red, velvety, papillary excrescences

that vary in size from 1 to several mm in greatest dimension (look for them also in the anal region)

- **Micro**—branching, papillary connective tissue stroma covered by a hyperplastic (thickened) epidermis

  - The epidermal nuclei focally typically show enlargement and hyperchromasia with irregular outlines and perinuclear halos (these cells are known as koilocytes)

— *Giant condyloma of Buschke-Lowenstein*

- Some feel this is a low-grade (well differentiated) squamous cell carcinoma

- **Gross**—usually a single, large, exophytic lesion that may cover and destroy much of the penis; is associated with HPV infection (especially types 6 and 11); it is locally invasive and may recur after excision

- **Micro**—similar to condyloma acuminatum with additional feature of hyperplastic epithelium penetrating into subjacent dermis along a broad front

  - Rarely, if ever, metastasizes

    - **Therefore, in clinical behavior, it appears to occupy a position intermediate between a routine, strictly benign condyloma acuminatum, on the one hand, and squamous cell carcinoma on the other. It should be noted, however, that some authors do refer to this lesion as a low-grade variant of squamous cell carcinoma called "verrucous carcinoma."**

- Malignant

  — *Carcinoma in situ (Bowen's disease)*

  - Full thickness epidermal dysplasia (disorderly maturation) but no evidence for invasive malignancy
    - Clinical (gross) appearance of the lesions may vary widely

  — *Invasive squamous cell carcinoma*

  - Represents 1% of all cancers in American males; usually seen in men 40 to 70 years of age
  - Circumcision appears to offer protection from this type of cancer
  - **Gross**—varies from a papillary (exophytic) lesion to an ulcerating/invasive lesion
  - **Micro**—rather typical squamous cell carcinoma; histologically, nests and cords of malignant squamous cells infiltrating the dermis; may see keratinization
  - **Clinical course**—tend to be rather slow-growing carcinomas that may metastasize to regional (inguinal and iliac) lymph nodes; distant metastasis are uncommon, unless the lesion is far advanced

TESTIS

■ Cryptorchidism (Undescended Testis)

- In fetal life, the testes arise within the coelomic cavity and then (through differential growth of the body and disproportionate growth of the caudal end of the urogenital ridge) they eventually come to lie in the low abdomen/pelvic brim (internal descent).

- They normally next proceed into the inguinal canal and, ultimately, the scrotal sac (external descent).

  - **Testes may be abnormally positioned anywhere along this route.**

    - Most cases of cryptorchidism are idiopathic but some are caused by genetic defects (Trisomy 13 or hormonal deficit [luteinizing hormone releasing hormone, LHRH]).
    - Most cases are unilateral but up to 25% are bilateral.
    - 0.3% to 0.8% of adult male population suffers from cryptorchidism.

- Why is cryptorchidism important?

  - Histologic changes begin by 2 years of age and include loss of germ cell production and tubular fibrosis (scarring) that eventually produces a small, fibrotic testis. **Sterility is therefore a major complication.**
  - When the testis lies in the inguinal canal, it is more susceptible to traumatic injury than when it lies in the scrotal sac.
  - **Cryptorchidism is associated with 7 to 11 times increased risk of developing testicular cancer.**

■ **Atrophy (Loss of Testicular Seminiferous Tubules with Resultant Infertility)**

- Causes of testicular atrophy
  - Atherosclerosis
  - Cryptorchidism
  - End-stage orchitis
  - Hypopituitarism
  - Generalized malnutrition
  - Obstruction to outflow of semen
  - Irradiation
  - Administration of estrogen-like compounds (e.g., diethylstilbestrol [DES] for metastatic prostate cancer)
  - Exhaustion atrophy caused by persistently high levels of follicle-stimulating hormone (FSH)
  - Sex chromosomal abnormality (e.g., Klinefelter's syndrome—XXY)
  - Heavy androgen use

■ **Inflammatory Processes**

- Testis is much less often affected by inflammatory processes than is the case for the epididymis.
- Chlamydia trachomatis
- Neisseria gonorrhoea
  - May cause suppurative orchitis, but more often causes severe acute inflammation in epididymis
- Mumps
  - In the typical age group to be affected by mumps, there is usually no testicular involvement.
  - However, when post-pubertal males develop the infection, 20% to

30% will suffer from mumps orchitis, which is unilateral about 70% of the time.

   • Inflammatory cell process features lymphocytes, plasma cells, macrophages.

   • Most patients with this do heal with no resultant infertility, but sterility is the outcome in some patients.

● **Tuberculosis**

   • This infection almost always begins in the epididymis and may spread to the testis: look for granulomatous inflammation and acid-fast bacillus (AFB) organisms.

● **Syphilis**

   • Unlike most other infections that involve both the testis and the epididymis, syphilis typically involves the testis **first.**

   • Look for gummas *or* a diffuse interstitial chronic inflammatory cell response with lymphocytes and plasma cells and an arteritis with prominent plasma cell cuffing.

   • Organisms are demonstrable with silver stain (e.g., Warthin-Starry).

● **Granulomatous (?autoimmune) orchitis**

   • This condition, presumed autoimmune in nature, is a rare disorder seen mostly in middle-aged men.

   • One must rule out tuberculous orchitis before making this diagnosis.

● **Others**

   • In males older than 35 years, look for common urinary tract pathogens (especially *Escherichia coli* and *Pseudomonas* organisms). These usually do not involve testis but are typically limited to epididymis.

■ **Testicular Neoplasms**

   • **Testicular neoplasms** are the most important cause of firm, painless enlargement of the testis.

   • Nearly all testicular neoplasms are malignant and 95% arise from germ cells.

   • Most of the remaining neoplasms arise from Leydig and Sertoli cells (gonadal stromal tumors).

● **Epidemiology**

   • Average incidence in the United States is approximately 2 per 100,000 males.

   • Testicular neoplasms account for 1% of all cancers in males.

   • Their peak incidence is in the 15- to 34-year-old age group.

   • Incidence rates are 6 to 10 times higher in Caucasians than in African Americans.

   • Genetic influences are suggested in rare cases involving twins or fathers and sons.

   • Cryptorchidism is a predisposing factor.

   • The vast majority (95%) of testicular neoplasms are germ cell tumors, and about 60% feature more than one histologic pattern.

● **Classification of germ cell neoplasms**

—   *Seminoma*

     • It is the most common **pure,** germ cell neoplasm.

- Seminoma presents grossly with grey-white, lobulated tumor; hemorrhage and necrosis usually *not* conspicuous.

- Histologically, in its classical (typical) form, it is composed of sheets of uniform, large, polygonal cells, with central round nuclei and clear cytoplasm.

- Fibrous stroma may contain syncytiotrophoblastic giant cells (which produce human chorionic gonadotropin [HCG]) and lymphocytes.

- The two other types of seminoma are spermatocytic seminoma (good prognosis), and anaplastic seminoma (poor prognosis).

— *Embryonal carcinoma*

- Appears grossly as a grey-white, poorly demarcated mass, often with **extensive areas of hemorrhage and necrosis**

- Histologically, these neoplasms are composed of anaplastic, large cells with a high mitotic rate; this carcinoma may assume solid, tubular, or papillary microscopic growth patterns

- *Note:* Some element of embryonal carcinoma is seen in 45% of *all* germ cell cancers.

— *Teratoma*

- Typically, teratomas are multicystic and partly solid neoplasms, enlarging the testis in a nodular configuration.

- Hemorrhage and necrosis are not prominent.

- Tissues from all three germ cell lines (ectoderm, mesoderm, and endoderm) may be present.

- The fully differentiated variant, called mature teratoma, is composed entirely of benign adult types of tissue.

- The immature teratoma contains similar elements, which are incompletely differentiated but can be identified as embryonic tissues.

- In addition, there are teratomas with frank sarcoma or carcinoma (the latter being typically squamous cell carcinoma or adenocarcinoma) developing in them.

— *Yolk sac tumor (infantile embryonal carcinoma or endodermal sinus tumor)*

- Grossly, these lesions are similar to embryonal carcinoma.

- In its pure form, it is rare. However, it is the most common neoplasm affecting the testes of children under 3 years of age.

- Yolk sac tumors recapitulate the embryonic mammalian yolk sac and typically produce alpha-fetoprotein (AFP).

- Tumor cells vary from flattened to cuboidal to columnar cells and may be arranged in glandular, papillary, or solid formations.

- Other features include Schiller-Duval bodies (resemble glomeruli) and hyaline globules that contain AFP.

— *Choriocarcinoma*

- Highly malignant, metastasizing via the blood stream early and widely; produces HCG

- Grossly, choriocarcinoma is an ill-defined mass or nodule that is hemorrhagic and necrotic appearing

Table 28.1   *Staging of Testicular Cancer*

STAGE	EXTENT
Stage I	Confined to testis
Stage II	Distant spread confined to retroperitoneal nodes below the diaphragm
Stage III	Metastases outside the retroperitoneal lymph nodes or above the diaphragm

- Interestingly, these lesions are often quite small, giving no discernible testicular enlargement in many cases
- Represents differentiation to extraembryonic structures (placenta) and is composed of cytotrophoblasts and syncytiotrophoblasts

— *Mixed germ cell tumor*

- This shows a mixture of two or more of the above histologic patterns and **accounts for 60% of all testicular germ cell neoplasms.**
- In general, the prognosis of a mixed germ cell tumor is determined by the most malignant element.
- **The combination of embryonal carcinoma with teratoma is called *teratocarcinoma*.**

- Clinical parameters of testicular neoplasms

- Most present as painless testicular enlargement; any testicular mass should be considered neoplastic until proven otherwise.
- By convention and for therapeutic reasons, we divide neoplasms of the testis into seminoma and nonseminomatous germ cell tumors (NSGCT).

  - The latter lesions often present with distinctive clinical features and differ from seminomas with regard to therapy and prognosis.

- In general, testicular malignancies spread by the lymphatics.

  - Usually, this spread occurs first to the retroperitoneal and paraaortic lymph nodes and, later on, to mediastinal and supraclavicular lymph nodes.
  - Hematogenous spread may also occur, however, and this is primarily to lungs, liver, brain, and bones. **Although most metastases are similar to the primary cancer, in some cases one sees a different histologic appearance in the metastasis as compared to the primary testicular lesion.**

- Staging of testicular neoplasms is shown in Table 28.1.
- Neoplastic ("tumor") markers in the serum

  - AFP is produced by yolk sac tumors, embryonal carcinoma (also by hepatocellular carcinoma)
  - β subunit of HCG is produced by choriocarcinomas, some embryonal carcinomas

- Placental alkaline phosphatase (PLAP) is produced by seminomas
- *Note:* Elevations of AFP, β-HCG, or both are seen in nearly 90% of NSGCTs.

— *Three major uses of these markers*

- In the initial evaluation of the testicular mass
- In the staging of testicular germ cell neoplasms
- In monitoring response to therapy as part of recurrence assessment

— *Points regarding seminoma vs. NSGCTs*

- Seminomas tend to be confined to testis for a longer period of time than is the case for NSGCTs.

  - In fact, 70% of seminomas are stage I at the time of diagnosis, whereas 60% of NSGCTs are stages II and III at the time of diagnosis.

- Seminoma metastases typically involve lymph nodes, and hematogenous metastases from seminoma tend to occur late. For NSGCTs, metastases occur earlier and are more often hematogenous.
- Seminomas are extremely radiosensitive, whereas NSGCTs are relatively radioresistant.
- **Summary** is as follows: NSGCTs are more aggressive cancers with poorer prognosis than is the case for seminoma. The most aggressive of the NSGCTs is choriocarcinoma.

— *Therapy and prognosis*

- Surgery
- Radiotherapy
- Chemotherapy
- Most patients with seminoma can be cured; among patients with NSGCTs, 80% to 85% can achieve complete remission with chemotherapy. Unfortunately, a substantial number of these eventually relapse and die of their NSGCTs.

● **Other testicular neoplasms**

— *Leydig cell tumors*

- Arise from the interstitial cells of Leydig (which normally produce testosterone)
- Neoplastic cells may produce androgens, androgens and estrogen, or even corticosteroid
- Uncommon lesions (2% of all testicular neoplasms); seen mainly between ages of 20 and 60 years
- Usually present with testicular mass, but may first exhibit gynecomastia
- **Gross**—yellow-brown homogeneous mass
- **Micro**—large, round, or polygonal cells with abundant eosinophilic cytoplasm and a central round nucleus; crystals of Reinke seen in cytoplasm in 25% of cases
- 90% are benign

— *Sertoli cell tumors (androblastoma)*

- Composed of Sertoli cells or granulosa cells
- Androgens or estrogens produced, but usually in insufficient quantities to produce precocious masculinization or feminization; occasionally see gynecomastia
- **Gross**—firm, small, grey-white-yellow nodules
- **Micro**—tall, columnar, polyhedral cells that grow in cords, reminiscent of spermatic tubules
- 90% are benign

— *Malignant lymphoma*

- Accounts for 5% of all testicular neoplasms
- **Malignant lymphoma is the most common testicular cancer in men over age 60 years**
- In most instances, is disseminated by the time of detection of testicular mass
- Almost always is of the diffuse, large cell type
- Prognosis—poor

DISEASES OF THE PROSTATE

- The prostate gland is derived from endodermal buddings of the urethra.
- In the adult male, this compound tubuloalveolar gland weighs approximately 20 g; it is retroperitoneal, lies at the bladder neck, and encircles both the bladder neck and the urethra.
- Although the prostate gland has five discernible lobes (anterior, median, posterior, and two lateral) at the embryonic developmental stage, the distinctions between these are lost over the course of time so that, by adulthood, only three distinct lobes are seen (median and two lateral).
- Testicular-derived androgens stimulate prostatic growth.

■ Histologic "Game Plan" of Prostate

- Large, serpiginous glands lined by **two** cell layers (inner or columnar mucus secreting; outer or low cuboidal; the latter is *not* composed of myoepithelial cells)

  - Stroma—fibromuscular (fibroblasts, collagen, smooth muscle bundles)
  - Striated skeletal muscle sphincter

- **Prostatitis (three categories—acute, chronic bacterial, chronic "abacterial")**

  - In all of them, look for more than 15 leukocytes per high-power field (HPF) in prostatic secretions.

  — *Acute* Either a focal or a diffuse acute inflammatory process featuring numerous polymorphonuclear leukocytes (PMNs)

    - Most cases caused by typical urinary tract infection (UTI) type organisms, including *E. coli* and *Klebsiella, Proteus, Enterobacter,* and *Pseudomonas* organisms
    - Other candidate organisms include *Staphylococcus aureus* and *Enterococci* organisms

- Clinically, acute prostatitis patients exhibit fever, chills, dysuria, and a **painful gland** upon digital rectal examination (DRE)
- Look for greater than 15 leukocytes per HPF and a positive culture in prostate secretions

— *Chronic* Look for lymphocytes, plasma cells, macrophages and PMNs in prostate tissue.

- **Chronic bacterial**—same organisms as cause acute prostatitis; may present with back pain, dysuria, and suprapubic discomfort
  - These patients often have a history of recurrent UTIs.
- **Chronic abacterial**—most common type of prostatitis seen today; clinically similar to chronic bacterial form, but no history of UTI
  - Cultures are negative for typical urinary tract pathogens.
  - It is suspected that *Chlamydia trachomatis* and/or *Ureaplasma urealyticum* may be responsible pathogens in some cases.
- *Note:* Antibiotics penetrate the prostate gland very poorly; organisms can "set up shop" there and continuously seed the urinary tract on a long-term basis.

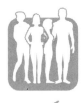

- **Nodular prostatic hyperplasia (benign prostatic hyperplasia [BPH]) (Fig. 28.1 and Fig. 28.2)**

  — *Epidemiology*

  - Beginning in the fifth decade of life, there is a progressive increase in incidence of nodular hyperplasia, until about 75% of men beyond the age of 80 years are affected.

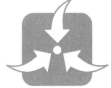

  — *Etiology*

  - The exact cause is not well established, but evidence strongly indicates that dihydrotestosterone, the active metabolite of testosterone, has a role in the origin of nodular hyperplasia.
    - **BPH develops only in men with an intact testis.**

  — *Pathology*

  - Nodular hyperplasia is characterized by nodules that originate around the urethra in the median lobe and more central portions of the lateral lobes.
    - In contrast, prostatic carcinoma usually involves the posterior aspect of the gland.
  - These expanding nodules distort and compress the urethral lumen.
  - Total gland weight is often in 60 to 100 g range and may become as great as 200 g.

  — *Microscopy*

  - Hyperplasia results from a proliferation of glands, smooth muscle, and fibroblasts in variable proportions.
  - Often one sees areas of infarction, squamous metaplasia and active inflammation.

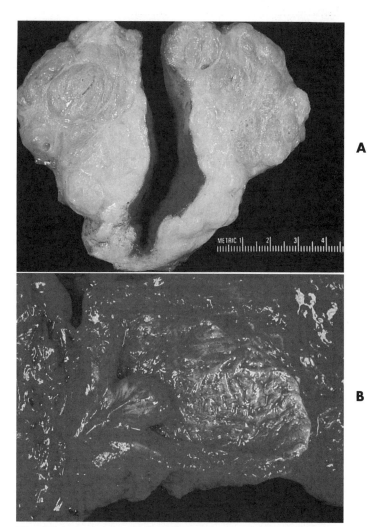

Fig. 28.1 Benign prostatic hyperplasia. **A,** Bulging nodules are observed in this gross photograph of an enlarged prostate gland. **B,** Gross photograph shows polyploid protrusion of prostate tissue involving glands of the bladder neck; this protrusion may act as a ball valve and result in severe urinary tract obstruction. (*From Damjanov I, Linder J:* Anderson's pathology, *ed 10, vol 2, St Louis, 1996, Mosby.*)

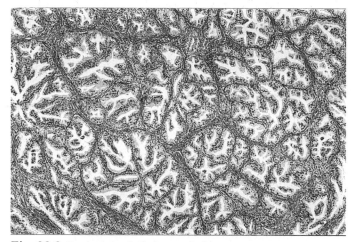

Fig. 28.2 Benign prostatic hyperplasia. (*From Damjanov I, Linder J:* Anderson's pathology, *ed 10, vol 2, St Louis, 1996, Mosby.*)

— *Clinical course*

• The clinical significance of BPH lies entirely in its tendency to produce urinary tract obstruction by impinging upon the urethra.

• Symptoms include urine dribbling, frequency, nocturia, and difficulty starting the urinary stream.

• Secondary changes observed in the urinary bladder include hypertrophy, smooth muscle trabeculation, and diverticulum formation.

• Acute urinary retention, hydronephrosis, and infection may occur secondary to obstruction.

• Treatment is necessary in only about 10% of men and may involve transurethral resection of the prostate (TURP) or suprapubic prostatectomy.

• Other, newer treatments include laser ablation and medical management (5 alpha-reductase inhibitors and $alpha_1$-adrenergic inhibitors).

• BPH is *not* considered to be a premalignant lesion.

● **Prostatic carcinoma**

— *Epidemiology*

• Among men, carcinoma of the prostate is the most common cancer and the second most common cause of death from cancer in the United States.

• In 1995, approximately 250,000 men were diagnosed with prostatic cancer and nearly 40,000 died from the disease in the United States.

• It is a disease of men over the age of 50 years, reaching a peak incidence around 75 years of age.

• **Note: More than 30% of men over 50 years old and 60% of men past the age of 80 years (none with clinical evidence of prostate cancer) are shown to have prostate cancer at autopsy.**

• Prostatic cancer rates are high in Scandinavian countries, low in Japan, and intermediate in the United States, suggesting a role for environmental factors (such as a high-fat diet).

• In the United States, African-Americans are affected more frequently than Caucasians.

• Genetic influences may also be involved, since there is a tendency toward familial aggregation.

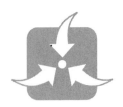

— *Etiology—unknown*

• As with nodular hyperplasia, its incidence increases with age, and it is speculated that the endocrine changes of old age are related to its origin.

• Also, androgens control normal prostate growth, and malignant prostatic epithelial cells, like their normal counterparts, possess steroid (androgen and estrogen) receptors, which would suggest responsiveness to hormones.

• Also, inhibition of these cancers can be often achieved with orchiectomy or estrogen therapy.

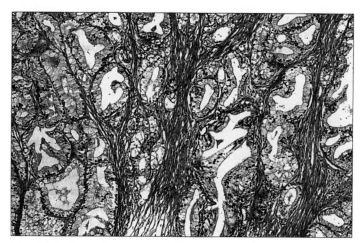

Fig. 28.3 Prostatic adenocarcinoma. Compare these glands to their benign counterparts in Fig. 28.2. (*From Stevens A, Lowe J:* Pathology, *London, 1995, Times Mirror International.*)

— *Pathology*

- Gross pathology indicates that prostatic cancer usually (70% of the time) begins in the peripheral zones of the prostate (classically in a posterior locale) but can arise anywhere in the gland, usually in multiple foci, which fuse to form a single mass.

- Irregular yellow-white or greenish indurated areas may be seen grossly and often the lesion blends imperceptibly into the background of the gland.

— *Microscopy*

- **The overwhelming majority of prostate cancers are adenocarcinomas, with varying degrees of differentiation (Fig. 28.3).**

- **Well-differentiated cases can be difficult to distinguish from nodular hyperplasia.**

- Poorly differentiated lesions exhibit little gland formation.

- Perineural invasion is a common feature.

■ Clinical Features

● Clinical presentation

- Dysuria, slow urinary stream, or urinary retention; local pain; symptoms or signs of metastasis; elevated serum prostatic specific antigen (PSA)

● Diagnosis

- DRE, transrectal ultrasound (TRUS), TRB (transrectal biopsy), serum PSA

- *Note:* Serum PSA alone does not detect many early stage cancers and is therefore not a good screening test for prostate cancer.

● Modes of spread

- The neoplasm may extend beyond the prostate to involve adjacent structures (i.e., seminal vesicle, bladder, and rectum).

- Distant spread of prostate cancer occurs via both lymphatics and vascular routes.
- Metastases to the regional lymph nodes occur early and often precede vascular spread.
- **Bone mets are the most common site of hematogenous spread.**
- Metastatic lesions in the bones, involving mainly the axial skeleton, may be osteoclastic (destructive) or **more commonly osteoblastic (bone forming).**
- Order of decreasing frequency for prostatic carcinoma bony metastases are lumbar spine, femur, pelvis, and thoracic spine.

● Prognostic factors

- In general, there is an excellent correlation between the cancer grade, anatomic extent (stage), and prognosis.

— *Tumor grade*

- Several grading schemes exist that are based on either glandular architecture or extent of cytologic atypia.
- Gleason's Score is gaining popularity.

— *Staging*

- Evaluation of the extent of carcinoma in the body (TRUS, computed tomography [CT], magnetic resonance imaging [MRI]); staging system—four clinical stages are defined

    - Stage A tumors are asymptomatic and discovered on histologic examination of clinically benign prostate specimens.
    - Stage B cancers are palpable by digital rectal examination and are confined to the prostate.
    - Stage C represents local invasion beyond the prostate but without metastases.
    - Stage D indicates the presence of regional lymph node metastases and/or more distant metastases.
    - **Unfortunately, 75% of patients with clinically significant prostate cancer present with stage C or stage D disease.**

— *Ploidy status*

- Diploid carcinomas have better prognosis.

● Treatment options

- Watchful waiting
- TURP
- Cryosurgery
- Radical prostatectomy
- Radiotherapy (sometimes in conjunction with surgery)
- Hormonal manipulation (in cases with metastatic disease)

    - Orchiectomy
    - Estrogens (e.g., DES)
    - Agonists of LHRH

- *Note:* Critical problem in dealing with prostate carcinoma is determining which cases need to be aggressively treated and which ones could be safely handled with "watchful waiting."

● **Prostatic intraepithelial neoplasia (PIN)**

- About 70% of prostate carcinomas feature a type of epithelial dysplasia analogous to cervical intraepithelial neoplasia of the uterine cervix.

- PIN features epithelial cells with substantial nuclear atypia, but these cells are still enveloped by a basal cell layer *and* an intact basement membrane.

MULTIPLE CHOICE
REVIEW QUESTIONS

1. The vast majority of testicular neoplasms are derived from which of the following?

    a. Squamous cells
    b. Leydig cells
    c. Sertoli cells
    d. Germ cells
    e. Endothelial cells

2. The combination of teratoma with which other neoplastic element is known as teratocarcinoma?

    a. Yolk sac tumor
    b. Choriocarcinoma
    c. Seminoma
    d. Embryonal carcinoma
    e. Malignant lymphoma

3. Acute prostatitis is most likely to be caused by which of the following pathogens?

    a. *Mycobacterium tuberculosis*
    b. *Escherichia coli*

    c. *Treponema pallidum* (syphilis)
    d. Cytomegalovirus (CMV)
    e. Herpes simplex virus

4. A 65-year-old man presents to your office with increased urinary frequency, nocturia, urinary "dribbling," and difficulty starting his urinary stream. This clinical scenario is most compatible with which of the following underlying diseases?

    a. Prostate cancer
    b. Urinary bladder cancer
    c. Urethral obstruction by a calculus
    d. Prostatic nodular hyperplasia
    e. Urinary bladder infection

5. Prostatic intraepithelial neoplasia (PIN) refers to which of the following basic pathologic processes?

    a. Dysplasia
    b. Invasive carcinoma
    c. Metaplasia
    d. Atrophy
    e. Hyperplasia

Chapter 29

Eye

■ **Degenerative Lesions**

- Figure 29.1 provides an overview of ocular architecture.

● **Arcus senilis of the cornea**

- A degenerative change associated with aging; may also be seen in certain hyperlipidemic states
- Deposition of lipid material in corneal stroma (about periphery of cornea), thereby giving rise to a milky ring about the periphery of the cornea

● **Pinguecula**

- Solar damage to conjunctival subepithelial soft tissue (substantia propria) results in proliferation of fibroblasts and accumulations of abnormal, often basophilic material that has the staining properties of elastic fibers (but is *not* actually composed of elastic fibers); epithelial changes also may be seen.
- Pinguecula clinically appears as raised, yellow, often bilateral lesions, characteristically on the nasal aspect of the conjunctiva.

● **Pterygium**

- Solar degeneration of corneal stroma with destruction of Bowman's membrane; corneal epithelial changes (proliferation) common
- Clinically appears as a winglike projection of tissue onto the cornea, thereby potentially interfering with normal vision
- May recur after excision

● **Retinitis pigmentosa**

- Hereditary lesion (may be autosomal dominant, autosomal recessive, or sex-linked recessive)—characterized by progressive loss of rods and cones (especially rods) and pigment dispersal into neural (inner) retina
- Progressive disease with clinical onset in early adulthood, eventually leading to blindness

● **Corneal dystrophies**

- A varied group of uncommon (sometimes hereditary) disorders characterized by deposition of material within the cornea
- **Major types** (all of these may result in a cloudy, opacified cornea)

  - **Macular dystrophy**—mucopolysaccharide deposited in stroma
  - **Lattice dystrophy**—amyloid deposited in stroma
  - **Fuchs' dystrophy**—loss of endothelial monolayer and deposition of glycoprotein material, with subsequent thickening of Descemet's membrane; accompanied by stromal edema

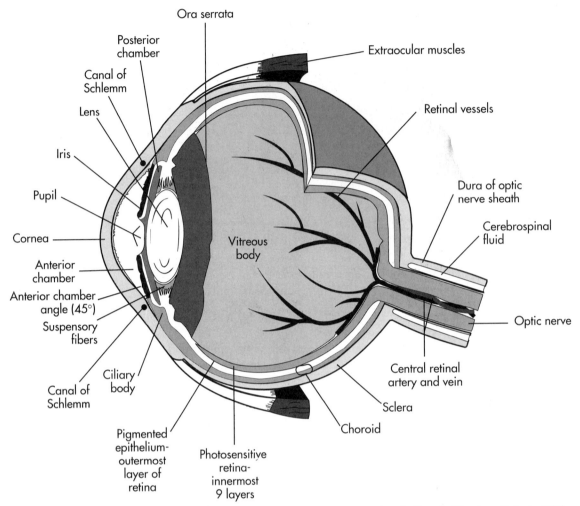

Fig. 29.1 Schematic showing ocular architecture. (*From Burns R, Cave D:* Ace the Boards: Histology, *St Louis, 1996, Mosby.*)

- ● Xanthelasma
  - • Common lesion consisting of yellow plaquelike lesions
  - • Microscopically, lipid-filled histiocytes within the dermis
  - • May sometimes be manifestation of underyling hyerlipidemic state
- ■ **Inflammatory Lesions**
- ● Hordeolum (stye, abscess)
  - • Acute inflammatory process (polymorphonuclear leukocytes [PMNs]) with abscess formation centered about skin adnexal structures (i.e., sweat glands, hair follicles)
- ● Chalazion
  - • A granulomatous inflammatory response initiated by lipid released from eyelid sebaceous glands (keep in mind that the eyelid has a high concentration of sebaceous glands); may clinically mimic sebaceous carcinoma (and vice versa) (Fig. 29.2)

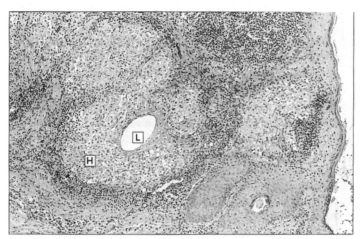

Fig. 29.2 Photomicrograph of chalazion depicts characteristic granuloma forming histiocytes (*H*) responding to lipid material (*L*) released from damaged sebaceous glands. (*From Stevens A, Lowe J: Pathology, London, 1995, Times Mirror International.*)

- **Trachoma**

    - Probably the leading cause of blindness in the world; affects principally the conjunctiva and the cornea

        - Caused by the bacterium *Chlamydia trachomatis*

        - Characterized by benign lymphoid hyperplasia in the conjunctiva and scarring in the cornea (pannus) with corneal intracytoplasmic epithelial inclusion bodies; followed by conjunctival and eyelid scarring

        - Eventually, process subsides, but only after considerable corneal damage with scarring, resultant opacification, and visual impairment

- **Granulomatous inflammation (mainly uveal)**

    - May be caused by bacteria (tuberculosis, leprosy, syphilis, tularemia); viruses (herpes zoster, cytomegalovirus); fungi (histoplasmosis, blastomycosis, candidiasis, aspergillus, cryptococcus, coccidioidomycosis); parasites (toxoplasmosis, onchocerciasis); sarcoidosis; sympathetic ophthalmia; and various autoimmune disorders (granulomatous inflammation in autoimmune disorders mainly centered in sclera)

    - Look for proliferation of histiocytes, with or without giant cells, to form granulomata

- **Congenital rubella syndrome (Greig's syndrome)**

    - Consists of cataracts, cardiovascular defects, mental retardation, and deafness

    - If maternal infection occurs during first month of gestation—50% of infants will be affected

    - **Ocular abnormalities**

        - Cataracts

        - Glaucoma

        - Iris abnormalities (including abnormal iris dilation with scarring later in life)

        - Retinopathy

- ● Congenital syphilis
  - • Not often seen today, but could soon see more (with the increase in syphilis we are witnessing today)
  - • May complicate primary, secondary, or tertiary syphilis (but much more likely to complicate primary or secondary stages)
  - • **Hutchinson's triad**—tooth abnormalities, deafness, and corneal stromal abnormality
  - • Corneal stromal inflammation (interstitial keratitis) followed by scarring with new blood vessel formation (neovascularization)

- ■ **Neoplastic Lesions**
  - ● Eyelid neoplasms
    - • Eyelid neoplasms include many types; **of the primary malignant eyelid neoplasms, the most common (>90%) is basal cell carcinoma.**
    - • Less common are squamous cell carcinoma, sebaceous gland carcinoma, and malignant melanoma.
    - • In addition to these primary malignancies, metastatic cancer is **uncommonly** seen, led in frequency by lung and breast carcinoma.
    - • For complete descriptions of basal cell carcinoma, squamous cell carcinoma, and melanoma, see Skin chapter).

  - ● Sebaceous carcinoma
    - • This malignant neoplasm arises from eyelid sebaceous glands (meibomian glands [found in tarsal plate] and the glands of Zeis [associated with eyelashes], more commonly the former, and from sebaceous glands in the caruncle).
    - • **Upper lid is a more common site for sebaceous carcinoma than is the lower lid.**
    - • Clinically, it often presents as a lesion easily mistaken for a **chalazion.**
      - • It may also resemble blepharitis and cutaneous horn.
      - • **Interestingly, sebaceous carcinoma is seldom seen in sites other than the eyelid.**

    - • **Microscopically,** its malignant cells have a foamy, vacuolated cytoplasm (because of contained lipid). An oil red O stain on fresh tissue (*not* on paraffin embedded or alcohol fixed tissues) should be done.
      - • Nuclei are bizarre and often feature mitotic figures.
      - • May see pagetoid spread, which is an overlying epithelium infiltrated by individual or small groups of malignant cells with abundant cytoplasm and bizarre nuclei.

  - ● Uveal malignant melanoma (keep in mind that uveal tract includes iris, ciliary body, and choroid)
    - • **Melanomas are undoubtedly the most common primary intraocular malignancy of adults** (Fig. 29.3 and Fig. 29.4).
      - • This lesion is rare in non-Caucasians.
      - • Most patients are over 50 years of age at the time of diagnosis.
      - • Most are mixed spindle and epithelioid cell types; other types are pure spindle cell, pure epithelioid cell, and necrotic type.

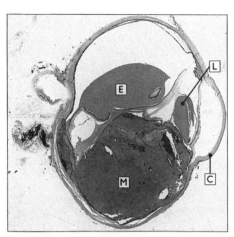

Fig. 29.3 Malignant melanoma. Photomicrograph depicts a large uveal melanoma (*M*) involving choroid and ciliary body. Also shown are cornea (*C*), lens (*L*), and detached retina with associated exudate (*E*). (*From Stevens A, Lowe J:* Pathology, *London, 1995, Times Mirror International.*)

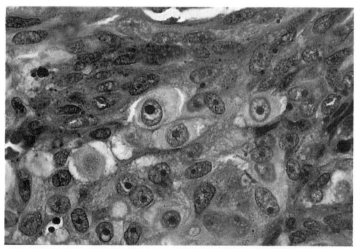

Fig. 29.4 Photomicrograph of uveal melamoma featuring a mixture of epithelioid (large cells with abundant pink cytoplasm and round nuclei, toward center of field) and spindle cells (cells with cigar shaped nuclei best seen in upper left of field). (*From Damjanov I, Linder J:* Anderson's pathology, *ed 10, vol 2, St Louis, 1996, Mosby.*)

- Therapy includes enucleation in some; also radiation, delivered either by proton beam or radioactive scleral plaque.
- Metastases, when they occur, **almost always involve the liver.**
- Prognosis is 55% 15-year survival for "all comers."
- Prognosis is affected by cell type (pure epithelioid is the worst, pure spindle is the best); greatest dimension of lesion; scleral extension; mitotic activity; and location (iris melanomas have a better prognosis than choroidal and ciliary body melanomas).

● Retinoblastoma

- Most common intraocular malignant neoplasm of **childhood;** may

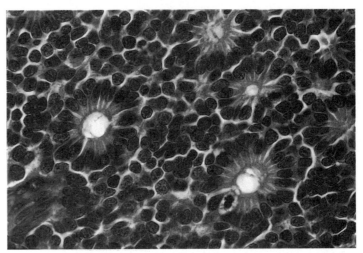

Fig. 29.5 Photomicrograph depicts retinoblastoma, replete with characteristic Flexner-Wintersteiner rosettes (circular structures with central clear spaces). (*From Damjanov I, Linder J:* Anderson's pathology, *ed 10, vol 2, St Louis, 1996, Mosby.*)

present with red, painful eye and leukocoria (white light reflex, instead of the normal red light reflex), strabismus (squint).

- 90% of all cases occur during first 3 years of life.
- ⅓ of retinoblastoma cases are bilateral.
- Retinoblastoma (Rb) gene is found on the long arm of chromosome 13.

    - Deletions or mutations in this locus result in loss of the protein material coded by the retinoblastoma gene.
    - This protein acts as a tumor-suppressing agent.
    - In its absence, there is definitely an increased risk of developing retinoblastoma and other neoplasms (see following).

- **6% of cases are hereditary.**

    - **Key point: Higher** incidence of bilaterality and multicentricity in hereditary cases.

- *Note:* Patients with inherited retinoblastoma are also at increased risk for other malignant neoplasms, especially osteogenic sarcoma, Ewing's sarcoma, and pineal-blastoma.

- **Primitive photoreceptor cells tend to invade optic nerve and seed the cerebrospinal fluid.**

- Look for fleurettes and **Flexner-Wintersteiner rosettes,** but these are *not* prerequisites for a diagnosis of retinoblastoma (Fig. 29.5).

    - Therapy

        - Enucleation
        - Radiation therapy

- Prognosis is 90% long-term survival in most series (1% of all cases show **spontaneous regression**).

    - When metastasis occurs, it is to central nervous system, bone, lymph nodes.

- "Tumors" of the lacrimal gland

  - Lacrimal gland lies in the superolateral orbit and, histologically, has an appearance essentially identical to that of the parotid gland.

    - ½ of lesions are lymphoid
    - ½ of lesions are epithelial

  - Of the epithelial lesions, approximately ½ are pleomorphic adenomas (90% of these are benign) and the remaining ½ are adenoid cystic carcinoma.

    - One looks for "down and in" proptosis (protrusion of the globe).

  — *Pleomorphic adenoma (benign mixed tumor)*

    - **Most common** benign neoplasm of salivary glands and lacrimal gland
    - May involve orbit and lids but will be discussed in depth here
    - Male:female—2:1
    - Locally invasive, **may recur after incomplete excision**
    - Do not do incisional biopsy when suspecting this lesion
    - **Microscopically**—marked variation in appearance, not only between cases, but even within the **same** lesion

      - Tubular structures, lined by two cell layers; inner one is secretory (but may undergo metaplasia to squamous epithelium), while outer layer is myoepithelial
      - Foci of fibrous tissue, cartilage, bone, and fat supplement myxoid stroma; derived from the myoepithelial cells
      - Pseudocapsule

    - If at all possible—resect completely

      - Carcinoma (including adenoid cystic carcinoma) may complicate long-standing and/or recurrent pleomorphic adenoma.

  — *Lymphoid pseudotumors*

    - Benign lymphoepithelial lesion
    - Encountered mainly in middle-aged women and is part of Sjögren's syndrome
    - Microscopically

      - Acinar (secretory) components of the lacrimal gland drop out consequent to a brisk inflammatory cell infiltrate featuring plasma cells and lymphocytes.
      - Duct cells proliferate, to give islands of cells (epimyoepithelial islands).

    - Clinically, dry mouth and dry eyes is called **Mikulicz's disease**, but term is outdated, as these findings can be seen in a number of diseases (sarcoid, lymphomas, Sjögren's syndrome, idiopathic); thus, the term *Mikulicz's* comments upon the clinical findings, not a specific etiology

  — *Adenoid cystic carcinoma (cylindroma)*

    - Age group—mid- to late adulthood (median age—38 years)
    - More rapid clinical course than benign mixed tumors

- Pain, problems with extraocular muscle function
- Account for 60% of all malignant epithelial neoplasms of lacrimal gland
- May arise de novo or from preexisting pleomorphic adenoma
- Microscopically

    - Usually not encapsulated
    - Constituent cells—basaloid with high nuclear/cytoplasmic ratio
    - Cells are arranged into columns, nests with holes, thereby giving a so-called cribriform (Swiss cheese) appearance
    - Look for an eosinophilic, hyaline, basement membranelike substance around aggregates of neoplastic cells
    - Perineural and blood vessel invasion are often seen

- Prognosis

    - Overall poor prognosis because of perineural invasion, local recurrence, and distant metastases

● Metastatic neoplasms

- These are the **most common of all intraocular neoplasms in adults.**
- In men, lung carcinoma is most common site of origin, while, in women, it is breast carcinoma.
- **Most common site in the eye for involvement by metastatic cancer is choroid** (the richly vascular coat just external to the retina).

■ **Manifestations of Systemic Diseases**

● Diabetic ophthalmopathy

- The critical defect in diabetes mellitus is angiopathy involving capillaries, arterioles, and arteries.
- Effects of long-term insulin-dependent diabetes mellitus on the eye

    - Accelerated cataract formation (cortical, nuclear, snowflake)
    - Increased incidence of glaucoma
    - Increased incidence of keratitis (inflammation of the cornea)
    - Diabetic retinopathy (Fig. 29.6)

- Approximately 80% to 90% patients develop some degree of retinopathy 15 to 20 years into their disease.

    - Capillary basement membrane thickening
    - Loss of pericytes (cells that support and nourish the endothelial cells)
    - Capillary microaneurysms
    - Excessive capillary permeability leading to leakage of serum proteins (exudates)
    - Cotton wool spots (infarcts of nerve fiber layer; clinically have a fluffy white appearance)
    - Hemorrhages
    - Neovascularization and fibrosis leading to retinal detachment

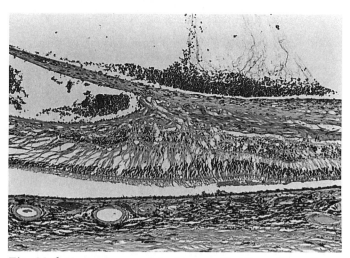

Fig. 29.6 Photomicrograph features proliferative retinopathy as is commonly encountered in long-standing diabetes mellitus. Note the anterior retinal neovascularization (toward top of field) and associated vitreal cavity hemorrhage. Early traction retinal detachment is also evident (lower left of field). (*From Damjanov I, Linder J:* Anderson's pathology, *ed 10, vol 2, St Louis, 1996, Mosby.*)

- Orbital infection (increased propensity of diabetics to suffer from infection)

● Hypertension

- When we speak of hypertensive effects on the eye, we really are addressing **hypertensive retinopathy.**

    - **Grade I**—generalized arteriolar narrowing
    - **Grade II**—generalized arteriolar narrowing *plus* focal arteriolar spasm
    - **Grade III**—same as above two grades, plus hemorrhages and exudates (splinter [flame] hemorrhages in nerve fiber layer; "cotton wool spots"; waxy exudates in outer plexiform layer)
    - **Grade IV**—all of the above, *plus* optic disc edema

■ **Miscellaneous**

● Cataracts

- Refers to **alterations in the lens** that result in interference with normal light transmittance

— *Nuclear (most common type of cataract)*

- Really a concomitant of aging; consists of compression of the lens fibers in the central aspect of the lens; caused by dehydration of nuclear protein and accumulation of urochrome pigment there

— *Cortical*

- Caused by any number of stimuli
- Denaturation of cortical proteins with subsequent liquefaction change and formation of **Morgagni's globules**
- **Mature cortical cataract**

    - Nucleus "sinks" in liquefied cortex (Morgagnian cataract)

- Hypermature cataract
    - Low molecular weight materials escape through degenerating lens capsule of mature cortical cataract; results in a small, shrunken lens with a "wrinkled" capsule

— *Posterior subcapsular*

- Most are idiopathic.
- Subcapsular cortical cells degenerate.
- Lens epithelial cells move posteriorly to become bladder cells of Wedl.

— *Anterior subcapsular cataract*

- Usually result of trauma or inflammatory process
- Scarring of lens cortex beneath capsule anteriorly

- Glaucoma
    - Glaucoma refers to a group of "diseases" characterized by an elevated intraocular pressure sufficient to cause either transient or permanent damage to ocular tissue.
    - Ocular hypertension is a term used to describe elevated intraocular pressure in the **absence** of tissue injury or visual impairment
    - Normal anterior chamber angle is 45° (see Fig. 29.1).

— *Primary open angle glaucoma*

- Accounts for nearly ⅔ of glaucoma seen in Caucasians
    - Hypersecretion—rare cause
    - **Impaired outflow—accounts for the vast majority of primary open angle glaucoma**
    - Exact mechanism not well delineated, but involves a **defect in trabecular meshwork aqueous filtration,** most likely caused by some sort of degenerative process

— *Secondary open angle glaucoma (angle is normally formed and open)*

- Hemorrhage
- Phacolysis
- Melanomalytic
- Uveitic
- Tumor seeding
- Increased episcleral venous pressures

— *Primary angle closure glaucoma (rare)*

- Caused by a congenital abnormality, in that the anterior chamber angle is not properly formed in the first place

— *Secondary angle closure glaucoma*

- Neovascular membrane (rubeosis iridis)
- Epithelial downgrowth
- Endothelial downgrowth
- Organization of inflammatory debris in angle

— *Key effects of prolonged elevation in intraocular pressure*

• Neural retinal atrophy (nerve fiber layer and ganglion cell layer) and optic nerve damage (optic disc cupping and atrophy)

• Other effects on the eye—corneal edema and stromal scarring; cataracts; rubeosis iridis (neovascularization on anterior surface of iris); uveal necrosis; and bulging of the cornea and sclera

● **Chromosomal anomalies**

• Many different chromosomal anomalies are associated with ocular problems, but just one of them is addressed here and that is trisomy 21 (Down syndrome).

— *Trisomy 21 (Down syndrome)*

• **Ocular features**

• Eyes set farther apart than normal (hypertelorism)
• Lid abnormalities
• Abnormalities in iris
• Cataracts
• Retinal dysplasia (disordered retinal structure)
• Keratoconus—cone-shaped cornea (pointing anteriorly) with central thinning and focal scarring
• Chronic conjunctivitis
• Severe myopia (nearsightedness)
• Abnormal optic disc region vascular pattern

MULTIPLE CHOICE
REVIEW QUESTIONS

1. A 65-year-old man comes to you for a general physical examination and no specific complaints. When examining his eyes, you notice a "milky ring" around the periphery of each cornea. This represents deposition of what type of material in the corneal stroma?

   a. Mucopolysaccharide
   b. Protein
   c. Lipid
   d. Cartilage
   e. Bone

2. Which of the following small round cell tumors of childhood is the most common *primary* intra-ocular malignant neoplasm (cancer) of *childhood*?

   a. Retinoblastoma
   b. Medulloblastoma
   c. Malignant lymphoma
   d. Rhabdomyosarcoma
   e. Neuroblastoma

3. Cotton wool spots represent which of the following?

   a. Neoplastic cell deposits
   b. Nerve fiber layer infarction
   c. Retinal neovascularization
   d. Cataract formation

4. One of the possible ocular features associated with Down syndrome (Trisomy 21) is a cone shaped cornea ("pointing" anteriorly) with central stromal thinning and scarring. This lesion is referred to as which of the following?

   a. Keratoconus
   b. Pterygium
   c. Hordeolum
   d. Arcus senilis
   e. Retinitis pigmentosa

Chapter 30

Endocrine Diseases

- **Multiglandular Endocrine Disorders**
  - Abnormalities of hypothalmic/anterior pituitary axis
    - Can affect thyroid, adrenal cortex, gonads
  - Multiple endocrine neoplasia (MEN) syndromes
    - Autosomal dominant neoplasia or hyperplasia of several endocrine organs
    - MEN, type 1—parathyroid hyperplasia, pituitary adenoma, pancreatic islet cell neoplasms
    - MEN, type 2—medullary thyroid carcinoma and pheochromocytoma
  - Polyglandular autoimmune syndromes
    - Malfunction, usually hypofunction, of several endocrine organs
    - *Pathogenic features*
      - Abnormal autoimmunity (including autoantibodies) directed against the affected endocrine glands
      - Other evidence of disturbed immune function
    - *Type I polyglandular autoimmune syndrome*
      - Childhood onset; usually only siblings affected (not multigenerational); no human leukocyte antigen (HLA) association
      - Most common manifestations
        - Hypoparathyroidism—82%
        - Mucocutaneous candidiasis—70%
        - Primary Addison's disease (primary adrenocortical insufficiency)—67%
    - *Type II polyglandular autoimmune syndrome*
      - Adult onset; affects multiple generations in same family; HLA-DR3 and HLA-DR4 associated
      - Most common manifestations
        - Primary Addison's disease, 100%
        - Autoimmune thyroid disease, 70%
        - Type 1 diabetes mellitus, 50%

- **Pituitary**
  - Overview
    - *Gross anatomy*
      - Sits in the sella turcica, a space in the sphenoid bone
      - Connected to hypothalamus by pituitary stalk

— *Adenohypophysis (anterior pituitary)*
A derivative of the oral ectoderm (Rathke's pouch)
Makes up approximately 75% of the weight of the adult pituitary
Light microscopic appearance

- Divided into lobules by fibrovascular septae
- Mosaic of cell types

  - 40% eosinophils (acidophils)—bright red
  - 10% basophils—deep purple
  - 50% chromophobes—pink to light purple

Immunocytochemical-ultrastructural classification

- Distinct cell types classified by hormone content

  - Hormones in secretory granules
  - Each cell-type functions separately, regulated by hormones from target tissues and from hypothalamus

- Growth hormone (GH) cells most numerous
- Prolactin (PRL) cells
- GH-PRL cells
- Adrenocorticotropic hormone (ACTH) cells
- Gonadotropin cells contain both luteinizing hormone (LH) and follicle-stimulating hormone (FSH)
- Thyroid-stimulating hormone (TSH) cells
- Unclassified

— *Neurohypophysis (posterior pituitary)*

- Neuroectodermal derivative
- Consists of nerve terminals and fibers originating in the hypothalamus and glial cells
- Contains antidiuretic hormone (ADH) and oxytocin

— *Normal pituitary function depends on normal function of the hypothalamus*
Releasing factors and release-inhibiting factors control adenohypophysis

- Reach anterior pituitary by hypophyseal-portal system
- Each factor affects function of specific cell types

  - Proliferation and differentiation
  - Hormone synthesis and secretion

- Overall effect of the hypothalamus—stimulatory

  - Inhibits PRL and (before puberty) gonadotropins

Neurons in the supraoptic and paraventricular nuclei of the hypothalamus

- Synthesize the neurohypophyseal hormones
- Give rise to the axons and terminals that make up the neurohypophysis

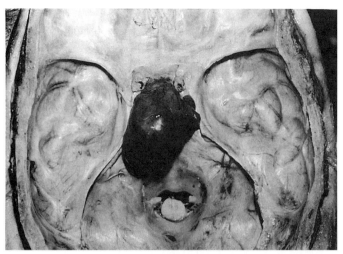

Fig. 30.1 Pituitary macroadenoma. Note the large vascular mass extending above the sella in this postmortem specimen. (*Damjanov I, Linder J:* Anderson's pathology, *ed 10, vol 2, St Louis, 1996, Mosby.*)

● Lesions

— *Pituitary adenoma*

Benign neoplasm of the adenohypophysis

Prevalence

- Found in up to 20% of autopsies in which the pituitary is examined microscopically
- 10% of brain neoplasms, according to neurosurgeons

Morphology

GROSS

- Microadenoma— <10 mm in greatest diameter
- Macroadenoma— ≥10 mm

    - Can damage pituitary; extend into hypothalamus; erode bone (Fig. 30.1)

HISTOLOGY

- Distortion of usual lobular architecture
- Cells arranged in sheets or nest; sometimes form papillae
- Usually consist of one cell type (e.g., chromophobe)

Classification by hormone content

- GH producing—14%
- PRL producing (prolactinomas)—27%
- GH-PRL producing—8%
- ACTH producing—14%
- Others (mostly gonadotropin producing)—12%
- Undifferentiated (sparsely granulated; oncocytomas)—25%

Clinical features

- Secretion of excessive amounts of hormone by the neoplasm
- Hypopituitarism

- Decreased hormone secretion because of damage to the normal pituitary and/or hypothalamus
- Associated with increased prolactin with hypothalamic damage

    - Neurologic—central nervous system (CNS) damage by macroadenomas extending above the sella turcica

— *Craniopharyngioma*

- Benign neoplasm apparently arising from Rathke's pouch remnants
- Three percent of intracranial neoplasms in clinical series

Morphology

- Typically occur above the sella
- Can be solid or cystic; often calcified
- Histology—does not resemble normal pituitary

    - Composed of nest of columnar and squamous epithelium, cholesterol clefts, necrotic debris, foam cells
    - Does not contain endocrine cells—does not produce hormones

Clinical features

- Hypopituitarism
- Neurologic

— *Anterior pituitary infarction*

- Infarction of >25% of anterior pituitary found in 2% to 3% of autopsies
- Causes

    - Increased intracranial pressure
    - Shock
    - Obstetrical hemorrhage (Sheehan's syndrome—postpartum pituitary necrosis)
    - Pituitary neoplasm

- Clinical consequences

    - Infarction >60% can cause hypopituitarism

— *Primary empty sella syndrome*

Enlargement of sella turcica without erosion of bone

Etiology-pathogenesis

- Herniation of arachnoid through defect in diaphragma sellae
- Sella fills with cerebrospinal fluid

Clinical features

- Most often found in obese, multiparous women with headaches

    - 30% hypertensive

- Endocrine effects rare

— *Other lesions that can affect the pituitary and/or hypothalamus*

- Granulomas (tuberculosis, sarcoidosis)
- Primary CNS neoplasms

- Metastases
- Lymphocytic hypophysitis
  - Rare autoimmune disorder

- **Clinical syndromes**
  - *Hypopituitarism*
    - Subnormal amounts of one or more adenohypophyseal hormones

    Causes

    - Destructive lesions of anterior pituitary
      - Neoplasm, surgery, radiation, trauma, infarction, inflammation
      - Usually >60% of gland must be damaged
    - Destructive lesions of hypothalamus
    - Inherited

    Clinical features

    - Growth hormone deficiency
      - Short stature in children
      - Effects in adults subtle (decreased muscle mass, possibly increased cardiovascular mortality)
    - Cortisol deficiency (secondary Addison's disease); see section on Adrenals later in the chapter
    - Central hypothyroidism; see section on Thyroid later in the chapter
    - Hypogonadism

  - *Hyperprolactinemia*

    Many physiologic, pharmacologic, or pathologic causes

    - Excessive secretion of PRL by a prolactinoma
    - Destructive pituitary stalk or hypothalamic lesions (including pituitary adenomas)
      - Excessive secretion by normal, but disinhibited, PRL cells
    - Other causes—pregnancy, estrogens, dopamine antagonists, hypothyroidism, cirrhosis, chronic renal failure

    Clinical effects

    - Females—amenorrhea or other menstrual disturbances; sometimes galactorrhea
    - Males—decreased libido, impotence, and infertility

  - *ACTH excess—a cause of cortisol excess (Cushing's syndrome); see section on Adrenals later in the chapter*
  - *Growth hormone excess*
    - Almost always because of GH-producing pituitary adenoma
    - Approximately 95% of cases occur in adults
    - Acromegaly
      - GH excess occurring after epiphyseal fusion
      - Soft tissue overgrowth, bone deformities, arthropathy, various metabolic abnormalities, increased risk of cardiovascu-

lar disease and possibly cancer, and decreased life expectancy

- • Gigantism
    - • GH excess occurring before epiphyseal fusion
- — *Posterior pituitary syndromes*
  Central diabetes insipidus (DI)
    - • Excess free water excretion caused by insufficient ADH
    - • Etiology
        - • Autosomal dominant (some because of mutations in gene encoding ADH)
        - • Acquired lesion of hypothalamus or pituitary stalk
  Nephrogenic DI
    - • Excess free water excretion because of renal resistance to ADH action
    - • Etiology
        - • X-linked because of mutations in V2 receptor
        - • Acquired
  Syndrome of inappropriate ADH (SIADH)
    - • Hyponatremia and water retention
    - • Etiology
        - • Excess secretion from pituitary caused by CNS disease
        - • Ectopic production (usually from lung)
- — *Neurologic manifestations associated with pituitary and suprasellar masses*
    - • Visual field defects
    - • Oculomotor palsies
    - • Headache
    - • Others (seizures, hydrocephalus, hyperphagia, abnormalities of temperature regulation)

- ■ **Thyroid**
  - ● Overview

    - — *Follicular epithelium*
        - • Concentrates iodide
        - • Synthesizes and secretes thyroxine (T_4) and triiodothyronine (T_3)
        - • TSH—stimulates follicular epithelial growth, iodide uptake, and hormone synthesis and secretion
        - • T_4 inhibits TSH
    - — *Small numbers of calcitonin-producing C cells*
        - • Can be within or outside follicles
    - — *Thyroid function*
      Tests of thyroid function
        - • TSH
            - • Single most useful test

- Total T_4 and T_3
  - Free hormones—biologically active
  - Almost all T_4 and T_3 circulate bound to plasma proteins (thyroid binding globulin, transthyretin, albumin)
  - Many conditions that alter levels of thyroid binding proteins alter total T_4 and T_3 levels, but do not affect clinical thyroid function
  - T_4 generally more useful than T_3
  - Nonthyroidal factors alter T_3 level

- Free T_4 and T_3
  - Clinical use limited by slowness or unreliability

- T-uptake
  - Measure plasma protein capacity to bind thyroid hormones

- Free thyroxine index (FT_4I).
  - Product of T_4 and T-uptake
  - Reliable estimate of free T_4
  - Similarly, can calculate FT_3I, if needed

Thyrotoxicosis—too much thyroid hormone
Caused by hyperthyroidism

- Definition—thyroid hyperfunction
  - Increased iodide uptake and production and secretion of T_4 and T_3
- Graves' disease (by far the most common)
- Toxic multinodular goiter
- Toxic adenoma
- Rare causes—increased pituitary; TSH production trophoblastic neoplasm (human chorionic gonadotropin [hCG] has weak TSH-like activity); iodine induced

Not associated with hyperthyroidism

- Ingestion of thyroid hormones
- Thyroiditis
- Rarely causes ostruma ovarii, functioning metastatic thyroid cancer

Signs and symptoms caused by hypermetabolism

- Common symptoms—nervousness, increased sweating, increased sensitivity to heat, palpatations, fatigue, weight loss, increased appetite
  - Common signs—tachycardia, tremor, thyroid bruit, eye signs
  - Thyrotoxic crisis (thyroid storm)
    - Usually occurs in undertreated patient subjected to additional medical stress
    - Fulminant increase in signs and symptoms of thryotoxicosis
    - Potentially fatal

LABORATORY FINDINGS

- Low TSH, elevated T_4 and T_3 are typical
- T_3-toxicosis—elevated T_3; normal T_4
- Hyperthyroidism from elevated TSH—rare

Euthyroid—just right

Hypothyroid—too little

SIGNS AND SYMPTOMS FROM SLOWING OF METABOLISM

- Weakness, lethargy, slow speech, sensation of cold, decreased sweating, cold skin, thick tongue, impaired memory, weight gain, and constipation

  - Additional manifestations in children

    - Infants—impaired mental and physical development (cretinism)
    - Older children—impaired linear growth

  - Myxedema coma

    - Hypothermia, stupor in severely hypothyroid patient
    - Potentially fatal

USUALLY BECAUSE OF THYROID DISEASE (PRIMARY HYPOTHYROIDISM)

- Iodine deficiency
- Autoimmune thyroid disease (common in United States)
- Surgeons, antithyroid medication, radiation (common in United States)
- Congenital anomalies of thyroid development
- Autosomal recessive deficiencies of enzymes of T_4 synthesis

CENTRAL HYPOTHYROIDISM (SEE PRECEDING, HYPOPITUITARISM)

- Secondary hypothyroidism—pituitary
- Tertiary hypothyroidism—hypothalamic

LABORATORY FINDINGS

- Primary hypothyroidism—elevated TSH; decreased T_4
- Central hypothyroidism—decreased TSH; decreased T_4

— *Goiter (enlarged thyroid)—occurs in many different diseases*

- Average weight of thyroid (adult)—15 to 20 g
- Goiter can be diffuse or nodular
- Patient can be thyrotoxic, euthyroid, hypothyroid

● **Autoimmune thyroid disease**

— *Demography*

- Common, although true prevalence unknown

  - Probably present in greater than 1% of population

- More common in females than in males (threefold to tenfold)

— *Immunopathology*

Certain HLA types increased in persons with autoimmune thyroid diseases

Probably both cellular and humoral immunity involved

- Activated self-reactive CD4$^+$ lymphocytes stimulate autoreactive B lymphocytes

Antithyroid antibodies

- Present in almost all patients with autoimmune thyroid disease
- Present in many persons without clinically apparent thyroid disorder (about 15% of adult women have detectable antithyroid antibodies)

    - Antithyroid peroxidase antibodies (antimicrosomal antibodies)

        - Cytotoxic—might be pathogenically important
        - Measured in clinical labs for diagnosis

    - Antithyroglobulin antibodies

        - Measured in clinical laboratories

    - Anti-TSH receptor-related antibodies

        - Can be agonist (mimics TSH) or antagonist (blocks TSH)
        - Measured in (some) clinical laboratories

Autoimmune thyroid disease can be manifestation of polyglandular autoimmunity

Patients commonly have family history of autoimmune thyroid disease

— *Graves' disease*

Multisystem disease hyperthyroid goiter, infiltrative ophthalmopathy, and dermopathy

Immunologic aspects

- Anti-TSH receptor-agonist antibodies pathogenically important
- Ophthalmopathy probably from cross-reaction between some antithyroid antibodies and orbital components
- HLA associations—DR3 and B8 (whites); BW46 (Chinese); BW35 (Japanese)

Morphology

THYROID

- Diffuse goiter (usually not much larger than 100 g)
- Histopathology (Fig. 30.2)

    - Follicular epithelium—hyperplasia (papillae) and hypertrophy (cuboidal or columnar, instead of flat)
    - Colloid depleted

INCREASED RETROORBITAL MASS (INCREASED GROUND SUBSTANCE AND CONNECTIVE TISSUE)

INFLAMMATION (MOSTLY T LYMPHOCYTES) AND FIBROSIS OF EXTRAOCULAR MUSCLES

Clinical course

ONSET BETWEEN 20 TO 40 YEARS MOST COMMON (BEFORE 10 YEARS, RARE)

THYROID DISEASE

- 97% have goiter
- Signs and symptoms of thyrotoxicosis
- Can remit spontaneously

— *Infiltrative ophthalmopathy*

- Clinically apparent in 50%

    - Almost all have increased orbital contents

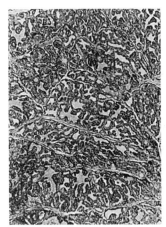

Fig. 30.2 Grave's disease. Note the diffuse hyperplasia with papillary infoldings of the epithelium. *(Damjanov I, Linder J:* Anderson's pathology, *ed 10, vol 2, St Louis, 1996, Mosby.)*

- Clinical course independent of that of thyroid disease
  - Rare, ophthalmopathy only (euthyroid Graves' disease)
- Signs and symptoms
  - Loss of motion of extraocular muscles
  - Exposure and damage to cornea
  - Involvement of optic nerve
- Infiltrative dermopathy (induration of skin over pretibial area)—5% to 10%
- Thyroid acropachy (clubbing of digits)—rare

— *Hashimoto's thyroiditis*

Chronic thyroiditis with hypothyroid goiter

Immune aspects

- Antithyroid peroxidase (present in 90% in high titre); antithyroglobulin; growth-promoting antibodies
- HLA associations—DR5 and B8

Morphology

- Goiter
- Lymphoplasmocytic infiltrate with germinal center formation (Fig. 30.3)
- Fibrosis and parenchymal destruction
- Atypical follicular epithelium and Hürthle cells (large cells with abundant eosinophilic cytoplasm)

Clinical features

- Most commonly present age 30 to 50 years
- Goiter—a common manifestation (often presenting problem)
- Thyroid function
  - Occasionally transient thyrotoxicosis (early)
  - Usually euthyroid or hypothyroid when diagnosed
  - Patients—usually become permanently hypothyroid

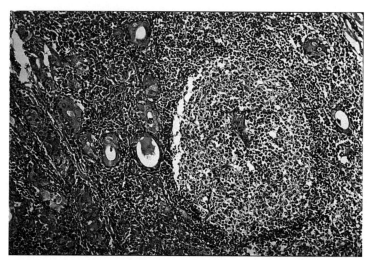

Fig. 30.3 Hashimoto's thyroiditis. Histology. Note the infiltration by lymphocytes and formation of a germinal center. (*Damjanov I, Linder J:* Anderson's pathology, *ed 10, vol 2, St Louis, 1996, Mosby.*)

— *Primary thyroid atrophy*

- Immune aspects

  - Anti-TSH receptor-antagonist antibodies important in some cases
  - HLA-DR3 associated

- Morphology—small, fibrotic thyroid
- Clinical aspects—hypothyroidism

● Other forms of thyroiditis

— *Painless thyroiditis*

- Seems to be common, although exact incidence unknown

  - Probably the second most common cause of thyrotoxicosis

- Etiologic and pathogenic features

  - About ⅔ cases in women, often immediately postpartum
  - Might be immunologically mediated

- Clinical features

  - 40% have goiter
  - Can be thyrotoxic (release of stored T_4) or euthyroid at time of presentation
  - With progressive damage to the gland—thyroid function declines
  - About 40%—develop transient hypothyroidism
  - Most patients—recover within a year of onset

— *Subacute thyroiditis (granulomatous thyroiditis)*

- Relatively uncommon
- Could be a sequel to viral infection
- Morphology

- Acute inflammation
- Granulomas and giant cells, often adjacent to colloid
- Fibrosis, parenchymal damage
- Often see mixture of these
  - Clinical features
    - Variable thyroid function, as in painless thyroiditis
    - Pain in neck
    - High erythrocyte sedimentation rate; a nonspecific indicator of inflammation
    - Patients usually recover
— *Riedel's thyroiditis*
  - Actually fibrosis, not inflammation
  - Rare
  - Etiology and pathogenesis unknown
  - Morphology
    - Fibrous replacement of thyroid
    - Extension of fibrosis outside thyroid
  - Clinical features
    - Hypothyroidism
    - Extremely hard gland
    - Often associated with fibrosis in other sites

- **Other forms of goiter (in addition to autoimmune thyroid diseases discussed previously)**
  — *Goiter caused by iodine deficiency*
  Epidemiology
    - Common in many parts of world
      - >100 million at risk
    - No longer a problem in the United States
  Etiology and pathogenesis
    - Insufficient iodine in diet
    - Dietary goiterogens
    - Decreased $T_4 \rightarrow$ elevated TSH $\rightarrow$ goiter formation
  Goiter development
    - Epithelial hyperplasia
      - Increased cell numbers with papillary projections
      - Many small, colloid-depleted follicles
      - Accompanied by increased vascularity
    - Involution
      - Reversal of hyperplasia
      - Formation of large colloid-distended follicles
    - Often apparently diffuse but with repeated cycles of hyperplasia, goiter becomes progressively nodular
    - Recently found that some nodules in some goiters are clonal

Clinical features

- Multinodular goiter (sometimes enormous)
- Hypothyroidism
- Cretinism in some children

— *Dyshormonogenic goiter*

- Rare
- Etiology and pathogenesis

  - Autosomal-recessive deficiency of one of the enzymes involved in thyroid hormone synthesis
  - Decreased $T_4 \rightarrow$ elevated TSH $\rightarrow$ goiter formation

— *Idiopathic goiter*

Epidemiology

- Clinically detected in about 4% of United States population
- Found in 50% of autopsies

Etiology and pathogenesis—uncertain

- TSH normal

Morphology

- Similar to goiter in iodine deficiency

  - Tends to be smaller

Clinical features

- Multinodular goiter or thyroid nodule(s) without apparent thyroid enlargement
- Thyroid function—usually normal
- Toxic multinodular goiter

  - Development of hyperthyroidism in patient with longstanding multinodular goiter

● **Hypothyroidism with reduced thyroid mass**

— *Central hypothyroidism*

- Disorder of anterior pituitary (secondary hypothyroidism) or hypothalamus (tertiary hypothyroidism)
- TSH deficiency $\rightarrow$ decreased functioning thyroid mass

— *Development anomalies of thyroid*

- Complete absence
- Failure to migrate normally during embryogenesis
- Responsible for most cases of neonatal hypothyroidism in United States

  - Screening programs—check thyroid function at birth and treat hypothyroidism

— *Postablative hypothyroidism—common in United States*

● **Thyroid neoplasms**

— *Adenoma*

- Benign neoplasm—derived from thyroid follicular epithelium

Morphology

- Solitary
- Fibrous encapsulation
- Uniform appearance different from the rest of thyroid
- Compression of surrounding nonneoplastic follicles
- Differential diagnosis

  - Nodule in multinodular goiter
  - Well-differentiated follicular carcinoma

Clinical features

- Presents as solitary thyroid nodule
- Function poorly—thyrotoxicosis rare

— **Carcinoma**

Incidence

- 97% of thyroid malignancies—carcinomas
- Epidemiology of thyroid malignancy

  - Estimated about 15,600 new cases diagnosed per year in the United States in 1996
  - Estimated 1200 deaths in the United States in 1996
  - 75% of cases and 65% of deaths in females

Usually presents as thyroid mass

Papillary

- Account for >65% of cases
- Estimated 10% to 15% in United States radiation induced
- Fusion between PTC and RET genes
- Histologic characteristics (Fig. 30.4)

  - Papillae
  - Psammoma bodies
  - Optically clear nuclei

- Lymphatic metastases
- Compatible with long survival

  - >90% 10-year survival
  - Survival for >30 years—common

Follicular

10% TO 20% OF THYROID CARCINOMAS

HISTOLOGIC FEATURES

- Absence of features of papillary carcinoma (papillae, clear nuclei)
- Follicular architecture

BLOOD-BORNE METASTASES

CLINICAL FEATURES

- 10-year survival

  - High (up to 90%) with small, localized lesions
  - Low (20% to 30%) with large, invasive lesions

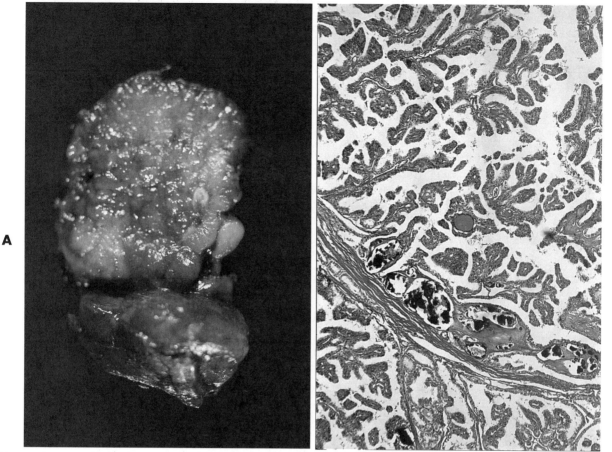

Fig. 30.4 Papillary carcinoma. **A,** Gross. Note the mass replacing one thyroid lobe. **B,** Histology. Note the branching papillae and psammoma bodies. *(Damjanov I, Linder J:* Anderson's pathology, *ed 10, vol 2, St Louis, 1996, Mosby.)*

- Rare thyrotoxicosis with widely metastatic disease

Undifferentiated (1% to 5%)

- >50% mortality within 6 months

Medullary carcinoma (5% to 10%)

DERIVED FROM C CELLS

ABOUT 10% TO 30%—FAMILIAL (ISOLATED FAMILIAL, MEN 2A AND 2B)

RET MUTATIONS

- RET

  - Receptor for glial-derived neurotopic factor with tyrosine kinase activity

- Germline mutations in familial cases

  - In extracellular domain in MEN 2A and isolated
  - In tyrosine kinase domain in MEN 2B

- Acquired mutations (in tumor) in tyrosine kinase domain in sporadic cases

MORPHOLOGY

- Usually polygonal or spindle cells arranged in nests or trabeculae

- Calcitonin demonstrated by immunohistochemistry
- Amyloid derived from procalcitonin in about 50%
- Multifocal tumors, C cell hyperplasia in familial cases

CLINICAL AND ENDOCRINE FEATURES

- Sometimes produce ectopic hormones (e.g., ACTH)
- Diagnosis by measurement of calcitonin (sometimes after stimulation with pentagastrin or calcium)
- Survival variable

  - 90% 10-year survival for isolated familial and MEN 2A
  - 30% to 50% 10-year survival for MEN 2B

— *Lymphoma (rare)*

- B cell neoplasm arising in thyroid
- Hashimoto's disease—may be risk factor
- 5-year survival—nearly 50%

— *Fine needle aspiration (FNA) biopsy*

- Useful technique for evaluation of clinically solitary thyroid nodule
- Distinguish between those with definitely benign masses (the overwhelming majority) who do not require surgery, and those with definitely or possibly malignant masses who do

■ **Parathyroids**

● Overview

- Parathyroid hormone (PTH) acts on the bone and kidney to increase serum Ca^{2+}, which down-regulates PTH
- Usually four parathyroid glands (PTGs), with a total mass of 120 to 150 mg
- Chief cells, oxyphil cells (in older persons), and variable amounts of interstitial fat

● Hyperparathyroidism—excess PTH

— *Primary hyperparathyroidism—malregulated PTH hypersecretion by the PTGs*

PTH elevated relative to calcium

- Relationship direct, rather than reciprocal

Primary hyperparathyroidism—a common cause of hypercalcemia

- Incidence in persons 60 years and older—1/500 to 1/1000

Morphology

ADENOMA

- Seen in approximately 80% of patients with primary hyperparathyroidism
- One of four glands is abnormal

  - Abnormal—increased weight
  - Microscopic examination—identify the sample as parathyroid

CHIEF CELL HYPERPLASIA

- Nearly 15% of patients with primary hyperparathyroidism
- Many cases familial—isolated, MEN 1, MEN 2A
- All four glands abnormal (enlarged; heavy), not necessarily equally so
- Histologically, a gland with chief cell hyperplasia often impossible to distinguish from a parathyroid adenoma

WATER CLEAR CELL HYPERPLASIA

- Rare
- Involves all glands (upper glands more than lower)
- Cells—almost clear cytoplasm with faint vacuoles

PARATHYROID CARCINOMA

- Rare
- Gross features

  - Usually involves one gland
  - Sometimes adherent to adjacent structures

- Histologic features

  - Dense, fibrous bands extending into capsule
  - Large cells
  - Invasion of blood vessels, capsule

Pathogenesis

- Cyclin D1 (PRAD) overexpressed in some nonfamilial adenomas

  - Chromosomal rearrangement places PRAD (11q13) under control of PTH gene promoter (11p15)

- 11q13 deletions observed in other sporadic adenomas and MEN 1 parathyroids

Clinical features

- Most patients with primary hyperthyroidism are asymptomatic.

  - Laboratory testing reveals mild hypercalcemia in an apparently healthy older individual.

- Probably 20% to 25% will develop symptoms within 5 years, if not treated

- Most common manifestations are renal stones, bone disease, and peptic ulcers.
- Parathyroid carcinoma

  - Often present with bone disease and high calcium
  - Recurrence rate 40% to 50%
  - Can be fatal because of uncontrolled hypercalcemia

— *Secondary hyperparathyroidism*

- Chief cell hyperplasia secondary to sustained hypocalcemia
- Causes—chronic renal failure, vitamin D deficiency

— *Parathyroid hormone-related peptide*

- Properties

  - Has most of the biologic activities of PTH
  - Immunochemically distinct, although has some amino acid sequence similarity
  - Produced by a number of normal tissues

- Secretion by a number of neoplasms—a cause of hypercalcemia

  - Examples—breast carcinoma, squamous cell carcinoma of lung and esophagus

- Ectopic PTH—extremely rare

— *Bone disease in patients with hyperparathyroidism (see Bone, Joint, and Soft Tissue Disorders chapter)*

● Hypoparathyroidism

- Decreased secretion of PTH

  - Idiopathic (autoimmune)
  - Damage or removal during surgery
  - Congenital absence (DiGeorge syndrome)
  - Decreased magnesium

- Resistance to PTH action (pseudohypoparathyroidism)
- Hypocalcemia, hyperphosphatemia, and sometimes tetany

■ **Thymus**

● DiGeorge syndrome

- Developmental abnormality involving third and fourth pharyngeal pouches

  - Disruption or deletion of gene on 22q11.2

- Thymic hypoplasia or aplasia with deficient cell-mediated immunity
- Other manifestations

  - Parathyroid hypoplasia or aplasia
  - Conotruncal cardiac abnormalities
  - Abnormal facial features

● Hyperplasia

- Presence of follicles
- Seen in about 65% of patients with myasthenia gravis

  - Removal of thymus used in treatment of myasthenia gravis

- Also seen in persons with immune disorders (Graves' disease, systemic lupus erythematosus [SLE], rheumatoid arthritis)

● Thymoma

— *Neoplasm of the thymic epithelium*

- Not other types originating in thymus (lymphoma, carcinoid)

— *Morphology*

- Benign thymoma (70%)

- Epithelium resembling normal medulla with some nonneoplastic lymphocytes
- Malignant thymoma, type 1 (20% to 25%)
  - Cytologically benign, but invades capsule
- Malignant thymoma, type 2 (thymic carcinoma)
  - Cytologically malignant (often, squamous cell carcinoma)
— *Clinical features*
  - Common—asymptomatic incidental finding, local effects, association with myasthenia gravis
  - Less common—metastases, association with other disorders (pernicious anemia, dermatomyositis, Graves' disease)

■ Adrenals

● Overview

- Each consists of a cortex and a medulla.
- Each weighs 4 ± 2 g.

● Cortex

— *Overview*

Approximately 80% of the adrenal mass in normal adults

Zona glomerulosa

- Produces mineralocorticoids (e.g., aldosterone)
- Angiotensin (regulated by renin) and potassium—stimulate aldosterone production

Zona fasiculata and zona reticularis—function together

- Produces glucocorticoids (e.g., cortisol) and androgens (e.g., dehydroisoandrosterone)
- ACTH
  - Maintains and stimulates proliferation of fasiculata and reticularis
  - Stimulates cortisol and androgen synthesis and secretion
  - Inhibited by cortisol

— *Cushing's syndrome*

Clinical syndrome from cortisol excess

Etiologic and morphologic categories

Excess pituitary ACTH (Cushing's disease)

- 65% to 70% of cases
- Bilateral adrenal hyperplasia, often multinodular (Fig. 30.5)
- >70% of the patients—documentable pituitary adenoma (usually a microadenoma) producing ACTH
  - ACTH-cell hyperplasia (possible hypothalamic disorder) seems to cause the remaining cases.

Ectopic ACTH

- 10% to 12% of cases
- Bilateral adrenal hyperplasia

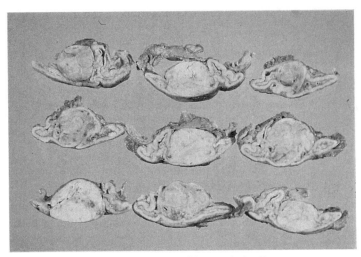

Fig. 30.5 Bilateral nodular adrenal hyperplasia. Transverse sections through the glands show multiple cortical nodules. (*Damjanov I, Linder J:* Anderson's pathology, *ed 10, vol 2, St Louis, 1996, Mosby.*)

- Causes—small-cell lung carcinoma (50%), carcinoids, islet cell neoplasms, medullary thyroid carcinoma, pheochromocytoma, inflammatory masses (rare)
- Most patients have obvious metastases before Cushing's syndrome becomes apparent

  - Occasionally Cushing's syndrome is an early and prominent manifestation of the underlying disorder.

- Rare ectopic corticotropin-releasing factor production clinically similar

ADRENOCORTICAL NEOPLASMS

- About 18% of cases
- Composed of adrenal cortical cells capable of ACTH-independent growth and steroid production
- Morphologic aspects

  - >90% unilateral
  - Reduction in mass of nonneoplastic ACTH-dependent portions of the cortex lose mass
  - Approximately 50% adenomas and 50% carcinomas

- Adenomas

  - Composed of relatively normal appearing clear and compact (eosinophilic) cells

- Carcinomas

  - Tend to be larger than adenomas
  - Histologic features favoring malignancy—dense fibrous bands; diffuse growth pattern; >5 mitoses/50 high-power field; abnormal mitoses; vascular invasion

ACTH-INDEPENDENT HYPERPLASIA—1% OF CASES

Clinical features

- Most common in 20- to 60-year-old females; occurs in others
- Abnormal metabolism—impaired glucose tolerance; abnormal distribution of body fat; net protein catabolism
- Impaired immune function
- Hypertension
- Psychiatric disorders
- Androgen excess—hirsutism or virilization of children or females
- Potentially fatal

Laboratory evaluation

LABORATORY RESULTS CONFIRMING DIAGNOSIS OF CUSHING'S SYNDROME

- Elevated plasma or urine cortisol
- Failure to suppress cortisol with low dexamethasone

LABORATORY RESULTS DISTINGUISHING DIFFERENT ETIOLOGIC CATEGORIES

- Pituitary Cushing's syndrome (Cushing's disease)

  - Cortisol usually suppressed by high-dose dexamethasone (especially if microadenoma)
  - ACTH elevated

- Ectopic ACTH

  - Cortisol not suppressed by high-dose dexamethasone
  - ACTH elevated, often markedly

- Adrenal Cushing's syndrome

  - Cortisol not suppressed by high dose dexamethasone
  - ACTH suppressed

Note: Therapeutic administration of synthetic glucocorticoids for chronic inflammatory diseases (rheumatoid arthritis, chronic inflammatory bowel disease) has similar clinical effects to diseases discussed previously and is much more common.

— *Primary (low renin) aldosteronism*

Usually caused by single adenoma of adrenal cortex (Conn's syndrome)

- Contains cells resembling those of normal cortex (small cells similar to glomerulosa, clear and compact cells resembling fasciulata and reticularis, and some intermediate types (Fig. 30.6)

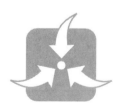

Other causes

- Idiopathic, with bilateral zona glomerulosa hyperplasia
- Carcinoma of the adrenal cortex
- Glucocorticoid remediable hyperaldosteronism (autosomal dominant)
- Ovarian sex cord-stromal neoplasm

Clinical and laboratory features

- Hypertension
- Accounts for less than 1% of all cases of hypertension
- Hypokalemia (low potassium)

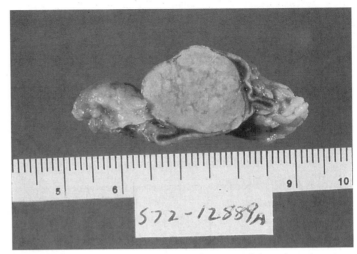

Fig. 30.6 Aldosterone producing adenoma of the adrenal cortex.
(*Damjanov I, Linder J:* Anderson's pathology, *ed 10, vol 2, St Louis, 1996, Mosby.*)

- Elevated aldosterone, low renin, failure to suppress aldosterone by saline

— *"Nonfunctional" adrenocortical neoplasms do not produce enough bioactive hormones to cause endocrine symptoms*

- Carcinomas can be very large and/or metastasize and thus become clinically evident.
- Small adenomas are sometimes an incidental finding at autopsy.

— *Deficiency of adrenal steroid hormones—Addison's disease*
Primary (adrenal) Addison's disease

- Deficiency of cortisol and aldosterone caused by disease of the adrenal cortex
- Idiopathic (autoimmune)

  - Most common cause
  - Antibodies to cytochrome P450 enzymes involved in steroidogenesis
  - Can be component of polyglandular autoimmune syndromes
  - Small adrenal glands; marked reduction in cortex; chronic inflammation; preserved medulla

- Other causes

  - Infections (tuberculosis used to be the most common cause)
  - Metastatic carcinoma, rare
  - Hemorrhage (with disseminated intravascular coagulation; Waterhouse-Friderichsen syndrome), rare

- Manifestations of aldosterone deficiency

  - Hypotension, hyponatremia, hyperkalemia, acidosis
  - Low aldosterone, elevated plasma renin activity

- Manifestations of cortisol deficiency

- Altered mental status, decreased stress response, hypotension, hypoglycemia, anorexia, nausea and vomiting, weight loss, hyperpigmentation (from elevated ACTH)
- Elevated ACTH, low baseline cortisol and no response to synthetic ACTH

Secondary and tertiary Addison's disease

- Abnormality of anterior pituitary (secondary) or hypothalamus (tertiary) causing ACTH deficiency
- Cortisol deficient; aldosterone normal
- Manifestations

  - Cortisol deficiency with low ACTH
  - Sometimes other manifestations hypopituitarism, intracranial mass

Note: Treatment with synthetic glucocorticoids or Cushing's syndrome will suppress hypothalamic corticotropin-releasing factor (the hormone that stimulates ACTH). Sudden withdrawal of glucocorticoid therapy or cure of Cushing's syndrome without steroid replacement can precipitate tertiary Addison's disease.

— *Congenital adrenal hyperplasia*

- Autosomal recessive deficiencies in one of the enzymes involved in the biosynthesis of cortisol and sometimes aldosterone

Pathogenesis

- Enzyme deficiency blocks cortisol production, impairing cortisol-mediated negative feedback control of ACTH secretion
- Effects of increased ACTH

  - Bilateral adrenal hyperplasia
  - Increased production of hormones whose pathways are not blocked

- Accumulation of precursors in the blocked pathways

21-hydroxylase deficiency

DEMOGRAPHY

- Accounts for least 85% of cases of adrenal hyperplasia
- One of the most common autosomal recessive disorders

  - Overall, might occur in 1%
  - Much more common in some ethnic groups

GENETICS

- 21-hydroxylase gene located within the HLA gene cluster (6p21)

  - 21-hydroxylase deficiency associated with specific HLA types

- Most mutations because of recombination with adjacent pseudogene

  - Nearly equal to 15% deletions
  - Nearly equal to 75% gene conversions (deleterious sequences from pseudogene)

- Different mutations—different effects on the amount of enzyme activity, although relationship not exact
- Most patients heterozygous for different abnormal alleles

PATHOPHYSIOLOGY

- Pathways leading to the production of aldosterone and cortisol blocked
- Androgen synthesis (does not involve 21-hydroxylation)—increased

ELEVATED PLASMA 17-HYDROXYPROGESTERONE AND EXAGGERATED RESPONSE TO ACTH USED FOR LABORATORY DIAGNOSIS

CLINICAL PRESENTATION OF 21-HYDROXYLASE DEFICIENCY—VARIABLE, DEPENDING UPON THE SEVERITY OF THE ENZYME DEFICIENCY

- "Classical"
  - Clinically significant at or shortly after birth
  - Salt-wasting—life-threatening dehydration
  - Simple virilizing
- Nonclassic (late onset)
  - Accounts for most cases of 21-hydroxylase deficiency
  - Present with androgen excess in childhood or at puberty

11-β hydroxylase deficiency

SECOND MOST COMMON CAUSE OF CONGENITAL ADRENAL HYPERPLASIA

ABNORMALITIES

- Mineralocorticoid (deoxycorticosterone) excess
  - Hypertension and low potassium
- Cortisol deficiency
- Androgen excess

● **Medulla**

— *Overview*

- Neural crest derivative
- Makes catecholamines
- Similar tissue found outside the adrenal gland, in paraganglia

— *Pheochromocytoma*

- Catecolamine-producing neoplasm of adrenal medulla

Morphology

- About 15% bilateral
- 10% to 15% occur outside of adrenal
  - More likely to be malignant

CHROMAFFIN REACTION

- Turns brown in potassium dichromate solution
  - Caused by oxidation of catecholamines

HISTOLOGY

- Usually nests of cells resembling normal medulla

ABOUT 10% OF CASES ARE MALIGNANT (THAT IS, METASTASIZE)

About 10% cases are inherited

- Usually autosomal dominant
- Isolated or part of syndrome (MEN 2A or 2B, von Hippel-Lindau disease, von Recklinghausen's neurofibromatosis, Sturge-Weber syndrome)
  - Inherited cases—differ from sporadic
    - Higher incidence of bilaterality (50% to 70%) than sporadic
    - Often preceded or accompanied by adrenomedullary hyperplasia
    - Lower risk of malignancy than sporadic

RET mutations

- Germline in inherited cases
- Acquired (in tumor) in some sporadic cases

Clinical and laboratory features

- Usually diagnosed between ages of 30 and 50 years

PRESENTATIONS

- Hypertension resistant to usual medical management
- Hypertensive crisis
- Paroxysm
  - Headache, sweating, palpatations, apprehension, sometimes with hypertensive crisis

HYPERTENSION

- About 60% pheochromocytoma patients have sustained hypertension.
  - About half of these also have hypertensive crises.
- About 25% have paroxysmal hypertension only.
- About 0.3% of hypertensives have pheochromocytoma.
- Laboratory diagnosis is made by measurement of urine catecholamine metabolites (metanephrines, vanillylmandelic acid).

— *Neuroblastoma*

- Childhood malignant neoplasm—derived from presumptive neuroblasts

Pathogenesis

- Amplification of N-myc gene
  - Produces double minutes chromosomes and homogeneously staining regions
  - Overexpression of N-myc mRNA
- Deletion of 1p36
- Triploidy or tetraploidy

Morphology

- 80%—originate in or near adrenal
- Histology

- Small, round blue cells
- Homer-Wright rosettes (pale fibrillar material surrounded by cells)
- Sometimes shows ganglionic differentiation with abundant Schwann cell stroma

Clinical features

USUALLY OCCURS EARLY IN CHILDHOOD

- Mean age of presentation—2 years
- Can be congenital

OFTEN PRESENT BECAUSE OF ABDOMINAL MASS

STAGING

- Stage I—confined to site of origin
- Stage II
    - Extends beyond site of origin, but continous with it
    - Does not cross midline
    - ± involved regional lymph nodes
- Stage III
    - Same as II, but crosses midline
- Stage IV
    - Involvement of viscera, distant lymph nodes, soft tissue, or bone
- Stage IVS
    - Primary same as stage I or II
    - Involvement of liver, skin, or bone marrow

FAVORABLE PROGNOSTIC FEATURES

- Early age of presentation
- Triploidy
- Ganglionic differentiation
- Stages I, II, or IVS

UNFAVORABLE PROGNOSTIC FEATURES

- Presentation after age 2 years
- Amplification of N-myc gene (most important)
- Stage III or IV
- 1p36 deletion

■ Islet Cell Neoplasms

● Endocrine pancreas

- Pancreatic endocrine cells—located in the islets of Langerhans
    - Small, circumscribed groups, scattered throughout the pancreas
    - About 1% to 2% of pancreatic mass
- Islet cells—classified by their hormone content
    - Beta (B) cells—contain insulin; 70% of the cells in most islets
    - Alpha (A) cells—contain glucagon; 20% of the cells of most islets
    - Delta (D) cells—contain somatostatin

- **General considerations**
  - — *Found in 0.5% to 1.5% of autopsies; clinically recognized neoplasms much less frequent*
  - — *Usually occur in adults*
  - — *Endocrine aspects*
    - Classified by the hormone produced
    - Can produce non-islet hormones
    - Nonfunctional neoplasms do not secrete enough hormone to cause clinical abnormalities
    - Islet cell hyperplasia can cause endocrine symptoms similar to those seen with neoplasms
  - — *Morphology*

    - Usually they are composed of nests and cords of cells resembling normal islet cells.
    - Some contain amyloid, derived from islet amyloid protein (amylin).
    - Malignant neoplasms can be identified by metastases or invasion across major tissue boundaries (blood vessels or nerves).
      - Metastases are usually found in regional lymph nodes or the liver.
      - Islet cell carcinomas generally grow slowly.
- **Insulinoma (beta cell neoplasm)**
  - — *By far the most common*
    - Many clinically nonfunctional neoplasms contain insulin.
  - — *Most are benign*
  - — *Clinically functional neoplasms produce high insulin levels and cause hypoglycemia*
    - Insulinoma is a relatively unusual cause of hypoglycemia.
      - Insulin overdose, liver disease, and alcohol are much more common causes.
  - — *Neonatal hypoglycemia*
    - Islet cell hyperplasia or nesidioblastosis (islets budding from ductal system)
    - Idiopathic or infants of diabetic mothers
- **Gastrinoma (Zollinger-Ellison syndrome)**
  - Second most common islet cell neoplasm
  - 67% malignant, 33% benign (sometimes multiple), 10% extrapancreatic
  - Many patients have MEN 1—>40% of MEN 1 patients have gastrinoma
  - — *Hypergastrinemia—causes secretion of large quantities of low pH gastric juice*
    - Causes severe peptic ulcer disease
      - Ulcers frequently occur in unusual locations (esophagus or jejunum).

- Ulcers tend to be resistant to usual medical therapy.
- About ⅓ of the patients have intractable diarrhea

■ Multiple Endocrine Neoplasia

- ● General
  - Autosomal dominant
  - Hyperplasia, often developing into neoplasia
  - Neoplasms sometimes multifocal

- ● Multiple endocrine neoplasia, type 1 (MEN 1)
  - MEN 1 gene
    - Tumor suppressor gene (anti-oncogene) on chromosome 11
    - 11q13 deletions in abnormal parathyroid and pituitary tissue from MEN 1 patients
  - Manifestations
    - 95% of MEN 1 families—have parathyroid abnormalities, usually chief cell hyperplasia
    - Islet cell neoplasia or hyperplasia (80%)
    - Gastrinoma most common
    - Pituitary adenomas—also common (50% to 80%)
    - Carcinoids, thyroid adenomas, and adrenocortical adenomas—less common

- ● Multiple endocrine neoplasia, type 2A (MEN 2A)
  - Point mutations in RET (chromosome 10q11.2) in extracellular domain
  - — *Manifestations*
    - Medullary thyroid carcinoma (almost all families)
      - Can be multifocal
      - Can be associated with or preceded by C cell hyperplasia
    - Pheochromocytoma (about 50%)
      - Often bilateral
      - Can be preceded or accompanied by hyperplasia
    - Parathyroid hyperplasia—20% to 30% of families

- ● Multiple endocrine neoplasia, type 2B (MEN 2B)
  - Occurs in different families than MEN 2A
    - Mutation in RET tyrosine kinase domain (different than those in MEN 2A)
  - Manifestations
    - Medullary thyroid carcinoma (almost all), pheochromocytoma (50%)
    - Parathyroid hyperplasia rare
    - Nonendocrinologic manifestations—thickened corneal nerves; ganglioneuromatosis of the intestine, with abnormalities of the

intestinal motility; poor muscle development; lax joints; and a marfanoid body habitus

■ Diabetes Mellitus

● Overview

— *Diabetes mellitus (DM)—a heterogeneous group of hyperglycemic disorders*

- Absolute or relative insulin deficiency

  - Usually absolute or relative glucagon excess

- A tendency to develop late complications, involving the eyes, kidneys, large and small blood vessels, and peripheral nerves

— *Idiopathic DM—nomenclature and definitions*

- Insulin-dependent diabetes mellitus (IDDM)

  - Requires daily injections of insulin to prevent ketoacidosis

- Non–insulin-dependent diabetes mellitus (NIDDM)

  - Does not require daily insulin injection to prevent ketoacidosis

- Type 1 DM

  - Immunologically mediated beta cell destruction

- Type 2 DM

  - NIDDM not caused by type 1 DM or secondary DM

- Common usage—IDDM = Type 1 DM; NIDDM = Type 2 DM.

— *Other forms of DM*
  Gestational DM

- Carbohydrate intolerance first recognized during pregnancy
- Common, but prevalence varies among location, ethnic background
- Glucokinase mutation found in small number of cases
- Clinical manifestations

  - Can cause morbidity, mortality for mother and child
  - Usually reverses itself after the end of gestation
  - Up to 60% eventually become diabetic

  Secondary DM

- Extensive destruction of pancreas

  - Chronic pancreatitis
  - Cystic fibrosis (CF)
  - Neoplasm

- Excess of hormones (GH, cortisol, catecholamines, glucagon) whose actions counter those of insulin can cause diabetes, usually mild
  - Drug induced
  - Insulin receptor defects
  - Rare genetic syndromes
  - Others

— *Laboratory diagnosis of DM*

- Sometimes needed in asymptomatic individual
- Plasma glucose >140 mg/dl after overnight fast on two separate occasions
- Oral glucose tolerance test
    - Give 1.75 g/kg body weight, up to 75 g
    - DM if plasma glucose >200 mg/dl at 2 hours and one other point
    - Impaired glucose tolerance if glucose 140 to 200 mg/dl at 2 hours and >200 mg/dl at one other point

● Type 2 DM (non–insulin-dependent diabetes mellitus [NIDDM])

— *Nearly 85% of primary DM*

— *High prevalence*

- >1% in many populations, including United States
- High-risk populations—30% in Micronesians; 40% in Pima Indians

— *Etiology—interaction between genetic and environmental factors*
Familial tendency

- About ⅓ of siblings or children of individuals with NIDDM— have either diabetes or abnormalities of glucose tolerance
- Concordance among identical twins, >90%

Genetic aspects

- Maturity onset diabetes of young (MODY)

    - Accounts for about 2% cases of type 2 DM
    - Autosomal dominant
    - 30% to 50% of cases caused by mutations in glucokinase gene
    - Other loci identified on chromosomes 20 and 12

- Mode of inheritance—not known (except for MODY)
- A number of genes postulated to play a role in the inheritance

    - Some implicated in rare types of DM or in certain populations
    - None proven responsible in the majority of cases
    - Glucokinase gene—MODY, gestational DM
    - Others implicated—proinsulin, insulin receptor, glucose transporters, glycogen synthase, glucagon receptor genes

Environmental influence

- Marked increase in NIDDM in recently urbanized groups
- Presumably the major factor—greater food availability, predisposing to obesity, converting normoglycemic subjects into hyperglycemic patients

— *Pathogenesis*
Impaired islet function

- Decreased insulin response to glucose

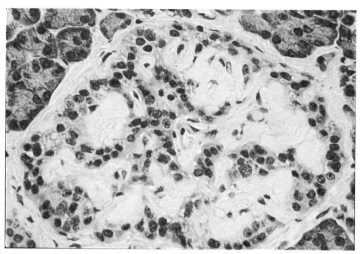

Fig. 30.7 Islet amyloidosis. Amyloid deposits replace some endocrine cells. (*Damjanov I, Linder J:* Anderson's pathology, *ed 10, vol 2, St Louis, 1996, Mosby.*)

- • Basal insulin level normal to elevated
- • Relative hyperglucagonemia

Insulin resistance

- • Often obesity related
  - • Correctable, at least partially, by weight reduction
- • Decreased skeletal muscle glycogen storage
- • Abnormalities in insulin receptor or glucose transporters

— **Pancreatic morphology**

- • Can be normal
- • Increased number of alpha (glucagon) cells relative to beta cells
- • Increased or decreased islet cell mass

Amyloidosis of islets

- • Amyloid derived from islet amyloid protein (IAP; also called amylin)
  - • Beta cell hormone that inhibits insulin action and affects secretion of islet hormones secretion
- • Found in majority of patients with type 2 DM
  - • Also in others treated with insulin for long time and about 10% of aged, nondiabetics (Fig. 30.7)

— **Clinical features**

- • Typical patient—presents after age of 40 years (adult onset diabetes)
  - • Exception—MODY (usual onset by age 25 years)
- • Patients—often few or no symptoms
- • Patients—often obese

- Weight reduction helpful (for some, only treatment needed)
- Morbidity and mortality from long-term complications (see following)

● **Type 1 DM (insulin-dependent diabetes mellitus [IDDM])**

— *About 15% of primary DM*

— *Demography*

  - Type 1 DM—more common in Caucasians than in others
  - In the United States—prevalence by age 20 years is 0.26%

    - Incidence—approximately 1/10,000

— *Etiology and pathogenesis*

  Immunologically mediated destruction of beta cells in genetically susceptible individual

  Family studies

  - About 5% to 10% of siblings or parents of type 1 DM patients will have it.
  - About 50% of identical twins of type 1 DM patients will develop it.

  Susceptibility loci

  - Major locus on chromosome 6p21 (HLA DQα and β)

    - Different alleles confer high susceptibility, susceptibility, or resistance.

  - Second most important locus—on 11p, near insulin gene
  - Apparently many other less significant loci

  Evidence for autoimmunity in type I DM

  - Association with class II histocompatibility antigens

    - Especially HLA-DR3 and HLA-DR4

  - Occurrence in polyglandular autoimmune syndromes
  - Morphologic findings in endocrine pancreas
  - Anti-islet cell and anti-insulin antibodies

    - Often present years before onset of disease
    - Beta cell autoantigens—glutamic acid decarboxylase (GAD) and protein tyrosine phosphatases
    - Autoimmunity directed against GAD—might be pathogenically important

  - Recurrence of islet cell inflammation (distinct from rejection) in some pancreases transplanted into type 1 DM patients
  - Immunosuppressive therapy can induce remission

  Viruses—most likely environmental agent inducing type 1 DM in susceptible persons

  - Coxsackievirus B is most frequently implicated, but many others are also cited (mumps, measles, Epstein-Barr virus).
  - Viruses can cause islet cell inflammation and destruction in experimental systems.

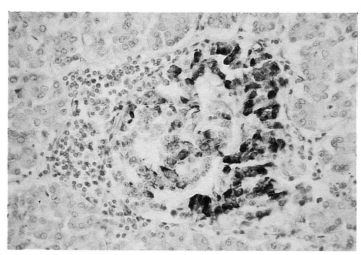

Fig. 30.8 Type I diabetes mellitus. Lymphocytes infiltrate an islet containing beta cells (shown by immunoperoxidase staining for insulin). *(Damjanov I, Linder J:* Anderson's pathology, *ed 10, vol 2, St Louis, 1996, Mosby.)*

— *Pancreatic morphology*

Changes within 1 year of onset

- Grossly normal
- Reduced beta cell mass
- Inflammation (mostly T lymphocytes) of islets containing beta cells (Fig. 30.8)

Later changes

- Reduction in pancreatic weight caused by loss of acinar mass
  - Caused by loss of growth promoting effect of insulin
- Further reduction of beta cell mass
- Resolution of inflammation with disappearance of beta cells
- Extremely high ratio of alpha cells-beta cells (Fig. 30.9)

— *Clinical features*

Typical clinical features of type 1 diabetes

- Present in adolescence (juvenile onset diabetes)
  - Average age, 13 to 14 years old
- Usual presenting symptoms
  - Polyuria, polydipsia, polyphagia, weight loss for several weeks
  - 10% present with ketoacidosis
- Insulin dependent (ketosis prone)—require daily insulin injection

Insulin-dependent diabetics—morbidity and premature mortality from long-term complications (see following)

- Median survival after diagnosis—36 years
- Median age at death—49 years

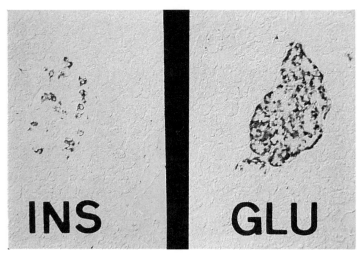

Fig. 30.9 Type I diabetes mellitus for 21 years. Immunoperoxidasae stains for insulin (*left*) showing few beta cells and glucagon (*right*) showing marked relative increase in alpha cells. (*Damjanov I, Linder J:* Anderson's pathology, *ed 10, vol 2, St Louis, 1996, Mosby.*)

Some type I diabetics—present later in life with NIDDM

- Differ from type II diabetics

  - Lean
  - Hypoinsulinemic
  - Have anti-islet cell antibodies
  - Sometimes become insulin dependent

● **Long-term complications of DM**
  — *Overview*

    - Complications occur in patients with all types of DM
    - Occurrence relates, in part, to length and severity of disease
    - Some unique to DM (retinopathy, nephropathy)
    - Others not unique, but more common in diabetics (atherosclerosis)
    - Causes substantial amount of morbidity and early mortality in patients with DM

      - Greater than twentyfold increased risk of blindness, end-stage renal disease, and amputation (usually of a foot)
      - At least twofold increased risk of stroke, myocardial infarction

  — *Pathogenesis*

    - Unlikely to be a single mechanism for all complications
    - Probably a causal relationship between severity and length of hyperglycemia and development of complications

    Polyol pathway

    - Aldose reductase catalyzes glucose reduction to sorbitol
    - Occurs in tissues not dependent on insulin for glucose transport (lens, nerve, blood vessels, kidney)

- Effects

  - Lens—swelling from osmotic effect
  - Schwann cells and retinal pericytes— increased sorbitol → decreased myoinisitol → decreased phosphoinositide → decreased diacylglycerol → decreased protein kinase C → decreased Na^+ ATpase → further decreased myoinositol

- In experimental animal models—aldose reductase inhibitors prevent myoinositol decrease and peripheral neuropathy

Nonenzymatic protein glycation

- Steps

  - Addition of hexose to protein, usually at valine or lysine
  - Hexose reversibly forms Schiff's reagent (hours)
  - Schiff's reagent can reversibly rearrange to form Amadori product (days)

- Glycated proteins hemoglobin, albumin, collagen, lens crystal, lipoproteins, fibrinogen

  - Glycation can alter function, metabolism of these proteins
  - Clinical measurement of glycated hemoglobin (HbA_{1C}), glycated albumin

- Glycated proteins can form advanced glycation end products (AGEs)

  - AGEs can undergo irreversible cross-linkage

- AGEs bind to receptors on many cell types (monocytes and macrophages, endothelium, lymphocytes, mesangium)
- Effects of AGEs potentially related to diabetic complications

  - Macrophage release of cytokines and growth factors
  - Increased endothelial permeability
  - Fibroblast and smooth muscle cell proliferation and synthesis of extracellular matrix
  - Increased endothelial and macrophage procoagulant activity

Angiotensin converting enzyme (ACE)

- Variants in ACE gene independent risk factor for

  - Nephropathy in IDDM patients
  - Coronary artery atherosclerosis (high-grade lesion or transmural myocardial infarction) in NIDDM patients

- ACE levels higher in IDDM subjects with nephropathy

Therapeutic implications

- Value of tight control of plasma glucose
- Aldose reductase inhibitors
- Aminoguanidine (inhibitor of AGE cross-linking)
- ACE inhibitors for diabetic nephropathy

— **Diabetic microangiopathy (microvascular disease)**

- Basement membrane thickening

- Most apparent in capillaries of skin, skeletal muscle, retina, renal glomeruli
- Probably related to glycation of basement membrane collagen
- Morphology—homogeneous or multilayered, periodic acid-Schiff (PAS) positive
- Capillaries more permeable than normal—leakage of plasma proteins

- Increased hyaline arteriolosclerosis

  - Nonspecific—also increased by aging, hypertension
  - Amorphous hyalinization with lumenal narrowing

— *Atherosclerosis*

Diabetes greatly increases risk and severity

Pathogenic factors probably related to protein glycation

- Hyperlipidemia
- Decreased high density lipoproteins
- Increased uptake of low density lipoproteins
- Increased platelet response to aggregating agents and increased adhesion

Effects

- Coronary artery disease and myocardial infarction

  - DM eliminates protective effect of being female
  - Earlier onset than in nondiabetics, especially if nephropathy present
  - Higher mortality than nondiabetics from myocardial infarctions

- Increased risk of stroke
- Markedly increased risk of gangrene of feet

— *Retinopathy and other eye manifestations (see Eye chapter)*

— *Nephropathy and other renal manifestations*

Nephropathy develops in 35% of IDDM patients, 20% of NIDDM patients

- ⅓ new dialysis patients have diabetic nephropathy.

Natural history of nephropathy

- Protein (mostly albumin) in urine increases in amount over years.
- Hypertension, nephrotic syndrome, and renal failure eventually develop.
- Typically takes >20 years for chronic renal failure.

Morphology of nephropathy

- Glomerular basement membrane thickening, increased mesangial matrix
- Diffuse glomerulosclerosis
- Nodular glomerulosclerosis (Kimmelstiel-Wilson disease)

- Specific for DM
- Round hyaline masses in periphery of glomerulus
- Usually diffuse glomerulosclerosis in other glomeruli

Other renal manifestations

- Infections
- Papillary necrosis
- Vascular changes of hypertension

    - Hyaline arteriolosclerosis

— *Neuropathy*

- Peripheral, symmetric sensorimotor neuropathy—most common

    - Complicates foot care
    - Occasionally can cause extreme pain

- Autonomic neuropathy

    - Gastroparesis
    - Impotence—common in diabetic men
    - Incontinence
    - Tachycardia, postural hypotension

- Mononeuropathy

    - Involvement of single peripheral or cranial motor nerve

- Mononeuropathy probably caused by microvascular disease; others related to hyperglycemia

— *DM and infection*

- Pathogenic aspects

    - Decreased neutrophil and macrophage function
    - Disruption of skin

- Infections more frequent and/or severe in diabetics
- Infections related to DM

    - Malignant external otitis
    - Rhinocerebral mucormycosis
    - Emphysematous cholecysitis
    - Emphysematous myelonephritis

Multiple Choice
Review Questions

1. The environmental factor most likely to induce type 1 diabetes mellitus in a genetically susceptible individual is which of the following?

   a. Coxsackievirus B infection
   b. Excess caloric intake
   c. Insufficient dietary iodine
   d. Insulin injection
   e. Therapeutic use of synthetic glucocorticoids

2. A 31-year-old woman with unexplained weight gain resulting in central obesity, mild hypertension, impaired glucose tolerance, and reduced bone mass has elevated morning plasma cortisol not suppressed by low dose (1 mg) dexamethasone. This patient has which of the following?

   a. Addison's disease
   b. Alport's syndrome
   c. Caplan's syndrome
   d. Conn's syndrome
   e. Cushing's syndrome

3. Further evaluation of the patient described in the Question 3, shows slight elevation of the plasma ACTH and suppression of cortisol by high dose (8 mg) dexamethasone. These findings are most compatible with which of the following?

   a. Adrenocortical adenoma
   b. Adrenocortical carcinoma

   c. Pheochromocytoma
   d. Pituitary adenoma
   e. Small cell lung carcinoma

4. A 42-year-old woman notes fatigue, lethargy, weakness of several months' duration and a gain of 10 pounds despite decreased appetite. Her physician detects an enlarged thyroid. The thyroid stimulating hormone (TSH) is markedly elevated and the free thyroxine index is low. It is most likely that the patient has which of the following?

   a. Pituitary adenoma
   b. Papillary thyroid carcinoma
   c. Hashimoto's thyroiditis
   d. Graves' disease
   e. Reidel's thyroiditis

5. Infiltrative ophthalmopathy is characteristic of which of the following?

   a. Graves' disease
   b. Hashimoto's thyroiditis
   c. Type 1 diabetes mellitus
   d. Type 2 diabetes mellitus
   e. Pituitary adenoma

Answers and Explanations to Multiple Choice Review Questions

CHAPTER 1: CELLULAR INJURY AND ADAPTATION

1. **Answer c:**

    Caseous necrosis is a distinctive subtype of coagulative necrosis usually seen in infection with *Mycobacterium tuberculosis.* Grossly, caseous necrosis is white and cheesy (hence the name); microscopically it has an amorphous granular appearance and is usually accompanied by granulomatous inflammation.

    a: Infection with most bacteria (e.g., *Pseudomonas aeruginosa*) causes liquefactive necrosis.

    b: Infection with most bacteria (e.g., *Staphylococcus aureus*) causes liquefactive necrosis.

    d: Interruption of the blood supply, usually by blockage of a blood vessel, usually causes typical coagulative necrosis that is distinct from caseous necrosis.

    e: Loss of innervation can cause atrophy of skeletal muscle.

2. **Answer d:**

    Systemic hypertension increases the workload of the myocytes. They respond by enlarging (hypertrophy), which can increase their functional capacity.

    a: Amyloid deposition in the left ventricular interstitium will cause enlargement of the chamber, but it is not an adaptive response to hypertension.

    b: Hemosiderosis is the presence of iron in macrophages. It is caused by systemic (e.g., from multiple transfusions) or local (e.g., from hemorrhage) increases in iron

concentration. It is not an adaptive response to systemic hypertension.

    c: Fatty change can occur in cardiac myocytes, but it is a form of reversible injury (usually caused by ischemia) and is not the typical adaptive response to hypertension.

    e: Cardiac myocytes cannot replicate, so the heart does not increase its size and functional capacity by hyperplasia.

3. **Answer a:**

    Apoptosis is a type of cell death in which a calcium-sensitive endonuclease specifically degrades DNA into a series of fragments that are multiples of about 180 to 200 base pairs.

    b: In dysplasia, DNA synthesis can be greater than in corresponding normal cells.

    c: Metaplasia is a reactive change, not associated with DNA breakdown.

    d: In coagulative necrosis DNA is randomly degraded.

    e: In liquefactive necrosis DNA is randomly degraded.

4. **Answer e:**

    The activity of phospholipase A_2 promotes degradation of membrane phospholipids.

    a: Catalase is involved in cell defenses against damage (including that to cell membranes) by activated oxygen species and free radicals.

    b: Superoxide dismutase is involved in cell defense against damage by activated oxygen species and free radicals.

c: Sodium/potassium-dependent ATPase is an ion pump; its normal activity is necessary for maintaining normal cell electrolyte and water homeostasis.

d: Glutathione peroxidase is involved in cell defense against damage by activated oxygen species and free radicals.

5. **Answer d:**

A stable cell is one that ordinarily does not divide but can do so with the appropriate stimulus. Hepatocytes, epithelium of endocrine organs and many mesenchymal and connective-tissue cells (e.g., endothelial cells, smooth muscle cells, fibroblasts) are stable cells.

a: Cardiac myocytes are permanent cells (i.e., they cannot divide).

b: Central nervous system neurons are permanent cells (i.e., they cannot divide).

c: Hematopoietic stem cells are labile cells (i.e., they divide continuously).

CHAPTER 2: INFLAMMATION AND REPAIR

1. **Answer a:**

The initial extracellular matrix of granulation tissue is rich in fibronectin and proteoglycan. Fibronectin is a chemoattractant for cells making up granulation tissue—fibroblasts, myofibroblasts, endothelium, lymphocytes, and macrophages.

b: Tenascin appears during the second week of granulation tissue formation.

c: Type I collagen appears in the second week of granulation tissue formation and subsequently becomes predominant. The mature, dense, fibrous scar contains dense collagen bundles.

d: Type III collagen appears during the first week of granulation tissue formation.

e: Type IV collagen is found in basement membranes and does not play an obvious role in granulation tissue formation.

2. **Answer b:**

The acute-phase protein response appears to be regulated primarily by interleukin 6.

a: Interleukin-3 is a colony-stimulating factor that promotes myeloid and erythroid differentiation.

c: Interferon alpha, like other interferons, is an antiviral agent and an activator of leukocytes.

d: Interferon gamma, in addition to its antiviral and leukocyte-activating activity, also induces expression of major histocompatibility antigens.

e: Prostaglandin E_2 might promote fever, but it does not mediate acute-phase protein synthesis.

3. **Answer a:**

Oxygen-dependent mechanisms are considered to be the principal means by which phagocytes kill microbes. The activities of NADPH oxidase and myeloperoxidase generate hypohalous acids from oxygen and halides.

b: Nitric oxide is produced by endothelium, neurons, and macrophages. It is a vasodilator. Its role in killing of microorganisms is uncertain.

c: Perforin is a product of cytotoxic T-lymphocytes involved in killing virally infected cells.

d: Prostaglandin E_2 increases blood flow and vascular permeability; it may inhibit some effector activities of phagocytes.

e: Serotonin is found in platelets; it increases vascular permeability.

4. **Answer e:**

Parasites and/or their eggs often elicit a granulomatous inflammation or eosinophil-rich response. Sometimes granulomas with many eosinophils are seen.

a: Allergic reactions are characterized by eosinophilic infiltration but not granulomas.

b: The granulomas of cat scratch disease often contain abscesses but not eosinophils.

c: The granulomas of chlamydial infections often contain abscesses but not eosinophils.

d: The granulomas of mycobacterial infections often show caseous necrosis but not eosinophils.

5. **Answer c:**

Antigen-antibody complexes containing IgM or IgG (especially IgG2) activate C1, initiating the classical complement pathway.

a: Aggregated IgA2 can initiate the alternative complement pathway.

b: IgE is involved in initiating histamine release from mast cells and basophils; it is not related to complement.

d: Plasminogen activator converts plasminogen to plasmin, which can activate C3.

e: Plasmin activates C3.

CHAPTER 3: HEMODYNAMIC DISTURBANCES

1. **Answer a:**

Fainting results from a transient fall in arterial pressure caused by a temporary reduction of venous return—in this instance, resulting from rapid postural change. Shock is the result of sustained, inadequate perfusion that does not meet the metabolic requirements of the tissue.

b: Sepsis results in shock by the actions of lipopolysaccharide from the bacterial cell wall and release of tissue necrosis factor by monocytes.

c: Saddle pulmonary embolus results in sudden cardiac failure (pump failure).

d: Massive hematemesis can result in hypovolemic shock if rapid blood loss exceeds 15% of the total blood volume.

e: Myocardial infarction results in pump failure, a cause of shock.

2. **Answer e:**

Virchow's triad consists of altered blood flow (stasis or turbulence), endothelial damage, and increased blood coagulability.

a: Leukocytosis, thrombocytosis, and erythrocytosis, if caused by myeloproliferative diseases, may be associated with increased thrombosis. For reactive causes

they would only carry the risk of the cause for the increased counts.

b: Increased plasminogen, protein C, and protein S are protective against thrombosis as they are *anti*coagulant proteins.

c: Occult cancer (by a multifactorial mechanism) and heart failure (stasis), but not jaundice, are risk factors for thrombosis. Jaundice may be associated with increased risk of bleeding if liver failure or vitamin K malabsorption occurs.

d: Hyperglycemia, hyperlipidemia, and hypertension are examples of etiologies for vascular endothelial damage.

3. **Answer c:**

A decrease in albumin production by the liver lowers the plasma oncotic pressure, leaving more fluid in the interstitial space.

a: Hyponatremia (low serum sodium) results from the increased renal water retention mechanisms evoked by the loss of fluid from the vascular space secondary to the hypoalbuminemia.

b: Hypergammaglobulinemia (increased serum gammaglobulins) helps to preserve intravascular fluid.

d: Anemia (low hemoglobin) does not have a major effect on maintaining intravascular volume.

e: Hypocalcemia (low serum calcium) does not have a major effect on maintaining intravascular volume.

4. **Answer a:**

While all sites are possible, by far the most common site of origin for systemic emboli is from mural thrombi post myocardial infarction. The highest risk period is in the first 1 to 2 weeks.

b: Systemic emboli arising in atrial fibrillation are uncommon because of a lower prevalence relative to myocardial infarction.

c: Systemic emboli arising from valvular vegetations are uncommon because of a low prevalence of vegetations.

d: Pulmonary venous thrombi are virtually nonexistent.

e: Ulcerated atherosclerotic plaques are the most common sites of emboli, but these are regional, as for example central nervous system strokes.

5. **Answer b:**

Widespread fat emboli of the lung, brain, and kidney are the finding for fat embolus. The history is classic for this disorder.

a: The classic history for pulmonary emboli would be sudden death and would not include confusion and petechia.

c: Aspiration pneumonia is unlikely in anyone with normal airway control.

d: Myocardial infarction would occur in older individuals.

e: Occult endocarditis is unlikely without a history of rheumatic fever or heart murmur.

CHAPTER 4: IMMUNITY

1. **Answer c:**

Selective IgA deficiency is the most common form of inherited immunodeficiency. Common variable immunodeficiency is the next most common form.

a, b, d, e: Severe combined immunodeficiency, chronic variable immunodeficiency, ataxia-telangiectasia, and x-linked agammaglobulinemia are all uncommon.

2. **Answer b:**

60% of severe combined immunodeficiency is caused by a defect in the interleukin 2 gamma chain located at Xq13.

a: Adenosine deaminase defects are a cause of non–X-linked severe combined immunodeficiencies or disorders that resemble SCID.

c: MHC class I and II expression defects are a cause of immunodeficiency resembling non–X-linked severe combined immunodeficiency.

d: A deficiency of btk is the cause of X-linked agammaglobulinemia (Bruton's agammaglobulinemia).

e: Nucleoside phosphorylase defects are a cause of non–X-linked severe combined immunodeficiency.

3. **Answer a:**

Dense dermal fibrosis, in addition to vascular obliteration and epidermal atrophy with loss of adnexal structures, are typical features of scleroderma.

b: Linear bandlike immunofluorescence for immunoglobulin deposition at the basement membrane of lesional and nonlesional skin (the lupus band test) is typical of SLE.

c: Follicular plugging is caused by epidermal thickening.

d: The basement membrane thickening is best seen with special stains to highlight the basement membrane.

e: This is not specific for SLE but can be seen.

4. **Answer b:**

HLA DR4 is most prevalent in rheumatoid arthritis.

a: SLE is associated with HLA B8, DR2 and DR3.

c: CREST is associated with various HLA types depending on the ethnic background.

d: Ankylosing spondylosis is associated with B27.4.

e: Sjögren's syndrome is associated with HLA B8 and DR3.

CHAPTER 5: INFECTIOUS DISEASE

1. **Answer d:**

Staphylococcus aureus is notorious for its ability to induce abscess formation.

a: CMV characteristically produces a chronic inflammatory cell response and not abscess formation.

b: Prions do not elicit any inflammatory cell response.

c: *Treponema pallidum* elicits a chronic inflammatory cell response especially rich in plasma cells.

2. **Answer c:**

N. gonorrhoeae is the only choice that is a significant cause of pelvic inflammatory disease. Another pathogen commonly implicated as a cause of pelvic inflammatory disease is *Chlamydia trachomatis*.

a, b, d, e: This pathogen is capable of producing sexually transmitted (venereal) disease, but not pelvic inflammatory disease.

3. **Answer b:**

Studies have shown that this risk is finite but only approximately 0.3%.

a, c, d, e: Risk of infection is approximately 0.3%.

4. **Answer a:**

Bacillary angiomatosis is commonly encountered in AIDS patients and has recently been shown to be caused by *Bartonella henselae* and *Bartonella quintana*.

b: Infection with *Pneumocystis carinii* commonly causes pneumonia in AIDS patients.

c: Infection with *Mycobacterium avium-intracellulare* could cause widespread infection but not angiomatosis.

d: Infection with *Toxoplasma gondii* typically causes CNS infection.

e: Infection with *Aspergillus fumigatus* could cause widespread infection but not angiomatosis.

5. **Answer c:**

Secondary tuberculosis is caused by either exogenous or endogenous reexposure to the tuberculosis bacillus, and its most common sites of involvement are the highly oxygenated apical and posterior lung segments.

a: The spleen is not a common location for endogenous reexposure.

b: The pleural space is not a common location for involvement by secondary tuberculosis.

d: The brain is not a common site for secondary tuberculosis involvement.

e: The GI tract is not a common site for secondary tuberculosis involvement.

CHAPTER 6: NEOPLASIA

1. **Answer a:**

Ultraviolet light is a major contributory factor in the development of the primary skin malignancies: basal cell carcinoma, squamous cell carcinoma, and malignant melanoma.

b: Squamous cell carcinoma of the lung, as well as other histologic types, is most often related to cigarette smoking; exposure to ionizing radiation (e.g., from radon) can also contribute.

c: Chronic infections with hepatitis B virus or hepatitis C virus, alcoholic cirrhosis, and ingestion of aflatoxin B1 are among many agents contributing to hepatocellular carcinoma.

d: Some cases of papillary thyroid carcinoma of leukemia are caused by exposure to ionizing radiation.

e: Exposure to ionizing radiation and some mutagenic chemicals (including anticancer chemotherapeutic agents) can induce acute myelogenous leukemia.

2. **Answer e:**

Human papillomavirus types 16, 18, 31, and 33 are associated with squamous cell carcinoma of the uterine cervix.

a: *Aspergillus flavus* produces aflatoxin B1, associated with hepatocellular carcinoma.

b: Infection with *Helicobacter pylori* is related to carcinoma and lymphoma of the stomach.

c: *Schistosomiasis hematobium* infection contributes to squamous cell carcinoma of the urinary bladder.

d: Infection with Epstein-Barr virus is related to Burkitt's lymphoma and neoplasms in immunosuppressed individuals.

3. **Answer c:**

Lung cancer is by far the leading cancer killer of women, accounting for about 24% of such fatalities in 1995

a: Breast cancer is second leading cancer killer of women, accounting for about 18% of such fatalities in 1995.

b: Colorectal cancer is third leading cancer killer of women, accounting for about 11% of such fatalities in 1995.

d: Skin cancers, although extremely common, cause only a small percentage of cancer fatalities.

e: Uterine malignancies account for about 5% of female cancer deaths, making them far from the leading cancer killer.

4. **Answer b:**

Hypophosphorylated pRb binds and sequesters some members of the E2F transcription factor family; the activity of these transcription factors is necessary for entrance into the S phase of the cell cycle.

a: p53 is a transcription factor.

c: bcl-2 protein is predominantly located in mitochondrial membrane and is unlikely to interact directly with transcription factors that are found in the nucleus.

d: The protein encoded by Ki-ras is cytoplasmic and involved in signal transduction. It does not directly interact with nuclear transcription factors.

e: c-sis encodes a subunit of platelet-derived growth factor, a secreted growth factor that does not directly interact with nuclear transcription factors.

5. **Answer c:**

Most chemical carcinogens require metabolic activation. Most carcinogens that require activation (called procarcinogens, or indirectly acting carcinogens) are activated by cytochrome P450 cyclooxygenases.

a: Myeloperoxidase, an enzyme of neutrophil granules, catalyzes the conversion of hydrogen peroxide to $HOCl^-$, an agent involved in killing of microbes.

b: Many protooncogenes and growth factor receptors have tyrosine kinase activity, which catalyzes the addition of phosphate to tyrosines in many substrates; tyrosine kinases are not involved in metabolism of procarcinogens.

d: Superoxide dismutases catalyze conversion of hydrogen peroxide to water and oxygen; this reaction is important in protecting cells from oxidative injury.

e: Cathepsin D is a protease. Its role in cancer involves its ability to catalyze extracellular matrix components, promoting invasion and metastasis.

Chapter 7: Genetic Diseases

1. **Answer b:**

Clinically, the infant has Down syndrome.

47,XY, +21 (trisomy 21) accounts for about 95% of cases of Down syndrome.

a: Although 46,XY, −14, +t(14q21q) results in Down syndrome, it accounts for only about 4% of cases.

c: 45,XO causes Turner's syndrome; affected individuals are female.

d: 46,XXY results in Klinefelter's syndrome.

e: Deletion of the short arm of chromosome 5 (5p−) causes cri du chat (cat cry) syndrome.

2. **Answer e:**

The characteristic lung manifestation of alpha$_1$-antitrypsin deficiency is panacinar emphysema. Liver disease in alpha$_1$-antitrypsin deficiency is caused by excess accumulation of the protein in hepatocytes; this occurs in persons expressing PiZZ, not in those homozygous for null alleles, who produce no alpha$_1$-antitrypsin.

a: Chronic bronchitis is not characteristic of alpha$_1$-antitrypsin deficiency. Along with bronchiectasis and recurrent pneumonia, chronic bronchitis is one of the pulmonary manifestations of another genetic disease, cystic fibrosis. Meconium ileus occurs in a small number of infants with cystic fibrosis.

b: Chronic bronchitis is not characteristic of alpha$_1$-antitrypsin deficiency. Along with bronchiectasis and recurrent pneumonia, chronic bronchitis is one of the pulmonary manifestations of another genetic disease, cystic fibrosis.

c: Panacinar emphysema is the pulmonary manifestation of alpha$_1$-antitrypsin deficiency, but meconium ileus is a manifestation of cystic fibrosis.

d: Liver disease alpha$_1$-antitrypsin deficiency is caused by excess accumulation of the protein in hepatocytes; this occurs in persons expressing PiZZ, not in those homozygous for null alleles, who produce no alpha$_1$-antitrypsin.

3. **Answer a:**

Most Down syndrome patients who survive to age 40 years have at least neuropathologic evidence of Alzheimer's disease.

b: Individuals with Edwards' syndrome (trisomy 18) rarely survive past age 1 year, so they do not develop Alzheimer's disease.

c: Familial hypercholesterolemia causes premature atherosclerosis; affected individuals are at increased risk of stroke.

d: Marfan syndrome can affect the eyes (ectopia lentis is highly suggestive of the syndrome), but it does not have an obvious relationship to Alzheimer's disease.

e: Patau's syndrome (trisomy 13) patients do not usually survive past age 1 year, so they do not develop Alzheimer's disease.

4. **Answer d:**

Genomic imprinting is a normal process involving preferential expression of nuclear genes derived from one parent. DNA methylation (typically involving the genes whose expression is inhibited) is the postulated mechanism.

a: Expansion of trinucleotide repeats appears to occur in oogenesis to a much greater extent than spermatogenesis, but this is not related to imprinting.

b: Expansion of trinucleotide repeats occurs in the nuclear genome. The mitochondrial genome is of maternal origin; imprinting does not occur.

c: Imprinting is a normal process. Deletion of specific chromosome would be lethal or result in a specific syndrome. An interstitial deletion involving a region of a chromosome that is imprinted can result in disease, if the active region is deleted. This occurs in Prader-Willi syndrome and Angelman's syndrome where both involve a deletion in 15q11-13. In the former, the deletion is in the paternally-derived chromosome, and in the latter, it is in the maternally-derived chromosome.

d: An individual's mitochondrial genome is all of maternal origin; imprinting does not occur.

CHAPTER 8: ENVIRONMENTAL AND NUTRITIONAL DISEASES

1. **Answer c:**

Kwashiorkor is caused by severe deficiency of protein, and occurs even if caloric intake is high.

a: Marasmus is a deficiency of all nutrients, i.e., total starvation.

b: Lead intoxication causes neither protein deficiency nor obesity.

d: In infants born of mothers who drank heavily during pregnancy, there may be growth and mental retardation, microcephaly or other malformations of the nervous system, facial abnormalities, and cardiac and skeletal abnormalities.

e: Rickets is caused by a deficiency of vitamin D.

2. **Answer b:**

Unenriched white flour, polished white rice, and refined white sugar may be high in calories, but these foods specifically contain very little thiamin (vitamin B_1), which is removed during processing.

a: Partially true, but polished white rice, unenriched white flour, and refined white sugar have had almost all vitamin B_1 removed in processing.

c: Some vitamin C is present in grains, but polished white rice, unenriched white flour, and refined white sugar have had almost all vitamin B_1 removed in processing.

d: Grains contain ergosterol, a precursor of vitamin D. However, polished white rice, unenriched white flour, and refined white sugar have had almost all vitamin B_1 removed in processing.

e: Vitamin E is abundant in grains. But polished white rice, unenriched white flour, and refined white sugar have had almost all vitamin B_1 removed in processing.

3. **Answer c:**

Isoniazid therapy is often associated with pyridoxine (vitamin B_6) deficiency, so supplements should be given.

a: Isoniazid therapy for tuberculosis is not complicated by vitamin A deficiency.

b: Thiamin deficiency does not occur with isoniazid therapy; pyridoxine deficiency does.

d: Ascorbic acid (vitamin C) deficiency does not occur with isoniazid therapy; pyridoxine deficiency does.

e: Niacin deficiency is not associated with isoniazid therapy; pyridoxine deficiency is.

4. **Answer b:**

With further depletion of the ozone layer and an increase in the amount of ultraviolet radiation striking the earth's surface, microscopic phytoplankton, food for many sea creatures, may be killed and the entire aquatic food chain may be severely damaged.

a: The atmospheric ozone layer has no effect on surface temperature; it does help to screen out ultraviolet radiation, preventing it from reaching the earth's surface. Increases in atmospheric "greenhouse gases," however, will lead to global warming. Significant global warming has already occurred.

c: The incidence of lung cancer is influenced by atmospheric pollution, including ozone polluting the air we breathe, but not by the ozone layer in the upper atmosphere.

d: Although an increase in ultraviolet radiation striking the earth because of depletion of the ozone layer will damage certain species of plant life, possible damage to rain forest areas is problematic.

e: Increases in chlorofluorocarbon compounds in the atmosphere damage the ozone layer; damage to the ozone layer does not increase the atmospheric content of these gases.

5. **Answer b:**

Posterolateral degeneration of the spinal cord is caused by vitamin B_{12} deficiency and is *not* associated with alcohol abuse.

a: Wernicke's encephalopathy is associated with alcohol abuse.

c: Central pontine myelinolysis is often (but not necessarily) associated with alcohol abuse. It is caused by rapid shifts in Na concentration in the blood.

d: Marchiafava-Bignami syndrome, a degeneration of the central portion of the corpus callosum, is linked to drinking large quantities of Italian red wine.

e: Korsakoff's psychosis usually occurs in alcoholics, and, like Wernicke's encephalopathy, is caused by deficiency of thiamin.

Chapter 9: Diseases of Childhood

1. **Answer b:**

Most organs form during weeks 3 to 9. Exposure to teratogens during this period can cause major organ malformations.

a: Exposure before week 3 tends either to cause death or to have no effect, depending upon the number of cells injured.

c: Exposure after week 9 causes less serious malformations or physiologic abnormalities, or results in the fetus being small for gestational age.

d: Exposure after week 9 causes less serious malformations or physiologic abnormalities, or results in the fetus being small for gestational age.

e: Exposure after week 9 causes less serious malformations or physiologic abnormalities, or results in the fetus being small for gestational age.

2. **Answer c:**

Cortisol is the principal stimulus to surfactant synthesis. It increases synthesis of both protein and lipid components of surfactant.

a: Aldosterone regulates water and electrolyte balance.

b: Chorionic gonadotropin is not obviously related to surfactant synthesis; its production is greatest earliest in pregnancy.

d: Insulin is an important inhibitor of surfactant synthesis. Fetal hyperinsulinemia, such as is seen in maternal diabetes mellitus, increases the risk of infant respiratory distress syndrome.

e: Somatostatin inhibits secretion of several hormones, but does not have an obvious relationship to surfactant synthesis.

3. **Answer c:**

Bronchopulmonary dysplasia and necrotizing enterocolitis are complications of prematurity, as is hyaline membrane disease.

a: Bronchopulmonary dysplasia and necrotizing enterocolitis are complications of prematurity, not components of a genetic disease such as cystic fibrosis.

b: Bronchopulmonary dysplasia and necrotizing enterocolitis are complications of prematurity, not components of a chromosomal disorder such as Down syndrome.

d: Bronchopulmonary dysplasia and necrotizing enterocolitis are complications of prematurity and are not directly related to malformation such as renal agenesis.

e: SIDS is the sudden death of an infant not expected from history and not explained by a thorough autopsy: This diagnosis would not be compatible with findings of bronchopulmonary dysplasia or necrotizing enterocolitis.

CHAPTER 10: AMYLOIDOSIS

1. **Answer a:**

This is an example of secondary amyloidosis, consisting of AA fibrils. AA derives from the acute phase reactant SAA whose concentration is elevated as a result of inflammation. Persons with chronic inflammatory disorders are predisposed to secondary amyloidosis.

b: This case appears to represent secondary amyloidosis. AL, derived from an immunoglobulin light chain of a paraprotein, is found in myeloma-associated and primary amyloidosis.

c: This case appears to represent secondary amyloidosis. AGel, derived from gelsolin, a cytoskeletal actin-binding protein, is found in rare familial amyloid polyneuropathy.

d: This case appears to represent secondary amyloidosis. Aβ is found in the senile plaques and blood vessels in Alzheimer's disease patients, as well as in older Down syndrome patients and some normal elderly individuals.

e: This case appears to represent secondary amyloidosis. Aβ2M, derived from β_2-microglobulin, is found in the synovium, joints, tendon sheaths of some patients on chronic hemodialysis.

2. **Answer d:**

This is an example of senile systemic amyloidosis. This entity primarily involves the heart (it was formerly called *senile cardiac amyloidosis*) and blood vessels. ATTR derived from apparently normal transthyretin (TTR) makes up the amyloid fibrils in senile systemic amyloidosis.

a: Amyloid P component is found in all types of amyloid; it is bound to the amyloid fibrils.

b: Amylin, or islet amyloid peptide, gives rise to AIAP, the amyloid fibril protein in the amyloid found in islets of most Type II diabetics and within some islet cell neoplasms.

c: Atrial natriuretic peptide (also called atrial natriuretic factor) gives rise to AANF, which makes up the amyloid fibrils in isolated atrial amyloid, a common but apparently not clinically significant finding in many elderly individuals.

e: Retinol binding protein, which is bound to TTR in plasma, is not known to be amyloidogenic.

CHAPTER 11: BLOOD VESSELS

1. **Answer c:**

When blood coagulates within the vascular tree, it is referred to as a thrombus, but when this occurs outside the vascular tree, it is referred to as a clot (coagulum).

a: When blood coagulates within the vascular tree it is called a thrombus.

b: An embolus occurs when a mass of material (solid, liquid, or gaseous) is carried by the bloodstream to a site distant from its origin.

d: An infarct represents tissue death caused by insufficient vascular supply.

e: An organized thrombus occurs when fibroblasts begin to grow into a thrombus, laying down collagen and forming the equivalent of a scar.

2. **Answer c:**

Although any of these materials can constitute emboli, the most common one is a thrombus.

a: Fat (especially that derived from bone fracture sites) forms emboli, but it is not their most common cause.

b: Air may form emboli, but it is not their most common cause.

d: Amniotic fluid may form emboli, but it is not the most common cause.

e: Cholesterol may form emboli, but it is not the most common cause.

3. **Answer a:**

Most examples of vasculitis in the United States present as a skin rash resulting from hypersensitivity. They primarily involve capillaries and venules; the vast majority of vasculitis cases are caused by a drug reaction, but some are associated with bacteremia, viremia, serum sickness, and cryoglobulinemia, as well as Schönlein-Henoch purpura.

b: Autoimmune disease is often associated with vasculitis, but this vasculitis is not as commonly observed in the United States as is hypersensitivity vasculitis.

c: Polyarteritis nodosa is a form of vasculitis but is not as common as hypersensitivity vasculitis in the United States; it is characterized by involvement of small to medium-sized arteries by intramural acute inflammation.

d: Wegener's granulomatosis is a form of vasculitis but is not as common as hypersensitivity vasculitis in the United States.

e: Giant cell arteritis is a form of vasculitis but is not as common as hypersensitivity vasculitis in the United States.

4. **Answer d:**

This is a classical presentation for giant cell arteritis, also known as temporal arteritis.

a: Clinical features of Wegener's granulomatosis may include sinusitis, skin rash, pulmonary lesions, and renal disease.

b: Polyarteritis nodosa is characterized by a vasculitis of small to medium-sized muscular arteries of the kidneys and abdominal viscera.

c: Hypersensitivity vasculitis should be considered, especially if the patient

has recently been taking medication(s).

e: Buerger's disease is characterized by acute inflammation of small to medium-sized arteries (and sometimes veins) of the lower extremities; it is seen mostly in middle-aged males who are cigarette smokers.

5. **Answer b:**

This is a classic description for Kaposi's sarcoma, most likely arising in a patient with AIDS (HIV infection).

a: Bacillary epithelioid angiomatosis is an infection mediated vascular proliferation caused by *Bartonella henselae* and *Bartonella quintana,* the same organisms responsible for cat-scratch disease and peliosis hepatis.

c: Adenocarcinoma consists of malignant glands.

d: Squamous cell carcinoma is characterized by a proliferation of malignant squamous cells.

e: Melanoma consists of malignant melanocytes and mainly arises from skin, although it may originate in mucous membranes.

CHAPTER 12: HEART

1. **Answer c:**

Discrepant blood pressure from upper to lower limb is the classic clinical finding in coarctation of the aorta. This usually results in death in severe cases before age 40 years.

a: Tetralogy of Fallot is the most common cyanotic congenital heart disorder.

b: Ventricular septal defect does not produce systemic hypertension but, if sizable, may cause pulmonary hypertension.

d: Patient ductus arteriosus typically causes a machine-like precordial murmur and would produce a left-to-right shunt that could not result in systemic hypertension.

e: ASDs of the ostium secundum type are characterized by a left-to-right shunt that could not produce systemic hypertension.

2. Answer e:

Cyanosis is the result of right-to-left shunting. Coarctation of the aorta produces no shunting.

a: The abnormal turbulence and high-velocity jet present in a tight coarctation predisposes to the development of infective endocarditis (aortitis).

b: Cerebral hemorrhage, headaches, and epistaxis are the result of sustained upper body hypertension.

c: Congestive heart failure occurs with ventricular hypertrophy and accelerated atherosclerosis secondary to the increased workload of hypertension.

d: Cystic median necrosis and aortic rupture occur from hypertension and are caused by high-velocity jet flow aortic wall damage and postobstructive dilation.

3. Answer e:

Almost all patients with myocardial infarctions will suffer some type of arrythmia, and they account for up to 50% of deaths.

a: Ventricular rupture is seen most often in older patients, with their first infarction at about 1 week. It is virtually always fatal.

b: Pericardial tamponade is a rare complication associated with ventricular rupture or hemorrhagic pericarditis.

c: Ventricular aneurysms are formed of scar tissue that fails to contract, bulging out, with systole, and is a rare complication of myocardial infarction.

d: Pulmonary emboli are produced in the leg veins, and cardiac failure, as well as bed rest, predispose to their formation because of increased venous stasis. Prophylactic anticoagulation is used, and many emboli are silent.

4. Answer a:

S. pyogenes still accounts for two thirds of community-acquired cases of endocarditis, followed by *S. aureus*.

b: *S. viridans* is not the organism that most frequently causes endocarditis.

c: *P. aeruginosa* is not the organism that most frequently causes endocarditis.

d: *K. pneumoniae* is not the organism that most frequently causes endocarditis.

e: *C. albicans* is not the organism that most frequently causes endocarditis.

5. Answer a:

These are the findings of classic tetralogy of Fallot.

b: Tetralogy of Fallot consists of subpulmonary stenosis, ventricular septal defect, overriding aorta, and *right* ventricular hypertrophy.

c: Tetralogy of Fallot consists of *subpulmonary* stenosis, ventricular septal defect, overriding aorta, and right ventricular hypertrophy.

d: Tetralogy of Fallot consists of subpulmonary stenosis, *ventricular* septal defect, overriding aorta, and right ventricular hypertrophy.

e: Tetralogy of Fallot consists of subpulmonary stenosis, ventricular septal defect, *overriding aorta,* and right ventricular hypertrophy.

CHAPTER 13: LUNG

1. Answer e:

Left-sided heart failure is the most common cause of pulmonary edema.

a: Right-sided heart failure results in congestion of the systemic venous circulation, but not pulmonary edema.

b: Liver failure may lead to generalized soft-tissue (interstitial) edema, but generally not pulmonary edema.

c: Renal failure is not a common cause of pulmonary edema.

d: Pancreatic failure is not a common cause of pulmonary edema.

2. Answer b:

Bronchioloalveolar carcinoma is classified as a well-differentiated variant of adenocarcinoma. Pure bronchioloalveolar carcinoma has a better 5-year survival than "regular" adenocarcinoma or "regular" adenocarcinoma mixed with bronchioloalveolar carcinoma.

a, c, d, e: These choices represent types of carcinoma; squamous cell carcinoma, small
cell anaplastic carcinoma, and large cell
anaplastic carcinoma are well-recognized
types of primary lung cancer, whereas
transitional cell carcinoma is a histologic
type that much more commonly arises in
the urinary tract, especially the urinary
bladder.

3. **Answer a:**

These are the classic, characteristic findings for small cell anaplastic carcinoma.
Note: Small cell anaplastic carcinoma is
separated from the other types of carcinoma because its natural history is typically much more aggressive, and it is
usually widely disseminated at the time
of diagnosis. Chemotherapy and radiotherapy are the mainstream treatment for
small cell anaplastic carcinoma; surgery
has a very limited, but apparently growing, role in the treatment of this cancer.
Also, of all the primary cancers, small cell
anaplastic carcinoma is most often associated with ectopic hormone production
and other manifestations of the paraneoplastic syndrome, including neuromuscular deficits.

b: Squamous cell carcinoma is characterized
by sheets of cells with prominent intercellular bridges and often by keratinization.
c: Adenocarcinoma is characterized by the
formation of malignant glands.
d: Hamartoma is a benign lesion consisting
of hyaline cartilage admixed with respiratory epithelium.
e: Large cell anaplastic carcinoma consists
of large cells with abundant cytoplasm.

4. **Answer d:**

*Pseudomonas aeruginosa, Staphylococcus
aureus* and Burkholderia (formerly *Pseudomonas cepacia*) are the main pulmonary
pathogens in patients with cystic fibrosis.

a, b, c, e: Although these choices may infect the
lungs of cystic fibrosis patients, they do
so much less often than *Pseudomonas
aeruginosa, Staphylococcus aureus,* Burkholderia (formerly *Pseudomonas cepacia*).

5. **Answer b:**

Secondary spontaneous pneumothorax
refers to pneumothorax that occurs in
previously diseased lung tissue, such as
in this case; this patient has emphysema
caused by his long-term cigarette use.

a: Primary empyema refers to pus in the
pleural space.
c: Iatrogenic means caused by medical
intervention.
d: *Pleurisy* refers to inflammation of the
pleura.

Chapter 14: White Blood Cell Diseases

1. **Answer b:**

The clinical features and morphologic
findings are typical of lymphoblastic
lymphoma. This is a neoplasm of precursor T cells, and the distinction between
lymphoma and leukemia is usually based
on the extent of bone marrow involvement. Treatment is substantially different
only if the disease is stage I, and the lymphoma and leukemia have been united in
recent classification proposals under the
heading of precursor T cell neoplasm.
The finding of TdT in a lymphoma is
virtually diagnostic of a precursor lymphoid neoplasm.

a: Burkitt's lymphoma usually involves
extranodal sites, especially the abdomen;
morphologically consists of small cells
with distinct nucleoli; has a high mitotic
rate; and is TdT negative, immunophenotyping as a mature B cell.
c: Diffuse large B cell lymphoma may occur
at any site; is cytologically of large
nuclear size with clumped chromatin;
and is TdT negative, immunophenotyping as a mature B cell.
d: Hodgkin's disease may occur in the
mediastinum; must have diagnostic
Reed-Sternberg cells (giant cells with
multilobated nuclei or multinucleation
and huge inclusion-like nucleoli) and is
never TdT positive.
e: Small lymphocytic lymphoma/chronic
lymphocytic leukemia occurs in older

adults; more frequently has generalized lymphadenopathy; and is composed of small, mature-appearing lymphocytes that are typically of B immunophenotype.

2. **Answer d:**

SLL/CLL and MCL are the only indolent lymphomas listed. The remainder are all aggressive. SLL/CLL has a much longer median survival.

a: Burkitt's lymphoma is very aggressive, one of the fastest-growing neoplasms.

b: MCL has a distinctly short survival of about 3 years, being the shortest of all indolent lymphomas.

c: Lymphoblastic lymphoma is an aggressive lymphoma that rapidly spreads to the blood and bone marrow. It overlaps in all features with acute lymphoblastic leukemia.

e: Diffuse large B cell lymphoma, untreated, has a survival time of less than 1 year.

3. **Answer c:**

In North America this is the classic setting and findings. Although the differential diagnosis may include HIV, it is less likely. Confirmatory testing should include a mono test.

a: Chronic lymphocytic leukemia is a disease of older adults; the lymphocytes appear mature, and it is usually asymptomatic, detected by a blood count.

b: "Strep throat" produces a neutrophilic leukocytosis and local adenopathy.

d: Hodgkin's disease characteristically presents as isolated adenopathy, with no throat symptoms and a normal peripheral blood count or a neutrophilic leukocytosis.

e: Human immunodeficiency virus infection is very similar, with the acute early infection except the sore throat is unusual, systemic flulike symptoms being most common.

4. **Answer e:**

Auer rods are the lineage marker of AML. They are not seen in all cases but when they occur they ensure a myeloid lineage.

Auer rods represent crystalized components of myeloid granules.

a: Auer rods are never seen in acute lymphocytic leukemia.

b: Auer rods are never seen in chronic lymphocytic leukemia.

c: Auer rods are never seen in hairy cell leukemia.

d: Auer rods are never seen in chronic myelogenous leukemia.

5. **Answer d:**

The end stage, or burnt-out phase, of PV is characterized by myelofibrosis and myeloid metaplasia virtually indistinguishable from the idiopathic disorder.

a: Fibrosis of the marrow is not seen in chronic lymphocytic leukemia.

b: Fibrosis of the marrow can also occur with myelodysplasia, but this does not usually produce the extramedullary hematopoiesis and generalized fibrosis of myeloid metaplasia with myelofibrosis.

c: Fibrosis of the marrow can also occur with hairy cell leukemia, but this does not usually produce the extramedullary hematopoiesis and generalized fibrosis of myeloid metaplasia with myelofibrosis.

e: Fibrosis of the marrow can also occur with Hodgkin's disease, but this does not usually produce the extramedullary hematopoiesis and generalized fibrosis of myeloid metaplasia with myelofibrosis.

CHAPTER 15: RED BLOOD CELL DISEASES

1. **Answer b:**

Only anemia of chronic disease has all of these features.

a: Iron deficiency would have a hypochromic microcytic morphology and absent iron stores in the marrow. The serum iron and iron binding capacity will be low and high, respectively, in iron deficiency.

c: Malaria has a normochromic, normocytic morphology and should have parasites visible in the erythrocytes. The serum iron and iron binding capacity will be normal to high and normal, respectively, in malaria.

d: G6PD deficiency has a normochromic, normocytic anemia and may have heinz bodies on reticulocyte staining or occasionally blister cells in the peripheral blood. The serum iron and iron binding capacity will be normal to high and normal, respectively.

e: Beta thalassemia has a hypochromic microcytic morphology. Beta thalassemia usually has increased iron stores in the marrow. The serum iron and iron binding capacity will be high and normal, respectively.

2. **Answer a:**

Myelophthisic anemia is usually caused by significant bone marrow disease and is an indication for bone marrow examination. A replacement of the marrow is expected because of malignancy, fibrosis, or some other space-occupying disease such as ones producing granuloma or storge diseases. On a transient basis, similar changes of nucleated red cells and early white cells may be seen with hemolysis, significant hemorrhage, sepsis, and other acute marrow or physiologic stresses (pregnancy, severe hypoxia, and others).

b: Iron deficiency anemia alone is unlikely to produce these features unless associated with significant hemorrhage. Hypochromic microcytic red cell morphology is typical of iron deficiency.

c: Hereditary spherocytosis has a negative direct antibody (Coomb's negative) and a spherocytic red cell morphology.

d: Hemoglobin C disease is characterized by target red cells and occasional red cells with intracellular crystals.

e: Alpha thalassemia trait is typified by a hypchromic microcytic anemia with normal iron stores.

3. **Answer e:**

This is classic pernicious anemia, an autoimmune disease with the listed features, common in the elderly of northern European descent. B_{12} deficiency is a cause of megaloblastic anemia. The presence of antiparietal cell antibodies indicate autoimmune atrophic gastritis with diminished production of intrinsic factor

and B_{12} malabsorption. The finding of low serum B_{12} levels or the response to B_{12} administration would confirm the diagnosis.

a: Although folic acid deficiency can also cause megaloblastic anemia, the presence of antiparietal cell antibodies indicate autoimmune atrophic gastritis, diminished production of intrinsic factor, and B_{12} malabsorption. The neurologic findings of burning feet and unsteady gait are not part of folate deficiency.

b: Niacin deficiency causes pellagra, not anemia.

c: Thiamine deficiency causes beriberi, not anemia.

d: Vitamin C deficiency causes scurvy, not anemia.

4. **Answer d:**

Although hereditary spherocytosis may be caused by defects in spectrin, ankyrin, and protein 4.2 production or mutations, most will result in diminished spectrin, the major structural red cell membrane skeleton protein.

a: Decreased alpha hemoglobin causes alpha thalassemia trait with a hypochromic microcytic anemia.

b: Decreased beta hemoglobin causes alpha thalassemia trait with a hypochromic microcytic anemia.

c: Glucose 6-phosphate dehydrogenase deficiency causes a normochromic normocytic anemia without spherocytes.

e: Increased susceptibility to complement lysis is typical of paroxysmal nocturnal hemoglobinuria, which produces a normochromic normocytic anemia or iron deficiency anemia.

5. **Answer c:**

The thalassemias are diminished production of hemoglobin chains, resulting in lower hemoglobin and often hemolysis of red cells or intramedullary destruction from the excess of the normally synthesized reciprocal globin chain. Decreased beta chain production results in beta thalassemia.

a: Sickle cell anemia is caused by production of a mutant beta chain with a substitution of B_6 from glutamic acid to valine.

b: Alpha thalassemia results from decreased production of alpha chains usually caused by only two of the normal four alpha genes producing hemoglobin.

d: Hemoglobin C disease is caused by production of a mutant beta chain with a substitution of B_6 from glutamic acid to lysine.

e: Hemoglobin H disease results from severe underproduction of alpha chains, with only one of the usual four alpha chain's genes functioning.

CHAPTER 16: BLEEDING DISORDERS

1. **Answer a:**

Vitamin K is an important cofactor in the gamma carboxylation of the calcium binding coagulation factors of II, VII, IX, and XII that occurs in the liver.

b: Vitamin K has no effect on platelet function.

c: Vitamin K has no effect on platelet production.

d: Vitamin K has no effect on platelet survival.

e: Vitamin K has no role in vessel support or collagen synthesis.

2. **Answer d:**

Aspirin interferes with normal platelet function by preventing prostaglandin synthesis in the platelet, one of the aggregation pathways.

a: Only with aspirin overdose has diminished synthesis of the vitamin K factors been described.

b: Only with aspirin overdose has diminished synthesis of the vitamin K factors been described.

c: Aspirin has no effect on platelet production.

e: Aspirin inhibits the synthesis of prostacyclin (PGI_2) by the endothelial cell, but this pathway inhibition would serve to promote platelet action.

3. **Answer a:**

In addition to platelet function abnormalities, a bleeding time will be abnormal with some vessel abnormalities, thrombocytopenia, aspirin ingestion, and von Willebrand's disease.

b: This is the screening test for vitamin K–dependent factors and the extrinsic coagulation pathway; it does not test platelet function.

c: The thrombin time assesses the presence of adequate fibrinogen and thrombin inhibitors. Platelet function is not evaluated.

d: The activated partial thromboplastin time assesses the intrinsic coagulation pathway, not platelet function.

e: Although dysfibrinogenemia and hypofibrinoginemia could cause platelet dysfunction, they are extremely rare conditions. Fibrinogen levels do not actually test platelet function.

4. **Answer a:**

This prostaglandin is elaborated by the endothelial cell and is a very potent inhibitor of platelets.

b: Epinephrine is a platelet agonist.

c: ADP is a platelet agonist.

d: 5-Hydroxytryptophan has no effect on platelets.

e: Thrombin is a platelet agonist.

5. **Answer a:**

The conversion of prothrombin (factor II) to its active form of thrombin is central to coagulation and the production of fibrin through its cleavage of fibrinopeptides from fibrinogen.

b: Factor X has no effect on fibrinogen.

c: Plasminogen degrades fibrin at sites of formation and fibrinogen in pathologic fibrinolytic states.

d: Factor XIII cross-links fibrin to stabilize clot formation after the formation of fibrin by thrombin.

e: Thrombomodulin does not affect fibrinogen.

Chapter 17: Transfusion Medicine

1. Answer d:

The red cells in a group O unit would be compatible with the patient serum becaues they lack A antigens. Packed cells (most of the plasma removed) would contain the least amount of antiA, antiB, and antiAB that is found naturally in a group O donor that could react with the group B recipient's red cells.

a: Group A red cells would not be suitable because the naturally occuring antiA in the B recipient would cause hemolysis.
b: Group AB red cells would not be suitable because the naturally occuring antiA in the B recipient would cause hemolysis.
c: Group AB red cell would not be suitable because the naturally occurring antiA in the B recipient would cause hemolysis.
e: Group O red cells would not be compatible because they lack the A antigen that would react with naturally occuring antiA in a group B recipient's plasma. A unit of group O whole blood also contains about 200 ml of plasma. This plasma from the group O donor would have antiA, antiB, and antiAB present, which could react with a group B recipient's red cells. The group O packed cells, with a reduced amount of plasma, would therefore be a better choice.

2. Answer a:

The antibody screen serves to exclude the presence of unexpected (not naturally occuring) antibodies to clinically significant red cell antigens other than those of the ABO system. When these are not present, it can be assumed that a transfusion of group-specific blood will be compatible.

b: A patient's ABO type is determined by testing with specific antisera.
c: The patient's Rh phenotype is determined by testing with specific antisera.
d: Naturally occuring antiA and antiB are detected by testing the patient's serum against test red cells of known ABO

type. This also verifies the patient's ABO type.
e: A positive direct antiglobulin test indicating the presence of antibodies on a patient's own circulating red cells is not normally evaluated during pretransfusion testing.

3. Answer c:

The basic rule is that people with the antigen do not make the antibody.

a: Group O individuals will make both antiA and antiB because they lack these two antigens on their red cells.
b: Group B individuals will make antiA because they lack this antigen on their red cells.
d: Group A individuals will make antiB because they lack this antigen on their red cells.
e: Bombay phenotype is very rare and characterized by a lack of H substance, the precursor for both A and B antigens. They make antiA, antiB, and antiH naturally, and are incompatible with all blood groups except other Bombay individuals.

4. Answer b:

A father who is group AB must pass on either the A or B allele to his children, none of whom could be group O.

a: A group A father could genetically be either A/A or A/O, and therefore could father a group O child. Similarly, an Rh-positive father could be heterozygous at this locus and therefore father an Rh-negative child.
c: A group O father can have only group O children or group B children, given the mother's group B status. He could still father an Rh-negative child if he were heterozygous at the Rh locus.
d: A group O, Rh-negative father could only father group O or B, Rh-negative children given the mother's group B, Rh-negative status.
e: A group B father could genetically be either B/B or B/O, and therefore could father a group O child. Similarly, an Rh-positive father could be heterozygous at

this locus and father an Rh-negative child.

5. **Answer e:**

Antibodies to almost all of the blood group antigens except the ABO group occur after exposure to nonself red cells that express this antigen. This usually happens through transfusion or pregnancy.

a: A Jk^a positive individual would not normally make an antibody to this antigen unless it was an autoantibody. The general rule is that antibodies are produced only for antigens an individual lacks.

b: Jk^a is not a glycolipid antigen.

c: Antibodies are produced by plasma cells.

d: Antibodies directed towards blood group antigens, besides the naturally occurring ABO antibodies, are almost always of IgG type.

Chapter 18: Head and Neck

1. **Answer e:**

Corynebacterium diphtheriae may be a component of normal, healthy individuals' oral flora.

a: Uncontrolled diabetes decreases general resistance to infection.

b: Systemic antibiotic therapy upsets the local immunologic balance maintained by commensal oral flora, salivary flow, and immunoglobulin secretion.

c: IgA deficiency upsets the local immunologic balance maintained by commensal oral flora, salivary flow, and immunoglobulin secretion.

d: Sjögrens disease upsets the local immunologic balance maintained by commensal oral flora, salivary flow, and immunoglobulin secretion.

2. **Answer d:**

These histologically inflammatory lesions with a prominent vascular proliferation (granulation tissue) are of undetermined etiology and are frequent in pregnancy, when they are termed "pregnancy tumors."

a: Pyogenic granulomas are not associated with *S. pyogenes* or other specific infections.

b: This is typical of infective granuloma, typically seen with *Tuberculosis* sp. and some fungal infections.

c: Pyogenic granuloma are not associated with fungal or other specific infections.

e: Pyogenic granuloma are not seen in hyperparathyroidism.

3. **Answer b:**

Tobacco abuse, alcoholism, betel nut chewing, and chronic local physical and chemical irritants all predispose to squamous cell carcinoma, and leukoplakia as well.

a: Squamous cell carcinoma is the most frequent malignancy of the oral cavity.

c: Squamous cell carcinoma is not associated with aphthous stomatitis.

d: Squamous cell carcinoma is uncommon in females.

e: Squamous cell carcinoma often arises in multiple sites within the oral cavity.

4. **Answer d:**

This highly vascular benign tumor occurs almost exclusively in teenage males and may bleed profusely with surgical manipulations.

a: Nasopharyngeal angiofibroma is uncommon in infancy and childhood.

b: Nasopharyngeal angiofibroma is uncommon in elderly males.

c: Nasopharyngeal angiofibroma is uncommon in elderly females.

e: Nasopharyngeal angiofibroma is uncommon in teenage females.

5. **Answer c:**

Aphthous stomatitis consists of recurrent, painful shallow ulcers covered by a fibrinopurulent exudate, not white patches (leukoplakia).

a: Squamous cell carcinoma may have the clinical appearance of leukoplakia (white patches).

b: Thrush (oral candidiasis) may have the clinical appearance of leukoplakia (white patches).

d: Lichen planus may have the clinical appearance of leukoplakia (white patches).

e: Benign hyperkeratosis may have the clinical appearance of leukoplakia (white patches).

Chapter 19: Gastrointestinal Tract

1. Answer a:

Intraluminal masses frequently are the leading point of an intussesception. Adenomatous polyps are common and, by definition, intraluminal.

b: Intraluminal masses frequently are the leading point of an intussesception. However, in children no intestinal disease is the most frequent association with intussesception.

c: Intraluminal masses frequently are the leading point of an intussesception. Dysentry is not associated with intussesception.

d: Intraluminal masses frequently are the leading point of an intussesception. Crohn's disease is not associated with intussesception.

e: Intraluminal masses frequently are the leading point of an intussesception. Carcinoid tumors are usually intramural.

2. Answer c:

Peptic ulcers are most common in the duodenum, followed by the stomach.

a: The esophagus is the third most common site of peptic ulceration.

b: Peptic ulcers are most common in the duodenum, followed by the stomach.

d: Peptic ulceration only rarely occurs in the jejunum.

e: Peptic ulceration almost never occurs in the ileum.

3. Answer c:

Squamous cell carcinoma still accounts for about 60% of esophageal malignancies, but the incidence of adenocarcinoma seems to be rising.

a: Leiomyosarcoma is very rare in the esophagus.

b: Small cell carcinoma is very rare in the esophagus.

d: Adenocarcinoma is the second most common malignancy of the esophagus.

e: Metastases to the esophagus are very rare, but direct extension from the stomach or thoracic structures can occur.

4. Answer d:

Hamartomatous polyps are characteristic of Peutz-Jeghers syndrome.

a: Turcot's syndrome has adenomatous polyps.

b: Familila polyposis coli has multiple adenomatous polyps.

c: Gardner's syndrome has adenomatous polyps.

e: Lynch's syndrome is not associated with any polyps.

5. Answer d:

Peutz-Jeghers syndrome has hamartomatous polyps of the gastrointestinal tract that are not considered premalignant. Malignancies in other organs are seen with increased frequency in Peutz-Jeghers syndrome.

a: Longstanding ulcerative colitis has an increased risk of adenocarcinoma, especially if dysplasia is identified.

b: Familial adenomatmous polyposis has an almost 100% chance of carcinoma developing by age 40 years.

c: Gardner's syndrome and Turcot's syndrome are considered varients of familial adenomatous polyposis with an increased risk of colorectal carcinoma.

e: Gardner's syndrome and Turcot's syndrome are considered varients of familial adenomatous polyposis with an increased risk of colorectal carcinoma.

Chapter 20: Liver, Biliary Tract, and Exocrine Pancreas

1. Answer b:

Jaundice appears when the total serum bilirubin level exceeds 2.5 mg/dl.

2. Answer a:

Hepatitis E, like hepatitis A, is transmitted mainly by the feco-oral route.

b: Hepatitis B is transmitted parenterally (other than by mouth).

c: Hepatitis C is transmitted parenterally (other than by mouth).

d: Hepatitis D is transmitted parenterally (other than by mouth).

e: HIV is primarily transmitted by parenteral routes.

3. **Answer c:**

Cholesterol stones are the most common type of gallstone encountered in the United States.

a: Pigmented stones are a type of gallbladder stone, but not the most common type encountered in the United States.

b: Urate stones are a type of urinary tract stone.

d: Cystine stones are a type of urinary tract stone.

e: Magnesium ammonium stones are a type of urinary tract stone.

4. **Answer c:**

The gallbladder is *not* essential for life.

a: The gallbladder lacks a muscularis mucosa.

b: The gallbladder lacks a submucosa.

d: About 10% to 20% of the American population harbors gallstones.

5. **Answer e:**

High levels of bilirubin conjugated to glucuronic acid residues do *not* cause kernicterus in premature infants.

a: Conjugated bilirubin is water soluble.

b: Conjugated bilirubin is excreted into bile.

c: Conjugated bilirubin binds weakly to albumin.

d: Conjugated bilirubin is also known as direct bilirubin.

CHAPTER 21: SKIN

1. **Answer a:**

Munro microabscesses are collections of neutrophils and debris located with the stratum corneum.

b: Munro microabscesses are not seen in lichen planus.

c: Munro microabscesses are not seen in Herpes simplex type 2.

d: Munro microabscesses are not seen in mycosis fungoides.

e: Munro microabscesses are not seen in seborrheic dermatitis.

2. **Answer b:**

Epidermal maturation time in psoriasis is 3 to 5 days.

a: Epidermal maturation time in psoriasis is not 1 to 2 days.

c: Epidermal maturation time in psoriasis is not 10 to 15 days.

d: Epidermal maturation time in psoriasis is not 40 days.

e: Epidermal maturation time in psoriasis is not 50 days.

3. **Answer d:**

Staphylococcal scalded skin syndrome is mediated by a toxin known as *exfoliatin.*

a: Staphylococcal scalded skin syndrome is not mediated by granuloma formation.

b: Staphylococcal scalded skin syndrome is not mediated by abscess formation in the skin.

c: Staphylococcal scalded skin syndrome is not mediated by viral infection.

4. **Answer c:**

Depth of melanoma invasion is the most important prognostic factor in cutaneous melanoma.

a: Melanoma cell type is *not* the most important prognostic factor in cutaneous melanoma.

b: Melanoma cell mitotic index is not the most important prognostic factor in cutaneous melanoma.

d: Associated solar damage is not the most important prognostic factor in cutaneous melanoma.

5. **Answer c:**

Eosinophilic granuloma represents the least severe component of the Langerhans' Cell Histiocytosis spectrum.

a: The least severe component of Langerhans' Cell Histiocytosis spectrum is not
Hand-Schuller Christian disease.

b: Letterer-Siwe disease is actually the most
severe component of the Langerhans' Cell
Histiocytosis spectrum.

d: Lymphoma is not a component of the
Langerhans' Cell Histiocytosis spectrum.

e: Melanoma is not a part of the Langerhans' Cell Histiocytosis spectrum.

CHAPTER 22: KIDNEY AND LOWER URINARY TRACT

1. **Answer d:**

    The clinical history and findings indicate
    acute tubular necrosis. Crush injuries and
    shock produce a pattern of ischemic
    tubular necrosis characterized by multi-
    ple foci of tubular necrosis, rupture of
    tubular basement membranes, and casts
    in the tubular lumens.

    a: Crescents in most glomeruli are found in
    rapidly progressive glomerulonephtis.

    b: Pus within the tubules and interstitial
    abscesses indicates acute pyelonephritis.

    c: Infarctions are usually a result of embo-
    lization, most often from the heart; they
    usually do not cause shock and renal
    failure.

    e: Fibrinoid necrosis of arterioles and hyper-
    plastic arteriolitis, along with necrotizing
    glomerulitis, are the findings of malig-
    nant hypertension.

2. **Answer b:**

    Most nephrotic syndrome patients under
    the age of 16 years have minimal change
    disease. Synthetic glucocorticoid therapy
    will eliminate proteinuria, often within
    weeks. Relapses sometimes occur, but
    they can be treated with glucocorticoids.
    Development of more serious renal or
    systemic disorders is not part of the min-
    imal change disease.

    a: Patients with nephrotic syndrome are at
    increased risk for bacterial infections,
    which must be treated with the appro-
    priate antibiotic, but such treatment will
    not affect nephrotic syndrome itself.

    c: Usually only short-term therapy is re-

quired for pediatric patients with nephrotic syndrome.

d: Development of more serious renal
disease is not common in children with
nephrotic syndrome.

e: Nephrotic syndrome in children does not
evolve into systemic disorders like SLE,
although such disease can cause nephrotic
syndrome (especially in adults).

3. **Answer b:**

    The Goodpasture's antigen is a compo-
    nent of basement membrane (type IV)
    collagen.

    a: Membranous nephropathy can involve
    circulating immune complexes or
    immune complexes involving planted
    antigens or glomerular antigens, but not
    those in the basement membrane.

    c: The immunologic mechanisms (if any)
    involved in minimal change disease
    (lipoid nephrosis) are unknown.

    d: Nodular glomerulosclerosis is a mor-
    phologic finding specific for diabetes
    mellitus, and is related to the length
    and severity of hyperglycemia.

    e: The immune complexes of poststrep-
    tococcal glomerulonephritis include
    microbial antigens.

4. **Answer a:**

    Acute pyelonephritis is a bacterial in-
    fection of the kidney, 90% is caused by
    infections originating in the urinary
    bladder. Gram-negative enteric organ-
    isms cause about 85% of cases of urinary
    tract infections and, of this category,
    Escherichia coli predominates.

    b: Group A beta-hemolytic streptococci are
    responsible for most cases of postinfec-
    tious glomerulonephritis, but this rep-
    resents an immune-complex mediated
    disorder and not infection of the kidney.
    Streptococci are an uncommon cause of
    urinary tract infection.

    c: Another class of microorganisms causes
    most cases of urinary tract infection.
    Mycobacterium tuberculosis can affect the
    kidney but would be expected to cause
    granulomatous, rather than acute, in-
    flammation.

    d: *Schistosoma hematobium* can infect the

urinary bladder but does not cause acute pyelonephritis.

  e: *Neisseria gonorrhoeae,* a gram-negative diplococcus, is a common cause of urethritis; complications tend to involve the genital tract rather than the urinary tract.

5. Answer a:

  About 75% of renal stones are composed of calcium oxalate/phosphate.

  b: From 10% to 15% of renal stones are composed of magnesium ammonium-phosphate.

  c: About 6% of renal stones are composed of uric acid.

  d: About 1% to 2% of renal stones are composed of cystine.

  e: Less than 10% of renal stones are of unknown composition.

Chapter 23: Bone, Joint, and Soft Tissue Disorders

1. Answer c:

  The history is classic for osteoid osteoma whose histologic findings of a central nidus are typified by woven bone trabeculae in osteoid.

  a: Osteosarcoma occurs in this age group, but the x-ray film and history of aspirin relief are not consistent. The axial skeleton is a less common site than the ends of long bones in the appendicular skeleton.

  b: Enchondroma does not occur at this site.

  d: Metastatic adenocarcinoma would be very uncommon at this age.

  e: Chondrosarcoma would be very uncommon at this age and site.

2. Answer b:

  This x-ray film finding and history in an elderly individual are most common in multiple myeloma. Although not a primary tumor of bone origin, multiple myeloma is the most common nonmetastatic tumor arising at a bone site in this age group.

  a: Osteoporosis does not produce lytic lesions.

  c: Metastasis are the most frequent cause of a "bone tumor" in older adults, but lytic lesions are not typical of prostatic adenocarcinoma, which usually causes sclerotic/osteoblastic changes.

  d: Osteosarcoma is uncommon in the elderly.

  e: Paget's disease may be associated with fractures, but it produces an osteoblastic appearance rather than lytic lesions.

3. Answer a:

  This is the typical finding of osteoporosis.

  b: Expanded osteoid would be more typical of osteomalacia or rickets.

  c: A mosaic tile appearance is characteristic of Paget's disease.

  d: This is associated with a variety of metabolic bone diseases.

  e: This is associated with a variety of metabolic bone diseases.

4. Answer d:

  Although all sarcomas are uncommon, rhabdomyosarcoma is the most frequent in childhood.

  a: Malignant fibrous histiocytoma is the most common adult sarcoma.

  b: Synovial sarcoma occurs in childhood and teen years to young adulthood but is less common.

  c: Ewing's sarcoma occurs in childhood but is less common.

  e: Clear cell sarcoma occurs in teen years to young adulthood but is less common.

5. Answer a:

  This is the characteristic feature of hyperparathyroidism.

  b: Organizing hematoma is an early phase of fracture repair.

  c: Woven bone formation is a later phase of fracture repair.

  d: Fibroblastic callus is an intermediate phase of fracture repair.

  e: Osteonecrosis and osteoclastic resorption are activities seen in early fracture repair.

Chapter 24: Peripheral Nervous System and Muscle

1. Answer e:

  The disease process in Guillain-Barré

syndrome (GBS) is a delayed hypersensitivity T-cell mediated attack against peripheral (Schwann cell) myelin. Similar changes can be induced in laboratory animals by injecting them with peripheral nerve myelin ("experimental autoimmune neuritis," or EAN). In humans the trigger for the attack is unknown.

a: No infectious agent can be consistently demonstrated in cases of GBS.
b: Prion diseases are noninflammatory; GBS is characterized by lymphocytic infiltrates in the root ganglia, nerve roots, and nerves. In any event, no infectious agent can be demonstrated.
c: GBS is a disease process that affects peripheral nerves, nerve roots, and root ganglia. Also see the explanation for answers (a) and (b).
d: The autoimmune attack is directed against peripheral myelin, not the axon.

2. **Answer a:**
Varicella-zoster virus probably can reside in ganglia throughout life following a childhood case of chickenpox and reactivate later, often in the elderly but also if immune incompetence develops earlier in life.

b: In childhood chickenpox, the vesicular rash following the dermatomal distribution of cutaneous nerves—which is characteristic of shingles, a disease of adults—usually does not occur.
c: Adults who have never had chicken pox, if exposed to it, will usually develop severe chicken pox, sometimes accompanied by varicella pneumonia and other systemic manifestations. Death may occur. A localized shingleslike eruption may also be present, however. Shingles, while painful, is usually not life threatening.
d: Shingles affects cutaneous nerves and ganglia, but muscle pain and weakness are not a manifestation.
e: "Glove-and-stocking" numbness is characteristic of diabetic and other sensory neuropathies. Shingles is a painful cutaneous eruption.

3. **Answer c:**
Compression of the median nerve by the transverse carpal ligament at the wrist (carpal tunnel syndrome) is the most common entrapment neuropathy.

a: Compression of interdigital nerves in the foot does occur but is not as common as the carpal tunnel syndrome.
b: Compression of the peroneal nerve at the knee occurs but is less common than compression of the median nerve at the wrist.
d: The ulnar nerve is commonly and acutely traumatized by inadvertently striking the elbow area against a hard object ("hitting one's funny bone"), but neuropathy usually does not follow this painful but minor trauma.
e: Compression of the sciatic nerve may lead to painful sciatic neuropathy (sciatica), but this is not the most common cause of entrapment neuropathy.

4. **Answer d:**
The only condition listed in which there is no significant necrosis of muscle fibers is amyotrophic lateral sclerosis. This denervating disease, in which there is death of anterior horn cells, their axons, and muscle atrophy, is sometimes called Lou Gehrig's disease.

a: Muscle cell necrosis does occur in all the hereditary muscular dystrophies.
b: Occlusion of the vascular supply to a muscle will cause necrosis (infarction).
c: Significant muscle necrosis does occur in bacterial myositis and abscesses.
e: The autoimmune attack against muscle in polymyositis does result in necrosis of muscle cells.

5. **Answer a:**
The amount of acetylcholine released at the terminal axon in myasthenia gravis is normal. Autoantibodies against the acetylcholine block excitation at the motor end plate and damage the motor end plate; weakness results.

b: Myasthenia gravis is often associated with thymic hyperplasia or neoplasia.

c: The degree of weakness in myasthenia gravis is promptly reduced by the administration of an anticholinesterase drug.

d: Circulating antibodies against acetylcholine occur and are important in blocking the excitation of the motor end plate or damaging the endplate itself.

e: Damage to the motor end plate does occur.

CHAPTER 25: CENTRAL NERVOUS SYSTEM

1. Answer a:

The necrotic, infarcted brain material is removed by macrophages, leaving a cavity that never fills because of the paucity of fibroblastic activity and lack of collagen production in the central nervous system. The fiber-producing cells of the nervous system, the astrocytes, are unable to fill the cavity with their relatively specific glial fibrillary acidic protein fibers.

b: There is a general lack of fibroblastic activity and collagen production within the parenchyma of the central nervous system.

c: The microglial cell, a controversial cell, is not known to produce fiber of any kind, although it may have phagocytic properties.

d: Necrotic brain tissue is removed, primarily by monocyte-derived macrophages.

e: Amyloid is not associated with cerebral infarcts. A central core of amyloid surrounded by dystrophic dendrites describes a senile plaque in Alzheimer's disease.

2. Answer d:

Streptococcus pneumoniae is the most common cause of acute purulent leptomeningitis in both childhood and adulthood.

a: Although tuberculous meningitis does affect children, it is rare compared with many other bacterial meningitides.

b: Central nervous system abscesses are relatively rare; they are often secondary to infected emboli.

c: Although *Haemophilus influenzae* type B used to be the most common cause of acute purulent cerebrospinal leptomeningitis in children, an effective vaccine has now greatly reduced the incidence of meningitis caused by this organism.

e: Fungal infections of the nervous system in otherwise healthy patients are rare. Against a background of immunosuppression, however, they are much more common.

3. Answer d:

Collagen-producing cells are active in the leptomeninges, although not in the parenchyma. Slowly developing fibrosis of the leptomeninges may obstruct the foramina of Luschka and Magendie at the base of the brain, resulting in slowly developing obstructive hydrocephalus, which may not become apparent until many years after the infection has resolved.

a: Tuberculous meningitis readily affects children.

b: Drug-resistant stains of *Mycobacterium tuberculosis* are becoming increasingly more common.

c: Nervous system tuberculosis is always secondary to infection elsewhere in the body, usually the lungs.

e: Tuberculous meningitis, like most forms of tuberculosis, is a subacute to chronic disease, and the clinical course is usually prolonged.

4. Answer d:

Although astrocytomas of the cerebellum are slightly more common than medulloblastomas in the childhood period, they are usually located laterally in the cerebellar hemispheres and typically do not grow within the fourth ventricle. Ependymomas, which do typically grow within the fourth ventricle, are much less common than medulloblastomas in this age group.

a: Glioblastomas are rare in children and do not usually present as intraventricular neoplasms.

b: Although the ependymoma of the fourth ventricle is an important diagnostic consideration during the childhood period, it is much less common than the medulloblastoma.

c: Colloid cysts usually occur later in life in the third ventricle. Colloid cysts of the fourth ventricle are extremely rare at any age.

e: Although astrocytomas, cystic or solid, are the most common brain neoplasm of the childhood period, they are usually located laterally in the cerebellum or within the brain stem as infiltrating neoplasms and usually do not grow within the fourth ventricle.

5. **Answer a:**

The senile plaque, which, in its mature form, consists of a ring of degenerating neuronal processes (mainly dendrites) surrounding a central mass of β-amyloid, is the most specific abnormality of Alzheimer's disease.

b: Although β-amyloid deposits in the walls of small cortical and leptomeningeal blood vessels frequently accompany Alzheimer's disease, they also occur in individuals without Alzheimer's disease.

c: Loss of neurons occurs in many neurologic diseases; astrocytic proliferation in response to loss of neurons is universal.

d: Intraganglionic neurofibrillary tangles are not specific for Alzheimer's disease and also occur in other neurodegenerative diseases.

e: Hirano bodies, which are brightly eosinophilic, often rectangular or trapezoidal-shaped collections of the filaments, are seen in Ammon's horn in many brains, including neurologically normal patients.

CHAPTER 26: BREAST

1. **Answer a:**

Staphylococcus aureus is a common cause of acute mastitis.

b: *Histoplasma capsulatum* rarely causes acute mastitis.

c: *Proteus vulgaris* rarely causes acute mastitis.

d: *Mycobacterium tuberculosis* rarely causes acute mastitis.

e: *Mycobacterium avium-intracellulare* rarely causes acute mastitis.

2. **Answer d:**

Lung cancer is the leading cause of cancer death in American women.

a: Breast cancer is not the most common cause of cancer death in American women.

b: Colon cancer is not the most common cause of cancer death in American women.

c: Ovarian cancer is not the most common cause of cancer death in American women.

e: Endometrial cancer is not the most common cause of cancer death in American women.

3. **Answer a:**

Intraductal carcinoma has the best prognosis.

b: Tubular carcinoma has a good prognosis, but not the best.

c: Papillary carcinoma has a good prognosis, but not the best.

d: Medullary carcinoma does not have the best prognosis.

e: Mucinous carcinoma does not have the best prognosis.

4. **Answer a:**

Bloody nipple discharge is the classical clinical complaint for intraductal papilloma.

b: Peau d'orange skin change is not characteristic of intraductal papilloma. It is a characteristic sign of underlying breast cancer.

c: Enlargement of ipsilateral (same side) axillary lymph nodes is not characteristic of the intraductal papilloma. It suggests carcinoma metastatic to axillary lymph node tissue.

d: Eczematoid skin changes are not characteristic of intraductal papilloma. They are often seen in mammary Paget's disease.

e: A red, firm, painful mass is not characteristic of intraductal papilloma.

5. **Answer e:**

Fat necrosis is *not* a feature of fibrocystic change.

a: Apocrine metaplasia is a feature that may be seen in fibrocystic change of the breast.

b: Cysts (benign) are a feature that may be seen in fibrocystic change of the breast.

c: Fibrosis is a feature that may be seen in fibrocystic change of the breast.

d: Sclerosing adenosis is a feature that may be seen in fibrocystic change of the breast.

CHAPTER 27: FEMALE GENITAL TRACT

1. **Answer d:**

Squamous cell carcinoma is the most common primary malignancy of the vagina.

a: Adenocarcinoma is a common malignancy of the endometrium.

b: Rhabdomyosarcoma, when seen in this site, usually occurs in young girls.

c: Clear cell carcinoma is a common malignancy of the endometrium and ovary.

e: Malignant melanoma is a common malignancy in sun exposed skin.

2. **Answer b:**

Leiomyoma represents the most common type of uterine neoplasm.

a: Lipoma is common in subcutaneous tissue.

c: Endometrial adenocarcinoma is not likely in this case because of the patient's age.

d: Sarcoma botryoides is seen almost exclusively in young girls, where it involves the vagina and/or urinary bladder.

3. **Answer e:**

The lung is the most common site of metastatic gestational choriocarcinoma.

a: Periaortic lymph nodes do not represent the most common site for gestational choriocarcinoma metastasis.

b: Deep pelvic lymph nodes do not repre-sent the most common site for gesta-tional choriocarcinoma metastasis.

c: The kidney is not the most common site for gestational choriocarcinoma metas-tasis.

d: The liver is not the most common site for gestational choriocarcinoma metas-tasis.

4. **Answer a:**

Serous cystadenocarcinoma has the high-est rate of bilaterality among any of the ovarian cancers.

b: Mucinous cystadenocarcinoma does not have the highest rate of bilaterality.

c: Malignant Brenner tumor is uncommon and does not have the highest rate of bilaterality.

d: Clear cell carcinoma does not have the highest rate of bilaterality.

e: Endometrioid carcinoma does not have the highest rate of bilaterality.

5. **Answer c:**

Adenocarcinoma is the most common type of *primary* malignancy of the fal-lopian tube.

a: Squamous cell carcinoma is almost never a primary malignancy at this site. It is common in the vulva, vagina and uterine cervix.

b: Malignant lymphoma is rarely a primary malignancy at this site. It is common in lymph nodes and certain extra-nodal sites (especially the GI tract).

d: Rhabdomyosarcoma is not a primary malignancy at this site.

e: Fibrosarcoma is not a type of primary malignancy at this site.

CHAPTER 28: MALE REPRODUCTIVE SYSTEM

1. **Answer d:**

Most testicular neoplasms are derived from germ cells.

a: Most testicular neoplasms are not derived from squamous cells. However, terato-carcinoma sometimes features malignant squamous cells.

b: Most testicular neoplasms are derived from germ cells.

c: Most testicular neoplasms are derived from germ cells.

e: Most testicular neoplasms are derived from germ cells.

2. **Answer d:**

The combination of teratoma and embryonal carcinoma is called teratocarcinoma.

a: A yolk sac tumor is a distinct histologic type of germ cell cancer.

b: Choriocarcinoma refers to a distinct histologic type of germ cell cancer.

c: Seminoma refers to a distinct histologic type of germ cell cancer.

e: Malignant lymphoma refers to a cancer composed of lymphoid cells.

3. **Answer b:**

E. coli is most likely to cause acute prostatitis.

a: *Mycobacterium tuberculosis* is rarely seen clinically at this site and is likely to cause granulomatosus, rather than acute prostatitis.

c: *Treponema pallidum* is rarely seen clinically at this site and is likely to cause gumma formation rather than acute prostatitis.

d: CMV is likely to cause chronic inflammation, rather than acute prostatitis.

e: Herpes simplex virus causes acute inflammation but only rarely causes acute prostatitis.

4. **Answer d:**

Increased urinary frequency, nocturia, urinary dribbling, difficulty starting the urinary stream, as well as this man's age are all indicators of prostatic nodular hyperplasia.

a: Prostate cancer typically presents as a firm mass on rectal examination; although obstructive symptoms may be seen, they are usually not prominent.

b: Urinary bladder cancer typically presents with hematuria.

c: Urethral obstruction by calculus would most likely result in total urinary stoppage.

e: Symptoms of urinary bladder infection include dysuria and pus in the urine.

5. **Answer a:**

Prostatic intraepithelial neoplasia (PIN) is considered a premalignant lesion but is not in and of itself malignant. It represents a form of dysplasia.

b: Invasive carcinoma refers to a type of malignant neoplasm.

c: Metaplasia refers to a reversible change from one adult cell type to another cell type.

d: Atrophy refers to tissue shrinkage.

e: Hyperplasia refers to an enlargement of a tissue caused by an increased number of cells in that tissue.

CHAPTER 29: EYE

1. **Answer c:**

This man has arcus senilis which is caused by lipid deposition and characterized by a milky ring around the periphery of each cornea.

a: Mucopolysaccharide deposition occurs in macular corneal dystrophy.

b: Deposition of protein material occurs in certain corneal dystrophies.

d: Deposition of cartilage in the cornea is essentially unknown in clinical practice.

e: Deposition of bone in the cornea is highly unlikely without prior specific trauma.

2. **Answer a:**

Retinoblastoma is the most common primary intraocular malignant neoplasm of childhood.

b: Medulloblastoma is a cancer that arises from the cerebellum typically during the second decade of life.

c: Malignant lymphoma is mostly seen in adults.

d: Rhabdomyosarcoma is a common neoplasm of childhood but only rarely arises within the eye.

e: Neuroblastoma is not an intraocular malignancy. It arises from the sympathetic nervous system and adrenal medulla.

3. **Answer b:**

Cotton wool spots represent nerve fiber layer infarction.

a: Neoplastic cell deposits are characterized by "floaters" in the vitreous cavity.
c: Retinal neovascularization is characterized by new blood vessel formation.
d: Cataract formation is characterized by a clouded, opacified lens.

4. **Answer a:**

A cone shaped cornea (pointing anteriorly) with central stromal thinning and scarring is the classic description of keratoconus.

b: Pterygium refers to solar damage to corneal stromal tissue.
c: Hordeolum refers to an abscess of the eyelid.
d: Arcus senilis refers to a "milky ring" around the periphery of each cornea.
e: Retinitis pigmentosa is characterized by progressive loss of rods and cones in the retina.

CHAPTER 30: ENDOCRINE DISEASES

1. **Answer a:**

Viruses are a likely initiator of type 1 diabetes mellitus. Viral infection predisposes to subsequent immunologically mediated injury in a genetically susceptible individual. Coxsackievirus B has often been implicated; others mentioned include Epstein-Barr virus, mumps virus, and measles virus.

b: Excess caloric intake leading to obesity is likely to be a contributing factor in type 2 diabetes mellitus.
c: Insufficient dietary iodine can cause multinodular goiter, often with clinically significant hypothyroidism, but is not known to be related to diabetes mellitus.
d: Insulin injection lowers blood glucose.
e: Therapeutic use of synthetic glucocorticoids can cause secondary diabetes mellitus.

2. **Answer e:**

These are typical clinical and laboratory features of Cushing's syndrome. Further

evaluation is needed to determine the cause.

a: Decreased cortisol, sometimes with hypotension and hypoglycemia, is characteristic of Addison's disease.
b: Alport's syndrome (hereditary nephritis with deafness) is not directly related to abnormal adrenal function.
c: Caplan's syndrome (rheumatoid arthritis and pneumoconiosis) is not directly related to abnormal adrenal function.
d: Conn's syndrome is primary (low renin) hyperaldosteronism caused by an adrenocortical adenoma.

3. **Answer d:**

The laboratory findings indicate excess pituitary ACTH; in the majority of such cases a pituitary adenoma can be found.

a: In adrenocortical neoplasms causing Cushing's syndrome, ACTH is low, and high-dose dexamethasone rarely suppresses cortisol.
b: In adrenocortical neoplasms causing Cushing's syndrome, ACTH is low, and high-dose dexamethasone rarely suppresses cortisol.
c: The major secretory products of pheochromocytoma are catecholamines, not steroids. Pheochromocytoma is a rare cause of ectopic ACTH syndrome, but in that syndrome ACTH usually is markedly elevated and not suppressed by high-dose dexamethasone.
e: Small-cell carcinoma is the most common cause of ectopic ACTH syndrome, but in that syndrome ACTH usually is markedly elevated and not suppressed by high-dose dexamethasone.

4. **Answer c:**

The elevated TSH, in combination with the other findings, indicates that this patient has primary (thyroidal) hypothyroidism, Hashimoto's thyroiditis is a common cause of primary hypothyroidism with goiter.

a: A large pituitary adenoma can cause central hypothyroidism—the TSH is low. A pituitary adenoma producing central hypothyroidism would not cause a goiter, but could be associated with other manifestations of hypopituitarism in addition to hypothyroidism and/or neurologic findings.

b: Papillary thyroid carcinoma would cause a thyroid mass and would not usually cause hypothyroidism (at least not until a thyroidectomy was performed).

d: Graves' disease would cause hyperthyroidism with low TSH.

e: Riedel's thyroiditis is an extremely rare cause of primary hypothyroidism in which fibrosis involves the gland and the surrounding structures (raising the possibility of neoplasia).

5. **Answer a:**

Infiltrative ophthalmopathy in Graves' disease might be caused by cross reaction between anti-TSH receptor antibodies and extraocular muscle; an alternative view is that Graves' disease is a systemic autoimmune disease most prominently involving the thyroid, but also affecting striated muscle and connective tissue. Several common endocrine disease have eye manifestations that differ pathogenically and clinically from infiltrative ophthalmopathy.

b: Eye involvement is not typical of Hashimoto's disease.

c: Patients with diabetes mellitus can develop diabetic retinopathy.

d: Patients with diabetes mellitus can develop diabetic retinopathy.

e: By compression of cranial nerves, large pituitary adenomas can cause visual field defects and abnormalities of extraocular motion.

INDEX

Italic page numbers indicate figures; page numbers with *t* indicate tables.

Mosby's Reviews Series
Copyright © 1997,
Mosby–Year Book, Inc.

How to install this program—Windows users

1. Place the disk in Drive A: (or B:)
2. From Program Manager, select File, then Run, then enter:
   A:SETUP (or B:SETUP if your disk drive is B:)
3. Follow the instructions on screen.

How to run this program—Windows users

Open the MOSBY Program Group and select the Mosby's Reviews Series icon.

How to install this program—Macintosh users

1. Insert the disk into the disk drive. Double-click on the disk icon.
2. Double-click on the install icon. The program will be saved to your hard drive.

How to run this program—Macintosh users

Open the MOSBY folder and select the Mosby's Reviews Series icon.

For complete instructions on using the program, please read the "How to use this Program" file.